Qw 504
SPI

Normal ranges

D1323043

Serum immunoglobulins (adults)

IgG	5.8–15.4 g/l
IgA	0.64–2.97 g/l
IgM (males)	0.24–1.90 g/l
IgM (females)	0.71–2.30 g/l

IgG subclasses (adults)

IgG$_1$	2.2–10.8 g/l
IgG$_2$	0.5–8.0 g/l
IgG$_3$	0.05–0.9 g/l
IgG$_4$	0.0–2.4 g/l

Antibacterial antibodies

Pneumococcal (Pneumovax® 23)	> 20 u/l
Tetanus (protective)	> 0.1 IU/ml
Haemophilus influenzae B (full protection)	> 1 mcg/ml

Complement

C3	0.68–1.80 g/l
C4	0.18–0.60 g/l

C1-esterase inhibitor (adult)

Immunochemical	0.18–0.54 g/l
Functional	80–120% of normal plasma

Total IgE (>14 years)

IgE	< 100 kU/l

Specific IgE

Grade 0	< 0.35 IU/ml
Grade 1	0.35–0.70 IU/ml
Grade 2	0.70–3.50 IU/ml
Grade 3	3.50–17.50 IU/ml
Grade 4	17.5–50.0 IU/ml
Grade 5	50–100 IU/ml
Grade 6	> 100 IU/ml

Lymphocyte subsets (adult values)

Total T cells (CD3$^+$)	690–2540 cells/mm^3
Total B cell (CD19$^+$ or CD20$^+$)	90–660 cells/mm^3
T helper cells (CD3$^+$CD4$^+$)	410–1590 cells/mm^3
T cytotoxic cells (CD3$^+$CD8$^+$)	190–1140 cells/mm^3
NK cells (CD16$^+$CD56$^+$)	90–590 cells/mm^3

NB normal total lymphocyte count for infant < 6 months is 3500–7000 cells/mm^3

OXFORD MEDICAL PUBLICATIONS

Oxford Handbook of
Clinical Immunology and Allergy

Published and forthcoming Oxford Handbooks

Oxford Handbook of
Clinical Immunology and Allergy

Fourth edition

Gavin Spickett

Consultant Clinical Immunologist
Regional Department of Immunology
Royal Victoria Infirmary
Newcastle upon Tyne
UK

OXFORD
UNIVERSITY PRESS

OXFORD
UNIVERSITY PRESS

Great Clarendon Street, Oxford, OX2 6DP,
United Kingdom

Oxford University Press is a department of the University of Oxford.
It furthers the University's objective of excellence in research, scholarship,
and education by publishing worldwide. Oxford is a registered trade mark of
Oxford University Press in the UK and in certain other countries

© Oxford University Press 2020

The moral rights of the author have been asserted

First Edition published in 1999
Second Edition published in 2006
Third Edition published in 2013
Fourth Edition published in 2020

Impression: 1

Published in the United States of America by Oxford University Press
198 Madison Avenue, New York, NY 10016, United States of America

British Library Cataloguing in Publication Data
Data available

Library of Congress Control Number: 2018965183

ISBN 978–0–19–878952–9

Printed and bound in China by
C&C Offset Printing Co., Ltd.

Dedication from first edition

To the memory of the late Charles Newman, who inspired me to continue with a career in medicine, when I was assailed by doubts about my chosen path.

Contents

Symbols and abbreviations

⮎	cross-reference
▶	important
❶	warning
℘	online reference
☼	emergency
>	greater than
<	less than
AA	aplastic anaemia
AAE	acquired angioedema
ABPA	allergic bronchopulmonary aspergillosis
ACA	anti-cardiolipin antibody
ACE	angiotensin-converting enzyme
ACH	acetylcholine
AChRAb	anti-acetylcholine-receptor antibody
ACP	Association of Clinical Pathologists
ACTH	adrenocorticotrophic hormone
ADA	adenosine deaminase
ADCC	antibody-dependent cell-mediated cytotoxicity
AECA	anti-endothelial cell antibody
AGA	anti-gliadin antibodies
AICAR	5-amino-imidazole-4-carboxamide ribonucleotide
AIDS	acquired immune deficiency syndrome
AIH	autoimmune hepatitis
AIHA	idiopathic autoimmune haemolytic anaemia
AIRE	autoimmune regulator
ALG	anti-lymphocyte globulin
ALL	acute lymphoblastic leukaemia
ALP	alkaline phosphatase
ALPS	autoimmune lymphoproliferative syndrome
AMA	anti-mitochondrial antibody
AML	acute myeloid leukaemia

ANA	anti-nuclear antibody
ANCA	anti-neutrophil cytoplasmic antibody
ANNA	anti-neuronal nuclear antibody
APC	antigen-presenting cell
$APCH_{100}$	alternate pathway haemolytic complement 100%
APECED	autoimmune polyendocrinopathy–candidiasis–ectodermal dysplasia
APGS	autoimmune polyglandular syndrome (also APS)
APP	amyloid-precursor protein
APS	autoimmune polyglandular syndrome (also APGS)
APS	anti-phospholipid syndrome
APTT	activated partial thromboplastin time
ARA	American Rheumatism Association
ARB	angiotensin-II receptor blocker
ARDS	adult respiratory distress syndrome
AS	ankylosing spondylitis
ASCA	anti-*Saccharomyces cerevisiae* antibodies
ASOT	antistreptolysin O titre
α_1-AT	α_1-antitrypsin
AT	ataxia telangiectasia
ATG	anti-thymocyte globulin
ATM	ataxia telangiectasia mutated protein
AZT	azidothymidine (zidovudine)
BACNS	benign angiitis of the CNS
BAL	bronchoalveolar lavage
BCG	bacille Calmette–Guérin
BCOADC	branch-chain 2-oxo-acid dehydrogenase complex
bd	twice a day
BIS	bias index score

BM	bone marrow
BMS	biomedical scientist
BMT	bone marrow transplantation
BSACI	British Society for Allergy and Clinical Immunology
BSI	British Society for Immunology
C4BP	C4 binding protein
CAH	chronic active hepatitis
CALLA	common acute lymphoblastic leukaemia antigen
CAMP	cyclic adenosine monophosphate
C-ANCA	cytoplasmic ANCA
CAR	cancer-associated retinopathy
CATCH-22	cardiac abnormalities, abnormal facies, thymic hypoplasia, cleft palate, and hypocalcaemia, associated with 22q11 deletions
CCD	cross-reactive carbohydrate determinant
CCP	cyclic citrullinated peptide
CCV	chosen coefficient of variance
2CDA	2-chloro-deoxyadenosine
CE	Conformité Européenne
CF	cystic fibrosis
CFS	chronic fatigue syndrome
CGD	chronic granulomatous disease
CH_{100}	classical pathway haemolytic complement 100%
CHAD	cold haemolytic disease
CHARGE	colobomata, heart disease, atresia of choanae, delayed growth, genital hypoplasia, ear anomalies
CHH	cartilage–hair hypoplasia
CHIMP	Commission for Health Improvement
CHS	Chediak–Higashi syndrome
CID	combined immunodeficiency
CIDP	chronic inflammatory demyelinating polyneuropathy
CJD	Creutzfeldt–Jakob disease
CK	creatine kinase
CLL	chronic lymphocytic leukaemia
CMC	chronic mucocutaneous candidiasis
CME	continuing medical education
CMI	cell-mediated immunity
CML	chronic myeloid leukaemia
CMV	cytomegalovirus
CNS	central nervous system
CONA	concanavalin A
COPD	chronic obstructive pulmonary disease
COSHH	Control of Substances Hazardous to Health
CPA	Clinical Pathology Accreditation
CPD	continuing professional development
CPSM	Council for Professions Supplementary to Medicine
CQC	Care Quality Commission
CR & E	creatinine and electolytes
CREST	calcinosis–Raynaud's–oesophageal dysmotility–sclerodactyly–telangiectasia
CRF	chronic renal failure
CRP	C-reactive protein
CSF	cerebrospinal fluid
CSF-1	colony-stimulating factor-1
CSS	Churg–Strauss syndrome
CT	computed tomography
CTD	connective tissue disease
CTL	cytotoxic T lymphocyte
CTLP	cytotoxic T-lymphocyte precursor
CV	coefficient of variation
CVA	cerebrovascular accident
CVID	common variable immunodeficiency
CXR	chest X-ray
CYA	ciclosporin (previously cyclosporin A)
DAF	decay accelerating factor
DATP	deoxyadenosine triphosphate
DBPC	double-blind, placebo-controlled
DCT	direct Coombs' test

DGTP	deoxyguanosine triphosphate
DH	dermatitis herpetiformis *or* Department of Health
DIC	disseminated intravascular coagulation
DIF	direct immunofluorescence
DM	dermatomyositis
DMARDs	disease-modifying drugs anti-rheumatic drugs
DNA	deoxyribonucleic acid
DNA-PKCS	DNA protein kinase catalytic subunit
DOCK8	dedicator of cytokinesis 8
DPT	diphtheria–pertussis–tetanus
DRL	drug-related lupus
DRVVT	dilute Russell's viper venom test
dsDNA	double-stranded DNA
DTH	delayed-type hypersensitivity
DV	designated value
DVT	deep vein thrombosis
EA	early antigen
EAA	extrinsic allergic alveolitis
EBNA	EBV nuclear antigen
EBV	Epstein–Barr virus
ECG	electrocardiogram
ECP	eosinophil cationic protein
EDTA	ethylene-diaminetetraacetic acid
EGF	epidermal growth factor
EIA	enzyme-linked immunoassay
ELISA	enzyme-linked immunosorbent assay
EM	electron microscopy
EMA	endomysial antibodies
EMEA	European Agency for the Evaluation of Medicinal Products
EMG	electromyogram
ENA	extractable nuclear antigen
ENT	ear, nose, and throat
EPD	enzyme-potentiated desensitization
EPO	erythropoietin
EQA	external quality assessment

ESID	European Society for Immunodeficiencies
ESR	erythrocyte sedimentation rate
FAST	fluorescent allergosorbent test
FBC	full blood count
FCAS	familial cold autoinflammatory syndrome
FCR	Fc receptor
FCS	fetal calf serum
FDA	Food and Drug Administration
FEV_1	forced expired volume (in one second)
FFA	free fatty acid
FFP	fresh frozen plasma
FIA	fluorescent immunoassay
FISH	fluorescent *in situ* hybridization
FITC	fluorescein isothiocyanate
FLH	familial lymphohistiocytosis
FMF	familial Mediterranean fever
fMLP	*N*-formyl-methionyl-leucyl-phenylalanine
FSH	follicle-stimulating hormone
FT3	free triiodothyronine
FT4	free thyroxine
FVC	forced vital capacity
G6PD	glucose 6-phosphate dehydrogenase
GABA	γ-aminobutyric acid
GACNS	granulomatous angiitis of the CNS
GAD	glutamic acid decarboxylase
GBM	glomerular basement membrane
GBS	Guillain–Barré syndrome
GCA	giant-cell arteritis
G-CSF	granulocyte colony-stimulating factor
GDP	guanosine diphosphate
GFD	gluten-free diet
GFR	glomerular filtration rate
GGT	gammaglutamyl transferase
GI	gastrointestinal
GLP	good laboratory practice

GM-CSF	granulocyte–macrophage colony-stimulating factor
GN	glomerulonephritis
GP	general practitioner or glycoprotein
GPC	gastric parietal cell
GPI	glucosylphosphatidylinositol
GS-ANA	granulocyte anti-nuclear antibody
GTN	glyceryl trinitrate
GVHD	graft-versus-host disease
GVL	graft-versus-leukaemia
GVT	graft-versus-tumour
GWAS	genome-wide association study
HAART	highly active antiretroviral therapy
H & E	haematoxylin and eosin
HAE	hereditary angioedema
HAMA	human anti-mouse antibodies
HANE	hereditary angioneurotic oedema
HB	haemoglobin
HBsAg	hepatitis B surface antigen
HCC	Healthcare Commission
HCL	hairy-cell leukaemia
HCV	hepatitis C virus
HD	Hodgkin's disease
HDIVIg	high-dose intravenous immunoglobulin
HELLP	haemolysis–elevated liver enzymes–low platelets
HEP	histamine equivalent potency
HEp-2	human epithelial type 2
HES	hyper-eosinophilic syndrome
HGV	hepatitis G virus
HHV	human herpesvirus
HIB	*Haemophilus influenzae* type b
HIGE	hyper-IgE syndrome
HIGM	hyper-IgM
HIT	heparin-induced thrombocytopenia
HIV	human immunodeficiency virus

HLA	human leucocyte antigen
HR-CT	high-resolution CT
HRF	homologous restriction factor
HRT	hormone replacement therapy
HSCT	haematopoietic stem cell transplantation
HSE	Health and Safety Executive
Hsp	heat-shock protein
HSP	Henoch–Schönlein purpura
HSV	herpes simplex virus
5-HT	5-hydroxytryptamine (serotonin)
HTLP	helper T-lymphocyte precursor
HTLV-1	human T-cell leukaemia virus-1
HUS	haemolytic–uraemic syndrome
HUV	hypocomplementaemic urticarial vasculitis
ICA	islet cell antibodies
ICAM	intercellular adhesion molecule
ICF	immunodeficiency–centromeric instability–abnormal facies
ICOS	inducible co-stimulator
ID	intradermal
IDDM	insulin-dependent diabetes mellitus
IDT	intradermal test
IEF	immunoelectrophoresis
IF	intrinsic factor
IFN	interferon
Ig	immunoglobulin
IGF1-R	insulin-like growth factor-1 receptor
IIF	indirect immunofluorescence
IL	interleukin
IM	intramuscular(ly)
IMIg	intramuscular immunoglobulin
iNKT	invariant NK T cells
INR	international normalized ratio

IPEX	X-linked immune dysregulation with polyendocrinopathy
IPF	idiopathic pulmonary fibrosis
IPOPI	International Patient Organization for Primary Immunodeficiencies
IRAK-4	interleukin-1 receptor-associated kinase 4
ISCOMs	immunostimulatory complexes
ITP	immune thrombocytopenia
ITU	intensive care unit
IU	international units
IV	intravenous(ly)
IVIg	intravenous immunoglobulin
JCA	juvenile chronic arthritis
JDF	Juvenile Diabetes Foundation
JRCPTB	Joint Royal Colleges of Physicians Training Board
KIR	killer-cell Ig-like receptors
LAC	lupus anticoagulant
LAD	leucocyte adhesion defect
LAK	lymphokine-activated killer cell
LC	liver cytosol
LDH	lactate dehydrogenase
LE	lupus erythematosus
LEMS	Lambert–Eaton myasthenic syndrome
LFA	lymphocyte function antigen
LFT	liver function test
LG	lymphomatoid granulomatosis
LGL	large granular lymphocyte
LIF	leukaemia inhibitory factor
LKM	liver–kidney microsomal antibodies
LM	liver microsome
LP	lumbar puncture
LPS	lipopolysaccharide
LYDMA	lymphocyte-determined membrane antigen
mAbs	monoclonal antibodies
MAG	myelin-associated glycoprotein

MAOI	monoamine oxidase inhibitor
MAST	multiple allergosorbent test
MBL	mannan-binding lectin
MBP	mannan-binding protein
MCP	macrophage chemotactic peptide
MCTD	mixed connective tissue disease
MCV	mean corpuscular volume
MDP	muramyl dipeptide
MDS	myelodysplastic syndrome
'ME'	'myalgic encephalomyelitis'
MFE	materno-fetal engraftment
β_2MG	β_2-microglobulin
MG	myasthenia gravis
MGUS	monoclonal gammopathy of unknown significance
MHC	major histocompatibility complex
MI	myocardial infarction
MIS	misclassification score
MLA	medical laboratory assistant
MLR	mixed lymphocyte reaction
MLSO	Medical Laboratory Scientific Officer (Biomedical Scientist)
MMF	mycophenolate mofetil
MMR	measles, mumps, and rubella vaccine
MND	multiple nuclear dots
MOG	myelin oligodendrocyte glycoprotein
MPA	microscopic polyarteritis
MPGN	membranoproliferative glomerulonephritis
MPO	myeloperoxidase
MRA	magnetic resonance angiography
MRBIS	mean running bias index score
MRCP	Member of the Royal College of Physicians
MRCPATH	Member of the Royal College of Pathologists
MRA	magnetic resonance angiography

MRI	magnetic resonance imaging
MRVIS	mean running variance index score
MS	multiple sclerosis
MSA	mitotic spindle antigens
mTOR	mammalian target of rapamycin
MTX	methotrexate
MUD	matched unrelated donor
MUSK	muscle-specific tyrosine kinase
NADPH	reduced nicotinamide adenine dinucleotide phosphate
NAP	neutrophil alkaline phosphatase
NARES	non-allergic rhinitis with eosinophilia
NB	nota bene
NBT	nitroblue tetrazolium test
NCAM	neuronal cell adhesion molecule
NEQAS	National External Quality Assurance Scheme
NF-AT	nuclear factor of activated T cells
NHL	non-Hodgkin's lymphoma
NHS	National Health Service
NICE	National Institute for Health and Care Excellence
NIDDM	non-insulin-dependent diabetes mellitus
NK	natural killer
NMR	nuclear magnetic resonance
NOMID	neonatal-onset multisystem inflammatory disease
NQAAP	National Quality Assurance Advisory Panel
NRL	natural rubber latex
NSAIDs	non-steroidal anti-inflammatory drugs
NUMA	nuclear mitotic apparatus protein
OCP	oral contraceptive pill
od	once a day
OGDC	oxoglutarate dehydrogenase complex
OMIS	overall misclassification score

OMPC	outer membrane porin C
P450scc	P450 side-chain cleavage enzyme
PA	pernicious anaemia
PACNS	primary angiitis of the CNS
PAF	platelet-activating factor
PAN	polyarteritis nodosa
P-ANCA	perinuclear ANCA
PANDAS	paediatric autoimmune neuropsychiatric disorders associated with Streptococcus
PBC	primary biliary cirrhosis
PCNA	proliferating cell nuclear antigen
PCP	Pneumocystis jirovecii (carinii) pneumonia
PCR	polymerase chain reaction
PDC	pyruvate dehydrogenase complex
PDGF	platelet-derived growth factor
PE	pulmonary embolism or phycoerythrin
PEFR	peak expiratory flow rate
PEG	percutaneous endoscopic gastrostomy or polyethylene glycol
PFAPA	periodic fever with aphthous ulcers, pharyngitis, and cervical adenopathy
PGE2	prostaglandin E2
PHA	phytohaemagglutinin
PID	primary immunodeficiency
PLL	prolymphocytic leukaemia
PM	polymyositis
PMA	phorbol myristate acetate
PMR	polymyalgia rheumatica
PNH	paroxysmal nocturnal haemoglobinuria
PNP	purine nucleoside phosphorylase
PNU	protein nitrogen units
POEMS	polyneuropathy–organomegaly–endocrine abnormalities–monoclonal gammopathy–skin changes

POTS	postural orthostatic tachycardia syndrome
PPD	purified protein derivative (of tuberculin)
PPV	positive predictive value
PR3	proteinase 3
PRP	prion protein
PRU	Protein Reference Unit
PSC	primary sclerosing cholangitis
PSS	progressive systemic sclerosis
PTH	parathyroid hormone
PTLD	post-transplant lymphoproliferative disease
PUO	pyrexia of unknown origin
PUPP	pruritic urticaria and plaques of pregnancy
PUVA	photochemotherapy using psoralens with ultraviolet A irradiation
PV	pemphigus vulgaris
PWM	pokeweed mitogen
QA	quality assurance
QC	quality control
QMS	quality management system
RANA	rheumatoid-associated nuclear antibodies
RAST	radioallergosorbent test
RBC	red blood cell
RFLP	restriction fragment length polymorphism
RFT	respiratory function test
RhA	rheumatoid arthritis
RhF	rheumatoid factor
RIA	radioimmunoassay
RID	radial immunodiffusion
RNA	ribonucleic acid
RNP	ribonucleoprotein
RRNP	ribosomal ribonucleoprotein
RS	Reed–Sternberg
RSCA	reference-strand-mediated conformation analysis
RSV	respiratory syncytial virus
SAA	serum amyloid A
SAC	*Staphylococcus* strain A Cowan

SAP	serum amyloid P
SAPHO	synovitis–acne–pustulosis–hyperostosis–osteitis
SBE	subacute bacterial endocarditis
SC	subcutaneous(ly)
SCAT	sheep-cell agglutination test
SCID	severe combined immunodeficiency
SCIG	subcutaneous immunoglobulin
SCL	scleroderma
SCLC	small cell lung carcinoma
SCT	stem cell transplantation
SD	standard deviation
SERPIN	serine protease inhibitor
SFLC	serum free light chains
SIFTR	service increment for teaching and research
SIRS	systemic inflammatory response syndrome
SLA	soluble liver antigens
SLE	systemic lupus erythematosus
SLVL	splenic lymphoma with circulating villous lymphocytes
SM	Smith antibodies
SMA	smooth muscle antibodies
SNP	single nucleotide polymorphism
SOP	standard operating procedure
SPET	single-photon emission tomography
SPS	stiff person syndrome
SPT	skin-prick test
SRP	signal recognition particle
SRSV	small round structured virus
SS	Sjögren's syndrome
SSC	systemic sclerosis
ssDNA	single-stranded DNA
SSOP	sequence-specific oligonucleotide probe
SSP-PCR	sequence-specific primer PCR
stat	immediate
STAT1 OR3	signal transducer and activator of transcription 1 or 3

SV40	simian virus 40
T3	triiodothyronine
T4	thyroxine
TAME	tosyl-L-arginine methyl ester
TB	tuberculosis
TC	transcobalamin
Tcr	T-cell receptor
TDT	terminal deoxytransferase
TFT	thyroid function test
TGF	T-cell growth factor
TGSI	thyroid growth stimulating immunoglobulins
Th1	T helper-1
Th2	T helper-2
Th17	regulatory T cells
THI	transient hypogamma-globulinaemia of infancy
TIA	transient ischaemic attack
TIL	tumour-invading lymphocytes
TLI	total lymphoid irradiation
TNF	tumour necrosis factor
TPMT	thiopurine methyltransferase
TPN	total parenteral nutrition
TPO	thyroid peroxidase
TRAB	thyrotropin receptor antibody
TRAPS	TNF receptor-associated periodic syndrome
TREC	T-cell receptor excision circle
Treg	regulatory T-cell
TSH	thyroid-stimulating hormone
TSH-R	thyroid-stimulating hormone receptor
TSI	thyroid-stimulating immunoglobulins
tTG	tissue transglutaminase
TTP	thrombotic thrombocytopenic purpura
UC	ulcerative colitis
UKAS	UK Accreditation Service
UK-PIN	UK Primary Immunodeficiency Network

UCTD	undifferentiated connective tissue disease
UNG	uracil-DNA glycosylase
USS	ultrasound scan
UV	ultraviolet
VCA	viral capsid antigen
VCAM	vascular cell adhesion molecule
VCF	velocardiofacial syndrome
VDRL	Venereal Disease Research Laboratory
VEGF	vascular endothelial growth factor
VGCC	voltage-gated calcium channel
VGKC	voltage-gated potassium channel
VI	variance index
VIP	vasoactive intestinal polypeptide
VIS	variance index score
VKH	Vogt–Koyanagi–Harada syndrome
VLA	very late antigen
VNTR	variable number tandem repeat
VWF	von Willebrand factor
VZV	varicella zoster virus
WAS	Wiskott–Aldrich syndrome
WASP	Wiskott–Aldrich-associated protein
WHIM	warts, hypogammaglobulinaemia, infection, myelokathexis (syndrome)
WHO	World Health Organization
XIAP	X-linked inhibitor of apoptosis
XLA	X-linked agammaglobulinaemia
XLPS	X-linked lymphoproliferative syndrome
XLT	X-linked thrombocytopenia
ZAP	zeta-associated protein

Introduction

Welcome to the fourth edition of the *Oxford Handbook of Clinical Immunology and Allergy*. Thanks are due to Michael Hawkes for his persistence in prodding me to work faster! As always, the errors are all mine. Despite being 'flexibly retired', i.e. retired but continuing to work part-time, I still enjoy the challenge of putting together the Handbook, and I hope that readers will also still find it useful.

Re-reading my introduction to the third edition, nothing that has happened in the intervening years has made me believe that anything that I said then was incorrect. As I have been writing, the NHS has celebrated its 70th birthday and like many elderly people it is beginning to show its age. There is a desperate need for new solutions. The NHS is no longer able to cope with winter demand, or even now summer demand. We have had a junior doctors' strike in the NHS against an imposed contract. The pyrrhic victory of the Health Secretary in this dispute has driven more and more junior doctors to leave the country or, worse, leave medicine altogether. We have seen a junior doctor convicted of medical negligence manslaughter, when in fact she was working in a failed system, with IT failures and staff shortages. We have seen an outpouring of anger against the GMC. We are seeing financial meltdown in the NHS, but also significant failures of private companies used to outsource NHS tasks such as GP records and payment of GP trainees.

We have had a referendum in the UK in favour of leaving the European Union (EU). This has further destabilized staffing in the NHS, with EU healthcare professionals either deciding to leave or not coming in the first place. The increasing rate of retirement of senior doctors, driven by the tax and pension system, means that the NHS faces an unprecedented skills shortage. This is not, as in the 1960s, going to be filled by migration from Asia, particularly in view of the Home Office's unhelpful cap on visas. How Brexit will affect drug licensing and regulation, drug supply, as well as key biomedical research collaboration and funding is still completely opaque.

We have had yet another iteration of junior doctor training in the UK, in the form of 'Shape of Training' which reinvents the old senior registrar position (although for political reasons this is now a junior consultant!). More trainees will be forced to do general medicine. As surveys by the RCP have shown that 60% of trainees would rather not do general medicine and 45% of consultants don't enjoy it either, there is clearly a problem. General physicians are sadly lacking now, but being a general physician is deemed synonymous with doing acute medicine, which it isn't. Training itself is driven by a tick-box mentality, rather than working on the basis that learning to be a good doctor is an apprenticeship!

Virtually no hospital trust in the UK is now able to operate at a profit, even the best run organizations. Temporary funding of £20 billion has been promised, but this in fact simply restores the £20 billion of 'efficiency savings' removed from the system over the last 5 years, and with inflation, probably doesn't even restore the position. The inflation of the cost of medical care outstrips general inflation and is compounded by the swathes of new therapies. Comparing the section on biologicals in the first edition of the Handbook with the chapter on immunotherapeutics today, there was just OKT3 and Campath®. Now there are literally hundreds of biological therapies with new ones being licensed all the time. Some of the new gene-based therapies of diseases such as cystic fibrosis are being marketed at $0.5 million per patient. The problem here is that the treatment is curative, so the pharma companies do not benefit from long-term retreatment, so must recover their development costs upfront. These treatments, needless to say, are currently unaffordable and a new funding model is required.

The biggest change over the last 5 years is the impact of genetic technology. Most of the revision of this edition has been to update the genetics of old diseases and incorporate information on the 'new' genetic diseases. This has applied particularly to the primary immune deficiencies and to the autoinflammatory diseases. Even during the writing process, dozens of new genetic immunological diseases have been described. So readers beware— you absolutely need to monitor the literature regularly! This Handbook contains as much as is practical, but is not encyclopedic in coverage. For PIDs, the IUIS publishes regular (now yearly) updates on the recognized immunodeficiencies.

So far, clinical immunology services have survived, although there is still no agreed funding model for providing primary immunodeficiency services. It has, however, just been announced that there will be support for transplantation services for adults with PIDs and neonatal screening for SCID will be introduced. However, we are still locked in to a system of 'individual funding requests' every time we want to use expensive drugs in rare conditions. These take a disproportionate amount of time to complete by the responsible clinician, followed by internal review processes by Trust senior medical and pharmacy staff, before being sent to yet more committees to review. It would be cheaper for the NHS just to fund the drug!

The amalgamation of laboratory services is still proceeding and the exodus of senior staff continues. The lack of finance means that it is harder than ever to develop and implement new tests. From the perspective of immunology, the massive advances in genetic testing are beginning to render some of our historical functional assays redundant, such as T-cell proliferation assay, which are no longer really needed for diagnosis of PIDs.

Since the last edition, UKAS has absorbed CPA and laboratory inspection is now under ISO15189, a typical compromise of competing international interests. This accredits tests not laboratories and as long as a laboratory states that a test is not accredited it can continue to offer that service. At least under UKAS there is an annual inspection, not just the 4-yearly CPA inspection. The bureaucratic paperchase has increased disproportionately.

The structure of the book remains the same, divided into a clinical section and a section on diagnostic tests and administrative information. In particular, readers are directed to Drew Provan's *Oxford Handbook of Clinical and Laboratory Investigation*, fourth edition, which covers non-immunological investigation (and a condensed section on immunological testing!). I remain grateful to my many clinical and laboratory colleagues who help both wittingly and unwittingly in improving my knowledge base. I am particularly grateful to my loyal and hard-working secretary, Jackie Rutherford, who doubtless is relieved that I now only work part-time.

As in the previous edition, this book is not referenced, specifically to encourage readers to seek out the most up-to-date information on topics. We have, however, included the URLs of useful websites, where these have either relevant clinical information or suitable material for patients.

Other general sources of detailed information are listed in the following sections. It is noteworthy that the internet has led to a marked decline in the publication of major textbooks. Wikipedia is an excellent source of medical information, although it needs to be cross-checked for accuracy!

Textbooks

Abbas, A.K., Lichtman, A.H. and Pillai, S. (2017). *Cellular and molecular immunology*, 9th edn. Elsevier.

Adkinson, N.F., Bochner, B.S., Burks, A.W., Busse, W.W., Holgate, S.T., Lemanske, R.F. and O'Hehir, R.E., eds (2014). *Middleton's allergy: principles and practice*, 8th edn. Mosby Elsevier.

Detrick, B, Hamilton, R.G. and Schnitz, J.L., eds (2016). *Manual of molecular and clinical laboratory immunology*, 8th edn. ASM Press.

Firestein, G.S., Budd, R.C., Gabriel, S., McInnes, I.B. and O'Dell, J.R., eds (2016). *Kelley's textbook of rheumatology*, 10th edn. Saunders Elsevier.

Metcalfe, D., Sampson, H.A., Simon, R.A. and Lack, G. (2014). *Food allergy: adverse reactions to foods and food additives*, 5th edn. Wiley-Blackwell.

Ochs, H.D., Smith, C.I.E. and Puck, J.M. (2014). *Primary immunodeficiency diseases*, 3rd edn. Oxford University Press.

Paul, W.E. (2012). *Fundamental immunology*, 7th edn. Lippincott Williams & Wilkins.

Rich, R.R., Fleisher, T.A., Shearer, W.T., Schroeder, H.W., Frew, A.J. and Weyand, C.M., eds. (2018). *Clinical immunology: principles and practice*, 5th edn. Mosby Elsevier.

Shoenfeld, Y., Meroni, P.L. and Gershwin, M.E., eds (2014). *Autoantibodies*, 3rd edn. Elsevier.

Stiehm, E.R., Ochs, H.D. and Winkelstein, J.A. (2004). *Immunologic disorders in infants and children*, 5th edn. Saunders Elsevier.

Useful handbooks

Protein Reference Units (2004). *Handbook of autoimmunity*, 3rd edn. PRU.

Protein Reference Units (2004). *Handbook of clinical immunochemistry*, 8th edn. PRU.

Sadly no new editions of these Handbooks have been produced but electronic versions are available from the PRU websites.

Journals

Advances in Immunology
Allergy
Annual Review of Immunology
Clinical and Experimental Allergy
Clinical and Experimental Immunology
Clinical Immunology
Current Opinion in Clinical Immunology and Allergy
Current Opinion in Immunology
Immunological Reviews
Journal of Allergy and Clinical Immunology
Journal of Clinical Immunology
Journal of Immunology
Nature Immunology
Nature Reviews Immunology
Trends in Immunology (formerly *Immunology Today*)

General websites

Clinical Evidence: ℘ www.clinicalevidence.org
Highwire: ℘ www.highwire.stanford.edu
e-medicine: ℘ www.emedicine.com
mdlinks: ℘ www.mdlinks.com
Medscape: ℘ www.medscape.com
PubMed: ℘ www.ncbi.nlm.nih.gov
Quackwatch: ℘ www.quackwatch.com
UK Pub Med: ℘ www.ukpmc.ac.uk
UpToDate: ℘ www.uptodate.com/index (requires a subscription)

Professional societies

Association for Clinical Pathology: ℘ www.pathologists.org.uk
British Society for Allergy and Clinical Immunology: ℘ www.basaci.org
British Society for Immunology: ℘ www.immunology.org
Clinical Immunology Society: ℘ www.clinimmsoc.org
European Academy for Allergology and Clinical Immunology: ℘ www.eaaci.net
European Society for Immunodeficiencies: ℘ www.esid.org

Training

JRCPTB: ℘ www.jrcptb.org.uk/
Royal College of Pathologists: ℘ www.rcpath.org
Royal College of Physicians: ℘ www.rcplondon.ac.uk
Laboratory and healthcare standards (UKAS): ℘ www.ukas.com
Department of Health: ℘ www.dh.gov.uk
NICE: ℘ www.nice.org.uk
Care Quality Commission: ℘ www.cqc.org.uk/

Part 1

Primary immunodeficiency

Introduction

In general, immunodeficiencies are divided into those of the specific immune system (e.g. T cells or B cells or combined) or those of the innate or non-specific immune system (e.g. complement and neutrophils). The age at which the patient presents gives good but not absolute clues as to the type of immune deficiency; for instance, severe combined immune deficiency (SCID) will present within the first 6 months of life. The type of infection also gives excellent clues as to the nature of the underlying immune defect. For example, recurrent meningococcal infection is a major feature of complement deficiency, while persistent respiratory syncytial virus infection in a small baby should raise the question of SCID. Other associated features also provide clues; for example, ataxia (unsteadiness on the feet) together with bacterial infections suggests ataxia telangiectasia.

Immunodeficiencies may also be divided into primary (usually genetic) and secondary, where the immune defect is caused by some other non-immunological disease; for example, a glycogen storage disease that causes a neutrophil defect, or a drug (e.g. phenytoin). Sometimes the distinction is blurred; for example, the AIDS virus (HIV-1) infects CD4+ T lymphocytes and macrophages and alters their functional capacity. This is usually referred to as a secondary immunodeficiency, despite the 'primary' effect on T cells (see ➔ Chapter 2 for a further discussion of secondary immunodeficiencies). There may be some overlap between groupings (e.g. adenosine deaminase has its immunological effect through a metabolic abnormality that is genetically determined). Some host defence disorders are covered in Chapter 2, e.g. cystic fibrosis.

There has been a massive expansion in the number of known inborn errors of immunity over the last few years. As of February 2017, the IUIS recognized 354 such conditions, and the number continues to grow month by month. It is clearly impractical to cover every single one of these in this Handbook, although I have endeavoured to mention as many as possible. The interested reader is advised to monitor the literature regularly. The IUIS regularly publishes updates. See ➔ 'Further reading' (but check regularly for updates).

▶All patients with primary immunodeficiencies should be under the care of an immunologist, who will be familiar with the range of complications.

Further reading

Picard, C. et al. (2018). International Union of Immunological Societies: 2017 Primary Immunodeficiency Diseases Committee Report on inborn errors of immunity. *J. Clin. Immunol.* 38:96–128.

Bousfiha, A. et al. (2018). The 2017 IUIS phenotypic classification for primary immunodeficidencies. *J. Clin. Immunol.* 38:129–143.

Classification of immunodeficiency

Immunodeficiencies affecting cellular and humoral immunity (severe combined immunodeficiencies, SCID, defined by CD3 T-cell lymphopenia)

- SCID T negative B positive.
- SCID T negative B negative.

Immunodeficiencies affecting cellular and humoral immunity (combined immunodeficiencies generally less profound than severe combined immunodeficiency)

- Low CD4, low MHC class II expression.
- Low CD8.
- Immunoglobulins normal.
- Immunoglobulins low.
- Normal immunoglobulins but poor specific antibody responses.

Combined immunodeficiencies with associated or syndromic features

- Congenital thrombocytopenia.
- DNA repair defects, not covered under SCID.
- Immuno-osseous dysplasia.
- Thymic defects with additional congenital abnormalities (22q11 deletion syndromes).
- Hyper-IgE syndromes.
- Dyskeratosis congenital.
- Defects of vitamin B_{12} and folate metabolism.
- Anhidrotic ectodermal dysplasia with immunodeficiency (includes NEMO deficiency).
- Others (includes PNP deficiency, calcium channel defects, Kabuki syndrome, STAT5b deficiency, hepatic veno-occlusive disease with immunodeficiency, Vici syndrome, Hennekam–lymphangiectasia–lymphoedema syndrome, HOIL1 and HOIP1 deficiency).

Predominantly antibody deficiencies (hypogammaglobulinaemia)

- B cells absent (X-linked agammaglobulinaemia).
- B cells > 1% (common variable immunodeficiency).
- Rare genetic hypogammaglobulinaemias.
- IgA deficiency.

Predominantly antibody deficiency (other antibody deficiencies)

- Hyper-IgM syndromes.
- Selective IgA deficiency.
- Transient hypogammaglobulinaemia of infancy.
- IgG subclass deficiency.
- Specific antibody deficiency with normal immunoglobulins.
- Heavy and light chain mutations.
- Selective IgM deficiency.
- CARD11 deficiency.

Disease of immune dysregulation (HLH and EBV susceptibility)

- Hypopigmentation syndromes (Chediak–Higashi, Griscelli, and Hermansky–Pudlak syndromes).
- Familial HLH.
- Susceptibility to EBV.

Disease of immune dysregulation (with autoimmunity)
- Autoimmune lymphoproliferation (ALPS and related syndromes).
- With and without regulatory T-cell defects (APECED, IPEX).
- Immune dysregulation with colitis.

Congenital defects of phagocyte numbers ± function (neutropenia)
- With syndromes (e.g. Shwachman–Diamond syndrome, Barth syndrome, Cohen syndrome, glycogen storage disease type 1b).
- Without syndromes, e.g. HAX1 deficiency (Kostman's syndrome).

Congenital defects of phagocytes (functional defects)
- LADI–III.
- Normal dihydrorhodamine test (GATA2 deficiency = MonoMac syndrome).
- Abnormal dihydrorhodamine test (chronic granulomatous disease, RAC2 deficiency, G6PD deficiency).

Defects in intrinsic and innate immunity
- Susceptibility to bacterial infections (IRAK4 deficiency, MyD88 deficiency, IRAK1 deficiency, congenital asplenia).
- Susceptibility to parasitic and fungal infections (chronic mucocutaneous candidiasis syndromes; trypanosomiasis—APOL1).
- Others (hidradentiis suppurativa, osteopetrosis).

Defects in intrinsic and innate immunity (Mycobacteria and viruses)
- Interferon gamma receptor defects.
- IL-12 defects.
- Epidermodysplasia verruciformis (HPV).
- Susceptibility to viral infections (STAT1, STAT2, CD16 deficiency).
- Herpes simplex (UNC93B1, TLR3).

Autoinflammatory diseases
- See ➋ Chapter 14.

Complement deficiencies
- Component and regulator deficiencies.

Phenocopies of primary immunodeficiencies
- Associated with somatic mutations (e.g. autoinflammatory conditions).
- Associated with autoantibodies (e.g. to interferon-gamma, C1-inhibitor, autoantibodies to factor H).

Secondary immunodeficiencies
- See ➋ Chapter 2.
- Viral infections (HIV, CMV, EBV, rubella).
- Chronic infections (TB, leishmania).
- Malignancy.
- Lymphoma/leukaemia.
- Extremes of age.

- Transfusion therapy.
- Drugs.
- Plasmapheresis; immunoadsorption.
- Radiation.
- Nutrition.
- Chronic renal disease (including dialysis).
- Toxins (including alcohol, cigarettes).
- Surgery (e.g splenectomy, thymectomy).

Clinical features of immunodeficiency

Recurrent infections
There is no universally accepted definition of what constitutes 'recurrent infection' and therefore it is difficult to be categorical about who should be investigated for immunodeficiency. The following should be used as guidance.
- Two major or one major and recurrent minor in 1 year.*
- Unusual organisms (*Aspergillus, Pneumocystis*).
- Unusual sites (liver abscess, osteomyelitis).
- Chronic infections (sinusitis).
- Structural damage (e.g. bronchiectasis).
- Other suspicious features.

Other features raising suspicion of an underlying immunodeficiency
- Skin rash (atypical eczema): Wiskott–Aldrich syndrome, hyper-IgE syndrome, Omenn's syndrome.
- Chronic diarrhoea: SCID, IPEX, antibody deficiencies.
- Failure to thrive: any immune deficiency in childhood.
- Hepatosplenomegaly: common variable immunodeficiency (CVID), Omenn's syndrome.
- Chronic osteomyelitis/deep-seated abscesses: chronic granulomatous disease.
- Mouth ulceration (?cyclical): neutropenia.
- Autoimmunity: CVID, hyper-IgM syndrome.
- Family history.

Features associated with specific immunodeficiencies
Some features are diagnostic of particular immunodeficiencies.
- Ataxia: ataxia telangiectasia, PNP deficiency.
- Telangiectasia: ataxia telangiectasia.
- Short-limbed dwarfism: X-linked immunodeficiency.
- Skeletal abnormalities: ribs in ADA deficiency.
- Cartilage–hair hypoplasia.
- Ectodermal dysplasia.

---

* A major infection is severe infection, usually requiring parenteral treatment in hospital, with objective evidence of infection (elevated CRP, positive culture). Minor infection is less severe, usually treatable in the community with oral therapy, but with objective evidence of infection.

- Endocrinopathy (particularly with hypocalcaemia): chronic mucocutaneous candidiasis.
- Partial albinism: Chediak–Higashi disease; Griscelli syndrome.
- Thrombocytopenia (particularly with small platelets): X-linked thrombocytopenia; Wiskott–Aldrich syndrome.
- Eczema: Wiskott–Aldrich syndrome; hyper-IgE syndrome; Omenn's syndrome.
- Neonatal tetany: 22q11 deletion syndromes (DiGeorge).
- Severe bowel disease: IPEX.
- Abnormal facies (leonine; fish-shaped mouth, low-set ears): hyper-IgE (leonine); 22q11 deletion syndrome (fish-shaped mouth, low-set ears); ICF syndrome (see ➲ 'Other chromosomal instability disorders', p. 53).
- Intellectual disability: 22q11 deletion syndromes, PNP deficiency; other genetic immunodeficiencies.[*]

Investigation of immunodeficiency

History
Must include the following.
- History of all infections: site, severity, need for antibiotics, hospitalizations.
- Operations (grommets, lobectomies, etc.).
- Immunization history.
- Family history, especially for serious infections, unexplained sudden deaths, diagnosed immunodeficiencies, and autoimmune diseases.
- Various organizations, including the Jeffrey Modell Foundation and the European Society for Immunodeficiencies have produced guidelines for non-specialists to encourage greater recognition of primary immunodeficiencies.[*]

Examination
Particular features to pay attention to include the following.
- Weight and height (failure to thrive).
- Structural damage from infections (ears, sinuses, lungs).
- Autoimmune features: vitiligo; alopecia; goitre.
- Other suspicious/diagnostic features, as previously noted.

Differential diagnosis
Formulate differential diagnoses in rank order and then investigate appropriately. The advances in genetic analysis mean that many cases of unusual immune deficiency are now amenable to genetic identification, with a huge increase in the number of genetically based rare disorders. The reader is advised to follow the literature carefully. This chapter will cover only those syndromes known at the time of writing: new syndromes are described on a monthly basis.

---

[*] ℘ http://www.esid.org/clinical-10-warning-signs-of-pid-general-339-0 and ℘ http://www.esid.org/clinical-6-warning-signs-for-pid-in-adults-175-0

Laboratory investigation

Use laboratory facilities wisely

- Target investigations to differential diagnosis.
- Do not blanket screen.
- Ensure basic tests are done before exotic tests.
- Think whether tests will contribute to diagnosis or management: if they will not then do not do them!

B-cell function

Full evaluation of the humoral immune system requires that all the parts are present *and* functioning. The latter usually requires *in vivo* test immunization, bearing in mind the caveat that no patient with suspected immunodeficiency should receive live vaccines. The following tests comprise a full screen of humoral function.

- Serum immunoglobulins (be sure to use low-level detection system for IgA to confirm absence).
- Serum and urine electrophoresis (evidence for bands and urinary loss).
- IgG subclasses.
- IgE.
- Antibacterial, antiviral antibodies (appropriate to immunization and exposure history).
- Immunization responses (protein and polysaccharide antigens).
- Isohaemagglutinins (IgM, dependent on blood group; thought to be less useful now).
- B-lymphocyte numbers (flow cytometry); class-switch memory B cells (CD27$^+$/IgD$^-$/IgM$^-$).
- Pokeweed mitogen (PWM) and antigen-stimulated antibody production *in vitro* (clinical indications limited).

T-cell function

Tests of T-cell function are less easy and less reliable than for B cells, where antibody provides a convenient read-out. 'Normal' ranges for *in vitro* proliferation assays are quite wide: know your own laboratory ranges. Use absolute T-cell counts, not percentages.

- T-cell numbers and surface phenotype.
- CD2, CD3, CD4, CD8, CD7, Tcr ($\alpha\beta$, $\gamma\delta$), CD40 and CD40 ligand, MHC class II; CD45RA and RO, CD27.
- CD40 ligand expression on activated T cells.
- T-cell proliferation to antigens, mitogens (OKT3, PHA, phorbol myristate acetate (PMA), calcium ionophore, cytokines).
- T-cell cytokine production *in vitro*.
- *In vivo* skin (delayed-type hypersensitivity, DTH) testing: the Multitest CMI is a convenient tool, but responses will depend on prior exposure. It is not widely used.

Neutrophil function

Neutrophil function tests are not widely available, so if there is suspicion of a neutrophil defect, specialist help should be sought. Interpretation is difficult and tests may be influenced by intercurrent infection and drug therapy.

- Neutrophil markers (CD11a, CD11b, CD11c, CD18, CD15).
- Upregulation of neutrophil markers (PMA, fMLP).
- Oxidative metabolism (quantitative and qualitative nitroblue tetrazolium reduction (NBT test); flow cytometric determination of oxidative burst, dihydrorhodamine).
- Phagocytosis.
- Bacterial killing (relevant organisms should be selected).
- Chemotaxis (difficult to standardize, with wide normal range: not widely used).

NK-cell function
This is an area of particular interest.
- NK-cell numbers by flow cytometry (absolute counts).
- K562 killing assay (radioimmunoassay, flow cytometry).
- Cytokine-stimulated killing (lymphokine-activated killer cell (LAK) assay).
- Perforin, granule release assays.

Complement assays
- Measurement of specific components.
- Functional assays (haemolytic assays).
- Complement breakdown components (C3a, C5a, C5b–C9).

Toll receptor assays
- Measurement of specific pathways.

Cytokine and interferon assays
- Measurement of specific components and receptors (see ⊃ Chapter 20).

Genetic studies
Genetic studies form an essential part of the investigation and management of primary immunodeficiencies. Many of the functional tests have been rendered redundant by new genetic testing strategies.
- Cytogenetics (deletions, translocations).
- Ig and Tcr gene rearrangements (clonality).
- X-linked gene studies.
- 22q11 microdeletions (FISH—fluorescent in situ hybridization).
- Protein expression studies (SAP, btk).
- MHC studies.
- Prenatal diagnosis.
- A number of centres now offer screening panels for common primary immunodeficiencies.
- Whole exome (WES) and whole genome sequencing (WGS) will be valuable in rare immunodeficiencies not identified on the standard screening panels.

Other investigations
The use of other investigative procedures depends very much on the clinical state of the patient.
- Detection of autoimmunity:
  - anti-red cell, platelet, neutrophil antibodies;
  - anti-endocrine autoimmunity (e.g. thyroid autoantibodies).

- Exclusion of secondary causes:
  - renal disease, bowel disease (loss of immunoglobulins ± lymphocytes);
  - malignancy (lymph-node biopsy; PET-CT);
  - nutritional deficiencies (zinc, vitamin B_{12}, iron);
  - drugs (cytotoxics, anticonvulsants).
- Detection of nodular lymphoid hyperplasia (CT scanning, barium follow-through, endoscopy, and biopsy).
- Lung function (including FEV_1, FVC, transfer factor).
- Imaging studies (HR-CT lungs, CT sinuses).
- Direct isolation of pathogens: bacteria, fungal, and viral (serology is usually unreliable—use PCR-based tests where culture is not possible).

Major B-lymphocyte disorders

- X-linked agammaglobulinaemia (Bruton's agammaglobulinaemia; XLA).
- Common variable immunodeficiency (acquired hypogammaglobulinaemia; CVID). Including P1K3CD gain- and loss-of-function mutations; PTEN deficiency.
- Selective IgA deficiency.
- IgG subclass deficiency.
- Specific antibody deficiency with normal immunoglobulins.

Rare antibody deficiency syndromes

Antibody deficiency, presenting as 'common variable immunodeficiency', has been associated with extremely rare genetically identified disorders.
- X-linked hyper-IgM syndrome (HIGM-1); CD40 ligand deficiency.
- Autosomal hyper-IgM syndromes (HIGM-2–4):
  - HIGM-2; autosomal recessive activation-induced cytidine deaminase deficiency;
  - HIGM-3; autosomal recessive CD40 deficiency;
  - HIGM-4; similar to HIGM-2, molecularly undefined;
  - HIGM due to uracil-DNA glycosylase (UNG) deficiency.
- INO80 deficiency.
- MSH6 deficiency.
- X-linked hypogammaglobulinaemia with growth hormone deficiency.
- Selective IgM deficiency.
- X-linked lymphoproliferative syndrome (Duncan's syndrome; XLPS).
- Hyper-IgE syndrome (Job's syndrome).
- Selective IgE deficiency.
- Transient hypogammaglobulinaemia of infancy.
- Mu-chain deficiency.
- Igα (CD79a) deficiency.
- Igβ (CD79b) deficiency
- BLNK deficiency.
- ICOS deficiency.
- λ5/14.1 (surrogate light chain, IGLL1, CD179B) deficiency.

- SWAP-70 deficiency.
- κ and λ light chain deficiency.
- CD19 deficiency.
- CD20 deficiency.
- CD21 deficiency.
- CD81 (TAPA1) deficiency.
- LRRC8A (leucine-rich repeat-containing protein 8A) deficiency.
- Thymoma with immunodeficiency (Good's syndrome).
- CD19 deficiency.
- P13KR1 deficiency.
- E47 transcription factor deficiency.
- TWEAK deficiency (TNFS12).
- MOGS deficiency (mannosyl-oligosaccharide glucosidase deficiency).
- TTC37 deficiency.
- IRF2BP2 deficiency.
- CARD11 gain-of-function mutation.
- NFKB1 and NFKB2 deficiency.
- IKAROS deficiency.
- ATP6AP1 deficiency (X-linked).

Identification of these rare syndromes requires a high index of suspicion. Some may be identifiable by flow cytometry, but in the main diagnosis will depend upon genetic studies.

X-linked agammaglobulinaemia (Bruton's disease)

This is the first described immunodeficiency (1952). It has an incidence of 1 in 100 000–200 000 and a prevalence of 1 in 10 000.

Cause

- Genetic disorder due to mutations on the X chromosome affecting the *btk* gene.
- *btk* codes for a tyrosine kinase involved in B-cell maturation.
- Defects in the gene prevent B-cell maturation from pro-B-cell to pre-B-cell.
- Gene is located at Xq21.3–22. Mutations include deletions and point mutations, either conservative or leading to premature termination.
- Phenotype correlates poorly with genotype.
- Mild phenotypes occur with some limited B-cell development.
- New mutations common, so a family history may be absent.
- The *xid* mutation in mice is similar, although some features differ.

Presentation

- Usually early in childhood, after 6 months of age, when maternal antibody has largely disappeared.
- Recurrent infections of lungs and ears (children of this age don't have sinuses):
  - *Haemophilus influenzae* and pneumococci (upper and lower respiratory tract, meningitis);

- meningococcus (meningitis);
- staphylococci (septic arthritis);
- *Giardia, Salmonella,* and *Campylobacter* infections of the gut.
- Rarely *Pneumocystis.*
- Milder phenotypes may present later.

Diagnosis—key features

- Early-onset bacterial infections in a male child with a family history.
- Family history often absent.
- Neutropenia very common at presentation but goes away with treatment and is probably due to chronic bacterial sepsis.
- Failure to thrive and chronic diarrhoea common.
- Distinction of milder forms, with some B cells and low but not absent IgG, from CVID is difficult and relies on the demonstration of abnormalities of the *btk* gene. Some patients previously classified as CVID will turn out to be XLA.
- Specific antibody deficiency only reported with *btk* mutations.
- XLA may rarely be associated with growth hormone deficiency (and short stature).
- Occasional females will be identified with the immunological features of XLA.
- Differential diagnosis will include coeliac disease and cystic fibrosis, although the laboratory tests will rapidly identify antibody deficiency.

Immunology

In the complete forms the immunology is fairly distinctive.
- All immunoglobulins are absent or very low.
- B cells are low or absent.
- Btk protein absent (confirm with genetic studies where there is a good history, to exclude production of non-functional protein).
- Lymph nodes show no germinal centres; no tonsils; pre-B cells in bone marrow (BM).
- T-cell numbers and function are normal.
- NK-cell numbers and function are normal.

Mild or incomplete variants may be difficult to distinguish from CVID.
- Variable numbers of B cells including normal.
- Variable immunoglobulins.
- Poor/absent specific antibodies to polysaccharide antigens.

Complications

The major complications relate to delay in diagnosis.
- Structural lung damage (bronchiectasis, sinusitis). Inadequate therapy will lead to progression of lung damage and the development of chronic sinus damage.
- Chronic meningoencephalitis due to echoviruses and coxsackieviruses may cause a progressive and fatal dementing illness; there is often muscle involvement, with a myositis and contractures. Diagnose by viral culture of CSF or by PCR-based techniques. Antiviral pleconaril is helpful (though not licensed by the FDA). This disease appears less often

since the introduction of intravenous immunoglobulin (IVIg) therapy as standard, but has not disappeared completely.
- *Ureaplasma*/*Mycoplasma* septic arthritis. This is difficult to diagnose without special culture facilities. It is a highly destructive chronic infection and requires prolonged treatment (6 months) with tetracyclines ± erythromycin.
- Haemophilus conjunctivitis.
- Crohn's-like disease of intestines. Possible increased risk of colonic cancer.
- Possible increase in malignancies (colorectal, gastric, squamous cell lung).

Treatment
- IVIg should be started at the earliest opportunity (see ➲ Chapter 16); dose of 200–600 mg/kg/month given at intervals of 2–3 weeks. Longer intervals do not give satisfactory replacement.
- Subcutaneous immunoglobulin given weekly or by daily push (same total dose) is an alternative.
- Trough IgG levels should be monitored regularly, with the aim of maintaining a level well within the normal range (6–9 g/dl). Early institution of IVIg and adequate trough levels preclude the development of bronchiectasis.
- Prompt antibiotic therapy (course of 10–14 days) for upper and lower respiratory tract infections together with physiotherapy and postural drainage if lung damage has already occurred. Ciprofloxacin is a valuable antibiotic (though not licensed for small children). Use cystic fibrosis approach of zero tolerance to cough.
- Prophylactic azithromycin 3×/week ± carbocisteine is valuable where there is established bronchiectasis—teach postural drainage and effective cough.
- As children get older and can comply, perform annual lung function testing, including transfer factor.
- High-resolution CT scanning (HR-CT) is useful for identifying subclinical bronchiectasis, but imposes a significant radiation burden and should not be overused.
- Do not give oral poliovaccine as patients often fail to clear it, which increases the risk of reversion to wild type, with consequent paralytic disease.
- Genetic counselling of the patient and family once genetic basis confirmed. Identify and counsel carriers.
- Long-term immunological follow-up (plus additional specialist input as required).

XLA with growth hormone deficiency
This is a very rare disorder with immunological features identical to XLA, in association with short stature (as opposed to failure to thrive). The disease maps the region of the X chromosome containing the *btk* gene, but not all cases appear to have mutations in the *btk* gene. Prognosis appears to be good. It is treated with IVIg and growth hormone.

Common variable immunodeficiency (CVID)

CVID is the commonest symptomatic antibody deficiency with an estimated incidence of 1 in 25 000–66 000, based on Scandinavian data.

Cause

• Cause of CVID is unknown: one hypothesis suggests that an environmental insult (virus infection?) in a genetically susceptible individual triggers the disease. No conclusive viral trigger has been identified.
• Some evidence for a genetic background (linked to MHC A1B8DR3C4Q0 and to polymorphisms in the TNFα gene).
• May be a family history of other antibody deficiencies (especially IgA deficiency and IgG subclass deficiency) in up to 50% of cases, although other family members may be entirely asymptomatic.
• Disease is heterogeneous in phenotype and immunological findings.
• Diagnosis is now one of exclusion, once other genetic diseases have been ruled out.
• Some CVID patients have been identified with mutations in TACI and BAFF-R—significance is uncertain: may not be disease-causing.
• SNPs in the gene *MSH5* have been reported with increased frequency in patients with CVID and IgA deficiency.
• CLEC16A has been associated with CVID and a mouse model also shows hypogammaglobulinaemia.
• Use of WES and WGS has identified gene defects in some but not all patients with CVID.

Presentation

• May present at any age from childhood through to old age, although the peak of presentation is in early childhood and early adulthood.
• Usual presentation is with recurrent bacterial infections, as for XLA.
• May present with autoimmune problems, especially thrombocytopenia, haemolytic anaemia, and organ-specific autoimmunity (e.g. thyroid, diabetes, vitiligo, and alopecia); these are common and may precede the development of recurrent infections.
• Nodular lymphoid hyperplasia of bowel (polyclonal hyperplasia of Peyer's patches) is unique to CVID. The cause is unknown, but it is possibly premalignant. This has characteristic features on small-bowel radiology.
• Granulomatous disease with lymphadenopathy and (hepato-)splenomegaly, and often involving the lung, is common in the severe form of CVID (about 25% of cases). Disease resembles sarcoidosis. Specifically associated with complete absence of class-switch memory B cells.
• More severe cases may develop opportunist infections (see ➲ 'Late-onset combined immune deficiency', p. 45).

Diagnosis

- History gives the clues. Clues are usually missed by general physicians and an average diagnostic delay of over 7 years is typical, by which time structural lung and sinus damage is severe and irretrievable.
- Immunoglobulin levels are variably low: test immunization and exclusion of secondary loss (gut, urine) may be required.
- Lymphopenia affecting predominantly the CD4+ T cells (CD45RA+ naïve cells in particular) and B cells is common.
- When splenomegaly is present it may be difficult to exclude lymphoma, without CT scanning, lymph node biopsy, and bone marrow examination.

Immunology

- Immunoglobulin levels are highly variable, and IgG may be only marginally reduced; specific antibodies are invariably low with poor/ absent immunization responses.
- IgM may be normal, which contrasts with lymphoma, when the IgM is the first immunoglobulin to drop (see ➔ Chapter 2).
- B cells may be normal or low but some cases in males may be late-presenting XLA.
- CD4+ T cells are low, with specific depletion of CD45RA+ T cells.
- T-cell function *in vivo* and *in vitro* to antigens and mitogens is poor and there is poor NK-cell function, with reduced NK-cell numbers.
- Abnormalities of 5'-nucleotidase activity on the lymphocyte surface have been described but this is not a separate syndrome as is sometimes stated. The significance of the abnormality is not known.

Classification

Three groups are identified on the basis of B-cell responses to IL-2 + anti-IgM *in vitro*.

- Group A: severe disease, with granulomata (hepatosplenomegaly); no IgG or IgM production *in vitro*.
- Group B: rare; IgM production only *in vitro* (?cryptic hyper-IgM).
- Group C: mild disease; IgG and IgM production *in vitro*.

This technique is unsuited to routine diagnosis; identification of class-switch memory B cells is more useful (group A patients lack class-switch memory B cells).

Clinical grouping by complications has been used as an alternative.

- No complications.
- Polyclonal lymphocytic infiltration.
- Enteropathy.
- Lymphoid malignancy.

83% of patients show a single clinical phenotype.

Phenotyping by flow cytometry has also been used (EUROclass trial): three patterns emerge.

- Nearly absent B cells (< 1%).

- Severely reduced class-switched memory B cells (< 2%)—may be seen in other PIDs: Wiskott–Aldrich syndrome, XLPS, idiopathic CD4 lymphopenia, and CGD.
- Expansion of CD21^{low} B cells (associated with lymphoproliferative disease and splenomegaly) > 10%. CD24 may also be helpful in analysing this subset; calcium signalling is also abnormal.

Reduction of regulatory T-cells (Tregs) is associated with an increase in autoimmune disease.

CVID: complications and treatment

Complications

- Major complications of CVID relate to the delay in diagnosis with structural damage from infection: bronchiectasis and chronic sinusitis.
- Patients may also have unusual infections, such as *Campylobacter* cholangitis, and *Mycoplasma/Ureaplasma* arthritis (see ➔ 'XLA', p. 12). Rarely, opportunist infections such as *Pneumocystis* occur (but this should suggest hyper-IgM syndromes).
- Malabsorption may occur due to a coeliac-like enteropathy, with villous atrophy.
- Inflammatory bowel disease may occur with strictures.
- Chronic norovirus has been reported and may be a cause of villous atrophy.
- Nodular regenerative hyperplasia of the liver is seen.
- Granulomatous disease may affect any organ (brain, lungs, liver, spleen, lymph nodes, skin, eye).
- In group A patients with splenomegaly, hypersplenism may occur with marked thrombocytopenia: splenectomy may be required.
- A 40-fold increase in the risk of lymphoma, including intestinal lymphoma. Any patient with lymphadenopathy should have a lymph node biopsy and BM examination to exclude the diagnosis. Lymphomas are often high grade and respond poorly to treatment.
- Increase in gastric carcinoma, not related to *Helicobacter pylori* colonization.
- Autoimmune disease is common and patients should be monitored for the development of overt disease (hypothyroidism, pernicious anaemia, diabetes).
- Thymomas (benign or malignant) are also associated with CVID: this is Good's syndrome. These frequently give rise to myasthenia gravis and haematological problems such as aplastic anaemia and immune thrombocytopenia (ITP). It is not clear that this is a separate diagnostic entity.

Treatment

- The earlier the diagnosis is made, the better the prognosis.
- Treatment is identical to that of XLA, with IVIg/SCIg, antibiotics, and physiotherapy for chest disease.
- Prophylactic antibiotics should be considered if there is an inadequate response to optimal immunoglobulin therapy.

- Patients with complete IgA deficiency may have a higher risk of developing anti-IgA antibodies to IVIg therapy, and a product low in IgA should be selected for them; most IVIg products now have reduced IgA content. The value of monitoring anti-IgA antibodies is questionable.
- Patients with splenomegaly may catabolize IgG faster and may require larger doses or more frequent doses (weekly).
- Regular lung function tests (volumes and transfer factor) and HR-CT scanning is required. Deteriorating lung function requires more aggressive therapy.
- Chronic sinus disease requires ENT review, with endoscopic inspection.
- Granulomatous disease responds well to steroids (alkaline phosphatase and angiotensin-converting enzyme (ACE) are good markers); these are essential if there is interstitial lung disease (reduced transfer factor). They are not necessary for asymptomatic splenomegaly. Steroid use is associated with an increased risk of disseminated shingles. Splenectomy may be necessary for hypersplenism: such patients must have prophylactic penicillin, but immunizations are of little value. There is, however, an additional risk of infection post-splenectomy in CVID patients and caution is required.
- Treat inflammatory bowel disease as for Crohn's disease.
- Chronic norovirus has been treated with oral immunoglobulin, nitazoxanide, and ribavirin.
- Liver disease may cause portal hypertension and hepatic encephalopathy—shunting may be required.
- Gluten-free diet may help if there is coeliac-like disease.
- Monitor for the development of malignant disease. Review frequency of cervical smears.
- Consider need for bone mineral density monitoring (malabsorption); treat appropriately if low.

Experimental therapy
- Anti-TNF agents have been used in severe granulomatous disease.

Selective IgA deficiency

Selective IgA deficiency is the most common primary immunodeficiency, but mostly passes unnoticed. Depending on the racial group, 1 in 400–800 individuals will be affected.

Cause
- Cause is unknown, although it forms part of the spectrum of disease with CVID and shares the MHC type (A1, B8, DR3, C4Q0). It occurs in relatives of patients with CVID in 50% of cases.
- Rarely due to a gene deletion, which may include genes for IgG_2/IgG_4.
- Defects of class switching have been identified in a few patients.
- Selective deficiencies of IgA_1 or IgA_2 have been reported (all due to gene deletions).
- May be associated with other chromosomal abnormalities, usually involving chromosome 18 (18q syndrome and ring chromosome 18).

Also with variant Turner's syndrome (XO), multibranched chromosomes, Klinefelter's syndrome, and α_1-antitrypsin (α1-AT) deficiency.

- Associated with drug therapy, particularly with phenytoin and penicillamine, although in many reports it is not clear whether the defect was present before drug therapy was introduced.
- IgA-bearing B cells are present. IgA is synthesized but not secreted.
- In terms of mucosal protection, there is evidence that IgG and IgM may substitute as secretory immunoglobulins.

Presentation

- Most cases are asymptomatic.
- There is an increased incidence of allergic disease, including food allergies and intolerances.
- Connective tissue diseases (SLE, rheumatoid arthritis, and juvenile chronic arthritis), coeliac disease, inflammatory bowel disease, pernicious anaemia, and other organ-specific autoimmune diseases.
- Nodular lymphoid hyperplasia.
- Increased presence of a range of autoantibodies.
- False-positive pregnancy tests due to heterophile antibodies.
- Infections are rarely a problem unless there are additional humoral defects present.
- Occasional cases will come to light as a result of adverse reactions to blood products. This is deemed to be very rare (incidence 1 in 15 million transfusions). Blood Transfusion Services in the UK no longer recommend any specific precautions unless there has been a previous blood transfusion reaction.

Diagnosis

- Requires the demonstration of undetectable IgA, *not* just a low IgA. Automated analysers do not read low enough to ascertain this beyond doubt. Ideally check with low-level radial immunodiffusion or Ouchterlony double-diffusion assays.
- *Beware* of the presence of anti-animal antibodies in IgA deficiency, which give false readings in immunoassays using antisera derived from sheep, goats, and horses.
- Patients should be screened for evidence of other humoral defects: IgG subclasses and specific antibodies if there is a history of infections. If there is doubt, then test immunization should be undertaken.
- Anti-IgA antibodies can be measured but current assays detect IgG and IgM antibodies and therefore do not identify risk of anaphylaxis. The significance of IgG and IgM anti-IgA antibodies is uncertain: high levels may be seen in the absence of reactions. There is only one report of detection of IgE anti-IgA antibodies.

Immunology

- The IgA will be undetectable (< 0.05 g/l), but total IgG and IgM will be normal. IgG subclasses may be reduced (G_2 and G_4). Secreted IgA will be absent (secretory piece deficiency is vanishingly rare), but testing for this is of little clinical value.
- T-cell function is normal (PHA and antigens).

- Autoantibodies may be present (NB anti-IgA antibodies). There will be an increased IgE in the presence of atopic disease.
- In the absence of IgA, IgM and IgG appear on mucosal surfaces.

Complications
- Major problem with IgA deficiency is through related illnesses.
- Transfusion reactions are now thought to be extremely rare and specific precautions are not required unless there has been a prior reaction.
- Malignancy may be increased, although this may depend on other diseases present in association with IgA deficiency, especially lymphoma and gastric adenocarcinoma.
- It is possible that there may be progression to more significant humoral immunodeficiency with time.

Treatment
- Treatment is directed at the presenting disease.
- Avoid IgA-containing products if possible: The National Blood Authority no longer routinely provides blood products from IgA-deficient donors. Use an IVIg/SCIg (if required) with a low IgA content.
- Where immunoglobulin replacement therapy is required for recurrent infections, this has been shown to be safe.
- In view of the low risk of reactions, the wearing or carrying of an alert card is now of doubtful value.

Selective IgA$_2$ deficiency
- Cases have been reported with selective IgA$_2$ deficiency, with normal IgA$_1$. This does not appear to be due to heavy chain gene deletions affecting the α_2 gene in all cases.

IgG subclass deficiency

Cause
- Cause of IgG subclass deficiency is unknown, but it too forms part of the spectrum with CVID and IgA deficiency. It is possible that some cases represent CVID in evolution. Rarely, cases may be due to gene deletions, but these individuals may be entirely healthy.
- IgG subclass levels are related to allotypes of IgG (Gm allotypes); different racial groups may therefore have different 'normal' ranges, depending on the prevalence of different allotypes. This should be taken into account when diagnosing IgG subclass deficiency.

Presentation
- Presentation, as for CVID, can be at any age. Recurrent infections may be a feature, particularly for IgG$_2$ ± IgG$_4$ deficiency. IgG$_4$ deficiency occurring alone has also been associated with bronchiectasis.
- Other conditions associated with subclass deficiency include: asthma (IgG$_3$ deficiency); sinusitis (IgG$_3$ deficiency); intractable epilepsy of childhood (though this may be due to anticonvulsants); and autoimmune disease (SLE).

Diagnosis

- Measurement of IgG subclasses on more than one occasion is required and it is important to check that appropriate age-specific normal ranges are used (preferably related to the racial background).
- Detection of low levels of IgG_4 may require more sensitive assays to detect true absence: earlier normal ranges using less-sensitive assays found a significant number of individuals with undetectable IgG_4. Most of these have detectable IgG_4 on sensitive assays.
- There is a poor correlation of specific anti-pathogen responses and IgG subclass levels. All patients should have specific antibodies measured and be test immunized.
- Detection of low or absent subclasses does not necessarily correlate with clinical disease.

Immunology

- A normal total IgG is entirely compatible with subclass deficiency, although low IgG_1 usually reduces the total IgG (this behaves like CVID for practical purposes). The IgA is normal or low; IgM is normal.
- B- and T-cell numbers are usually normal.
- Poor specific antibody responses to bacterial and viral antigens may be present in some patients.

Complications

- Long-term progression to CVID is a possibility.
- Bronchiectasis may occur in IgG_4 deficiency.

Treatment

- Treatment is controversial: only symptomatic patients should be treated. If recurrent infections are a problem, then the first step might be to use continuous prophylactic antibiotics, followed by IVIg if infections are not controlled.
- IVIg has been shown to be of benefit in asthma due to IgG_3 deficiency (and, interestingly, a low IgG_3 preparation worked), and in chronic sinusitis.
- It is theoretically possible to bypass IgG_2 deficiency using protein-conjugated polysaccharide vaccines to generate a protective IgG_1 response.

Specific antibody deficiency with normal serum immunoglobulins

This syndrome is probably much more common than hitherto realized.

Cause

- Cause is unknown. It is unrelated to IgG subclass deficiencies. There is usually a failure to respond to polysaccharide antigens (T-independent) and possibly other protein antigens (HBsAg?).
- In small children, it may be due to a maturational delay that resolves spontaneously.

Presentation

- Recurrent bacterial infection of upper and lower respiratory tract (*Haemophilus, Pneumococcus, Moraxella*) is the usual presentation.
- In immunization programmes for hepatitis B, about 5% of individuals fail to respond to the standard three-dose schedule; a fourth dose still leaves 1–2% who fail to make a serological response. These patients clearly have some form of specific immune deficit (see ➋ Chapter 2 for the approach to management of these individuals).

Diagnosis

- There is a history of recurrent typical infections with normal immunoglobulins and IgG subclasses.
- Proof requires demonstration of failure to respond to specific antigens (test immunization).

Immunology

- Immunoglobulins and IgG subclasses are normal, but there are low specific antibodies, especially to capsulated organisms, and poor responses to test immunization, especially to polysaccharide antigens (Pneumovax® 23).
- The use of serotype-specific responses may add confidence to the diagnosis.
- *Salmonella typhi* Vi antigen has also been evaluated as a test antigen.
- Meningococcal polysaccharide vaccines may be used but the serological responses are less well established.
- For all vaccines, a normal response is a rise in titre into the protective range AND a 4× increase over pre-immunization level; ideally pre-and post-vaccine samples should be run on the same assays as the inter-assay coefficient of variation (CV) of specific antibody assays is high.
- Children under the age of 2 years do not respond to Pneumovax® 23. However, the inability to respond to polysaccharide antigens in infants may be bypassed by conjugation of the polysaccharide to a protein, for example, the Hib-conjugate vaccines and Prevenar 13®, the heptavalent pneumococcal polysaccharide vaccine.
- T- and B-lymphocyte numbers and T-cell function are normal.

Complications

❶Long delay in diagnosis leads to structural lung damage: may be of the order of 15–20 years because clinicians fail to recognize immunodeficiency in the presence of normal total immunoglobulins.

Treatment

Treatment is still controversial. Conjugate vaccines should be tried to by-pass defect—if this is ineffective then:

- First step should be prophylactic antibiotics (azithromycin 250–500 mg od 3×/week, adult dose); tetracycline 500 bd is an alternative, but is less effective. Remember to warn regarding possible ototoxicity with azithromycin and obtain baseline ECG.

- Continuous antibiotics are inadequate for patients with established lung disease: these should be managed on IVIg/SCIg as for XLA. No randomized placebo-controlled trials.
- In small children, spontaneous improvement may occur, and continuous prophylactic antibiotics and close supervision may be sufficient.

❶*Remember.* Normal serum immunoglobulins and IgG subclasses do NOT exclude humoral immune deficiency!

X-linked hyper-IgM syndrome (HIGM-1)

Originally this was thought to be a B-cell disorder, but the demonstration in the X-linked form of a primary T-cell defect means that this form should be reclassified as a T-cell defect. The predominant effect, however, is of a humoral immune deficiency.

Cause

- X-linked form has now been shown to be due to a deficiency of the CD40 ligand (CD154) on T cells (gene located at Xq26–27), required for B-cell immunoglobulin class switch.
- CD40 is also expressed on monocyte–macrophages and the interaction with CD40 ligand is integral to antigen presentation.

Presentation

- Presentation is with recurrent bacterial infections; this may include *Pneumocystis jirovecii* pneumonia.
- There is often neutropenia and thrombocytopenia. Autoimmune disease of all types is common.

Diagnosis

- There is usually an early onset; the diagnosis should always be considered when *Pneumocystis* pneumonia is the presenting illness. The differential diagnosis includes SCID and HIV infection.
- There will be a normal or high IgM, with low IgG and IgA.
- Most cases can be identified by failure to upregulate expression of CD154 on activation of T cells; this does not identify cases where point mutations permit expression of non-functional CD154.
- Genetic confirmation is required.

Immunology

- IgM (and IgD) are normally raised with a low IgG and IgA. However, the IgM may be normal in the absence of infection. There will be high isohaemagglutinins. Specific IgM responses are present but may be short-lived. IgM$^+$ and IgD$^+$ B cells are present.
- T-cell function may be normal or poor. Some patients have reduced cell-mediated immunity, as evidenced by the occurrence of *Pneumocystis* infection. The expression of CD40 ligand on activated T cells may be defective (use PMA + ionophore).
- Mild variants exist, compatible with minimal disease and survival into adult life.

Complications

- Opportunist pneumonias. There appears to be a particular risk of cryptosporidial infection of the biliary tree, leading to a severe cholangitis and liver failure.
- Autoimmune diseases including haemolytic anaemia, thrombocytopenia, and neutropenia; parvovirus-induced anaemia.
- Increased risk of lymphomas (IgM+, due to chronic overstimulation), hepatocellular, bile duct, and neuroendocrine carcinomas.
- Long-term prognosis without transplantation is poor (infections and liver disease).

Treatment

- IVIg/SCIg should be started at the earliest opportunity: the IgM returns to the normal range with adequate therapy. Doses should be in the range 0.4–0.6 g/kg every 2–3 weeks.
- Prompt antibiotics are required for infections, as for other antibody deficiencies.
- Consideration should be given to the use of PCP prophylaxis (co-trimoxazole 480 mg bd, 960 mg od, or 960 mg three times per week; azithromycin and atovaquone are alternatives where co-trimoxazole cannot be tolerated).
- All drinking water, even if bottled, should be boiled, as domestic supplies cannot be guaranteed to be free of *Cryptosporidium*.
- Bone marrow/stem cell transplantation (BMT/SCT) is the treatment of choice, where the diagnosis is made early in life and where compatible donors are available. Gene therapy is now also being evaluated.
- Liver transplantation may be required for liver disease secondary to *Cryptosporidium* infection.

Autosomal hyper-IgM syndromes

Four rare types of autosomal hyper-IgM have now been identified.

HIGM-2

- Caused by defects in the activation-induced cytidine deaminase gene (*AID* gene, 12p13).
- Intrinsic B-cell defect with failure to class-switch. B cells express CD19, sIgM, and sIgD.
- T-cell function is normal: opportunistic infections such as *Pneumocystis* do not occur.
- T-cell expression of CD154 is normal.
- Lymphoid histology is abnormal with hyperplasia and giant germinal centres.
- Presentation is with recurrent bacterial and gastrointestinal infections from early in childhood.
- Treatment is with IVIg/SCIg.

HIGM-3

- Caused by deficiency of CD40 expression on B cells, due to a genetic defect (20q12–13.2).

- Clinical features are identical to those of HIGM-1, and opportunist infections can occur.
- Class-switch memory B cells are markedly reduced or absent.
- Monocyte function is also defective (CD40 is expressed on monocytes). CD40 is also expressed on endothelial cells.
- Neutropenia may occur.
- Increased risk of lymphomas, hepatocellular, bile duct, and neuroendocrine carcinomas.
- Treatment is the same as for HIGM-1 with IVIg/SCIg, prophylaxis against PCP, and consideration of BMT/SCT, although the latter will not completely restore CD40 expression in non-haematopoietic cell lineages.

HIGM-4
- Clinically a mild variant of HIGM-2, but with normal AID levels.
- The molecular defect is unknown.
- Some IgG production may occur.

HIGM-5
- Due to defects in uracil-DNA glycosylase (UNG).
- Clinically resembles HIGM-2. Enlarged lymph nodes and germinal centres are noted.
- From the limited clinical experience, IVIg/SCIg would appear to be the treatment of choice.

X-linked ectodermal dysplasia with HIGM (NEMO deficiency; IκBα deficiency)
- Cases have been reported of X-linked ectodermal dysplasia with HIGM due to loss-of-function mutations in the *NEMO* gene (Xq28), coding for IKK-γ, which block the release of NF-κB on cellular activation.
- Not all patients with *NEMO* mutations have extodermal dysplasia.
- Gain-of-function mutations in IκBα, with which IKK-γ interacts, have been reported to produce an autosomal dominant ectodermal dysplasia similar to *NEMO* deficiency.
- IL-10 production is lacking.
- Patients with *NEMO* mutations have impaired polysaccharide responses.
- IgA levels may be increased more than IgM.
- Patients with IκBα mutations have hypogammaglobulinaemia, reduced CD4⁺ and CD8⁺ T cells, and absent T-cell proliferation to anti-CD3.
- Clinical features include early-onset severe bacterial and viral infections, atypical mycobacterial infections, chronic diarrhoea, bronchiectasis, and failure to thrive.
- Hypomorphic *NEMO* mutations have also been associated with ectodermal dysplasia associated with osteopetrosis and lymphoedema, and incontinentia pigmenti.
- Prophylactic antibiotics are required.
- Anti-herpes prophylaxis may be required.
- Treatment with IVIg is helpful.
- HSCT has been used in both *NEMO* and IκBα mutations, with successful outcomes.

X-linked lymphoproliferative disease type 1, SAP deficiency (Duncan's syndrome, XLP-1)

This is a very rare genetic disorder, leading to failure to handle EBV correctly.

Cause

- Genetic defect has been localized to Xq26, and the gene has now been cloned.
- Gene product, SAP (SLAM-associated protein, SH2D1A) controls the activation of T and B cells via SLAM (signalling lymphocyte activation molecule), a surface protein. SLAM is involved in γ-IFN production and the switch from Th2 to Th1.
- Reason for the failure to handle EBV appropriately is not yet known.

Presentation

- Patients are fit and well until EBV is encountered. Upon infection with EBV, five outcomes are possible.
  - Fulminant EBV infection (58%); mortality is 96%!
  - Haemophagocytic lymphohistiocytosis (HLH).
  - EBV⁺ non-Hodgkin's lymphoma (30%); risk of lymphoma is 200-fold greater than the normal population.
  - Immunodeficiency, usually profound hypogammaglobulinaemia (30%). Some cases have been misdiagnosed as CVID.
  - Aplastic anaemia, often associated with hepatitis (3%).
  - Vasculitis, lymphomatoid granulomatosis (3%).
- Overall mortality was 85% by the age of 10 years, but is now improving especially for patients with HLH and lymphoma.
- Survival is only 18.6% for untransplanted patients with HLH.
- Overall survival is now 62.5% for untransplanted patients on Ig replacement.
- Mild cases are recognized.

Diagnosis

- Diagnosis is difficult, especially if there is fulminant EBV infection.
- Flow cytometric tests for intracellular proteins can demonstrate the presence of protein, but does not exclude mutations causing the production of non-functional proteins.
- Follow-up genetic testing for both SAP and XIAP is required.

Immunology

- Immunology is usually normal before infection, but it is rarely checked unless there is a family history. Carriers may have subtle immunological abnormalities, such as unusually high anti-EBV VCA antibodies.
- After infection, in those who survive, there are reduced immunoglobulins (all three classes). T-cell proliferation to mitogens and antigens is poor, and there is reduced γ-IFN production. NK-cell function is also poor. CD8⁺ T cells may be persistently elevated.
- Antibodies to EBV may be poor or even absent.

Treatment

- IVIg/SCIg should be used for the hypogammaglobulinaemia.
- HSCT may be an option, as part of the treatment of lymphoma. Survival after HSCT with good immune reconstitution is 81%.
- Prophylactic use of aciclovir in at-risk family members is of unproven value.
- During acute fulminant EBV, therapy directed against the abnormal CD8⁺ T cells (alemtuzumab (Campath®)) and transformed B cells (rituximab, anti-CD20) may be valuable.

X-linked lymphoproliferative disease type 2, XIAP deficiency (XLP-2)

XIAP is an (X-linked) inhibitor of apoptosis, also known as BIRC4, and stops cell death triggered by viral infection or excess caspase production.

Cause

- Genetic defect has been localized to Xq24–25.
- XIAP binds to and inhibits caspases 3, 7, and 9.

Presentation

- Mutations in XIAP have been associated with severe inflammatory bowel disease.
- Similar presentations to XLP-1 may occur.
- Asymptomatic cases are described.

Diagnosis

- Is based on clinical suspicion followed up by genetic testing.
- Flow cytometric tests for intracellular proteins can demonstrate the presence of protein, but does not exclude mutations causing the production of non-functional proteins.

Immunology

- XLP-2 patients have increased lymphocyte apoptosis in response to CD95.
- iNKT cells are normal and NK-mediated cytotoxicity is normal.

Treatment

- As for XLP-1.

Other rare causes of EBV susceptibility

Other rare genetic causes of increased susceptibility to EBV have been described:

- CD27 deficiency (TNFRSF7). Associated with aplastic anaemia, low iNKT cells, lymphoma, and hyphogammaglobulinaemia.
- FAAP24 deficiency. EBV-driven lymphoproliferation, and failure to kill EBV-transformed B cells.

- RASGRP1 deficiency. Recurrent pneumonia, herpes virus infections, EBV-driven lymphoma.
- CD70 deficiency. Hodgkin's lymphoma, hypogammaglobulinaemia.
- CTPS1 deficiency. Recurrent bacterial and viral infections. EBV lymphoma.
- RLTPR (CARMIL2) deficiency. Recurrent viral, fungal, bacterial, and mycobacterial infections. EBV lymphoma and malignancy. Atopic disease.
- ITK deficiency. Hypogammaglobulinaemia and EBV lymphoma.
- MAGT1 (XMEN, X-linked, magnesium transporter) deficiency. EBV infection and lymphoma, hypogammaglobulinaemia, and/or specific antibody defects. Reduced CD4$^+$ T cells, impaired T-cell activation, decreased NK- and CD8$^+$ T-cell cytotoxicity.
- PRKCD deficiency. Recurrent infections, SLE-like autoimmune disease. Hypogammaglobulinaemia. Lymphoma.

Transient hypogammaglobulinaemia of infancy (THI)

Cause
- THI is thought to be due to a delay in immune development, leading to a prolongation of the physiological trough of antibody after the age of 6 months, when maternal antibody has largely disappeared.
- Common in the families of patients with other antibody deficiencies.
- Diagnosis excludes hypogammaglobulinaemia by reasons of prematurity.

Presentation
- Usual presentation is with recurrent bacterial infections, typically of the upper and lower respiratory tract, occurring after 6 months of age. It may last up to 36 months before spontaneous recovery takes place.
- Transient neutropenia and thrombocytopenia have been reported.

Diagnosis
- There will be an early onset.
- Presence of normal B-cell numbers differentiates THI from XLA. IgM is frequently normal, and there may be evidence of specific antibody responsiveness.
- Check for btk expression, to exclude XLA.
- No specific diagnostic features and the diagnosis can only be made for certain after full recovery of immune function has taken place.

Immunology
- IgG and IgA are low for age; IgM is usually normal. B cells are present; T-cell numbers and function are normal. IgG must be reduced on more than one occasion. A reduction to < 2 SD below the lower end of the normal range has been suggested by some authorities.
- Vaccine responses may be normal or reduced.

Treatment

- Mild cases may be managed with prophylactic antibiotics.
- IVIg/SCIg treatment may be required in more severe cases, used for a fixed period, and be withdrawn at intervals to check for spontaneous recovery.
- By definition all recover! If there is no recovery, then the patient has an alternative diagnosis.

Hyper-IgE syndrome (Job's syndrome)

It is frequently classified with neutrophil defects, but the neutrophil defects are secondary to the dysregulation of T- and B-cell function and the very raised IgE.

Cause

- Autosomal dominant form is associated with dominant negative mutations in the DNA-binding domain of signal transducer and activator transcription (STAT3).
- Autosomal recessive inheritance has also been described and is due to mutations in tyrosine kinase 2 (TYK2); similar clinical features may be seen in dedicator of cytokinesis 8 (DOCK8) deficiency, also autosomal recessive.

Presentation

- Patients present with atypical eczema and recurrent invasive bacterial infections. Staphylococci and *Haemophilus* are usual pathogens. Invasive candidiasis and *Pneumocystis* may occur.
- Pneumatocoeles due to staphylococcal infection are a diagnostic feature. These may become colonized with *Aspergillus* or *Pseudomonas*.
- Non-tuberculous mycobacterial infection may occur in STAT3-deficient patients.
- Dominant form may be associated with invasive fungal infections and *Pneumocystis carinii*.
- Osteopenia, probably due to abnormal osteoclast function, is a feature and may lead to recurrent fractures, and scoliosis. Primary dentition may be retained.
- Coarse 'leonine' facies, but not all patients have red hair as originally described.
- There is an increased risk of lymphoma.

Diagnosis

- The clinical history is typical, especially the occurrence of pneumatocoeles.
- IgE levels are massively elevated and are usually much higher than in atopic eczema.
- Occurrence of invasive as opposed to cutaneous infections distinguish HIGE from atopic eczema.

Immunology
- IgE is massively elevated (> 50 000 kU/l) and there may be IgG subclass and specific antibody deficiencies, with poor/absent immunization responses.
- Class-switched and non-class-switched memory B cells may be reduced.
- BAFF expression increased.
- Eosinophilia may be present, especially during infection.
- Variable abnormalities of neutrophil function, affecting chemotaxis, phagocytosis, and microbicidal activity have been reported, but are likely to be due to inhibition by the high IgE or defects in cytokine production.
- Both STAT3 and TYK2 mutations lead to defective Th17 function. There may be defects in the production of γ-IFN, IL-12, IL-17, and IL-18.
- Absent CD45RO on T cells has been reported.

Treatment
- IVIg/SCIg should be used for the antibody deficiency. Cimetidine (as an immunoregulatory agent) has been recommended, although the value appears to be limited.
- γ-IFN is used in severe fungal infections (no randomized trials).
- Omalizumab has been tried, but may not be appropriate where there is very high IgE (unlicensed indication).
- Surgery for pneumatocoeles and deep-seated abscesses may be required.
- Stem cell transplantation has been tried in some cases, with benefit.

Hyper-IgE syndrome (rare causes)

Hyper-IgE is associated with:
- SPINK5 deficiency (see → 'Netherton's syndrome', p. 77).
- PGM3 deficiency, characterized by severe atopy, autoimmunity, immune-osseous dysplasia, recurrent pneumonia, boils, cognitive impairment. Eosinophilia is present; reduced B cells and CD8 and CD4 T cells.

Severe combined immunodeficiency (SCID)

SCID involves both the T-cell arm and the B-cell arm. Often the major defect is on the T-cell side: B cells may be present, but, in the absence of T cells, fail to respond or develop appropriately. The diagnosis is frequently missed at first, which reduces the chance of a successful outcome from treatment. It is estimated that the incidence is 1 per 50 000 births. Almost all cases are now accounted for by identified genetic defects.

Successful management of SCID requires a multidisciplinary team used to dealing with very sick small infants. Management should be restricted to centres experienced in the diagnosis and care of SCID. It should not be undertaken in haematology–oncology bone marrow transplant units as the requirements are very different from those of leukaemic patients.

Presentation

Most cases of SCID present with common clinical features, no matter what the underlying defect.
- Typical features include:
  - early-onset infections (bacterial, viral, fungal, opportunist);
  - persistent candidiasis;
  - chronic enteric virus excretion;
  - failure to clear vaccines (BCG, oral polio);
  - failure to thrive;
  - maternofetal engraftment, with graft-versus-host disease (GvHD), causing erythroderma (often with eosinophilia);
- (see p. 134 for an example) ❗lymphopenia: an absolute lymphocyte count of $< 2 \times 10^9/l$ in a baby less than 6 months old is pathological and indicates SCID until proven otherwise. Looking at the differential white count is therefore mandatory in all babies with recurrent infections.
- If SCID is suspected, investigation is **URGENT**—seek advice at once from a paediatric immunologist.

Infections in SCID

There is onset of infections soon after birth.
- These include:
  - recurrent bacterial infections (pneumonia, otitis media, sepsis);
  - persistent thrush;
  - persistent viral infections (RSV, enteroviruses, parainfluenza, CMV, other herpesviruses, rotavirus, small round structured virus (SRSV));
  - opportunist infections (PCP; fungal infections, including aspergillus).
- There are very significant risks from the administration of live vaccines especially BCG and polio.

❗BCG should not be given to babies where there is a family history of SCID.

Other features of SCID

These include:
- Failure to thrive.
- Diarrhoea (consider chronic enteroviral infection, rotavirus, SRSV).
- Skin rash (Omenn's syndrome, maternofetal engraftment).
- Bone abnormalities (flared ribs—ADA deficiency; malabsorption—rickets).
- Short-limbed skeletal dysplasia.
- Hepatosplenomegaly (BCGosis, GvHD from maternofetal engraftment (MFE) or blood transfusions; Omenn's syndrome).

SCID: investigations in suspected cases

On suspicion, first-line investigations
- Lymphocyte subpopulations (T-, B-, NK-, and T-cell subpopulations, with absolute numbers).
- Immunoglobulins.

- If the results are suspicious, then the baby should be referred at the earliest opportunity to a specialist centre with facilities for managing SCID.

Further investigations in the specialist referral centre
- T-cell proliferation.
- Cytokine assays.
- NK-cell function.
- Protein studies.
- Specific antibodies.
- Biochemical (exclusion of ADA deficiency).
- Genetic studies.
- HLA typing as part of work-up for BMT.

Aims of the initial investigations
- To confirm the diagnosis of SCID.
- To identify unusual variants, as this may affect the conditioning protocol used prior to HSCT.
- To provide evidence for subsequent genetic counselling of the family.
- To provide a baseline against which success of BMT can be measured.

Patterns of lymphocyte subpopulations in SCID and variants
- It cannot be stressed too often how important a low total lymphocyte count is as a marker of SCID: low lymphocyte counts should never be ignored.
- Typical pattern is of very low/absent T cells with normal or absent B cells; immature T cells may be present in low numbers (CD3$^+$, CD2$^+$, CD4$^-$, CD8$^-$).
- SCID with MFE: T cells are present but are usually CD8$^+$ and activated (CD25$^+$, DR$^+$); B cells are usually low or absent. Maternal origin of the cells may be confirmed by genetic studies.
- Omenn's syndrome (leaky SCID): T cells may be present, including CD4$^+$ T cells; clonal restriction with limited Tcr $\alpha\beta$-chain repertoire (this requires genetic analysis).
- Bare lymphocyte syndrome (see ➔ 'SCID: MHC class I deficiency (bare lymphocyte syndrome type I)', p. 42, and 'SCID: MHC class II deficiency (bare lymphocyte syndrome type II)', p. 43): absence of marked reduction of MHC class II antigen expression with variable MHC class I antigen expression; T cells are normal or low.
- ZAP-70 kinase deficiency and ζ-chain deficiency (see ➔ 'SCID: ZAP-70 kinase deficiency and ADA deficiency', p. 39 and p. 40): marked reduction/absence of CD8$^+$ T cells; low normal CD4$^+$ T cells.
- Absence of CD3/Tcr complexes (CD3 γ-, δ-, or ε-chains) variable expression of CD3: T-cell numbers are usually normal.

Proliferation assays
- Functional studies are useful in cases when T cells are present.
- PHA response: invariably absent in all major forms of SCID, including Omenn's and SCID with MFE; may be low–normal in ZAP-70 kinase deficiency.

- Phorbol esters (PMA) ± calcium ionophore: will be normal where there is a membrane defect (e.g. ZAP-70 kinase or CD3 complex) that can be bypassed (PMA acts intracellularly on protein kinase C).
- Anti-CD3 ± IL-2: abnormal when the defect involves the CD3/Tcr complex (e.g. CD3 deficiency, ZAP-70 kinase deficiency). The normal newborn anti-CD3 response is lower than in adults.
- Reconstitution of proliferation to mitogens with IL-2 may suggest a failure to produce this cytokine.

Cytokine assays
- Rarely used: IL-2 deficiency has been reported but is exceptionally rare.

Immunoglobulins
- If the diagnosis is made within the first few weeks of life, maternal antibody will still be present.
- Even if the child has B$^+$ SCID, immunoglobulins and specific antibody are not produced.
- It may be worth checking for specific antibodies if there is late presentation and the child has been immunized.

Biochemistry and genetics
- Check for ADA deficiency: abnormal metabolites (dATP, S-adenosyl homocysteine) will be present.
- Genetic testing is required to pinpoint the exact defect, e.g. X-linked SCID (common cytokine receptor γ-chain gene), Jak-3, IL-7Ra, RAG-1/RAG-2 MHC class II deficiency (*CIITA* or *RFX-5* genes), ZAP-70 kinase deficiency, CD3γ-, δ-, ε-chain deficiency.
- The genetics department will be able to assist in the distinction of Omenn's syndrome from SCID with MFE: skin biopsies are helpful. Cytogenetics can be used if it is a male baby; otherwise molecular genetics are required.

Screening
- Screening is possible using a multiplex immunoassay on the standard Guthrie blood spot, or through measuring TRECs.
- Pilot studies have confirmed the utility of screening and it has been introduced in some countries, states in the USA, but not yet in the UK.

SCID: treatment and outcomes

Treatment
The approach to treatment is also common to all types.
- Isolation to prevent further infection.
- Do not give any live vaccines.
- Irradiate all cellular blood products, to prevent engraftment of any donor lymphocytes.
- Ensure all blood products are from CMV-negative donors.
- Identify and treat all infections: use direct culture and PCR-based techniques.

- Transfer immediately diagnosis is suspected to nearest specialist paediatric immunodeficiency centre with facilities for definitive treatment.
- Do not initiate investigations for underlying cause.

❶Delay in transfer significantly reduces the chances of a successful outcome (90% success rate for babies diagnosed and treated immediately after birth, compared to 40% where treatment is delayed).

Once in the tertiary centre, management will include the following.
- Isolation in laminar flow.
- Establish venous access and commence nutritional support (enteral or parenteral) if required.
- Initiation of diagnostic tests: T- and B-cell numbers; baseline T-cell function; serum immunoglobulins; screen for pathogens (nasal secretions, bronchial lavage, stool, urine, blood). Biopsies as required (lymph nodes, skin for GvHD).
- Undertake genetic testing to identify gene defect, if possible.
- Tissue typing of baby and family; initiation of search for matched unrelated donor on bone marrow registries or consider SCT.
- Counsel family about diagnosis and treatment.
- Initiation of IVIg replacement.
- Use PEG-ADA as a temporizing measure in ADA-deficient SCID (see ➲ 'SCID: ADA deficiency', p. 40).
- Initiate aggressive treatment for identified infections with antibacterials, antivirals, and antifungals as appropriate—good microbiological and virological control is essential.
- Cytoreductive conditioning of recipient (to prepare space for incoming stem cells).
- T-cell depletion and stem cell enrichment of donor marrow (for mismatched grafts).
- Undertake BMT, SCT as appropriate; consider gene therapy. BMT may be:
  - sibling (identical);
  - parent (haploidentical);
  - matched unrelated donor (MUD);
  - stem cell.
- Undertake post BMT/HSCT immunological monitoring, treating infection and GvHD as appropriate.
- Gene therapy is increasingly available.

Outcomes
- Outcome is dependent on the promptness of the diagnosis and what infections are present at the time of diagnosis. Poor prognostic indicators are late diagnosis and chronic viral infections (especially parainfluenza pneumonitis).
- Meticulous care is required during the aplastic phase between conditioning and engraftment: this will require cell support (platelets, red cells), infection prophylaxis and treatment (fungi, viruses, and bacteria), management of the complications of conditioning (veno-occlusive disease of the liver; pneumonitis) and of GvHD (mismatched donors).

- Survival should be > 80% with early diagnosis, good matching of donors, and no pre-transplant infections. This falls to < 40% with late diagnosis, chronic infections, and poorly matched donors.

Regular monitoring post-HSCT is required to follow engraftment and development of immune function. This should include the following.
- Lymphocyte subpopulations: the return of T and B cells, expression of activation markers in association with GvHD, effectiveness of immunosuppression.
- T-cell proliferation: this is only valuable when T cells have returned to the circulation. The return of a PHA response defines probable safety for release from laminar flow confinement.
- NK-cell function and numbers may correlate with graft survival.
- Immunoglobulins: adequacy of replacement IVIg therapy, return of IgA and IgM synthesis, IgG subclass development (off IVIg).
- Specific antibodies: return of functional antibodies—isohaemagglutinins; immunization responses.
- Genetic studies: chimerism of lymphocytes (DNA studies on separated T and B cells).
- Biochemical reconstitution (ADA deficiency; enzyme deficiencies, e.g. ZAP-70 kinase).

T⁻B⁻NK⁺SCID: RAG-1/RAG-2 deficiency and Omenn's syndrome

RAG-1/RAG-2 deficiency

Cause
- Autosomal recessive. Mutations in *RAG-1/RAG-2* genes, required for V(D)J recombination of the T- and B-cell antigen receptors. Located at 11p13.
- Now known to account for Omenn's syndrome ('leaky SCID').

Presentation
- As a typical SCID; see ➲ 'Severe combined immunodeficiency (SCID)', pp. 30–33.
- There is no radiation sensitivity.

Diagnosis
- Typical presentation with recurrent infections and lymphopenia on full blood count.
- Confirmed by immunological and genetic studies.

Immunology
- Low/absent serum immunoglobulins, severe lymphopenia (T⁻B⁻ SCID).
- NK cells are present and comprise the majority of circulating lymphocytes.
- MFE is common.

Omenn's syndrome

Cause
- Autosomal recessive. Mutations in *RAG-1/RAG-2* genes, required for V(D)J recombination of the T- and B-cell antigen receptors. Located at 11p13.
- Partial activity present, allowing the development of oligoclonal, peripherally expanded T-cell clones.

Presentation
- Presents with erythrodermic rash, lymphadenopathy, and hepatosplenomegaly; must be distinguished from MFE.
- Cytogenetics of the peripheral blood cells may identify maternal cells.

Diagnosis
- May be difficult.
- Cytogenetics is required to exclude MFE.
- Immunological tests are variable.
- Oligoclonal T-cell pattern is distinctive.

Immunology
- Eosinophilia.
- Leucocytosis, variable CD4$^+$ and CD8$^+$ T-cell numbers; high level of activation marker expression (DR, CD25, CD45RO).
- B cells absent; hypogammaglobulinaemia usual.
- Oligoclonal Tcr usage.
- Abnormal lymph node histology: excess eosinophils, lymphocyte depletion.

Artemis deficiency

This defect causes a T$^-$B$^-$NK$^+$ radiation-sensitive phenotype of SCID, similar to RAG-1/RAG-2 deficiency. It is present in the Athabascan-derived population (Navajo and Apache Indians).

Cause
- Mutation in the Artemis gene (*DCLRE1C*), located on chromosome 10p13, involved in DNA repair probably through interaction with DNA-PKcs.

Presentation
- As for SCID, but prone to oral and genital ulcers.
- May cause Omenn-like phenotype.

Diagnosis
- Should be considered in cases of T$^-$B$^-$NK$^+$ SCID, where RAG-1/RAG-2 mutations are not found.

Immunology
- Profound T- and B-cell lymphopenia with normal NK cell numbers and function.
- MFE common.

Cernunnos/XLF deficiency

This defect causes a T⁻B⁻NK⁺ radiation-sensitive phenotype of SCID or sometimes CID, similar to RAG-1/RAG-2 deficiency.

Cause
- Mutation in the *Cernunnos/XLF* (*NHEJ1*) gene, involved in DNA repair probably through interaction with XECC4/DNA ligase IV complex.

Presentation
- As for SCID, but with developmental delay, microcephaly.

Diagnosis
- Should be considered in cases of T⁻B⁻NK⁺ SCID, where RAG-1/RAG-2 mutations are not found.

Immunology
- T cell absent with progressive loss of B cells.

DNA ligase IV (LIG4) deficiency

This defect causes a T⁻B⁻NK⁺ radiation-sensitive phenotype of SCID or CID, similar to RAG-1/RAG-2 deficiency. For milder cases treatment with IVIg may be enough. High risk of lymphoma.

DNA-PKcs deficiency

One child with T⁻B⁻NK⁺ SCID with radiation sensitivity has been shown to have a mutation in DNA-PKcs preventing its binding to Artemis. Mutation also reported in horses and dogs, which develop SCID with opportunistic infections.

T⁻B⁺NK⁺SCID: Jak-3 kinase deficiency, common gamma chain deficiency, and IL-7Rα deficiency

Jak-3 kinase deficiency (autosomal recessive T⁻B⁺NK⁺ SCID)
This form, in which T cells are absent but B cells are present in normal numbers, accounts for about 10% of all cases of SCID.

Cause
- Mutations in the gene encoding Jak-3 kinase (19p12–13.1), which prevent signalling through the surface cytokine receptors containing the common gamma chain. Signals from IL-2, IL-4, IL-7, IL-9, IL-15, and IL-21 are blocked.
- T-cell but not B-cell differentiation is blocked.

Presentation
- Presents with typical SCID features.
- Mild cases occur, presenting later with increased infections, but not SCID.
- May also present with lymphoproliferative disease (compound heterozygote).

Diagnosis
- Typical SCID presentation or high index of suspicion.
- Absent T cells with normal or increased B and decreased NK cells; overall total lymphocyte count may be normal.
- Western blotting of lymphocyte lysates may identify the absence of Jak-3 protein and genetic studies will confirm the gene defect.

Immunology
- T cells are very low or absent; NK cells are reduced, B cells are normal or increased; absent mitogenic responses.
- Mild variants may exist with significant numbers of poorly functioning T cells.
- Hypogammaglobulinaemia is usual.

Treatment
- Gene therapy has been attempted, but immune reconstitution was not achieved.

Common gamma chain deficiency (X-linked T⁻B⁺NK⁺ SCID)
This accounts for 50–60% of SCID.

Cause
- Mutations in the common cytokine receptor gamma chain CD132; signals from IL-2, IL-4, IL-7, IL-9, IL-15, and IL-21 are blocked.
- Gene is located at Xq13.1–13.3.
- Missense mutations may lead to the expression of a mutant non-functional gamma chain.

Presentation
- Typical SCID features in male infant.

Diagnosis
- Pattern of infections.
- Low/absent T cells, NK cells; normal or increased B cells.
- Demonstration of absent common gamma chain and genetic mutations. As levels of common γ-chain on lymphocytes are low, demonstration of absence is difficult, and may be confused if there is MFE.
- Flow cytometry can be used to identify the absence of the common gamma chain (CD132).
- Functional STAT5 phosphorylation assay, using flow cytometry to detect tyrosine phosphorylated STAT5 after stimulation with IL-2 can distinguish between JAK-3 and XL-SCID.

Immunology
- Low serum immunoglobulins.
- Normal or increased B cells, low/absent T cells and NK cells (dependent on IL-15).

- Poor mitogen responsiveness. B cells may make IgE *in vitro* via a common γ-chain independent IL-4 receptor.

Interleukin-7 receptor-α deficiency
Accounts for 1–2% of SCID patients.

Cause
- Autosomal recessive mutation in IL-7Rα.
- Gene is located at 5p13.
- Missense mutations may lead to the expression of a mutant non-functional protein that binds IL-7 poorly.

Presentation
- Typical SCID features in infant.

Diagnosis
- Pattern of infections.
- Low/absent T cells, normal or increased B cells, and normal NK-cell numbers.
- Demonstration of absent IL-7Rα and genetic mutations. Should be sought in atypical cases of B⁺ SCID, not accounted for by Jak-3 and common γ-chain mutations.

Immunology
- Low serum immunoglobulins.
- Normal or increased B cells, low/absent T cells, and normal NK cells.
- Poor mitogen responsiveness.

SCID: ZAP-70 kinase deficiency
This is a rare cause of autosomal recessive SCID.

Cause
- Autosomal recessive mutation in CD3 zeta-associated protein, ZAP-70.
- Gene is located at 2q12.
- Mutations cluster in region of gene encoding the site for enzymatic activity.
- ZAP-70 is involved in signal transduction from the membrane CD3 complex to the internal cascade.
- ZAP-70 is crucial in thymic development, especially in the development of CD8⁺ T cells from double-positive precursors.

Presentation
- Typical SCID features in infancy, with (usually) an early presentation.
- Later presentation with mild CID phenotype may occur.
- Inflammatory bowel disease and autoimmune cytopenia have been described.
- Omenn-like and HLH syndromes may occur.
- Lymph nodes and thymic shadow may be present.

Diagnosis
- Pattern of infections.
- Characteristic selective absence of circulating CD8+ T cells.
- Demonstration of absence of ZAP-70.
- Thymic biopsy may show double-positive cells in the cortex but only CD4+ T cells in the medulla.

Immunology
- Serum immunoglobulins may be normal.
- Normal or increased B cells, absent CD8+ T cells, normal/low CD4+ T cells, and normal NK cells.
- Failure of response to membrane acting mitogens, PHA, and anti-CD3 monoclonal antibodies, with normal responses to phorbol esters and ionophores (acting at the level of protein kinase C).

Treatment
- Gene therapy may be possible.
- Otherwise treat as for SCID.

SCID: purine metabolic disorders—ADA and PNP deficiencies

Adenosine deaminase (ADA) deficiency
This was the first genetically identified cause of SCID. It accounts for 20% of cases of SCID.

Cause
- Mutations in the *ADA* gene on chromosome 20q13.11. This gene has now been cloned and sequenced.
- Gene product is involved in purine metabolism.
- In the absence of ADA, there is a progressive reduction of T and B cells due to toxic effects of dATP and S-adenosyl homocysteine, with increased lymphocyte apoptosis.

Presentation
- Typical SCID features in infancy, with (usually) an early presentation.
- Liver enzymes are often raised.
- There is abnormal flaring of the rib ends, pelvic dysplasia.
- Neurological features, including cortical blindness; deafness; cognitive defects.
- Pulmonary alveolar proteinosis.
- Presentation with mild form in adult life has been reported; presentation is with recurrent bacterial infections and opportunist infections such as PCP; evidence of immune dysregulation (autoimmunity and allergy).
  - Lymphoma is a complication for late presenters.
- Relatives may show reduced levels of red cell ADA activity.
- Lymphocytes may be normal at birth (due to maternal ADA), but fall rapidly after delivery.

Diagnosis
- Pattern of infections (in early childhood); diagnosis of adults may be difficult.
- Lymphopenia.
- Bone changes are not specific, although suggestive in the context of the immunological abnormalities.
- Measurement of ADA in erythrocytes, together with serum levels of toxic metabolites is essential (Purine Research Laboratory, Guy's Hospital, London).

Immunology
- Serum immunoglobulins may be normal initially, but fall rapidly.
- Progressive severe lymphopenia, affecting all cell types.
- Poor/absent responses to all mitogens.

Treatment
- HSCT is treatment of choice, as for other types of SCID.
- Red cell transfusions restore ADA levels and improve immune function; PEG-ADA is available and is highly effective in restoring immune function (although this makes HSCT harder!).
- Antibodies to PEG-ADA may occur.
- Gene therapy has been used successfully, but has been complicated in several cases by acute leukaemia, due to insertion of the retroviral vector into known oncogenes.

SCID: purine nucleoside phosphorylase (PNP) deficiency
This is a rare genetic deficiency of another purine metabolic enzyme, PNP, which leads to a combined immune deficiency of slower onset than ADA deficiency.

Cause
- Absence of PNP leads to a build-up of the toxic metabolite dGTP, which preferentially damages T cells in the early stages, but later damages B cells also.
- Disease is autosomal recessive; gene is located at 14q13.1.
- Disease is rare (about 50 cases worldwide).

Presentation
- Onset tends to be later than for other forms of SCID, and in this respect it behaves more as a combined immunodeficiency.
- Neurological signs (spasticity, tremor, ataxia, and intellectual disability) occur early.
- Infections are common, especially disseminated varicella, but also other bacterial, viral, and opportunist pathogens.
- Haemolytic anaemia, ITP, and thyroiditis are also common.

Diagnosis
- Combination of progressive neurological signs and infections should raise suspicion.
- A low serum urate is a useful marker.
- Diagnosis is made by enzymatic studies and by detection of elevated levels of the metabolite dGTP (Purine Research Laboratory, Guy's Hospital, London).

Immunology
- Immunoglobulins are normal or low, but some patients have elevated levels with monoclonal gammopathies.
- Poor specific antibody responses to immunization.
- Autoantibodies may be detected.
- B cells are normal in numbers until late disease, but there is a progressive decrease in T-cell numbers with time.
- Mitogen responses are variably reduced.

Treatment
- Optimum treatment is unknown, due to rarity of the condition. BMT or HSCT is probably best. If an HLA-identical sibling marrow is available, infusion without conditioning may be possible, as the defect causes a form of auto-conditioning.

SCID: MHC class I deficiency (bare lymphocyte syndrome type I)

This is a rare cause of combined immunodeficiency.

Cause
- Deficiency of either TAP-1 or TAP-2 (transporter associated with antigen presentation).
- Causes unstable peptide/MHC class I/β2M complex, which rapidly dissociates and cannot be expressed on the cell surface.

Presentation
- Recurrent bacterial sinopulmonary infections.
- Granulomatous skin lesions, with ulceration.
- Presentation at any age.
- SCID-like presentation in early life may occur.
- May be asymptomatic.

Diagnosis
- Symptoms plus failure of class I expression on cells.

Immunology
- Minor abnormalities of humoral immunity only.
- Lymphocyte subsets may be normal; abnormalities when present are minor and inconsistent.

Treatment
- Unsatisfactory; chest and sinus disease treated similarly to cystic fibrosis with aggressive antibiotics and physiotherapy.
- Skin disease is difficult to treat: immunosuppressive therapy and interferons may make the condition worse.
- Role of HSCT undefined (but class I expression occurs on all nucleated cells, so this is not a pure stem cell disorder).

SCID: MHC class II deficiency (bare lymphocyte syndrome type II)

This rare disease is found predominantly in North Africa and Mediterranean area (80 cases worldwide). It is autosomal recessive, but genetically complex.

Cause

- Mutations can occur in any of the following transcription factors: CIITA (16p13), RFX-5 (1q21.1–21.3), RFXAP (13q14), RFXANK (19p12, commonest).
- Patients with CIITA mutations have normal expression of regulatory factor X (RFX), while the other defects do not.

Presentation

- Presentation is usually early (first 6 months of age) with severe diarrhoea, hypogammaglobulinaemia, and malabsorption.
- Recurrent bacterial and viral chest infections.
- Viral infections of the nervous system (HSV, enteroviruses).
- Haemolytic anaemia.
- Hepatitis, cholangitis.
- Rarely, it is asymptomatic.

Diagnosis

- Diagnosis is made on clinical suspicion (differential diagnosis includes IPEX syndrome—see ➔ 'X-linked immune dysregulation with polyendocrinopathy syndrome (IPEX) due to FOXP3 deficiency', p. 58).
- Absence of MHC class II expression on lymphocytes.

Immunology

- Immunoglobulins are normal or low.
- B-cell numbers are normal; T-cell numbers may be normal but there may be low CD4$^+$ T cells and increased CD8$^+$ T cells, reversing the normal ratio.
- MHC class I expression is variable.
- MHC class II expression will be absent (DR, DP, DQ) but may be inducible with γ-IFN.
- Poor but variable mitogen responses.

Treatment

- BMT/HSCT is the treatment of choice, but is surprisingly difficult to do successfully.

SCID: reticular dysgenesis—adenylate kinase 2 (AK2) deficiency

This is a rare defect of the maturation of stem cells for both lymphoid and myeloid lineages, caused by mutations in the gene for adenylate kinase 2 (AK2), a mitochondrial enzyme. There is marked granulocytopenia, lymphopenia, and thrombocytopenia (sometimes no cells at all!). It presents with early overwhelming infections and often death before the diagnosis is made. MFE is common. HSCT is required.

Other rare forms of SCID/CID

Nezelof's syndrome

Mainly a T-cell deficiency, with no identified molecular cause(s), presenting with recurrent sinopulmonary and gastrointestinal infections and malabsorption, warts, allergic disease autoimmunity (haemolytic anaemia, ITP, neutropenia, hepatitis). Unclear whether this is a discrete diagnostic entity or represents earl-onset CVID. T lymphopenia, variably reduced immunoglobulin levels, poor humoral function, autoantibodies. Prognosis seems to be poor despite prophylactic antibiotics, antifungals, and IVIg: BMT/HSCT suggested.

CD3 ζ-chain deficiency

Presented as T⁻B⁺NK⁺ SCID; partial deficiency has also been reported with CID and coeliac disease and autoimmune disease.

CD3 deficiency

Deficiencies of CD3 γ-, δ-, and ε-chains have been described in small numbers of patients; there is variable expression of CD3. Cases present as severe combined immunodeficiency, recurrent sinopulmonary infections, and autoimmune phenomena. Reduced expression of the CD3 complex on T cells is suspicious; proliferative responses to mitogenic anti-CD3 monoclonal antibodies are absent, but responses to phorbol esters and ionophore are normal. CD3δ-deficient patients have markedly reduced T cells BMT/HSCT is probably the treatment of choice. IVIg is helpful in mild cases.

CD25 (IL-2 receptor-α) deficiency

A small number of patients have been reported with this condition, but presentations variable. Single patient reported presenting with severe T lymphopenia and diffuse lymphocyte infiltrates associated with mutation in *CD25* gene—similar in presentation to autoimmune lymphoproliferative syndrome (see ➌ 'Autoimmune lymphoproliferative syndromes (ALPS; Canale–Smith syndrome)', p. 60). Recurrent viral, bacterial, and opportunist infections occur. One patient had phenotype similar to IPEX syndrome (see p. 58), but had defective IL-10 production (unlike FOXP3 deficiency).

CD45 deficiency
Presents with SCID-like illness due to complete absence of surface CD45, due to mutations in the *CD45* gene 1q31–q32.

P56lck deficiency
Presents early with infections, panhypogammaglobulinaemia, reduced CD4⁺ T cells, and poor responses to surface acting mitogens. May be a cause of idiopathic CD4⁺ T cell lymphopenia or mimic CVID. Suggested treatment is IVIg and antibiotics; HSCT in one case unsuccessful.

Actin-regulating protein coronin 1A deficiency
Coronin 1 (*CORO1A*, 16p11.2) is involved in the correct formation of the actin cytoskeleton. Appears to be important in T cell emigration from the thymus. Mutations in *CORO1A* lead to absence of peripheral T cells and a SCID phenotype, but with a normally developed thymus.

DOCK8 deficiency
• Dedicator of cytokinesis 8 (DOCK8) deficiency (autosomal recessive) has been associated in a number of families with a combined immunodeficiency, with features similar to the hyper-IgE syndrome (see ➲ 'Hyper-IgE syndrome', p. 29).
• Patients had recurrent upper and lower respiratory tract infections, severe herpes zoster or simplex, persistent molluscum contagiosum, HPV infection.
• Severe atopic disease and anaphylaxis, with raised IgE and eosinophilia was present in most patients.
• Squamous cell carcinoma and lymphoma occurred.
• Immunoglobulins were reduced; T- and B-cell numbers were low. Reduced NK-cell numbers and function. Low CD27⁺ B cells.

Late-onset combined immune deficiency (LOCID)
A small subset of patients with CVID are recognized who go on to develop opportunist infections, more typical of a combined immune deficiency. Often from consanguineous families. CD4⁺ T cells usually < 200 × 10⁶/l, with decreased naïve T cells and B cells. Increased incidence of spleno-megaly, granulomata, and lymphoma. At present no genetic lesion has been identified.

Winged-helix nude phenotype, FOXN1 (*whn* mutation)
One Italian family with complete alopecia, nail dystrophy and neural tube defects, and SCID-like syndrome reported, associated with winged-helix nude mutation, similar to nude mouse. Thymic structure and function impaired. Reduced CD4⁺ T cells. T-cell proliferative function reduced. One patient successfully received HSCT.

STAT5b deficiency
Patients present with growth hormone insensitivity, short stature, skin problems (eczema, ichthyosis), recurrent chest infections, *Pneumocystis*, and viral infections (severe herpes zoster and simplex). Deficiency of STAT5b impairs signalling via receptors for IL-2, IL-4, CSF-1, and growth hormone. CD4⁺CD25⁺ regulatory T cells are reduced.

Calcium flux defects

Mutations in the genes *ORAI1/CRACM1* (calcium release-activated calcium modulator 1), involved in calcium channels and *STIM1* (stromal interaction molecule 1) which senses calcium release, affect lymphocyte activation. Both mutations lead to autosomal recessive immunodeficiency with increased susceptibility to bacterial and viral infections. Lymphocyte counts are slightly reduced, immunoglobulin levels normal but with poor T cell proliferative responses, and poor specific antibody responses. Ectodermal defects (teeth) and hypotonia occur. Lymphoproliferative disease occurs. Treatment is by HSCT.

CD8 deficiency

Single symptomatic patient described with homozygous mutation in CD8α chain (2p12). Presented with recurrent bacterial infections of chest and sinuses. CD8⁺ T cells completely absent. Two sisters had same defect but were asymptomatic (parents consanguineous). Presents later than ZAP-70 deficiency.

CD70 deficiency

These patients either lack CD70 or have frameshift mutations preventing CD70 binding to CD27. They present with increased susceptibility to EBV, varicella, EBV-associated lymphoma, and hypogammaglobulinaemia. EBV-specific memory CD8⁺ T cells are reduced.

Tripeptidylpeptidase 2 (TPP2) deficiency

Early-onset Evans syndrome (immune thrombocytopenia and auto-immune haemolytic anaemia) has been associated with mutations in TPP2. Associated mild immunodeficiency. Premature T- and B-cell senescence (CC7R⁻CD127⁻CD28⁻CD57⁺) and poor proliferative responses. Fibroblasts affected.

Other rare defects

- MAGT1 deficiency (X-linked, XMEN)—see ➲ 'Other rare causes of EBV susceptibility', p. 27.
- UNC119 deficiency.
- MST1 deficiency.
- Moesin deficiency (X-linked, CD8⁺ T cells express senescence marker CD57).
- OX40 deficiency.
- IL-21 deficiency.
- MALT1 deficiency.
- LAT deficiency.
- BCL11B deficiency.
- RIPK1deficiency (SCID with arthritis and intestinal disease).
- TCrα deficiency.
- PRKDC mutations (T⁻B⁻NK⁺ SCID)—also a cause of susceptibility to EBV.
- β₂-microglobulin deficiency.

Disorders with predominant T-cell disorder

- DiGeorge syndrome.
  - Including all the variants: CATCH-22 (see ➲ 'DiGeorge (22q11 deletion complex) syndrome', p. 47).
- Wiskott–Aldrich syndrome.
  - Also includes X-linked thrombocytopenia and GATA-1 deficiency.
- Ataxia telangiectasia.
- Other chromosomal breakage syndromes:
  - Nijmegen breakage and Seemanova syndrome;
  - Bloom's syndrome;
  - Fanconi anaemia;
  - ICF syndrome;
  - xeroderma pigmentosa.
- Chronic mucocutaneous candidiasis.
  - *AIRE* gene deficiency.
  - APECED.
- IPEX syndrome.
  - FOXP3 deficiency.
- Idiopathic CD4 lymphopenia.
- Autoimmune lymphoproliferative syndromes:
  - fas deficiency;
  - fas-ligand deficiency;
  - caspase 8 and 10 deficiencies.
- Cartilage–hair hypoplasia.
- WHIM syndrome.
- γ-Interferon/IL-12 pathway syndromes:
  - γ-IFNR1 deficiency;
  - γ-IFNR2 deficiency;
  - IL-12-Rβ1 deficiency;
  - IL-12p40 deficiency;
  - STAT1 deficiency.

DiGeorge (22q11 deletion complex) syndrome

DiGeorge originally described one phenotype of what is now realized to be a broad and complex array of developmental defects, probably due to more than one genetic lesion.

The range of defects is large and includes the CATCH-22 syndrome (cardiac abnormalities, abnormal facies, thymic hypoplasia, cleft palate, and hypocalcaemia, associated with 22q11 deletions), Shprintzen syndrome, velocardiofacial syndrome (VCF), cono-truncal face anomaly syndrome, Opitz G/BBB syndrome, CHARGE (coloboma, heart defect, atresia choanae, delayed growth and development, genital hypoplasia, ear anomalies/deafness) associations, Kallman syndrome, and arrhinencephaly/holoprosencephaly. Similar features may also arise in the fetal alcohol syndrome, maternal diabetes, and retinoid embryopathy.

Cause

- Microdeletions at 22q11, possibly affecting a zinc-finger (DNA-binding) protein involved in early development, have been associated with many of the phenotypic variants.
- Candidate genes include the transcription factor *TBX1* (van gogh mutation in zebrafish!), *CRKL* (mouse knockout, not reported in humans), and *UFD1L*.
- Other mutations, including 10p deletions (10p13–p14), may give a similar phenotype.
- CHARGE syndrome has been associated with mutations in the *CHD7* (chromodomain helicase DNA-binding protein 7) gene located at 8q12.1; multiple mutations have been identified with no genotype–phenotype correlation. These mutations tend to be sporadic rather than familial (as in 22q11 syndromes).
- Abnormal development of branchial arch-derived structures, including heart, thymus, and parathyroid glands.

Presentation

- Hypocalcaemic tetany, often occurring in first 48 hours after delivery, and due to parathyroid gland maldevelopment.
- Cardiac abnormalities, typically those of a truncus arteriosus type, interrupted aortic arch, or tetralogy of Fallot. Severity of the cardiac abnormalities often determines outcome.
- Dysmorphic face with cleft palate, low-set ears, and fish-shaped mouth.
- Highly variable immunodeficiency, associated with absence or reduction of thymic size; this often improves with age.
- Severe forms may present as SCID with absent T cells (1% of cases).
- Partial syndromes may occur without any immunological features (VCF and Shprintzen syndromes).
- Infections are mainly viral (adenovirus, CMV, rotavirus).
- GvHD from non-irradiated blood transfusions may occur if the diagnosis is not thought of during surgery for cardiac abnormalities.
- Increased risk of autoimmune disease and B-cell lymphomas.
- 10% have cleft palates.
- Development delay common, especially language.

Diagnosis

- Diagnosis is by clinical suspicion, based on the facial features, typical cardiac abnormalities, and abnormally low calcium in full-blown cases. Partial variants may be more difficult to identify.
- All children with relevant cardiac abnormalities should be screened for 22q11 deletions by FISH and for other cytogenetic abnormalities. If positive, screen parents and refer for genetic counselling (50% of subsequent pregnancies will be affected).

- Patients with an identified 22q11 deletion should be screened for immunological defects, both humoral and cellular (immunoglobulins, IgG subclasses, specific antibodies, lymphocyte surface markers, and proliferation assays).

Immunology

- Immunology is highly variable and tends to improve with age; extra-thymic development of T cells may occur.
- SCID-like immunology is possible.
- Variable reduction in T cells, with normal or low T-cell proliferation to mitogens.
- Immunoglobulins may be normal or reduced and specific antibody production may be poor, with low/absent immunization responses.
- Deficiency of IgA increased, and associated with autoimmunity.
- CHARGE syndrome associated with reduced CD4$^+$ and CD8$^+$ T cells and near absent T cells in a few cases. Poor proliferative responses to mitogens. NK- and B-cell numbers usually normal. Variable immunoglobulin levels but poor vaccine responses.
- TRECs analysis gives an idea of thymic output.
- Tcr Vβ analysis may also be abnormal.

Treatment

- Optimum treatment is uncertain: the cardiac abnormalities define prognosis and repair of these takes priority.
- Irradiated blood should be used until it is known how severe the immunological abnormality is. Children with normal T-cell function are probably at very low risk of developing transfusion-related GvHD.
- Calcium supplementation for hypoparathyroidism.
- As mild immune defects may improve, simple measures such as prophylactic antibiotics may be all that is required. If there is evidence for significant humoral deficiency, then IVIg may be required.
- Severe defects, with absent T cells, should be considered for BMT/HSCT, although in the absence of a thymus it is probable that reconstitution is due to engraftment of mature T cells.
- Thymic transplants (inserted into muscle peripherally) have been tried and are said to be of value.
- Long-term monitoring for the development of autoimmune disease, hearing disorders, and support for learning difficulties.
- Adolescents and adults may be more at risk of developing major depression and schizophrenia.
- Surgery may be required for palatal defects.
- The safety of vaccination with live vaccines has not been fully evaluated in controlled trials, but may be considered if:
  - CD8$^+$ T cells > 0.3 × 10^9/l.
  - CD4$^+$ T cells > 0.5 × 10^9/l.
  - Proliferative responses to mitogens normal.
- Long-term maintenance of immunity may be worse than healthy individuals.

Wiskott–Aldrich syndrome (WAS), X-linked thrombocytopenia (XLT), and X-linked neutropenia (XLN)

Wiskott–Aldrich syndrome (WAS) is an X-linked disorder causing thrombocytopenia with small platelets, eczema, and a progressive immune deficiency. The same gene is also responsible for X-linked thrombocytopenia (XLT), a milder variant in which the eczema and immune deficiency is absent, and X-linked neutropenia (XLN).

Cause

- X-linked disease; the gene is located at Xp11.23 encoding WASP (Wiskott–Aldrich-associated protein). The same gene is responsible for XLT.
- WASP is a multifunctional protein, with GTPase binding activity. It is involved in intracellular actin polymerization, intracellular signalling, apoptosis, and phagocytosis.
- Carrier females show non-random X-inactivation, indicating that WASP expression carries a selective advantage in cell development.
- Abnormal O-glycosylation of surface proteins of both lymphocytes and platelets is well described. One such surface antigen is CD43 (sialoglycophorin). However, the gene for CD43 is normal in WAS. N-linked glycosylation is normal.
- Gain-of-function mutations in the GTPase (cdc42) binding domain of WASP impair the autoinhibitory ability of the molecule and increase actin polymerization, causing a mild congenital neutropenia. These patients also have lymphocyte abnormalities with poor lymphocyte proliferation of anti-CD3.

Presentation

- Presentation is early in childhood in males with severe eczema, which has an atypical distribution compared to atopic eczema. Molluscum contagiosum, warts, and HSV may infect eczematous skin.
- Abnormal bleeding is due to the low platelet count, and bleeding complications occur early.
- Infections develop more gradually, usually affecting the respiratory tract, and are bacterial.
- Opportunist infections: *Pneumocystis*, disseminated molluscum contagiosum, papillomavirus, systemic varicella, herpes simplex, and CMV. Fungal infections are uncommon, mainly candida.
- Autoimmunity (vasculitis and glomerulonephritis) is well described.
  - Vasculitic aneurysms may occur.
  - Inflammatory bowel disease.
- Allergic reactions to food may occur.
- There is often a family history.
- XLT, a mild variant with thrombocytopenia alone, but without eczema and immune deficiency is recognized.

- Two forms of WAS exist: a severe form culminating in early lymphoma, and a milder form compatible with survival to adult life. There is no phenotype–genotype correlation.
- Symptomatic female carriers have been reported (skewed X-inactivation).
- XLN patients present with mild congenital neutropenia.

Diagnosis

- Clinical features: there is thrombocytopenia (variable in range < −70) with abnormally small platelet volume (< 6.0 fl is diagnostic).
- Identification of low/absent WASP with subsequent mutation analysis is required.
- No absolutely diagnostic immunological features.
- Prenatal diagnosis is possible.

Immunology

- There is a progressive reduction of T cells with poor proliferative responses to CD3, CD43, and periodate (specific for O-linked sugars). Proliferation to galactose oxidase and neuraminidase, which act via N-linked sugars, is normal.
- There are reduced IgM and IgA with a normal or high IgG and elevated IgE. There is a progressive loss of antipolysaccharide responses (including isohaemagglutinins) with poor/absent responses to test immunization with polysaccharide antigens. B-cell numbers are normal.
- CD43 (sialophorin) on lymphocytes and GPIb on platelets are unstable and tend to fall off cells when they are kept in vitro. Abnormalities of the cytoskeleton in T cells and platelets, with failure of actin bundling, have also been described.
- Variable thymic hypoplasia.

Treatment

- Splenectomy may be beneficial for thrombocytopenia, which is usually resistant to steroids. XLT patients are highly susceptible to overwhelming sepsis if splenectomy is undertaken, even though normally they do not have a problem with infection.
- Platelet transfusions should be avoided unless essential to control bleeding. Ensure blood products are from CMV⁻ donors.
- IVIg should be used for patients with poor antipolysaccharide responses, if recurrent bacterial infections are a problem and after splenectomy, as responses to post-splenectomy vaccination schedules will be poor.
- Consider prophylactic antibiotics; mandatory post-splenectomy. Prophylactic aciclovir for HSV.
- Treat eczema.
- Avoid aspirin and related drugs (increased risk of bleeding).
- Rituximab may be required for autoimmune complications.
- Early (< 5 years of age) BMT/HSCT should be considered to prevent the development of lymphoma: it cures all the features of the disease, including eczema.
- The role of BMT/HSCT in adult patients is unclear: development of lymphoma is an indication for aggressive chemotherapy followed by

transplantation in first remission, with matched unrelated donor for the graft-vs-lymphoma effect.
- Gene therapy is undergoing clinical trials, and may be helpful.

Outcome
- Death may occur from infection or intracranial haemorrhage.
- Very significant risk of death in late adolescence/early adulthood from high-grade lymphoreticular malignancy, usually EBV+; this may be preventable by early HSCT.
- Mild variants exist and may have fewer problems with bleeding or infection in adulthood.
- XLT life expectancy appears to be near normal.
- XLN patients are at increased risk of developing myelodysplasia.

Related conditions
- WIP deficiency (WIPF1): WAS protein absent and platelets small otherwise similar features.
- ARPC1B deficiency: recurrent invasive infections, colitis, mild thrombocytopenia with normal-sized platelets.

Ataxia telangiectasia

Cause
- Cells from AT patients have a disorder of the cell cycle checkpoint pathway, resulting in extreme sensitivity to ionizing radiation. Lymphocytes show frequent chromosomal breaks, inversions, and translocations; the major sites affected are the genes for the T-cell receptors and Ig heavy chains.
- Disease is autosomal recessive; six genetic complementation groups (A, B, C, D, E, V1, V2) have been described and all but V2 map to 11q22–23.
- One of the genes has now been identified and is a DNA-dependent kinase related to phosphatidylinositol kinase-3 (ataxia telangiectasia mutated protein (ATM)). Function appears to be to sense double-stranded DNA breaks.
- ATM phosphorylates BRCA1 (may explain increased risk of breast cancer in carrier females).

Presentation
- Progressive cerebellar ataxia, with typical telangiectasia, especially of the ear lobes and conjunctivae.
- Accompanied by recurrent bacterial sinopulmonary infections.
- Opportunist infections uncommon, but extensive warts are not unusual.

Diagnosis
- Clinical history is usually diagnostic, although the disease may be difficult to identify in the early stage when signs are minimal.
- α-Fetoprotein in serum is usually raised.

- Genetic testing is difficult due to the large size of the gene and the lack of clustering of the mutations.
- Spontaneous cytogenetic abnormalities occur, and will be increased by radiation exposure.

Immunology

- Immunoglobulins are variable: there is often a reduction of IgG_2/IgG_4, IgA, and IgE, with poor anti-polysaccharide responses. There is an increased incidence of autoantibodies.
- T-cell numbers and function are usually reduced.

Treatment

- No treatment is effective in what is a relentless disease with progressive neurological deterioration.
- PEG feeding may be required in the later stages when bulbar function deteriorates, to prevent recurrent aspiration.
- IVIg reduces the incidence of infections and improves quality of life but does not affect the outcome.
- Minimize radiation exposure.

Outcome

- Ataxia is progressive and patients become wheelchair-bound early (late teens, early twenties).
- High incidence of malignancy, especially high-grade lymphoma, and the incidence of malignancy is raised in other family members (fivefold increase in breast cancer).
- Death usually ensues in early adult life from infections or neoplasia.
- Heterozygotes for abnormal *ATM* genes may have an increased risk of chronic lymphocytic leukaemia.

Other chromosomal instability disorders

Ataxia-telangiectasia-like disorder (ATLD)

An AT-like disorder, without telangiectasia, has been identified linked to a gene at 11q21, *MRE11A*, leading to deficient activation of ATM. α-Fetoprotein and serum immunoglobulin levels were normal. Patients are radiosensitive. Rate of neurodegeneration is slower than AT and ocular telangiectasia is absent.

Ataxia-ocular apraxia type 1 (AOA1)

This is an autosomal recessive disorder characterized by cerebellar ataxia, oculomotor apraxis, and a sensorimotor neuropathy. Telangiectasia is absent. It is caused by mutations in the *APTX* gene coding for aprataxin. Muscle co-enzyme Q10 may be deficient; there is hypoalbuminaemia and raised cholesterol.

Ataxia-ocular apraxia type 2 (AOA2)

This is an autosomal recessive disorder characterized by cerebellar ataxia, variable oculomotor apraxia, and sensorimotor neuropathy. It is caused by mutations in the *SETX* gene on chromosome 9q34 coding for senataxin, an RNA and DNA helicase. There is no radiosensitivity. α-Fetoprotein levels are increased.

Nijmegen breakage and Seemanova syndromes

- These are syndromes of severe microcephaly, intellectual disability (not in the Seemanova syndrome), bird-like face, and recurrent infections.
- Increased chromosomal sensitivity to ionizing radiation.
- Gene has been identified on chromosome 8q21, encoding a protein nibrin (NBS1), involved in DNA repair.
- Nibrin associates with MRE11 (see ATLD earlier in this topic) and RAD50, deficiency of which has also been reported to cause a similar syndrome.
- Most patients have reduced/absent immunoglobulins and lymphopenia.
- T-cell responses to mitogens are poor.
- Cytogenetic analysis shows chromosomal abnormalities, and the most commonly involved chromosomes are 7 and 14, where the Ig and Tcr genes are located.
- Thymus is dysplastic.
- Malignancy is increased (lymphoma, neural tumours), and is the major cause of death.
- There is no specific treatment.

Bloom's syndrome

- Autosomal recessive syndrome commonest in Ashkenazi Jews.
- Gene located at 15q26.1, coding for the BLM protein, a RecQ helicase, that maintains the stability of DNA when duplexes are unwound.
- Presents with marked sun sensitivity, short stature, patchy vitiligo, infertility, immunodeficiency, and very high incidence of cancer.
- Early in childhood vomiting and diarrhoea can lead to severe dehydration.
- Immunodeficiency is characterized by low IgM, normal or poor specific antibody responses, poor T-cell function, poor B-cell IgM production, and NK-cell defects.
- Malignancy is the major complication and is difficult to treat because of the inability to repair DNA damage.
- Carriers do not seem to have an increased cancer risk.
- Immunoglobulin replacement is helpful, together with prompt antibiotic treatment.
- Regular screening for cancer is essential.

Fanconi anaemia

- This is an autosomal recessive disease with chromosomal breaks.
- Seven genes (*FANCA–FANCG*) have been identified, on different chromosomes, with eight different complementation groups.
- There are multiple organ defects, bone marrow failure (pancytopenia), radial hypoplasia, abnormal face, and leukaemic transformation.
- Presentation is usually with short stature, abnormalities of pigmentation, and organ defects.

- Decreased T cells, NK cells, increased IgE, and low IgA, and poor responses to polysaccharides have been reported, but immunological abnormalities are not a major feature.

ICF (immunodeficiency, centromeric instability, and abnormal facies)

- Caused by abnormalities of chromosomes 1, 9, and 16 (multiradial chromosomes).
- Four genes have been identified (ICF-1 *DNMT3B*; ICF-2 *ZBTB24*; ICF-3 *CDCA7*; ICF-4 *HELLS*) involved in DNA methylation.
- Presents with dysmorphic face, intellectual disability, and malabsorption with failure to thrive.
- Immunodeficiency occurs in all patients and is mainly humoral, with severe hypogammaglobulinaemia, but T-cell numbers are usually reduced. *In vitro* functional tests of T cells are usually normal.

Cockayne syndrome

A disorder of nucleotide excision and repair, associated with extreme sun sensitivity. Associated with mutations in the genes *ERCC6* or *ERCC8*. Not normally associated with immunological abnormalities.

Trichothiodystrophy

Similar to Cockayne syndrome.

Xeroderma pigmentosa

Extreme sun sensitivity leading to bullae, keratoses, and squamous cell carcinoma are the features of this syndrome, which is a DNA repair defect. Multiple genes can cause the phenotype. There is an immunodeficiency with low CD4+ T cells and poor *in vitro* and *in vivo* T-cell function in some patients; low IgG levels may also occur.

DNA ligase I deficiency

A single patient reported with short stature, sun sensitivity, low IgG, absent IgA, poor specific antibody responses, and death from lymphoma. Genetic defect was identified as DNA ligase I deficiency.

Other DNA repair defects

- PMS2 deficiency: associated with cafe-au-lait spots, colorectal and brain tumours. Abnormal immunoglobulin responses and reduced B cells.
- MCM4 deficiency: viral infections and short stature; adrenal failure; abnormal NK cell function.
- RNF168 (Riddle syndrome): short stature, motor problems, and learning difficulty. Reduced IgG and IgA.
- POLE1 & POLE2: dysmorphism; recurrent infections, autoimmunity; hypopgammaglobulinaemia.
- NSMCE3 deficiency: lung disease, thymic hypoplasia, radiosensitivity; poor immune function.
- ERCC6L2 (Hebo) deficiency: dysmorphism; bone marrow failure.
- GINS1: intrauterine growth restriction; neutropenia; low NK cells.

Chronic mucocutaneous candidiasis syndromes

Multiple syndromes, presenting with mucocutaneous candidiasis; rarely with invasive candidiasis. Often in association with endocrinopathy.

Cause

- Cause of many cases of CMC is unknown.
- Cytokine abnormalities have been documented.
- Autosomal dominant and recessive forms as well as sporadic cases are all documented.
- *AIRE* on chromosome 21 (21q22.3) is abnormal in autoimmune polyglandular syndrome type I (APECED (autoimmune polyendocrinopathy–candidiasis–ectodermal dysplasia), see ➲ Chapter 4): may be associated with autoantibodies to IL-17A, IL-17F, and IL-22, impairing Th17 cells.
- Gain-of-function STAT1 mutations (autosomal dominant CMC), impairing IL-17, IL-22, and γ-IFN production, and impaired Th1 and Th17 function by inhibiting STAT3.
- CARD-9 (autosomal recessive CMC): impairs Dectin-1 signalling and reduces Th17 cells.
- Other mutations known to be associated with CMC-like illness include:
  - Lymphoid phosphatase, lyp (protein tyrosine phosphatase non-receptor type 22, PTPN22).
  - Dectin-1 (C-type lectin receptor which enhances TLR2/TLR4 cytokine production) deficiency: causes mucosal but not invasive candidiasis.
  - TLR3 L412F variant (dysfunctional receptor): candidiasis, nail dystrophy, and severe sinopulmonary infections, viral infections, and autoimmunity.
  - IL-12p40/IL-12Rβ1 (also mycobacteria and salmonella).
  - IL-17F/IL-17RA/IL-17RC (also staphylococcal infections with IL-17RA deficiency).
  - ACT1 deficiency (associated with blepharitis and macroglossia).

Presentation

- Early onset of superficial candidiasis affecting nails and mouth and occasionally the oesophagus; persistent; invasive candidiasis is very rare and should raise questions of other diagnoses.
- There may be a family history.
- May be associated with an endocrinopathy causing hypocalcaemia due to parathyroid insufficiency, hypothyroidism, and adrenal insufficiency (consider APECED).
- Other autoimmune phenomena may occur: vitiligo, alopecia, hepatitis, pernicious anaemia.
- Increased susceptibility to bacterial infections (particularly of the respiratory tract), tuberculosis, herpesviruses, and toxoplasmosis. Severe forms may progress to a more generalized combined immunodeficiency, similar to SCID.

- May be associated with thymoma.
- Autosomal dominant form presenting with CMC and cerebral vasculitis similar to Moyamoya disease (genetic basis unknown).

Diagnosis

- There is no unequivocal diagnostic test.
- *In vivo* and *in vitro* T-cell responses to *Candida* antigens are poor or absent but anti-*Candida* IgG antibodies are high.
- Acquired immunodeficiency and other risk factors for candidiasis (diabetes, steroid inhalers, Sjögren's syndrome, proton-pump inhibitor use) should be excluded.
- Presence of superficial candidiasis with an endocrinopathy, either overt or cryptic (autoantibody positive without symptoms), is highly suspicious: *AIRE* gene should be checked.

Immunology

- Anti-*Candida* antibodies (IgG) are raised, often with multiple precipitin lines on double diffusion tests.
- IgG_2/IgG_4 are often reduced and there are poor antipolysaccharide responses with low immunization responses.
- Poor *in vitro* proliferation to *Candida* antigens, with abnormal cytokine production (high IL-6). T-cell responses to mitogens are usually normal. Cutaneous reactivity to *Candida* is absent, although other DTH responses are often normal. T-lymphocyte subsets are usually normal.
- Abnormal production of IL-17, IL-22, and γIFN.
- Reduced Th17 cells are a key feature.
- Autoantibodies may be detectable to endocrine organs (parathyroid, adrenal, ovary, thyroid).
- Autoantibodies to IL-17 and IL-22 may be detectable and may give a phenocopy of CMC.
- Mannan-binding lectin deficiency has been suggested as a cofactor.

Treatment

- Treatment is difficult: *Candida* will respond well to antifungals (fluconazole or itraconazole) but inevitably relapses when the antifungal is withdrawn. Resistance to these antifungals may occur. Prolonged therapy is undesirable and increases the chances of hepatotoxicy. Newer antifungals are voriconazole and caspafungin.
- Avoid the use of proton-pump inhibitors as these increase the risk of oesophageal candidiasis.
- Ruxolitinib (JAK inhibitor) has been used in CMC caused by gain-of-function mutations in STAT1.
- IVIg should be considered for patients with recurrent bacterial infections. Continuous antibiotics tend to exacerbate the candidiasis.
- Interferon gamma-1b may have some beneficial effect.
- HSCT should be considered for severe forms but the procedure is difficult in heavily infected patients.
- Maintain regular surveillance for significant endocrine disease, in particular adrenal insufficiency, which may be insidious in its onset. Treat endocrine disease normally.

Outcome

- CMC is not as benign as the books would have you believe!
- Cases may die from overwhelming sepsis, in addition to deaths from unrecognized adrenal insufficiency.
- STAT1 gain-of-function mutation patients appear to be at significantly increased risk of progressive multifocal leukencephalopathy (PML) from JC virus, compared to other PIDs.

X-linked immune dysregulation with polyendocrinopathy syndrome (IPEX) due to FOXP3 deficiency

An X-linked disorder characterized by severe endocrine autoimmunity, diarrhoea, eczema, and serious infections.

Cause

- Gene defect identified as *FOXP3* gene, also responsible in the mouse for the scurfy phenotype. Gene is close to WASP on the X chromosome, Xp11.23.
- FOXP3 is a forkhead DNA-binding protein.
- Clinical phenotype has also been seen in patients without mutations in FOXP3, indicating that other genes may also be involved.
- Patients are described with the phenotype but without mutations in *FOXP3* (IPEX-like syndrome); CD25 deficiency and STAT5b deficiency may cause a similar syndrome.

Presentation

- Presentation early in life with severe watery diarrhoea and failure to thrive.
- Severe eczema.
- Endocrine autoimmunity (early-onset diabetes mellitus, thyroid disease).
- Autoimmune haemolytic anaemia, ITP, neutropenia, splenomegaly.
- Infections may include meningitis, osteomyelitis, and pneumonia.
- Interstitial nephritis in one-third of patients.
- Rarely interstitial lung disease.

Diagnosis

- Clinical features.
- Anaemia, thrombocytopenia.
- Eosinophilia.
- Multiple autoantibodies: TPO, islet cell, platelets, neutrophils, erythrocytes (positive Coombs' test).
- Enterocyte antibodies.
- Testing for Treg cells.
- Genetic testing is possible.

Immunology
- Markedly elevated IgE, with normal IgG, IgA, and IgM; normal specific antibody responses.
- Raised IgE with allergen-specific IgE.
- Autoantibody to small bowel antigen AIE-75.
- T and B cells usually normal.
- Reduced/absent Tregs by flow cytometry (CD4$^+$CD25$^+$FOXP3$^+$).

Treatment
- BMT/HSCT, preferably before organ damage occurs.
- Control of endocrine disorder and attention to nutrition: immunosuppression may be required (ciclosporin, tacrolimus, sirolimus).
- Female carriers require genetic counselling.

OKT4 epitope deficiency
- In this condition, the epitope on the CD4 molecule recognized by the monoclonal antibody OKT4 is absent.
- If OKT4 is used to identify T cells, CD4$^+$ T cells will be spuriously absent.
- The mutation appears not to affect CD4 and T-cell function.
- Occurs in 8.3% of black people; very rare in other racial groups.
- Most patients are asymptomatic.
- Heterozygotes have normal numbers of OKT4$^+$ T cells, with a 50% reduction in CD4 density on the surface, when measured with OKT4.
- Recognition of this is important to prevent misdiagnosis as a severe T-cell deficiency.

Idiopathic CD4⁺ T-cell lymphopenia

Initially recognized in adults presenting with AIDS-like opportunist infections but with no evidence of retroviral infection. Unclear whether this is a discrete immunodeficiency or secondary to an unidentified pathogen.

Cause
- Unknown.
- Some cases associated with p56lck and CD45 abnormalities.
- Cases have been reported with deficient expression of the chemokine receptor CXCR4.
- One case caused by ITK deficiency.

Presentation
- Presents with opportunist infections (PCP, mycobacteria, candida, papillomavirus).
- Bacterial sepsis with unusual organisms.
- Increased incidence of lymphomas and autoimmune disease.
- Increased in IV drug users and haemophiliacs.
- May occur in children.

Diagnosis
- Pattern of opportunist infections in the absence of identified retroviral infection.
- Reduced CD4$^+$ T-cell numbers, with reduced CD45RA$^+$ naïve T cells. Decreased CD127 expression.

Immunology
- Persistently reduced CD4$^+$ T-cell numbers on more than one occasion; OKT4 epitope deficiency excluded.
- CD8$^+$ T cells may also be reduced—represents a poor prognostic factor.
- B cell numbers may be reduced.
- Restricted Tcr repertoires.

Treatment
- Treat infections.
- IL-2 has been helpful in some cases.
- γ-IFN has also been used to reverse defective cytokine production and treat cryptococcal meningitis.
- HSCT has been recommended in some cases.

Autoimmune lymphoproliferative syndromes (ALPS; Canale–Smith syndrome)

A series of disorders characterized by failure of apoptosis (programmed cell death), leading to uncontrolled lymphoproliferation and autoimmunity.

Cause

Genetic defects have been identified in a number of genes encoding proteins controlling apoptosis:
- Fas (TNFRSF6, CD95, APO-1), chromosome 10q24.1, ALPS Ia.
- Fas-ligand (TNFSF6, CD95L), ALPS Ib.
- Caspase 8 and caspase 10 deficiency, ALPS II.
- FADD deficiency.
- Somatic KRAS mutation (G13D) associated with ALPS-like phenotype, without evidence of germline RAS mutations.
- Somatic mutation in TNFRSF6 gives rise to ALPS phenocopy.
- Penetrance of defects may be variable within families.

Presentation
- Occurs in males and females, but with skewing to males; usual onset in childhood.
- Occasionally may be asymptomatic.
- Persistent splenomegaly, lymphadenopathy (typically neck), hepatomegaly.

- Autoimmunity: haemolytic anaemia, ITP (made worse by hypersplenism), hepatitis, uveitis, Guillain–Barré syndrome.
- Increased incidence of lymphoma (Hodgkin's > non-Hodgkin's) and other malignancies (carcinoma).
- Grey platelet syndrome may mimic ALPS.

Diagnosis

- Unexplained lymphoproliferation with autoimmunity in a child is highly suspicious.
- Lymphocytosis, often with eosinophilia in peripheral blood.
- Abnormal expression of fas and fas-ligand or caspases (genetic testing is required but not widely available).
- Abnormal apoptosis assays (see ➲ Chapter 20).
- Raised vitamin B_{12} levels (also seen in lymphoma) and raised sFasL
- Histology of lymph nodes shows infiltration of double-negative T cells, with no evidence of EBV.
- PET scanning may be valuable in identifying lymphadenopathy and targeting biopsies.

Immunology

- Lymphocytosis, with increase in peripheral $Tcr\alpha\beta^+$, $CD45RA^+$ double-negative T cells ($CD4^-CD8^-$) > 1% of total lymphocytes.
- Increase in $Tcr\ \gamma\delta^+$ double-negative T cells.
- Poor T-cell proliferative responses and abnormal apoptosis.
- Increased $CD5^+$ B cells; reduced CD27 expression.
- Increased immunoglobulins.
- Multiple autoantibodies.

Treatment

- Splenectomy may be required but increases risks of infection.
- Autoimmune disease may require treatment with corticosteroids and immunosuppressive drugs (all available drugs have been tried!). Sirolimus appears best and can lead to durable remission. Vincristine and MMF may also be very useful.
- Rituximab has been used.
- Antimalarial drugs may be helpful (effects on TNF?).
- HSCT has been used successfully.

Outcome

- May improve spontaneously over time, with regression of lymphadenopathy and splenomegaly.
- Increased risk of lymphoma.

Cartilage–hair hypoplasia (CHH) syndrome

An autosomal recessive T-cell immunodeficiency associated with short-limbed dwarfism and distinctive fine sparse hair.

Cause
- Autosomal recessive and linked to chromosome 9p21.
- Gene is ribonuclease mitochondrial RNA processing gene (*RMRP*), involved in the metabolism of RNA primers.
- Occurs particularly in Finland and old-order Amish in America.
- Carrier frequency is 1 in 19 in old-order Amish.

Presentation
- Short-limbed skeletal dysplasia, with fine sparse hair and ligamentous laxity.
- Anaemia (macrocytic), neutropenia, ITP; other autoimmune diseases.
- Infections, especially varicella, a problem in one-third; may rarely present as SCID, with opportunist infections. Recurrent bacterial infections may occur.
- Megacolon (aganglionic).
- Impaired spermatogenesis.
- Increased incidence of malignancy (non-Hodgkin's lymphoma, squamous cell carcinoma, basal cell carcinoma, and leukaemia).
- Phenotype is highly variable.

Diagnosis
- Typical radiographic appearances of joints; sparse hair, and macrocytic anaemia.

Immunology
- Immunology is variable.
- IgA ± IgG subclass deficiencies are reported.
- Neutropenia, together with a T-cell lymphopenia. B-cell numbers may be normal.
- Poor proliferative responses to mitogens.

Treatment
- IVIg if infections are a problem.
- HSCT if presenting as SCID; will not cure dwarfism.
- Consider varicella vaccine.

Warts, hypogammaglobulinaemia, infection, myelokathexis (WHIM) syndrome

WHIM syndrome is a rare immunodeciency and is the first to be associated with deficiency of a chemokine receptor (CXCR4). CXCR4 is also the co-receptor for HIV.

Cause
- Deficiency of CXCR4 chemokine receptor for stromal-derived factor 1 (SDF-1).
  - SDF-1 essential for normal myeloid maturation and differentiation; absence of SDF-1 increases granulocyte apoptosis and causes myelokathexis (white blood cell retention).
- Autosomal recessive; gene located at 2p21.

Presentation
- Presents early in childhood with recurrent bacterial infections, developing into bronchiectasis.
- Warts (papillomavirus infection) develop later and are extensive and confluent; genital warts will predispose to cervical carcinoma.
- Rare patients have cardiac defects.
- Severe granulocytopenia and lymphopenia; bone marrow shows granulocyte hyperplasia.

Diagnosis
- Clinical and laboratory features.
- Protein and molecular diagnosis not yet routinely available.

Immunology
- Hypogammaglobulinaemia; reduced B-cell numbers, especially memory B cells.
- Neutrophil function is normal.

Treatment
- IVIg for bacterial infections.
- G-CSF may be helpful, even though levels may be raised in some patients, by increasing neutrophil emigration.

Mendelian susceptibility to mycobacterial disease (MSMD)

γ-Interferon/IL-12 pathway defects

Multiple defects have been identified in association with inherited susceptibility to mycobacterial infection, especially low-virulence mycobacteria (BCG, environmental mycobacteria), and salmonellosis. IFNGR and IFNGR2 deficiencies give the most severe phenotypes. Other infections are rare. Autosomal dominant, autosomal recessive, and X-linked inheritances have been reported.

Causes

Defined genetic disorders identified so far include:
- γ-Interferon receptor-1 mutations (*IFNGR1*, 5q23–24), leading to autosomal recessive loss of expression of the receptor or loss of γ-IFN binding; these map to the extracellular domains. Partial defects with reduced γ-IFN responses have been reported. Dominant defects have also been reported, involving mutations in the intracellular domain, leading to surface over-expression of a truncated receptor.
- γ-Interferon receptor-2 mutations (*IFNGR2*, 21q22.1–22.2), causing either complete or partial deficiency of the receptor.
- Autosomal dominant mutations in STAT1 (signal transducer and activator of transcription-1) that impair the intracellular signal transduction of γ-IFN (two types of mutations, preventing phosphorylation and DNA-binding).
- IL-12 p40 subunit mutations.

- IL-12R and IL-23R β1 deficiency due to mutations in the *IL12RB1* gene.
- Interferon regulatory factor 8 (IRF8, 16q24.1): may occur as autosomal recessive and autosomal dominant forms. Dominant form associated with selective absence of dendritic cells; recessive form lacks monocytes and dendritic cells.
- GATA2 deficiency (3q21.3): MonoMac syndrome (monocytes deficiency and mycobacterial disease).
  - See ➔ 'MonoMac syndrome (GATA2 deficiency)', p. 68, for details.
- An acquired autoimmune syndrome with autoantibodies against γ-IFN has also been described. May respond to high-dose IVIg, plasmapheresis, or anti-B cell therapies such as rituximab).
- Mutations in *CYBB* gene (coding for gp91phox, normally causing XL-CGD) has been reported as causing just mycobacterial infection: these patients have *normal* oxidative metabolism by flow cytometry using dihydrorhodamine.
- Other causes include Tyk-2, RORc, JAK-1, and ISG15 deficiencies.

Diagnosis
- Lack of surface γ-IFNR can be identified by flow cytometry; but loss-of-function mutations require genetic identification.
- IL-12R defects so far reported lack surface expression, amenable to detection by flow cytometry.
- Other abnormalities require specific assays backed up by genetic studies to diagnose them.

Treatment
- Interferon gamma-1b in high doses may be helpful in autosomal dominant γ-IFNR1 and IL-12R defects, in combination with conventional antimycobacterial treatment; infection tends to recur.
- BMT/HSCT has been used in γ-IFNR defects, but outcomes have been poor with GvHD, infections, and generalized granulomatous disease.
- IL-12-related defects appear not to lead to recurrent infections.

Toll-like receptor (TLR) defects

TLRs are part of the innate immune system. Testing for defects in these pathways is now available via flow cytometry (see ➔ Chapter 20).

IRAK-4 deficiency

Deficiency of interleukin-1 receptor associated kinase-4(a Toll-like receptor, IRAK4) has been reported in association with severe recurrent pyogenic infections, including *Pneumococcus*, *Staphylococcus*, and *Shigella*, and poor inflammatory response (absent inflammatory markers). Specific antibody responses are poorly maintained after immunization. Interestingly, infections seem to become less problematic with increasing age. Antibiotic therapy and immunoglobulin therapy have been used.

MyD88 deficiency

An autosomal recessive condition. Features are similar to IRAK-4 deficiency, since the two molecules are associated as part of TLR signalling. All TLRs except TLR3 signal via MyD88. Infections are mainly *Streptococcus pneumoniae, Staphylococcus aureus*, and *Pseudomonas aeruginosa, **and can be life-threatening***. There was normal resistance to other bacteria, viruses, and fungi. As with IRAK-4 deficiency, susceptibility to infection declines with age.

UN93B1 & TLR3 deficiencies

Deficiencies of UNC93B1 or TLR3 lead specifically to increased susceptibility to HSV-1 encephalitis. UNC93B1 is an endoplasmic reticulum protein involved in the transport of TLR7 and TLR9 to endolysosomes. In the absence of these receptors normal antiviral interferon production does not occur.

Other conditions

Deficiency of IRAK-1 (X-linked MECP2 deficiency, due to deletion at Xq28 that encompasses both *MECP2* and *IRAK1*) may predispose to bacterial infections.

Deficiency of TIRAP predisposes to staphylococcal infection during childhood.

Phagocytic cell defects

γ-Interferon/IL-12 pathway defects and Irak-4 deficiency.

Major defects of phagocytic cells

- Chronic granulomatous disease:
  - X-linked.
  - Autosomal recessive.
- Leucocyte adhesion defects (LAD):
  - LAD-1: defects of CD18, common β-chain for LFA-1, Mac-1, and CR4 (CD11a, CD11b, CD11c); defect in CD11c (?).
  - LAD-2: defects in synthesis of fucose from GDP-mannose; lack of expression of Lewis X ligand.
  - LAD-3: mutations in Kinlin-3.
- MonoMac syndrome (GATA2 deficiency).
- Glucose 6-phosphate dehydrogenase (G6PD) deficiency.
- Myeloperoxidase deficiency.
- Secondary granule deficiency.
- Cyclic neutropenia and severe congenital neutropenia.
- Shwachman–Bodian–Diamond syndrome.
- Chediak–Higashi and Griscelli syndromes.
- Familial lymphohistiocytosis and haemophagocytic syndromes.
- NK-cell deficiency.
- Rare causes: rac2 deficiency; pulmonary alveolar proteinosis (CSF2RA (autosomal recessive) and CFS2RB(X-linked), CARD9 deficiency.

Chronic granulomatous disease

This is the most significant neutrophil defect, although not the most common. It is also the easiest to diagnose.

Cause
- There is a defect of intracellular bacterial killing in neutrophils and monocytes, due to a failure of superoxide, oxygen radical, and peroxide production.
- X-linked and autosomal recessive forms are described. There is a deficiency of components of cytochrome $b558$: 91 kDa protein (CYBB, X-linked; Xp21.1), 22 kDa protein (CYBA, 16q24), or NADPH oxidase p47 (NCF1, 7q11.23) or p67 (NCF2, 1q25).
- As phagocyte hydrogen peroxidase is normal, organisms that are catalase-negative are killed normally, whereas catalase-positive organisms (*Staphylococcus aureus, Aspergillus, Nocardia*, and *Serratia*) cause major problems.
- Kell blood group antigens are encoded adjacent to the X-CGD locus.

Presentation
- Infections with catalase-positive organisms, especially deep-seated abscesses, osteomyelitis, and chronic granulomata (including orofacial granuloma).
- May mimic inflammatory bowel disease and lead to malabsorption and obstruction of the bowel.
- Liver abscess is a common first presentation, and any child with a liver abscess has CGD until proven otherwise.
- Usually presents initially in childhood but, rarely, first presentation may occur in adults.
- Is a cause of atypical hepatic granulomata in the absence of infection.

Immunology and diagnosis
- Neutrophil oxidative metabolism is abnormal (see Part 2).
- Easiest screening test is the nitroblue tetrazolium reduction (NBT test), but this may miss some cases. The preferred test is a flow cytometric assay using dihydrorhodamine (DHR): some patients may have abnormal DHR but normal NBT!
- Bacterial killing will be absent.
- X-linked CGD patients should be tested for deficiency of Kell antigens.
- Carriers of XL-CGD are at increased risk of discoid lupus and photosensitivity.
- Skewed X-inactivation may give rise to females with XL-CGD.

Treatment
- Long-term antibiotics (co-trimoxazole ± itraconazole) are the mainstay of treatment. Use the liquid formulation of itraconazole (better absorption) and monitor trough levels, adjusting dose accordingly.
- In the USA low-dose prophylactic interferon gamma-1b tends to be used instead.
- Acute infections should be treated promptly with intravenous antibiotics, supplemented with high-dose interferon gamma-1b.

- Drainage of large abscesses may be required.
- Inflammatory bowel disease may be significantly helped by high-dose steroids, particularly where there are obstructive lesions due to granulomata. This increases infection risk.
- BMT/HSCT is the treatment of choice and should be carried out early before infective complications become a threat to life. Results from transplantation in adults are now good.
- Kell-negative XL-CGD patients are a transfusion hazard, and need to be transfused with Kell-negative blood.
- Gene therapy has been used: long-term outcome is variable even when there has been initial engraftment of transfected cells.

Outcome

- Outcome has been much improved by use of prophylactic antibiotics and interferon gamma-1b, but it is still a life-shortening illness (death usually by fifth decade).

Leucocyte adhesion molecule deficiency (LAD-1, LAD-2, LAD-3)

Cause

- LAD-1 is due to a deficiency of the β-chain (CD18) for LFA-1 (ITGB2) (CD11a), Mac-1 (CD11b), and CR4 (CD11c).
- The gene is located at 21q22.3. There may be variable expression: the severe phenotype has < 1% expression, while in the moderate (incomplete) phenotype there may be as much as 10% of control expression.
- LAD-2 is caused by a defect in fucose metabolism, causing the absence of the sialyl-Lewis X ligand from phagocytes (SLC35C1, CD15a). Defect is due to mutations in the GDP-fucose transporter (FUCT1).
- LAD-3 is caused by mutations in Kinlin3 (FERMT3, required for integrin mediated leukocyte adhesion to endothelium).

Presentation

- Presentation is variable, depending on the phenotype. Infections are most marked in LAD-1 and LAD-3.
- Delayed umbilical cord separation is a significant feature (> 10 days).
- Skin infections, intestinal and perianal ulcers, and fistulae are typical.
- Periodontitis occurs in older children and may lead to loss of teeth.
- Immunizations may leave scarred nodules.
- Lack of inflammatory change at the sites of infection and an absence of pus formation.
- LAD-2 is accompanied by marked developmental abnormalities; growth retardation, facial dysmorphism, and periodontitis occur.
- LAD-3 causes a severe bleeding disorder, osteopetrosis, and severe bacterial infections.

Diagnosis and immunology
- Diagnosis is dependent on the demonstration of reduced/absent molecules on lymphocytes and granulocytes by flow cytometry.
- PMA stimulation of granulocytes may be necessary to identify the moderate phenotype in which some upregulation occurs.
- There is usually a peripheral blood neutrophilia, which is often extreme.
- Neutrophil rolling is impaired in LAD-2 but not LAD-1 or LAD-3; Neutrophil adherence is markedly reduced in LAD-1 and LAD-3 but less so in LAD-2.
- In LAD-2 the H blood group antigen is missing from red cells (Bombay phenotype) and the Lewis blood group antigens are also absent.

Treatment
- Prompt antibiotic therapy is required.
- BMT/HSCT is necessary for the severe phenotype of both LAD-1 and LAD-3: graft rejection is not possible in the absence of LFA-1. This observation led to the use of anti-LFA-1 monoclonal antibodies as anti-rejection therapy. Moderate phenotypes may be more difficult to transplant.
- LAD-2 has been treated with high-dose oral fucose with benefit, although not all patients respond.
  - One patient developed autoantibodies against re-fucosylated antigens .

MonoMac syndrome (GATA2 deficiency)

Cause
- Autosomal dominant syndrome, due to mutations in the GATA2 transcription factor gene (3q21.3).
- Somatic mutations may also occur.

Presentation
- Mycobacterial, fungal, and viral infections.
- Mutations in GATA2 are also found in myelodysplastic syndromes, aplastic anaemia, and acute and chronic myeloid leukaemia.

Diagnosis and immunology
- Key feature is the absence of macrophage/monocytes and dendritic cells when peripheral blood is studied by flow cytometry.
- B-lymphocyte and NK-cell numbers and function are reduced.
- Immunoglobulins are normal or increased.

Treatment
- BMT/HSCT is the preferred treatment.

Other phagocytic cell defects

Rac-2 deficiency

An autosomal dominant mutation in the rho-GTPase Rac-2 (22q12.13) has been associated with a presentation similar to that of LAD-1, with delayed umbilical cord separation, absence of pus, and perirectal ulceration. Chemotaxis was abnormal, and neutrophil granule exocytosis was impaired. BMT was curative.

CARD9 deficiency

Autosomal recessive defects in CARD9 lead to an increased susceptibility to invasive fungal infections, including CNS. Neutrophil function is significantly impaired (production of chemoattractants, impaired killing of *Candida*).

G6PD deficiency

Cause
- An X-linked (Xq28) condition; the gene is prone to frequent mutations (200 variants have been recorded).
- Absence of functional G6PD (1–5% of normal activity) impairs the NADPH system of oxidative metabolism, with effects similar to those of CGD. However, most variants have enzyme activity of 20–50% normal and have no phagocytic defect.

Presentation and diagnosis
- The presentation is similar to that of CGD, when < 5% enzyme activity is present.
- Haemolytic anaemia is often present, and can be triggered by certain foods (fava beans) and drugs (sulfones such as dapsone; primaquine, salicylates).
- The NBT test is diagnostic and the enzyme activity can be measured.

Myeloperoxidase deficiency

This deficiency is not uncommon (the gene is located at 17q21.3–q23). The prevalence is between 1/2000 and 1/4000 in the USA. Cases are usually asymptomatic, although occasional defects in killing *Candida* have been reported, and infection may occur, particularly if the patient is diabetic.

Glucose-6-phosphatase deficiency

Mutations in the *G6PC3* gene cause autosomal recessive severe congenital neutropenia, thrombocytopenia, and recurrent bacterial infections. It is accompanied by cardiac and urogenital malformations. Other clinical features include inflammatory bowel disease, pulmonary hypertension, endocrine abnormalities, lymphopenia, thymic hypoplasia, myelokathexis, and dysmorphic features.

Glutathione synthetase deficiency

Rare autosomal recessive. May be associated with haemolytic anaemia. Severe deficiency is associated with metabolic acidosis with increased 5-oxoproline levels, progressive neurological disease, and recurrent bacterial infections, due to impaired phagocytosis and intracellular killing. Glutathione reductase deficiency is associated with haemolysis but not infections.

Shwachman–Bodian–Diamond syndrome

This is an autosomal recessive syndrome of hereditary pancreatic insufficiency, accompanied by neutropenia, abnormal neutrophil chemotaxis, thrombocytopenia, anaemia, and growth retardation. Chondrodysoplasia may be present. NK-cell lymphopenia is common. The gene is *SBDS* (7q11)—precise function unknown, but thought to be involved in RNA metabolism. Hypogammaglobulinaemia with recurrent sinopulmonary infections may also occur. Responses to polysaccharide antigens may be absent. Exocrine pancreatic supplementation required. Treatment with IVIg may be helpful, and G-CSF has been used, although there is concern over potential risk of myeloid leukaemias. HSCT has also been tried: there appears to be an increased risk of GvHD.

Secondary granule deficiency

Neutrophil structure is abnormal with bilobed nuclei. Secondary (lactoferrin) granules are absent and there is a deficiency of other neutrophil enzymes (alkaline phosphatase). This leads to defective neutrophil oxidative metabolism and bacterial killing, resulting in skin and sinopulmonary infections. The diagnosis can be made by careful examination of the blood film, supplemented by cytochemical studies for neutrophil enzymes (NAP score). Some cases have been associated with defects in the *C/EBPE* gene (14q11.2), a CCAAT enhancer protein-binding protein, which acts as a transcription factor in myelopoiesis.

Cyclic neutropenia

This is a rare syndrome characterized by cyclic reductions in neutrophils, but it is perhaps more common than previously thought, with milder variants escaping notice.

Cause

- Autosomal dominant disorder due to mutations in *ELA2* gene (SCN1), encoding neutrophil elastase. Mutations affect whether elastase localizes to granules or to cell surface membrane. Membrane expression is associated with disease. Similar mutations in *ELA2* also cause severe congenital neutropenia.
- Similar disease in dogs (grey collie syndrome) is due to different gene defect (see Hermansky–Pudlak syndrome in ➋ 'Disorders of pigmentation and immune deficiency', p. 72) and has a 14-day cycle.
- The cycle is usually 21 days ± 2–3 days, but the molecular cause of cycling is unknown.

Presentation

- Mouth ulceration typically occurs at the neutrophil nadir; more significant invasive infection may occur.
- Mood change just before the nadir is often marked. Symptoms may improve with age.

Diagnosis

- The clue is usually a low neutrophil count during an infective episode.
- Diagnosis is confirmed by serial full blood counts with full differential, three times weekly over 4 weeks. Neutrophils may disappear completely. Symptoms usually occur if the count drops below 1×10^9/l.
- There is a compensatory monocytosis at the time of the neutrophil nadir.

Management

- G-CSF prevents a dramatic drop but does *not* abolish the cycle, which shortens to approximately 14 days.
- There is, however, a risk of myeloid leukaemia with chronic G-CSF therapy and this should be used with circumspection. Data suggest that *ELA2* mutations increase the risk of AML and MDS, and this may be increased further by G-CSF use.
- Prophylactic co-trimoxazole either side of the predicted nadir may be valuable in preventing infection.

Other neutrophil defects

Barth syndrome (3-methylglutaconic aciduria type III)

This X-linked disorder caused by mutations in the *TAZ* gene, also features cyclic neutropenia, as well as dilated cardiomyopathy and methylglutaconic aciduria. The gene product is an acyltransferase involved in the synthesis of cardiolipin.

3-methylglutaconic aciduria is associated with mutations in CLPB and causes developmental delay, microcephaly, hypotonia, ataxia, epilepsy, cataracts, and IUGR.

Cohen syndrome

This rare autosomal recessive syndrome is due to mutations in the *COH1* gene, whose product is involved in vesicle sorting and intracellular protein transport. Neutropenia is associated with dysmorphic features and intellectual disability.

Severe congenital neutropenia (SCN)

Four different genetic variants of SCN have been reported. The majority of cases have defects in the *ELA2* gene, as in cyclic neutropenia, and are at risk of developing myelodysplasia (MDS) and acute myeloid leukaemia (AML). The disorder is autosomal dominant and homozygous defects have not been reported. The neutropenia is, however, static. Mutations in HAX-1 and AK2 (see → 'SCID: reticular dysgenesis: (adenylate kinase 2 (AK2) deficiency)', p. 44) also cause severe congenital neutropenia. Rare cases have been associated with autosomal dominant mutations in the transcriptional repressor *GFI1* gene, causing overexpression of elastase and overflow on to the cell membrane: these cases also have lymphopenia. WASP mutations have been associated with X-linked neutropenia (XLN, see → 'Wiskott–Aldrich syndrome (WAS), X-linked thrombocytopenia (XLT), and X-linked neutropenia (XLN)', p. 50). Mutations have also been reported in the gene encoding the receptor for G-CSF: these cases do not develop MDS or AML. Other possible defects in the *ELA2* promoter region may also contribute to SCN cases.

Kostmann's syndrome

This is a congenital severe neutropenia due to a neutrophil maturation defect with arrest at the pro-myelocyte stage. This has only been reported in one family, with an autosomal recessive pattern of inheritance, probably due to HAX1 mutations. It presents with recurrent severe infections. Immunoglobulins are raised; there is a compensatory monocytosis, eosinophilia, and a thrombocytosis. BMT/HSCT may be used as treatment. Co-trimoxazole prophylaxis is necessary.

β-Actin deficiency

Patients with defective β-actin (ACTB) present with recurrent bacterial infections, including abscesses, intellectual disability, and joint problems. Neutrophil chemotaxis is abnormal.

Other syndromes

Abnormal neutrophil numbers and function have been reported with:
- G-CSF receptor deficiency (CSF3R): stress granulopoeisis affected.
- GFI1 deficiency: neutropenia with T- & B-cell lymphopenia.
- MKL1 deficiency: neutropenia with thrombocytopenia and lymphopenia.

Disorders of pigmentation and immune deficiency

There have been major advances in the understanding of the genetics of immune deficiencies that are associated with pigmentary disorders.

Chediak–Higashi syndrome

Cause
- An autosomal recessive disease, due to mutations in the *CHS1* gene (also known as *LYST*—lysosomal trafficking regulator), located at 1q42.1.
- *CHS* is the human equivalent of the beige mutant mouse.
- Exact function of the *LYST* protein is not known.

Presentation
- Benign and aggressive presentations occur.
- Characteristic features are partial oculocutaneous albinism (due to abnormal melanocytes), leading to silver streaks in the hair (prematurely!) and pigmentary changes in the iris and also the skin.
- Recurrent infections, especially periodontitis and pyogenic infections.
- CNS abnormalities: peripheral and central, with neuropathy, cranial nerve palsies, parkinsonian features, fits, and intellectual disability.
- Hepatosplenomegaly occurs frequently.

Diagnosis
- There are giant primary cytoplasmic granules in leucocytes and platelets.
- Hair shafts show diagnostic clumping of pigment granules.

Immunology
- Granulocyte and monocyte chemotaxis is abnormal with delayed intracellular killing (correctable by ascorbate *in vitro*).
- Defective NK-cell function is common.
- Neutropenia.

Prognosis
- Outcome is poor in the accelerated phase with neurological deterioration and a haemophagocytic syndrome like familial lymphohistiocytosis (see later in this topic).
- Expression of CTLA-4 has been associated with development of the accelerated phase.
- This should be treated with etoposide followed by BMT/HSCT.

Partial albinism (Griscelli syndrome)

This is similar to Chediak–Higashi syndrome but is distinguished from it by the absence of giant granules.
- Three types have now been identified, and mouse models exist for all types. The genes identified are all involved in the intracellular movement of melanosomes, mechanisms that are also used in granule-containing cells to undertake exocytosis.
  - GS type 1 due to mutations in the *MYO5A* gene (15q21.1) encoding myosin Va. This type presents with albinism and severe neurological disease with intellectual disability and developmental delay.
  - GS type 2 due to mutations in *RAB27A* gene (15q21.1), encoding a GTPase Rab27a involved in the secretory pathway. Patients have hypopigmentation and a severe immune defect, culminating in an accelerated phase of fulminant haemophagocytosis. Treatment is with BMT/HSCT.
  - GS type 3 due to mutations in the *MLPH* gene, coding for melanophilin, and leading to impaired interaction with Rab27a. This type has the best prognosis.
- Diagnosis can be confirmed by microscopy of hairs, to examine pigment deposition.
- Delayed hypersensitivity and NK-cell function are defective; reduced immunoglobulins and neutrophil problems have also been described.

Hermansky–Pudlak syndrome type 2 & type 10

Type 2 HPS is an autosomal recessive disorder associated with mutations in the *AP3B1* gene. The clinical features are severe congenital (non-cycling) neutropenia, defects of platelet dense bodies, with a bleeding tendency and oculocutaneous albinism. The equivalent gene defect in dogs causes the grey collie syndrome; the mouse mutant is pearl.

HPS type 10 causes oculocutaneous albinism, severe neutropenia with recurrent infections, epilepsy, hearing loss, and developmental delay.

Other forms of HPS are recognized with distinct gene defects but these do not have neutropenia and infections.

p14/LAMTOR2 deficiency
A single family has been described with deficiency of the endosomal adaptor protein p14 (*MAPBPIP*). Features include severe congenital neutropenia, short stature, hypopigmentation, coarse features, and recurrent bacterial chest infections. T- and B-cell abnormalities were also noted, including hypogammaglobulinaemia and reduced CD8 T-cell cytotoxicity.

Other pigmentary disorders
Other genetic disorders of pigmentation not associated with immune deficiency include:
• Piebaldism due to mutations in the *KIT* gene.
• Waardenburg syndrome, characterized by piebaldism with sensorineural deafness, caused by multiple gene defects: *PAX3, MITF, SLUG, EDN3, EDNRB, SOX10*.
• Oculocutaneous albinism (four genes: *TYR, P, TYRP, MATP*).
• Hermansky–Pudlak syndrome, types 1 and 3–6 (*HSP1,3–6*).

In the mouse, other genes have been identified causing defects of pigmentation, but human equivalents have yet to be identified.

Familial lymphohistiocytosis, haemophagocytic syndrome in other conditions, and NK-cell deficiency

Familial lymphohistiocytosis (FLH)
• FLH is an autosomal recessive disease of childhood, presenting with infiltrations of polyclonal CD8$^+$ T cells and macrophages into many organs following viral infections.
• Genetics is complicated. Five defects have been identified:
  • FLH1: no gene identified; locus at 9q21.
  • FLH2: Perforin deficiency (*PRF1*).
  • FLH3: Munc 13-4 (*UNC13D*, 17q25.1).
  • FLH4: Syntaxin 11 (*STX11*, mainly Kurdish cases).
  • FLH5: Munc 18.2 (*STXBP2*).
  • In addition XIAP deficiency is sometimes also classified as one of the FLH conditions.
  • Polymorphisms in *CTLA-4* in Japanese people with infection-triggered HLH.
• Majority of Turkish patients are FLH-2, -3 or -4.
• Presentation is with fever, hepatosplenomegaly, liver dysfunction, neurological disease, rash, and lymphadenopathy.
• Inflammatory bowel disease may be a feature.
• NK-cell and cytotoxic T-cell function is markedly reduced.
• sCD25 increased (highest levels associated with poorer prognosis).
• Ferritin levels markedly increased.
• Specific flow cytometric tests are available for some variants (see ➲ Chapter 20).

- Perforin deficiency is the main cause of rapidly fatal FLH.
- Failure of apoptosis has been suggested as a mechanism for the excessive cellular infiltrates.
- Treatment is with etoposide-containing regimens and HSCT (ideally not when there is florid HLH as this markedly reduces survival).

Haemophagocytic syndrome in other conditions

Haemophagocytosis has been reported to occur as part of the accelerated phase of type 2 Griscelli syndrome patients, Chediak–Higashi syndrome, and X-linked lymphoproliferative syndrome triggered by EBV exposure. It is also seen in SLE, adult-onset Still's, juvenile rheumatoid arthritis, and Castleman's disease. It has been suggested that IL-18 may be responsible in the autoimmune secondary cases. Macrophage activation syndrome is seen juvenile rheumatoid arthritis or SLE—it is similar to HLH.

NK-cell deficiency

- Primary NK-cell deficiency has been reported, causing severe or fatal infections with herpesviruses and varicella, usually presenting in the teens or early adult life.
- Both sexes are affected.
- Differential diagnosis includes XLPS.
- Homozygosity for a polymorphism in the FcRγIIIa receptor (CD16) on NK cells has been associated with increased susceptibility to herpesviruses; this change also interferes with the ability of certain anti-CD16 monoclonal antibodies to bind.
- One family showed linkage to a region of chromosome 8.

Immunodeficiency in association with other rare syndromes

Immunodeficiency has been described as a feature in a wide variety of other genetic syndromes. This is not an exhaustive list!

Other genetic syndromes

Seckel syndrome

An autosomal recessive syndrome characterized by 'bird-headed' dwarfism, intellectual disability, hypoplastic anaemia, and hypogammaglobulinaemia.

Down's syndrome

This is due to trisomy 21. There is a progressive decrease in IgM, dysplastic thymus, low NK activity, and an unusual sensitivity to γ-interferon, whose receptor is located on chromosome 21. There is an increase in Tcr γδ cells at the expense of Tcr αβ cells. T-cell proliferation to mitogens is reduced, with poor IL-2 production. There is an increase in infections and also in malignancy and autoimmune disease.

Turner's syndrome

The genetic abnormality is XO. 50% of patients have low IgG and IgM and poor specific antibody responses.

Chromosome 18 syndromes
Ring chromosome 18 and deletions of the long and short arms of chromosome 18 are associated with facial hypoplasia, intellectual disability, and low/absent IgA.

Immunodeficiency with generalized growth retardation

Schimke immuno-osseus dysplasia

An autosomal recessive syndrome characterized by nephropathy, skeletal dysplasia, and lentigenes. Intrauterine growth restriction (IUGR). There is a lymphopenia of CD4$^+$ T cells with poor T-cell mitogen responses. Pancytopenia is common. Immunoglobulin levels may be reduced. The gene is *SMARCAL1*, encoding a chromatin remodelling protein. This gene affects thymic function. Patients are prone to bacterial, fungal, and viral infections. HSCT has been reported to be helpful.

Immunodeficiency with absent thumbs (TAR syndrome)

There is radial dysplasia, ichthyosis, and anosmia in this syndrome. Recurrent infections and chronic mucocutaneous candidiasis occur. There are poor T-cell mitogen responses and absent IgA, with low IgG and IgM. Abnormalities have been reported in the Y14 subunit of the exon-junction complex involved in RNA processing (RBMSA).

Wolf–Hirschhorn syndrome

Caused by deletions on chromosome 4p, leading to a syndrome of growth retardation, intellectual disability, microcephaly, and multiple other abnormalities, affecting skeleton, teeth, heart, ears, and eyes. Recurrent bacterial infections are a feature. Humoral immune defects are variable from pan-hypogammaglobulinaemia to IgA, IgG$_2$, or specific antibody deficiency. Candidate gene is *WHSC1*, a histone methyltransferase.

Others

- Dubowitz syndrome (autosomal recessive); dwarfism, eczema, bone marrow failure; defects identified include LIG4 and PRKAR1A.
- Growth retardation, facial anomalies, and immunodeficiency.
- Progeria (Hutchison–Gilford syndrome): premature ageing. LMNA defects affecting nuclear lamin production.
- MYSM1 deficiency: short stature, bone marrow failure, skeletal abnormalities, T-cell lymphopenia, hypogammaglobulinaemia.
- MOPD1 (RNU4ATAC) deficiency: intrauterine growth restriction, recurrent bacterial infections, lymphadenopathy retinal dystrophy; dysmorphism. Variable decrease in specific antibody production.
- EXTL3 deficiency: skeletal dysplasia, kyphosis developmental delay. Hypogammaglobulinaemia and T-cell lymphopenia.

These syndromes have all been reported with variable immunodeficiencies.

Skin disease and immunodeficiency

Dyskeratosis congenita

Dyskeratosis congenita is characterized by cutaneous pigmentation, nail dystrophy, and oral leucoplakia, and is complicated by malignancy and bone marrow failure. Autosomal dominant or recessive and X-linked forms occur. The X-linked form is associated with mutations in the *DKC1* gene encoding dyskerin, a nucleolar protein. Autosomal forms include defects in *NOLA2, NOLA3, RTEL1, TERC, TINF2, TERT, TPP1, DCLRE1B, SNM1, APOLLO, PARN, WRAP53*. Variable immune defects are found: hypogammaglobulinaemia and poor delayed-type hypersensitivity. Thymic aplasia may occur.

The same gene defect (*DKC1*) also causes the Høyeraal–Hreidarsson syndrome (microcephaly, growth failure, and pancytopenia, which may mimic SCID).

Netherton syndrome

There is trichorrhexis, ichthyosis, and atopy; some patients have low IgG, raised IgE & IgA, reduced class-switched and non-class-switched B cells, abnormal neutrophil function, and poor T-cell mitogens responses. Mutations in the gene *SPINK5*, encoding a serine protease inhibitor, have been identified in some patients.

Acrodermatitis enteropathica

This is caused by zinc deficiency, leading to eczema, diarrhoea, malabsorption, and sinopulmonary infections. T-cell numbers and function are reduced and immunoglobulins are low. All the defects are correctable with supplemental zinc.

Anhidrotic ectodermal dysplasia

This family of diseases is associated with defective NF-κB signalling. Autosomal recessive or X-linked forms of this syndrome occur. Defects in the *NEMO* gene have been reported (see ➲ 'Autosomal hyper-IgM syndromes', p. 24) in the X-linked form, associated with significant immunodeficiency. Autosomal dominant and recessive forms have mutations in the *EDA1* gene encoding ectodysplasin (a TNF cytokine family member) or its receptor EDAR, a member of the TNF receptor superfamily, encoded by *EDA3*. EDAR mutations have been associated with autosomal recessive disease. Hypohydrosis and faulty dentition are the key features. Upper respiratory infections occur. There is variable T- and B-cell function; specific antibody responses may be poor.

Papillon–Lefèvre syndrome

Abnormal neutrophil chemotaxis and reduced neutrophil killing have been reported in this syndrome of hyperkeratosis and pyoderma, with periodontitis. The gene defect has been identified as mutations in cathepsin C (*CTSC*, also known as dipeptidyl peptidase I), an enzyme involved in protein degradation.

Clericuzio syndrome

Deficiency in C16ORFS7. Poikilodermia with retinopathy, developmental delay, facial dysmorphism, and neutropenia.

Epidermodysplasia verruciformis (Lewandowsky–Lutz dysplasia)

Rare autosmosomal recessive skin disorder with high susceptibility to papillomavirus infection (typically HPV types 5 & 8). Due to inactivating mutations in *EVER1* and *EVER2* genes on chromosome 17, which control access to zinc. Present with flat wart like papules and have high risk of developing skin cancer. Treatment with retinoids, interferons, and high-dose cimetidine has been suggested.

Extensive warts have also been associated with common variable immune deficiency, interferon-γ deficiency, and WHIM syndrome.

Immunodeficiency with metabolic abnormalities

ADA and PNP deficiencies are metabolic abnormalities causing immunodeficiency, but are covered in ➲ 'SCID: ZAP-70 kinase deficiency and ADA deficiency', and 'SCID: purine nucleoside phosphorylase (PNP) deficiency', pp. 39–40.

Transcobalamin II deficiency

Autosomal recessive deficiency of TC II (*TCNII*, 22q11.2), a vitamin B_{12}-binding protein essential for transport of vitamin B_{12}, has been reported in association with diarrhoea, failure to thrive, megaloblastic anaemia, lymphopenia, neutropenia, and thrombocytopenia. Abnormal neutrophil function and hypogammaglobulinaemia are present. All the features are reversible with vitamin B_{12} therapy.

Methylmalonic acidaemia

The features are similar to those of TC II deficiency. It is treated with folic acid. Gene defects have been identified in the vitamin B_{12}-dependent enzyme methylmalonyl-CoA mutase (*MUT*) and in the mitochondrial enzymes *SUCLA2* and *SUCIG1*.

Type I hereditary orotic aciduria

This is an autosomal recessive disease caused by defects in uridine-5-monophosphate synthase (UMPS). It causes delayed growth, diarrhoea, and megaloblastic anaemia. Fatal meningitis and disseminated varicella may be complications. There is a T-cell lymphopenia and impaired T-cell function.

Biotin-dependent carboxylase deficiency

An autosomal recessive condition characterized by convulsions, ataxia, alopecia, candidiasis, and intermittent lactic acidosis. The severe neonatal form presents with severe acidosis and recurrent sepsis. There is increased urinary β-hydroxypropionic acid, methyl citrate, β-methylcrotonglycine, and 3-hydroxyisovalerate excretion. Decreased T and B cells with low IgA are noted. It is treated with biotin.

Mannosidosis

This is a lysosomal storage disease that is associated with abnormal neutrophil (chemotaxis, phagocytosis, and killing) and lymphocyte function (hypogammaglobulinaemia and poor PHA responses).

Glycogen storage disease type Ib

Recurrent infections, including severe oral ulceration and abscesses, are associated with a neutropenia and neutrophil dysfunction in this syndrome.

Hypercatabolism of immunoglobulin and lymphoedema/lymphangiectasia

Familial hypercatabolism

Familial hypercatabolism of IgG has been associated with bone abnormalities, abnormal glucose metabolism, and recurrent infections. IgG is very low with a very short half-life; serum albumin may be normal or low.

Primary intestinal lymphangiectasia (Waldmann's disease)

This is due to a failure of normal lymphatic development in the bowel, with abnormally dilated lymphatics. Similar abnormalities may occur elsewhere, causing localized oedema, effusions, and ascites. There is enteric loss of lymphocytes and malabsorption, particularly of fats. The cause is unknown: many cases are sporadic but familial cases are known. There is a profound lymphopenia, with hypoalbuminaemia and hypogammaglobulinaemia; IgM may be in the normal range and infections may be less severe than the IgG level might predict. Specific responses may be normal but very short-lived. IVIg/SCIg may be given but weekly therapy may be required to maintain adequate levels. Fat malabsorption may be severe and medium-chain triglyceride supplements may be required long term. Octreotide may be helpful. Malignancy (lymphoma) may be a long-term complication.

Hennekam syndrome

This rare syndrome is characterized by widespread lymphangiectasia, lymphoedema, and intellectual disability. It has been associated with mutations in collagen and calcium-binding EGF domain-containing protein 1 (CCBE1) and FAT4.

Milroy disease

This is primary congenital lymphoedema, a rare autosomal dominant disease due to mutations in vascular endothelial growth factor receptor 3 (VEGFR3). The lymphoedema is usually confined to the lower limbs and is present from birth. In males hydrocoeles occur. Recurrent lower limb cellulitis may occur.

A more severe form of generalized primary lymphoedema, accompanied by intestinal and pulmonary lymphangiectasia, pleural and pericardial effusions has been associated with mutations in *PIEZO1* (which encodes an ion channel).

See also ➔ Chapter 2.

Immune TOR-opathies

The immune TOR-opathies represent a range of conditions caused by mutations in the genes for the phosphoinositide-3-kinase (PI3K)/AKT/mTOR/S6 kinase pathway. These mutations cause disease with variable immune deficiency, autoimmunity, and other manifestations.

Activated PI3Kδ syndrome (APDS)

Gain-of-function mutations in the *PI3Kδ* gene cause lymphadenopathy, immunodeficiency, with senescent T cells. Two types of mutations are recognized (APDS 1 & 2). Present with early-onset severe sinopulmonary infections with capsulated organisms, benign lymphoproliferation and autoimmunity, and B cell lymphomas. Specific PI3Kδ inhibitors are available: idelalisib (FDA approved for treating CLL) and leniolisib (undergoing trials).

Lipopolysaccharide-responsive beige-like anchor protein (LRBA) deficiency

LRBA belongs to the Beige and Chediak–Higashi (BEACH) domain-containing family. LRBA deficiency causes recurrent infections, organomegaly, inflammatory bowel disease, hypogammaglobulinaemia and autoimmunity, and an IPEX-like syndrome. Tregs are reduced in a majority of patients. Class-switched memory B cells are reduced. Apoptosis and autophagy are disturbed.

CARD-11/BCL-10/MALT1 mutations

Autosomal recessive mutations in these three genes cause immunodeficiency with recurrent sinopulmonary infections, abnormal T-cell proliferation, and B-cell dysfunction. Loss-of-function CARD-11 mutations may be associated with *Pneumocystis* infection. Other CARD-11 mutations have been associated with severe atopic dermatitis, chest and skin infections, eosinophilia, B-cell lymphopenia, and low IgM, with normal or raised IgA and raised IgE. Gain-of-function CARD-11 mutations have been associated with a congenital B-lymphoproliferative syndrome (BENTA = B-cell expansion with NF-κB and T-cell anergy), characterized by massive B lymphocytosis with splenomegaly and lymphadenopathy but no autoimmunity (cf. ALPS— see ➔ 'Autoimmune lymphoproliferative syndromes (ALPS; Canale–Smith syndrome)', p. 60).

Cowden's syndrome

Cowden's syndrome is a rare autosomal dominant disease caused by mutations in the PI3-kinase and phosphatase and tensin homologue gene (*PTEN*). It causes hamartomatous polyposis of the gut and skin with an increased risk of cancer. It may be associated with immune deficiency and auto-immunity. T-cell lymphopenia and poor specific antibody responses have been reported.

Splenic disorders

Congenital asplenia and Ivemark syndrome

Asplenia may occur alone or in association with partial situs inversus and cardiac defects.

X-linked, autosomal dominant, and autosomal recessive forms have been reported. The X-linked form has been associated with mutations in connexin 43 and Xic3, while the autosomal dominant form has been associated in some cases with mutations in RPSA.

Early infections, especially with capsulated organisms, are a typical feature. Sudden unheralded death from overwhelming sepsis may occur and the diagnosis may only be made at post-mortem. Survival into adult life is possible without serious infection. Blood film will show Howell–Jolly bodies; ultrasound will demonstrate absence of the spleen, which can be confirmed by absence of uptake on a labelled white cell scan or on a red cell clearance scan. Initial poor polysaccharide responses may improve after the first 3 years of life. However, there remains a risk of overwhelming sepsis and lifelong prophylactic antibiotics should be administered, together with regular immunizations against influenza, pneumococci, *Haemophilus influenzae* type b (Hib), and meningococci. Management is as for acquired asplenia.

See also ➔ 'Asplenia', p. 120, for further details on management.

Tuftsin deficiency

Tuftsin is a tetrapeptide released from the CH_2 domain of IgG by the actions of a membrane leucokinase and a splenic endocarbocypeptidase. It stimulates the bactericidal function of phagocytic cells. Primary tuftsin deficiency has been described in five patients, in association with increased infections. Administration of immunoglobulin replacement may be beneficial. Secondary tuftsin deficiency occurs in splenectomy, asplenia, and hyposplenia (coeliac disease). Tuftsin production may also be impaired by parenteral nutrition, probably by lipid.

Complement deficiencies

Cause

- Genetic deficiencies of all complement components have been described, including the regulatory inhibitors, C1 inhibitor, factor I, and factor H.
- Properdin deficiency is X-linked; all the others are autosomal recessives, except C1-inhibitor deficiency, which is autosomal dominant.
- Factors B, C2, and C4 form part of the extended MHC complex (short arm of chromosome 6, located between HLA-D and HLA-B loci).

- Complement deficiencies are common in South Africa and in the countries of the North African coast and eastern Mediterranean. C2 and C4 deficiencies are relatively common. An increasing number of C4 null alleles increases substantially the risk of developing lupus.

Presentation

- Increased susceptibility to pyogenic infections in C3, factor I, and factor H deficiencies.
- Increased susceptibility to neisserial infections in C5, C6, C7, C8a, C8b, C9, factor D, and properdin deficiencies.
- Recurrent neisserial infection, especially meningitis, should always prompt a screen for complement deficiency; the disease may be milder than in complement replete individuals.
- C9 deficiency is common in Japan and may be asymptomatic, as slow lysis through C5–C8 may take place without C9.
- Increased susceptibility to SLE-like syndrome in C1q, C1r/C1s, C4, C2, C5, C6, C7, C8a, and C8b. C2-deficient lupus is often atypical with marked cutaneous features.
- Factor H, factor I, and MCP deficiencies are associated with the non-diarrhoea-associated haemolytic–uraemic syndrome.

Diagnosis

- Diagnosis is by the screening for classic, alternate, and terminal lytic sequence by functional complement assays (classic and alternate pathway CH_{100}—see Part 2), followed by measurement of individual components, as indicated by the screening tests.

Treatment

- No specific treatment is available; use of FFP may make the acute problems worse.
- Recurrent neisserial infection may be prevented by prophylactic antibiotics and meningococcal vaccination may help, although there are concerns that disease may be more severe if it occurs in a complement-deficient person after vaccination.
- Prophylactic penicillin (phenoxymethylpenicillin 500 mg bd adult dose; erythromycin 250 mg bd if allergic to penicillin) is highly desirable.
- Autoimmune disease is treated in the normal way.

Ficolin-3 deficiency

- Ficolin-3 is a recognition molecule in the lectin pathway, encoded by the *FCN3* gene.
- An adult patient has been described with homozygous deficiency of ficolin-3, who presented with recurrent respiratory tract infections, including *Haemophilus* and *Pseudomonas*, and extensive bronchiectasis.
- No specific treatment has been identified.

CD55 deficiency

- Autosomal recessive CD55 deficiency has been associated with an early-onset hyperactivation of complement, angiopathic thrombosis, and protein-losing enteropathy (CHAPLE syndrome).

- Intestinal lymphangiectasia is present.
- This may be recognized in patients who lack the Cromer red blood cell antigen (Inab phenotype).
- Eculizumab appears promising as treatment.

Mannan-binding lectin (MBL) deficiency

MBL (10q11.2) is involved in the initiation of complement activation via the lectin pathway, triggered by binding to mannose residues on bacterial cells' surfaces. Although deficiency of MBL has been associated with infections, many mutations (the gene is highly polymorphic) reducing MBL levels have been identified in asymptomatic families, indicating that MBL deficiency alone is insufficient to cause disease, in the absence of other host defence problems.

- It has been estimated that up to 5% of the population lack functional MBL and this has led to suggestions that MBL deficiency may have a beneficial effect in later life.
- MBL deficiency in cystic fibrosis has been associated with a worse prognosis.
- The risk of infection in children with low MBL seems to be highest in the first 2 years of life, when specific polysaccharide responses are poor. MBL's value may therefore be early protection, before specific antibody production is optimum, with its role diminishing in later life, replaced by antibody.
- MBL deficiency may be a risk factor for infections during chemotherapy, and after SCT.
- Infections are usually due to encapsulated organisms.
- Opsonic failure is described.
- Reports associate low MBL with autoimmune diseases.
- Deficiency of MASP2 has been reported in association with pyogenic infections.

Hereditary angioedema and C4-binding protein deficiency

Hereditary angioedema

Cause
- Two main types of HAE are recognized: type I (85%; gene deletion, no protein produced) and type II (15%; point mutation in active site of enzyme). The *SERPING1* gene is located on chromosome 11.
- Condition is autosomal dominant as one normal gene is insufficient to protect against symptoms.
- Type III HAE has been associated with a gain-in-function mutation in factor XII, causing failure of inactivation of the complement and kinin systems. Angioedema is most likely to be due to the latter (bradykinin) rather than the former.
- Type III HAE with no FXII mutation has also been associated with an autosomal dominant mutation in the plasminogen gene, which seems to be particularly associated with tongue swelling.

- One family with inherited angioedema has been associated with mutations in the angiopoietin-1 gene (*ANGPT1*).
- Other cases of HAE have no currently identified gene defect.

Presentation
- There is an angioedema (deep tissue swelling) of any part of the body, including airway and gut; the latter presents with recurrent abdominal pain and repeated laparotomies may be undertaken before the diagnosis is made.
- There is usually *no* urticaria or itch, although patients often describe an uncomfortable prodromal tingling.
- Attacks begin in later childhood/teenage years and may be precipitated by trauma (beware dental work and operations) and infections.
- Frequency of attacks may be increased by oral contraceptives and by pregnancy. There is an increased risk of immune complex disease.
- Type III HAE occurs mainly in women, especially if oral contraceptives are used.
- Attacks in all types of HAE can be triggered by trauma, infections, and emotional stress.

Diagnosis
- Typically C4 and C2 are undetectable during an acute attack and low/ absent in between.
- However, there are numerous reports of normal C4 levels in patients with HAE: C4 cannot therefore be relied upon to exclude the diagnosis, and measurement of C1-inhibitor immunochemically and functionally should be carried out where there is high suspicion.
- In type I, there will be a low C1-inhibitor level immunochemically and this will become undetectable in an acute attack.
- In type II, there will be a normal or high level of inhibitor measured immunochemically, but function will be low or absent.
- As it is an autosomal dominant, children of affected individuals should undergo screening. Levels of C4 and C1-inhibitor (immunochemical and functional) may not be reliable in children under 1 year old. Genetic testing is helpful.
- Angioedema may be acquired secondary to SLE or lymphoma and these may be distinguished from HAE by the reduction in C1q, although this is not always reliable.

Treatment
- Treat major attacks with purified or recombinant C1 esterase inhibitor, Berinert® or Cinryze® (1000–1500 IU, i.e. 2–3 ampoules) by slow intravenous injection. Guidelines suggest 20 units/kg, but not all patients require this dose.
- Recombinant C1 inhibitor (conestat alfa (Ruconest®)) is effective but because it is derived from rabbit milk, it has a short half-life (2 hours). It is contraindicated in patients with rabbit allergy.
- Subcutaneous treatment with icatibant (Firazyr®, bradykinin B2 receptor antagonist) 3 ml, repeated after 8 hours if necessary is as effective, and may be given by self-administration at home. Main side-effect is injection site pain.

- Ecallantide Kalbitor®, a plasma kallikrein inhibitor, is licensed for subcutaneous use in the USA but not Europe. It is effective but 2.7% of patients developed anaphylaxis! An oral kallikrein inhibitor is undergoing clinical trials.
- Lanadelumab (DX-2930) is a human monoclonal antibody inhibitor of plasma kallikrein, that has been approved by the FDA for regular prophylaxis.
- Pooled virally inactivated fresh frozen plasma (FFP) may be an emergency alternative. Untreated single-unit FFP has the usual risks of transmitted infection and it is also possible for FFP to exacerbate attacks by providing more substrate.
- Tracheostomy may be required if there is significant laryngeal oedema.
- Recurrent severe attacks may mandate regular long-term prophylaxis with purified C1 inhibitor rather than on-demand treatment of attacks. 40–60 u/kg twice weekly is recommended. Subcutaneous treatment is possible.
- Long-term prophylaxis may also be required during pregnancy if there is an increase in the number of attacks.
- Home treatment is appropriate for some patients, particularly those on long-term prophylaxis with C1-inhibitor.
- Vaccination against hepatitis A and B is recommended for recipients of plasma-derived C1-inhibitor.
- Recording of batch numbers for plasma-derived C1-inhibitor is strongly advised, against the possibility of the need for recall.
- Prophylaxis may be obtained with modified androgens (danazol, 200–600 mg/day; or stanozolol, 2.5–10 mg/day). However, stanozolol may be difficult to obtain and oxandrolone is an alternative. Current guidance aims to keep the dose of danazol to 200 mg/day or less. Regular liver function tests and liver ultrasounds are required for monitoring therapy with all these agents. Long-term use may be associated with increased risk of hepatic adenomas. Virilization in females will limit use. They should not be used in pregnancy or during breast-feeding.
- Abnormalities of lipids may occur, but do not on the trial evidence available so far appear to increase coronary events or carotid atherosclerosis.
- The anti-fibrinolytic tranexamic acid is an alternative prophylactic agent (2–4 g/day in divided doses). It should not be used where there is a history of thromboembolic events. Regular liver function testing and ultrasound is advisable.
- Prophylactic purified inhibitor should be used before high-risk surgical procedures (either 1000 units or 20 units/kg), although modified androgens or tranexamic acid may be adequate for minor procedures (not recommended as first choice).
- Patients with frequent severe attacks may be managed with regular prophylactic C1-inhibitor: this can be given intravenously, or by self-administered subcutaneous manual slow push.

- Dental work should always be carried out in hospital in view of the risk of developing oral oedema and airway obstruction.
- Abdominal attacks respond poorly to purified inhibitor—treatment should be conservative: analgesia (NSAIDs), IV fluids, and avoidance of unnecessary laparotomies (unless there is good evidence for other pathology).
- Type III HAE is said to respond to standard HAE therapies.

C4-binding protein (C4BP) deficiency

C4BP inhibits the classical pathway of complement activation by blocking the formation of the C3 convertase C4bC2a. Deficiency of C4BP may cause angioedema and, because of its interaction also with protein S, may be a cause of purpura fulminans.

Angioetensin-converting enzyme (ACE) deficiency

Deficiency of ACE, with undetectable serum levels is associated with recurrent angioedema. Manage as for HAE.

Acquired angioedema (AAE)

Acquired C1 inhibitor deficiency occurs in association with lymphoproliferative disorders and more rarely in association with SLE. The commonest disorder is splenic villous lymphoma, presenting predominantly in an older population. Splenomegaly is usual. Also associated with MGUS, Hodgkin's lymphoma, and adenocarcinoma. There may be autoantibodies to C1-inh; pattern of complement consumption is said to be different (as previously noted). Attacks are triggered by similar stimuli to HAE. Gastrointestinal attacks are less common than HAE. Manage as for HAE; treat underlying cause.

Miscellaneous host defence disorders

Primary ciliary dyskinesia (PCD)
- See ⭕ Chapter 2.

Cystic fibrosis
- See ⭕ Chapter 2.

Lymphoedema syndromes
- See ⭕ Chapter 2.

Pulmonary alveolar proteinosis
- See ⭕ Chapter 2.

α_1-Antitrypsin deficiency (α_1-AT deficiency)
- See ⭕ Chapter 2.

Websites

Clinical Immunology Society: *www.clinimmsoc.org*
European Society for Immunodeficiencies: *www.esid.org*
UK Primary Immunodeficiency Network (protocols and guidelines): *www.ukpin.org.uk*
Joint Council of Allergy, Asthma, and Immunology (guidelines): *www.jcaai.org/pp/practice_parameters.asp*

Secondary immunodeficiency and other host defence syndromes

Introduction

Many disease states have been associated with immune dysfunction of varying degrees of severity and significance: some rare secondary disorders have already been covered in Chapter 1. In this and subsequent chapters, the immunological abnormalities will be discussed, together with the value of immunological tests (if any): there will not, however, be a detailed discussion of the clinical and non-immunological features of the diseases and the reader is advised to consult other standard textbooks.

Classification of secondary immunodeficiency

- Viral infections.
  - HIV, CMV, EBV, rubella, ?enteroviruses (echoviruses, coxsackieviruses), measles, influenza.
- Acute bacterial infections.
  - Septicaemia.
- Chronic bacterial and parasitic infections.
  - Tuberculosis, leishmaniasis.
- Malignancy.
- Plasma cell tumours and related problems.
  - Myeloma, plasmacytoma, Waldenström's macroglobulinaemia.
  - Amyloidosis (see ➋ Chapter 14).
- Lymphoma/leukaemia.
  - Hodgkin's disease, non-Hodgkin's lymphoma, chronic lymphocytic leukaemia, other chronic and acute leukaemias.
- Extremes of age.
  - Prematurity, old age.
- Transfusion therapy.
  - Whole blood; clotting factors.
- Drugs and biologicals.
  - As an undesirable side-effect; immunosuppressive drugs (see ➋ Chapter 16).
- Physical therapies.
  - Plasmapheresis and variants, radiation (see ➋ Chapter 16).
- Nutrition.
  - Starvation, anorexia (see also ➋ Chapter 1 for immunological effects of certain inborn errors that affect nutritional status); iron deficiency.
- Chronic renal disease.
  - Uraemia, dialysis, nephrotic syndrome.
- Gastrointestinal disease.
  - Protein-losing enteropathies; secondary to cardiac disease.
- Metabolic disease.
  - Diabetes mellitus, glycogen storage disease, mannosidosis.
- Toxins.
  - Cigarettes, alcohol, other chemicals.

- Splenectomy.
  - In conjunction with other diseases (lymphoma; coeliac disease; sickle-cell disease); traumatic (see ➔ Chapter 1 for congenital asplenia).
- Cardiac surgery (thymectomy).
- Other host defence disorders.
  - Cilial dyskinesia.
  - Cystic fibrosis.
  - Yellow nail syndrome.
  - Young's syndrome.
  - α1-AT deficiency.
- Burns.
- Myotonic dystrophy.

Human immunodeficiency virus 1 and 2

HIV-1 and HIV-2 are retroviruses, responsible for the acquired immuno-deficiency syndrome (AIDS); for more detailed information on clinical aspects see ➔ *Oxford Handbook of Genitourinary Medicine, HIV, and Sexual Health.*

Immunological features

- Virus enters the cells via a cognate interaction of the gp120 env with CD4 and a chemokine receptor, either CxCR4 or CCR5.
- It also infects other CD4+ cells (macrophages, dendritic cells) and other cells expressing CD4-like surface proteins (neuronal cells).
- Macrophage tropic viruses use CCR5, and infect T cells poorly; T-cell tropic viruses use CXCR4 for entry and form syncytia.
- Resistance to viral infection is associated with polymorphism in the chemokine receptors.
- A viral isolate entering T cells via CD8 has been described.
- Uptake of virus into phagocytic cells may be augmented by antibody, and complement. HIV activates complement.
- High levels of viral replication may take place in lymph nodes.
- Initial viraemia after infection is controlled by CD8+ cytotoxic T cells (increased cell numbers). The asymptomatic phase is characterized by strong cytotoxic responses, but viral replication still detectable intermittently, i.e. HIV is not a true latent virus.
- The antibody response to major viral proteins appears after a lag phase of up to 3 months and persists through the asymptomatic phase but declines in late-stage disease.
- Marked B-cell dysfunction with polyclonal increase in immunoglobulins and the appearance of multiple autoantibodies.
- In the seroconversion illness there is a dramatic fall in CD4+ T cells and rise of CD8+ T cells. The levels of CD4+ T cells may drop to a level at which opportunist infections may occur at this early stage (poor prognostic indicator). Levels then usually recover to within the low normal range. There is then a slow decline of absolute CD4+ T-cell count over time (years) following infection.

- Passage to the symptomatic phase is characterized by a rapid drop in CD4⁺ T cells, loss of cytotoxic activity, and switch of virus type from slow-growing, non-syncytial-forming strains to rapidly growing, syncytial-forming strains (quasi-species evolving through lack of replicative fidelity and under immunological selection pressure). This is accompanied by the occurrence of opportunist infections.
- Activation of T cells enhances viral replication and hence CD4⁺ T-cell destruction. Therefore, opportunist infections enhance the self-destruction of the immune system.
- Long-term non-progressors and patients responding to highly active antiretroviral therapy (HAART) show good proliferative responses to gag proteins. Progression has been associated with a switch from Th1 to Th2 responses.
- HIV preferentially infects CD45RO⁺ cells but the depletion of T cells affects principally CD45RA⁺CD62L⁺ naïve T cells.
- T-cell depletion is caused by increased apoptosis, impaired production (HIV effects on thymus), and destruction of both infected and uninfected cells.
- HIV replication is suppressed by natural CCR5 chemokine ligands, RANTES, MIP-1α, and MIP-1β, which are secreted by CD8⁺ T cells. SDF-1α is the natural ligand for CXCR4. High levels of chemokine production have been associated with resistance to infection.

Diagnosis and monitoring

- Diagnosis depends on the detection of antiviral antibody ± viral antigen, *not* on immunological markers. Screening tests for anti-HIV antibody are followed up by PCR-based tests. Informed consent must be obtained.
- The most accurate monitoring of disease is now available through measurements of viral load by quantitative PCR (viral load).
- (see p. 134 for an example) ❶Lymphocyte surface markers (CD4 count) must not be used as a way of HIV testing without consent.
- CD4⁺ T-cell numbers will be reduced and CD8⁺ T cells increased in most acute viral infections and in seriously ill patients in the ITU setting.
- In the acute seroconversion illness, there is a sharp fall in absolute CD4⁺ T-cell numbers and increase in CD8⁺ T-cell numbers with T-cell activation markers increased (IL-2 receptor (CD25) and MHC class II (DR)); this normally returns rapidly to normal as evidence of viral replication disappears. Persistent CD4⁺ T-cell lymphopenia after seroconversion illness is a poor prognostic sign indicating rapid progression to terminal illness.
- Sequential monitoring of the CD4⁺ T-cell numbers provides guidance on the rate of progression of disease and identifies levels at which therapeutic interventions may be indicated (e.g. *Pneumocystis* prophylaxis at $0.2 \times 10^9/l$ CD4⁺ T cells).
- Once the CD4⁺ T-cell count falls below $0.05 \times 10^9/l$, further monitoring is of little clinical value (except psychologically to patients, who view cessation of monitoring as doctors giving up).
- Successful treatment with HAART will lead to a rise of CD4⁺ T cells to within the normal range and suppression of viral load.

- Immune function will recover in patients with a good response to HAART.
  - Recovery is biphasic.
  - Rapid increase in $CD4^+$ T cells in first 3–6 months, mainly $CD45RO^+$ memory T cells (decreased apoptosis and redistribution?).
  - Second phase is due to slower increase in $CD54RA^+CD62L^+$ naïve T cells, due to increased thymic emigration.
  - Rapid increase in $CD8^+$ T cells initially followed by decline.
  - Return of cutaneous reactivity to recall antigens.
- Serum immunoglobulins are usually polyclonally elevated (IgG levels > 50 g/l may be recorded); serial measurements have no clinical utility. Most of the antibody is either 'junk' or relates to an anamnestic response.
- Autoantibodies may be detected (including anti-nuclear and dsDNA antibodies, anti-neutrophil cytoplasmic antibody (ANCA), and anti-cardiolipin). The presence of autoantibodies may cause serious diagnostic confusion, especially if the clinical presentation is atypical.
- Rare patients, usually children, may suffer from panhypo-gammaglobulinaemia or specific antibody deficiency, presenting with recurrent bacterial infections: these patients may derive significant benefit from IVIg. It has been more difficult to demonstrate specific antibody defects in adults, although a subpopulation of adult patients do have recurrent sinopulmonary infections with *Haemophilus* and *Pneumococcus*: IVIg seems to be less helpful.
- Serum β-microglobulin levels may be elevated, as a marker of increased lymphocyte turnover; however, the range of elevation in HIV^+ patients is small compared to that seen in lymphoproliferative disease, and its value (except where $CD4^+$ T-cell counts are unavailable) is small. Serum and urinary neopterin, a marker of macrophage activation, may also be elevated. There is little to choose between these two surrogate markers and viral load is much more clinically relevant.

Immunotherapy

- Mainstay of therapy at present is the use of antiretroviral agents. Mono or dual agent therapy is not recommended. Complex multi-agent regimens are now used. The reader is advised to consult the current HIV literature for information on the current state of therapeutic options. Many regimens require strict timing of administration and high levels of compliance.
- Even with the use of HAART, there is persistent dysregulation of inflammatory responses and AIDS-specific complications may still occur.
- While markers of T-cell activation may return to normal, evidence of monocyte/macrophage activation may persist.
- Multiresistant HIV strains have been reported.
- IVIg may be helpful in certain HIV^+ infants, although not in adults.
- Other immunotherapies (interferons, IL-2) have been uniformly disappointing and are not used routinely. α-IFN enjoyed a vogue in the treatment of Kaposi's sarcoma (due to HHV-8), but the latter responds better to cytotoxic therapy and radiation.
- Use of passive immunotherapy has been disappointing.

- No reliable vaccine is yet available, although trials are continuing on a number of candidate vaccines. Animal studies confirm that neutralizing antibodies can protect against infection, but generating these in humans has proven difficult.

Immune reconstitution inflammatory syndrome (IRIS)

- Occurs in HIV⁺ patients with very low CD4⁺ T cell counts, especially if on protease inhibitors.
- Good virological and immunological response to HAART.
- Temporal association with the introduction of HAART, although may be delayed.
- Associated with the presence of infection (either recognized or cryptic):
  - TB, *Cryptococcus*, CMV, JC virus, PCJ, VZV, hepatitis B & C, Kaposi's sarcoma.
- Features include:
  - infection-specific features (depending on organ infected);
  - fever;
  - lymphadenopathy;
  - likely to be due to excessive cytokine release as improved lymphocyte numbers interact with infection;
  - protease inhibitors increase macrophage IL-6 and TNFα production.
- Management is aggressive treatment of underlying infection.

Castleman's syndrome

- Occurs in association with HIV, especially with HHV-8 co-infection.
- Characterized by polyclonal lymphoproliferation causing lymphadenopathy, fever, weight loss, and leucopenia.
- Histology of lymph nodes shows typical 'onion-skin' change.
- Also seen in SLE, POEMS syndrome, and paraneoplastic pemphigus.
- Caused by excessive IL-6 production.
- May respond to antiviral drugs (HHV-8, HIV), rituximab, or possibly anti-IL-6 monoclonal antibodies.

Epstein–Barr virus

EBV is associated with infectious mononucleosis (glandular fever), Hodgkin's disease, Burkitt's lymphoma, and nasopharyngeal carcinoma. Rare EBV-positive T-cell lymphomas have also been described (T/NK-lethal midline granuloma).

Immunological features

- EBV is a transforming B-lymphotropic virus of the herpes family, binding to the cells via CD21 (C3d) receptor and MHC class II antigens. This receptor is also expressed on follicular dendritic cells and pharyngeal and cervical epithelium. All these tissues are targets. Pharyngeal epithelium is usually affected first, with infection spreading to B cells in the adjacent lymphoid tissue of Waldeyer's ring.
- Following infection there is a B lymphoproliferation, triggered by cross-linking of the CD21, CD19, CD81 complex by virus, which is controlled

rapidly by cytotoxic T cells, which form the 'atypical mononuclear cells' seen on smears. Both MHC-restricted and unrestricted cells are produced, with the latter directly recognizing a virally induced antigen on the cells (LYDMA, lymphocyte-determined membrane antigen). The viral BZLF1 protein is a major target antigen.

- Viral persistence occurs, with reactivation of infection in the immunocompromised (immunosuppressed patients, transplant recipients, HIV-infected patients), giving oral hairy leucoplakia, lymphocytic interstitial pneumonitis, and lymphoma. Nasopharyngeal carcinoma also occurs, although other cofactors are likely to be involved.
- In patients with a genetic predisposition (Duncan's syndrome (XLPS), NK-cell deficiency, and other rare PIDs, see ➔ Chapter 1), severe or fatal infection can occur on first exposure to EBV.
- Although infectious mononucleosis (glandular fever) is usually a self-limiting illness, some patients fail to clear the virus and develop an appropriate sequence of IgG antibodies: such patients have persistently positive IgM antibodies to EBV and have chronic symptoms (fatigue, malaise, sore throats).
- In the acute phase of EBV infection there is suppression of mitogen and allogeneic responses. NK function is also abnormal even though cell numbers are increased. It has been shown that EBV-transformed cells secrete a homologue of IL-10. Monocyte chemotaxis is also abnormal.
- EBV infection may cause severe B-cell lymphoproliferative disease in immunosuppressed patients, and in patients after BMT. It also causes B-cell lymphomas, especially in solid organ transplant recipients on long-term immunosuppression.

Immunological diagnosis

- Usual screening test (Monospot) for acute EBV infection relies on the production of heterophile antibodies that agglutinate sheep cells. This test may miss cases. IgM antibodies are detected and are then succeeded rapidly by IgG antibodies to early antigen (EA) and viral capsid antigen (VCA); antibodies to EBV nuclear antigen (EBNA) appear weeks to months after infection.
- Initial lymphopenia is followed by lymphocytosis of CD8$^+$ T cells, which give rise to the atypical lymphocytes seen on blood films. However, monitoring of lymphocyte subpopulations is of little value, except in unusual variants of EBV infection.
- There is usually an acute polyclonal rise in immunoglobulins, which may be associated with the production of autoantibodies.

Immunotherapy

- None is required normally. However, in patients with a persistent EBV syndrome, high-dose aciclovir (800 mg five times daily for 14 days) may lead to remission of symptoms and disappearance of the IgM anti-EBV antibodies.
- Vaccines are in development, including peptide vaccines.
- Adoptive immunotherapy with EBV-specific CTL is undergoing trials, especially in immunosuppressed or immunodeficient patients.

Other viral infections

Cytomegalovirus
- CMV behaves similarly to EBV.
- Early CD8$^+$ T-cell lymphocytosis giving atypical lymphocytes on a blood film.
- Proliferative responses are reduced during acute infections.
- CMV infection of monocytes with production of an IL-1 inhibitor may be important.
- Congenital CMV infection leads to a prolonged suppression of T-cell function; may also suppress antibody production.
- In BMT recipients, there may be prolonged suppression of myeloid differentiation.
- Reactivation of the disease may occur in the context of immunosuppression (e.g. HIV, drug therapy).
- High-titre anti-CMV antibodies in the form of IVIg may help to prevent infection.
- Once infection is established, treatment with antivirals (ganciclovir, foscarnet, cidofovir) is necessary. Valganciclovir is an oral prodrug.

Rubella
- Congenital rubella, but not acute infection, causes poor lymphocyte responses (reduced PHA proliferation) and may lead to long-term depressed humoral immune function.
- Hypogammaglobulinaemia and a hyper-IgM syndrome, with transiently reduced CD40 ligand expression, have been reported.
- Rubella appears to directly infect both T and B cells.

Measles
- Measles virus is capable of infecting both lymphoid and myeloid cells.
- Acute measles depresses cutaneous type IV reactivity (tuberculin reactivity); this is transient. Similar effects occur with measles vaccines.
- NK activity and immunoglobulin production suppressed.
- Acute measles may lead to reactivation of TB due to immunosuppression.
- Acute measles may cause:
  - transient lymphopenia;
  - PHA- and PPD-driven proliferation decreased.
  - transient decreased neutrophil chemotaxis (?significance).
- Early inactivated measles vaccines led to a response predominantly against viral haemagglutinin but not to the fusion protein, sometimes leading to an atypical wild-type infection due to inappropriate immune response.

Influenza virus
- Acute influenza may give a marked but transient lymphopenia, accompanied by poor T-cell proliferative responses.

Hepatitis viruses

- Non-specific immunosuppressive effects are seen, which may be due to liver damage or to virus.
- Congenital infection with HBV leads to tolerance of the virus and chronic carriage.
- 5% of normal subjects do not make a humoral response to HBV vaccines after the normal 3-dose course (> 100 u). Where evidence of full seroconversion is required for occupation try:
  - different brand of vaccine;
  - double dose may be given (40 µg);
  - double dose of vaccine with γ-IFN-1b 50 µg/m^2—in practice give 100 µg (1 vial): warn subjects of severe flu-like symptoms;
  - interleukin-2 (1 mU) has also been used successfully.

Disseminated warts (papillomavirus)

- May occur as discrete warts or as epidermodysplasia verruciformis (defects in *EVER1*/*EVER2* genes—see ➔ Chapter 1).
- May be seen in immune deficiencies (see ➔ Chapter 1).
  - Common variable immune deficiency.
  - Wiskot–Aldrich syndrome (WAS) and other combined immune deficiencies.
  - WHIM syndrome.
- Full immunological evaluation required.
- Some patients have no identifiable immunological defect.
- May respond to intralesional interferon alfa or systemic interferon gamma-1b.
- The potent contact sensitizer diphencyprone (diphenylcyclopropenone) may also be helpful, although it may not be possible to obtain this now.
- Cimetidine has been used: this is said to improve cell-mediated immunity by blocking T-cell H$_2$-receptors.
- Imiquimod is a topical agent believed to act by local cytokine induction.
- Irritant agents such as fluorouracil and tretinoin can be used.
- Intralesional skin test antigens (mumps, candida, and trichophyton) have been used.
- Laser surgery is useful, particularly in WAS, as it prevents excessive bleeding.
- Role of HPV vaccine is uncertain, but may be beneficial in some cases.

Post-viral fatigue syndromes

- Chronic fatigue syndromes, accompanied by muscle/joint pains and neurocognitive symptoms, may occur after a range of viral infections, including herpesviruses (EBV), enteroviruses, and vaccines.
- Immunological abnormalities include: variable lymphopenia; IgG subclass abnormalities; atypical anti-nuclear antibodies.
- May be transient or persistent.
- See ➔ Chapter 14 for a fuller discussion.

Acute bacterial infections

Acute bacterial sepsis may lead to profound changes in immune function on a temporary basis.

Immunological features

- Neutrophil migration and chemotaxis are increased, while phagocytosis is normal or decreased.
- Lymphopenia affecting CD4+ and CD8+ cells may be marked.
- Significant and temporary hypogammaglobulinaemia may be present (? release of immunosuppressive components from bacteria).
- Massive acute-phase response with elevation of C-reactive protein (CRP) and other acute-phase proteins (complement, fibrinogen, protease inhibitors, α_2-macroglobulin (IL-6 carrier)) and a reduction in albumin (negative acute-phase protein).
- Complement components will be consumed rapidly, but synthesis will be increased (all are acute-phase proteins), so measurements may be difficult to interpret. Functional assays of complement are usually highly abnormal.
- Toxic shock may follow certain types of bacterial infections (staphylococci, streptococci), due to release of 'superantigenic' toxins, which activate many clones of T cells directly, bypassing the need for MHC on antigen-presenting cells by binding directly to the T-cell receptor. Effects are likely to be due to cytokine excess.

Immunological investigation

- The most important investigations are microbiological, to identify the pathogen, by culture and rapid antigen or PCR tests.
- Monitoring of the acute-phase response (CRP) gives a good indication of response to therapy.

❶*Acute measurement of immunoglobulins and complement is usually misleading* and may lead to erroneous diagnoses of antibody or complement deficiency. It is best to leave these investigations until convalescence. Functional assays of complement may take 2–3 weeks to normalize after acute sepsis.

- Acute measurement of cytokines in toxic shock is currently impractical and the diagnosis is a clinical one.
- High-dose IVIg is supported for treatment of staphylococcal or streptococcal toxic shock. Be aware that there is an increased risk of renal failure and pulmonary oedema in this setting.

Chronic bacterial sepsis

Immunological features

- Hypergammaglobulinaemia is usual, often with small and sometimes multiple monoclonal bands developing, representing the immune response against the pathogen.
- Chronic antigenaemia will cause immune complex reactions and secondary hypocomplementaemia (e.g. subacute bacterial endocarditis (SBE)).

- The acute phase becomes a chronic phase: anaemia of chronic disease, iron deficiency due to sequestration (defence against pathogen); see ➲ 'Iron deficiency and nutritional status', p. 119. There is the risk of amyloid development (see ➲ Chapter 14).
- T-cell function may be significantly impaired.
- Mycobacterial infection causes anergy to PPD and third-party antigens. 10% of TB cases do not respond to tuberculin.
  - Mycobacterial products (arabino-D-galactan) interfere with *in vitro* proliferative responses to PHA, PWM, and PPD; the effect is possibly via macrophages and may involve prostaglandins (inhibitable by indometacin).
  - There is often a lymphopenia.
  - Persistently raised CRP may also be suppressive.
  - Miliary TB may cause neutropenia, generalized bone marrow suppression, and leukaemoid reactions.
- Untreated leprosy is a potent suppressor of cell-mediated immunity: T-cell responses to mitogens and antigens are reduced.
  - Defect disappears with appropriate antibiotic therapy and appears to be mediated by a glycolipid.
  - Underlying bias of the immune system towards either Th1 (cellular) or Th2 (antibody) responses determines whether the response to leprosy is tuberculoid (Th1) or lepromatous (Th2).
  - Other immunological features include the development of vasculitis (erythema nodosum) and glomerulonephritis (assumed to immune complex with IgG and complement).

Immunological monitoring

- Acute-phase markers provide the best guide to progress and response to therapy (but beware of elevations from drug reactions). The erythrocyte sedimentation rate (ESR) is less useful because of its long half-life.
- Low complement (C3) and elevated C3d indicates immune-complex reaction (renal involvement likely); monitoring of functional haemolytic complement is not valuable.
- Cryoglobulins may be present (type II or III).
- Immunoglobulins are usually high (polyclonal stimulation ± monoclonal bands). Electrophoresis also shows elevated α_2-macroglobulin, reduced albumin; beware apparent monoclonal 'bands' from very high CRP (use specific antisera on immunofixation to demonstrate this).
- Hypogammaglobulinaemia is rare: consider underlying immunodeficiency.
- Measurement of *in vitro* T-cell function and lymphocyte markers is not valuable unless there is a suspicion that the infections are due to an underlying immunodeficiency.

Immunotherapy

- γ-Interferon offers some possibilities for modifying the Th1:Th2 balance in chronic mycobacterial infections and in leishmaniasis.

Bronchiectasis

Clinical features

- Syndrome of chronic inflammatory/infective airway damage, leading to chronic cough with sputum production.
- Associated with deficiencies of host defence, but may be idiopathic.

Causes

- See Table 2.1.

Treatment

- Prophylactic azithromycin, 250–500 mg 3×/week (has anti-inflammatory activity as well as anti bacterial activity).
- Mucolytics (carbocisteine).
- Nebulized antibiotics (colistimethate sodium (Colomycin®)).
- Treat underlying cause.

❶Do not use IVIg without evidence of humoral immune deficiency (test immunization required); IgG levels should be increased in non-immune bronchiectasis: low normal IgG levels in patients with significant bronchiectasis is suspicious of an underlying immune defect.

Table 2.1 Causes of bronchiectasis

Primary	Secondary
Primary immune deficiencies: antibody deficiency, combined immune deficiency (see ➲ Chapter 1)	Tuberculosis
Cystic fibrosis (see this chapter)	HIV with secondary infections
α₁-antitrypsin deficiency (rare)	Rheumatoid arthritis/Sjögren's syndrome, especially if smokers
MBL deficiency (see ➲ Chapter 1)?	Allergic bronchopulmonary aspergillosis (see ➲ Chapter 3)
Cilial dyskinesia (see this chapter)	Inflammatory bowel disease (ulcerative colitis, Crohn's disease)
Young's syndrome (sinusitis-infertility syndrome)	Aspiration/obstruction
	Whooping cough

Fungal and parasitic infections

Fungal infections

Except for cutaneous infections, invasive fungal infections are usually the markers of, rather than the cause of, immunodeficiency, indicating defective neutrophil/macrophage and T-cell immunity.

Parasitic infections

Immunological features

- Malaria has no overt effect on cell-mediated immunity but reduces the humoral immune responses to bacterial antigens (tetanus toxoid, meningococcal polysaccharide, and *Salmonella* O antigen), presumably through effects on the spleen. There appears to be little interaction between HIV infection and malaria where the two diseases overlap. Tropical splenomegaly due to vivax malaria is associated with a CD8$^+$ T-cell lymphopenia and raised IgM.
- Trypanosomes suppress cellular responses, but there is often a polyclonal increase of non-specific immunoglobulin, especially IgM.
- Visceral leishmaniasis is characterized by a polyclonal hypergammaglobulinaemia, often massive, but with absent cell-mediated immunity until after treatment. Splenomegaly may be massive and there is often lymphopenia. The cachexia and lymphopenia are mediated by release of TNFα by infected macrophages.
- Many parasites, including malaria and trypanosomes, escape immunological surveillance by antigenic variation. This occurs under selection pressure from the immune system. Other avoidance mechanisms include shedding of surface antigen complexed with antibody.
- Autoimmunity may occur as a consequence of the chronic infection: schistosomiasis is associated with anti-nuclear antibodies including anti-calreticulin antibodies. Onchocerciasis is also associated with anti-calreticulin antibodies (which cross-react with an onchocercal antigen).
- Parasitic infections are associated with excess eosinophil and IgE responses.

Immunological monitoring

- There is little value in monitoring anything other than the acute-phase response.

Malignancy

Immunological features

- Malignancy, especially lymphoid, is very common in primary immunodeficiencies (Wiskott–Aldrich syndrome, CVID, DNA repair defects; see ➲ Chapter 1) and in secondary immunodeficiencies (HIV, EBV). Some viruses are directly oncogenic (hepatitis B, EBV).
- Malignancy is also increased in patients with autoimmune disease, possibly secondary to immunosuppressive drug therapy, and in transplant patients who are immunosuppressed (skin tumours, carcinoma of the anogenital tract).
- Abnormalities of T- and NK-cell function may be due to impaired surveillance or secondary to tumour/treatment.
- T-cell defects include reduction of IL-2 and TNFα production, and activation markers such as CD71 (transferrin receptor).

- Cancer cells may release of TGFβ, which reduces T-cell proliferative responses and macrophage metabolism, and through inhibitors of complement.
- Some tumours cause autoimmune responses due to inappropriate expression of antigens; these may lead to paraneoplastic phenomena, such as the Lambert–Eaton myasthenic syndrome (small cell lung carcinoma) due to an autoantibody against voltage-gated calcium channels, and neuronal and retinal autoantibodies in breast, ovarian, and colonic tumours.
- Major immunosuppression may result from radio- and chemotherapy. This may be prolonged and lead to secondary infective complications.

Immunological monitoring
- There is little value in immunological monitoring of aspects such as NK-cell numbers or function.
- Patients with significant and persistent infective problems post-treatment may warrant investigation of cellular and humoral immune function, depending on the type of infections. Lymphocyte surface markers, immunoglobulins, IgG subclasses, and specific antibodies to bacteria and viruses may be appropriate.
- Paraneoplastic phenomena may suggest a search for unusual autoantibodies (voltage-gated calcium channels, cerebellar Purkinje cells, retinal antigens)—see ♦ Chapter 5.

Immunotherapy
Immunotherapy of solid tumours has a chequered career.
- IL-2 therapy has been proposed for certain tumours (renal and melanoma) but there are no good controlled trial data to support this and it is very toxic.
- *In vitro* stimulation of non-specific killers (LAK cell therapy) by IL-2, using either peripheral blood cells or tumour-infiltrating cells, has also been claimed in small trials to be beneficial but is even more toxic.
- Other immunotherapies tried have included the use of non-specific immunostimulants such as BCG, *Corynebacterium parvum*, and *Bordetella pertussis*, often given intralesionally. Occasionally spectacular results have been achieved.
- Interferon alfa has been used with success in certain lymphoid disorders (hairy cell leukaemia, plateau-phase myeloma).
- Monoclonal antibodies are now being introduced, targeted against tumour-specific antigens, e.g. CD20 (rituximab) in lymphoma, anti-CD52 in CLL, and anti-Her-2 (trastuzumab) in breast cancer.
- Monoclonal antibodies have also been used to target radiopharmaceuticals to tumours where the antibody itself may kill tumour cells poorly (e.g. anti-CD20 monoclonals labelled with yttrium-90).
- A major benefit of immunotherapy has been in the use of colony-stimulating factors to protect the bone marrow, allowing higher doses of conventional cytotoxic agents to be used. This approach may increase the risk of secondary myeloid leukaemias.

Myeloma

Immunological features

- Myeloma is a tumour of plasma cells, leading to clonal proliferation. A single isolated lesion in bone is referred to as a plasmacytoma. Waldenström's macroglobulinaemia is a clonal proliferation of IgM-producing lymphocytes.
- > 10% plasma cells in bone marrow.
- Staging of disease depends on bone marrow features, paraprotein level, calcium, and haemoglobin.
- There may be a genetic background (HLA-Cw2, -Cw5) and IgA paraproteins may be associated with a translocation t(8;14). Other translocations may occur; Ig gene rearrangements are detectable (FISH is the preferred technique).
- Myeloma cells often express both lymphocyte and plasma cell antigens simultaneously. Abnormal B cells may be detectable in the peripheral blood, expressing high levels of CD44 and CD54. Cells also express CD56 (NCAM), an adhesion molecule, and soluble levels of NCAM are elevated in myeloma.
- IL-6 plays a key role as either an autocrine or paracrine factor stimulating proliferation. CRP may be raised in consequence. Osteoclast-activating factors are also produced, leading to bone destruction (IL-1, IL-6, TNFβ).
- Monoclonal immunoglobulin production parallels the frequency of B cells: 52% IgG; 22% IgA; 25% free light chain only; and 1% IgD. IgE myeloma is exceptionally rare and is found with plasma cell leukaemia. Biclonal myeloma and non-secreting tumours may be found.
- Synthesis of heavy and light chains is often discordant and whole paraprotein may be accompanied by excess free light chains. Free light chains are readily filtered but nephrotoxic. IgD myeloma often presents in renal failure.
- Hyperviscosity is common with high levels of IgM and IgA paraproteins but is rare with IgG and free light-chain paraproteins. IgA frequently polymerizes *in vivo* (dimers and tetramers).
- Paraproteins may have autoantibody activity and may be cryoglobulins (types I and II).
- Complexes of paraproteins (especially IgM) with coagulation factors may cause bleeding.
- Although myelomatous change probably arises in spleen or lymph nodes, these are unusual sites for disease, which is usually found in bone and bone marrow. Excess clonal plasma cells will be found in the bone marrow.
- Normal humoral immune function is impaired and there is suppression of non-paraprotein immunoglobulin (arrest of B-lymphocyte maturation). Specific antibody responses are poor.
- T-cell function is also impaired, leading to viral infections.
- Low levels of monoclonal paraproteins are found in other lymphoproliferative conditions, chronic infections, connective tissue diseases, and old age.

- Where a paraprotein is present without other features of myeloma (no increase in plasma cells in bone marrow), the term 'monoclonal gammopathy of uncertain significance' (MGUS) is applied. A proportion of these patients develop myeloma with time and all should be monitored at intervals.
- Heavy-chain disease is rare (μ, γ, and α). α-Heavy-chain disease is the most common. All are associated with lymphoma-like disease.
- POEMS syndrome (polyneuropathy, organomegaly, endocrine abnormalities, monoclonal gammopathy, and skin rashes) appears to be a plasma-cell variant of Castleman's disease, a hyperplasia of lymph nodes, which may occur with autoimmune diseases (see also ➔ Chapter 4). It is associated with high circulating levels of IL-1, IL-6, VEGF, and TNF.

Immunological diagnosis and monitoring

- Diagnosis of a paraproteinaemia depends on accurate electrophoresis of serum *and* urine, followed by immunofixation. Immunochemical measurements of immunoglobulin levels (by radial immunodiffusion (RID) or nephelometry) may be misleading due to polymerization or, in the case of IgM, monomeric paraprotein.
- Paraprotein levels are best determined by scanning densitometry, provided that the total protein in serum can be measured accurately. There are difficulties if the M-band overlaps the β-region.
- Urinary light-chain excretion may be helpful as a prognostic monitor of tumour cell burden, but there are difficulties in the calculation of this (see Part 2) and renal function affects the output.
- Measurement of serum free light chains is a more sensitive marker of clonality and tumour burden.
- Serum β_2-microglobulin is a marker of tumour-cell activity, but has fallen out of favour.
- CRP may be a surrogate for IL-6 production.
- Degree of humoral immunodeficiency should be assessed by measurement of exposure and immunization antibodies, followed by test immunization with protein and polysaccharide antigens.
- Light chain (AL) amyloid may be a complication.

Immunotherapy

The disease is probably not curable at present.

- Standard chemotherapy includes melphalan and prednisolone; other agents used include vincristine, doxorubicin (or related drugs), cyclophosphamide, and carmustine. Dexamethasone is usually added.
- Interferon alfa has a major effect in prolonging the plateau phase.
- Thalidomide (and newer derivative, lenalidomide) has been shown to be valuable—side-effects can be significant.
- Bortezomib (Velcade®) is a proteasome inhibitor which has produced excellent clinical responses. Neutropenia and neuropathy are significant side-effects.

- Daratumumab, an antibody against CD38 (over-expressed on myeloma cells) has been approved for resistant disease. This antibody binds to red cells as well and interferes with cross-matching. It also interferes with flow cytometry, causing an apparent lack of plasma cells.
- HSCT (allogeneic and autologous purged marrow) may also prolong remission but it is doubtful if it is curative. Colony-stimulating factors should be used with caution as they may enhance tumour cell growth.
- Waldenström's macroglobulinaemia may be treated with fludarabine or cladribine; rituximab is also helpful.
- Radiotherapy may be required for localized plasmacytomas.
- IVIg may be beneficial in dealing with secondary infective problems but should be used with great caution in patients with renal impairment and those with rheumatoid activity of their paraproteins (both may lead to renal failure). Prophylactic antibiotics may be an alternative.
- Plasmapheresis may be required to deal with hyperviscosity and/or cryoglobulinaemia.

Monoclonal gammopathy of uncertain significance (MGUS)
- Asymptomatic premalignant clonal plasma cell disorder.
- Found in 3% of population aged over 50.
- < 10% plasma cells in bone marrow.
- Chromosomal abnormalities in bone marrow common (FISH).
- Paraprotein < 15 g/l.
- IgG, IgA paraproteins account for 80%; IgM 17%; small number of light-chain only MGUS.
- Monitor paraproteins at regular intervals—often stable for years.
- Rising level indicates development of myeloma.
- Most MGUS will progress to myeloma, given long enough (20+ years in some cases).

Lymphoma: Hodgkin's disease

Immunological features
- Hodgkin's disease (HD) is a lymphoma seen predominantly in the young. It is characterized by the presence of typical Reed–Sternberg (RS) cells (CD15, CD30 positive).
- Three major types (nodular sclerosing, mixed cellularity, and lymphocyte depleted) are recognized. Lymphocyte predominant may well be a separate disease, as it occurs later and often relapses to non-Hodgkin's lymphoma. Staging depends on the number of sites affected and by the presence or absence of constitutional symptoms.
- EBV genome is often found in HD, and cells are usually positive. RS cells are thought to be the true neoplastic cell, possibly derived from interdigitating reticulum cells.
- T- and B-cell numbers are reduced. Immunoglobulins are often raised, especially IgE. 10% of patients will have hypogammaglobulinaemia (severe disease). There may be poor specific antibody responses; primary antibody responses are impaired, whereas secondary responses may be normal.

- T-cell proliferation is reduced (reversible by indometacin, suggesting a possible macrophage defect). Cutaneous anergy is common. Responses to Pneumovax® 23 may be present even if there is a lack of DTH responses.
- In some cases the defects have been shown to precede the development of the disease and also to persist long term after successful treatment (although the role of the cytotoxic regimens in this is poorly understood). It is difficult then to distinguish from a primary immunodeficiency complicated by lymphoma.
- Bacterial infections are common (*Pneumococcus* and *Haemophilus influenzae*), related to poor humoral function and possibly also to poor neutrophil function.
- Before CT scanning became widespread, splenectomy for staging was common. This is now only undertaken for symptomatic hypersplenism. Splenectomy has a very significant effect on immune function in lymphoma, and patients may become unresponsive to bacterial vaccines.

Immunological diagnosis and monitoring

- Diagnosis is made on histological examination of excised lymph node, supplemented by the use of immunocytochemistry to identify populations of cells. This may be useful in the identification of scanty RS cells. RS cells may also be found in association with:
  - glandular fever;
  - reactive hyperplasia;
  - some non-Hodgkin's lymphomas.
- There is usually a reactive expansion of CD4+ T-cells.
- Molecular techniques should be used to look for evidence of EBV genome.
- HD is associated with an acute-phase response, with elevated ESR, CRP, and caeruloplasmin. This may be a poor prognostic indicator.
- All patients with lymphoma should be monitored for evidence of humoral immune deficiency: serum immunoglobulins, IgG subclasses, and specific antibodies. Test immunization is appropriate. Particular attention should be paid to apparently cured patients, who may still have a persisting immunodeficiency.

Immunotherapy

- Treatment is with radiotherapy and/or chemotherapy. The latter is used for patients with constitutional ('B') symptoms. There are many regimens for combination chemotherapy.
- Most regimens are myelosuppressive and impose a temporary secondary defect through neutropenia.
- Relapse may be treated with autologous bone marrow transplantation (harvested in remission) or with a stem-cell transplant.
- Secondary neoplasms may occur (myelodysplasia, acute myeloid leukaemia) and the risk is related to the intensity of treatment.
- IVIg may be required for those with a persisting symptomatic humoral defect after treatment.

Non-Hodgkin's lymphoma

Immunological features

- This category includes all those lymphoid and histiocytic lymphoid malignancies that are not HD. There are many classifications, but the two used most often in the UK are Kiel and the Working Formulation. A WHO classification was introduced in 1999. Morphology and cellular origin play a major role in classification.
- Tumours are also divided on the basis of their clinical grade (= aggressivity). Low-grade B-cell tumours overlap with chronic lymphocytic leukaemia. Waldenström's macroglobulinaemia is often referred to as an immunocytic lymphoma. Both T- and B-cell lymphomas are recognized, as well as tumours derived from histiocytic elements.
- Retrovirus, HTLV-1, has been associated with T-cell lymphomas in areas where it is endemic (Japan and the Caribbean).
- EBV has been associated with certain B-cell lymphomas, particularly associated with immunosuppression and endemic Burkitt's lymphoma, which is found in malarial areas. This tumour, but also others, is associated with chromosomal abnormalities, normally translocations t(14;8).
- Many other translocations have been identified. It is thought that these translocations allow dysregulated activity of cellular oncogenes, such as bcl-2 and abl, by placing them in proximity to active promoters. In Burkitt's lymphoma it is the oncogene c-myc.
  - Often sites of translocations involve the heavy- and light-chain genes for immunoglobulin and the genes for T-cell receptors.
- Secondary lymphomas are usually non-Hodgkin's lymphoma (NHL). These are found with:
  - primary immunodeficiencies (WAS, CVID, AT, Chediak–Higashi, DNA repair defects);
  - connective tissue diseases (rheumatoid arthritis, Sjögren's syndrome, SLE);
  - phenytoin therapy;
  - post-transplant (ciclosporin therapy).
- In the case of primary immunodeficiency, it is likely that the chronic infections lead to an abortive immune response that predisposes to lymphoma. Perhaps earlier diagnosis and better treatment will prevent this.
- Studies of humoral and cellular function have shown abnormalities that have not always correlated with the type of lymphoma. Abnormalities are more likely in high-grade tumours. Both hypo- and hypergammaglobulinaemia may occur and may persist after treatment. Monoclonal bands, often IgMκ, may be found in association with B-cell tumours. Autoantibody activity may be noted.
- Acquired angioedema (AAE, see ➲ Chapter 1) is often associated with an underlying B-cell lymphoma with a paraprotein.
  - Paraprotein binds to and inhibits C1-esterase inhibitor.
  - Usual tumour in AAE is splenic villous lymphoma.

- As in Hodgkin's disease, splenectomy may have been undertaken in the past, imposing an additional immunological defect. These patients require careful supervision.

Immunological diagnosis and monitoring

- Diagnosis requires histological examination of lymphoid tissue, accompanied by immunohistochemistry, using panels of monoclonal antibodies to identify the predominant cell type.
- Clonality will be established by molecular techniques looking at Ig and Tcr gene rearrangements.
- Humoral immune function should be monitored, as for HD.
- Serial β_2-microglobulin measurements may be helpful as a marker of lymphocyte turnover.
- Electrophoresis will demonstrate the presence of paraproteins.
- If autoimmune phenomena are present, then association with the paraprotein can be shown by light-chain restriction on immunofluorescence.
- Sometimes abnormalities of immunoglobulins precede overt disease. In contrast to primary immunodeficiency, IgM disappears first, followed by IgG and IgA.

❶Finding an isolated but marked reduction of IgM in an older person should lead to a review for evidence of lymphoma (selective IgM deficiency is *vanishingly rare!*).

Immunotherapy

- Treatment depends on the type of treatment and its grade. Localized disease may be amenable to radiotherapy, while disseminated disease will require chemotherapy. Aggressive chemotherapy of high-grade tumours may result in some cures.
- Autologous bone marrow transplantation may be helpful in relapse. IVIg may be required if there are infective problems.
- The monoclonal antibody rituximab, with or without attached radioisotope, is valuable for treating CD20-positive lymphomas.
- Daratumumab (anti-CD38) is approved for use in some type of lymphoma.

Chronic lymphocytic leukaemia (CLL)

Immunological features

- CLL is a clonal proliferation of small lymphocytes. It is the most common form of lymphoid leukaemia. 95% are B-cell in origin; 5% are T-cell in origin. Other variants include prolymphocytic leukaemia (B-PLL), hairy cell leukaemia (HCL), and splenic lymphoma with circulating villous lymphocytes (SLVL). Cell counts may become very high (> 100 $\times$ 10^9/l). It is predominantly a disease of the elderly (95% of patients are aged over 50).
- Different variants may be distinguished by flow cytometry:

- B-CLL is usually CD5$^+$, CD23$^+$, FMC7$^-$, CD22$^\pm$, with weak surface Ig. Clonal restriction can usually be demonstrated with anti-light-chain antisera.
- B-PLL has the phenotype CD5$^+$, CD23$^-$, FMC7$^+$, CD22$^+$, sIg$^+$.
- HCL is CD5$^-$, CD23$^-$, FMC7$^+$, CD22$^+$, sIg$^+$.
- SLVL is CD5$^\pm$, CD23$^\pm$, FMC7$^+$, CD22$^+$, sIg$^+$.
- Circulating lymphoma cells may be distinguished because they often express CD10 (CALLA).
- T-PLL is rare: cells are usually CD4$^+$, CD8$^-$, but dual-positive or CD4$^-$, CD8$^+$ variants may occur.
- Large granular lymphocytic leukaemia has the phenotype CD4$^-$, CD8$^+$, CD11b$^+$, CD16/56$^+$, CD57$^+$. The cells may be highly active in an NK assay.
- Bone marrow examination shows an excess of lymphocytes.
- Chromosomal abnormalities are common: trisomy 12 and deletions of the long arm of chromosome 13 in B-cell disease, and chromosome 14 abnormalities (inversion or tandem translocation) or trisomy 8q in T-cell disease. Deletions of 17p affecting p53 expression have a poorer prognosis. Recent studies have demonstrated that some CLL patients have an abnormal *ATM* gene (ataxia telangiectasia mutated).
- Recurrent bacterial infections are a major problem.
- Humoral function is impaired and response to Pneumovax® 23 is a better predictor of infection than total IgG.
- Studies of normal B-cell function is difficult *in vitro* due to the predominance of the aberrant clone.
- Electrophoresis may show small bands (usually IgM). T-cell numbers may be increased (CD4$^+$ T cells), but function may be poor with low/absent PHA responses.
- Viral infections may be a problem (shingles with dissemination, HSV).
- Autoimmune phenomena are common: ITP and haemolytic anaemia. Splenectomy may be required and this exacerbates the immune deficit.
- Vaccine responses are frequently entirely absent in this situation and patients must have prophylactic antibiotics.
- HCL may be associated with vasculitis.

Immunological diagnosis and monitoring

- Diagnosis of straightforward CLL is usually possible from the white cell count and examination of the film. Confirmation requires flow cytometry and examination of the bone marrow.
- Studies of humoral immune function are necessary and should include test immunization with Pneumovax® 23. As these diseases are chronic, monitoring should be carried out at regular intervals to identify deterioration.

Immunotherapy

- Treatment is with cytotoxic agents. Chlorambucil is the usual agent but fludarabine, deoxycoformicin, and 2-chlorodeoxyadenosine are highly effective. The last named produces a state similar to ADA deficiency. This leads to a profound immunosuppression, with T-cell lymphopenia and a significant risk of opportunist infections. Patients treated with

these agents should have regular T-cell counts by flow cytometry and receive prophylactic co-trimoxazole and irradiated blood products (risk of engraftment).
• Interferon alfa is very effective in HCL. Rituximab or ofatumumab (anti-CD20) is valuable in combination with fludarabine and cyclophosphamide. The humanized monoclonal antibody alemtuzumab (Campath-1H®) has been used in resistant cases with success, but causes profound immunosuppression. Younger patients may be candidates for HSCT (autologous BMT is not curative).
• Recurrent infections may require prophylactic antibiotics or IVIg. Monthly treatment is usually adequate (dose 200–400 mg/kg).

Chronic myeloid leukaemia (CML) and myelodysplastic syndromes

Immunological features
• Chromosomal abnormalities occur in almost all cases of CML and myelodysplastic syndromes. The Philadelphia chromosome (t(9;22)) is the most common, but others have been described, including the 5q- syndrome, monosomy 7, trisomy 8, 19, or 20, and deletions on other chromosomes (12 and 20). The deletions of chromosome 5 are of interest because they map to the region containing the genes for IL-3, -4, -5, G-CSF, and GM-CSF.
• There is a high incidence of progression to acute myeloid leukaemia.
• Abnormal neutrophil function is well described: neutropenia is common in myelodysplasia. Even if the neutrophil count is normal, function is often not, with abnormalities of adhesion, chemotaxis, phagocytosis, and bacterial killing being well documented. This occurs particularly with monosomy 7 in childhood.
• Infections are common.

Acute leukaemias

Overview
• Acute leukaemia is a common malignancy of childhood, and accounts for about 30–40% of paediatric malignancy. 80% of cases are due to acute lymphoblastic leukaemia (ALL).
• Certain primary immunodeficiencies are risk factors for ALL (Bloom's syndrome, ataxia telangiectasia, Shwachman's syndrome, xeroderma pigmentosa—see → Chapter 1). Most ALLs are B cell in origin.
• T-ALL is associated strongly with HTLV-1 infection in areas where this virus is endemic.
• A number of chromosomal translocations have been described, including the Philadelphia translocation (t(9;22)), which is common in adult ALL. Other translocations are well described.

- T-ALL is often associated with translocations involving the T-cell receptor genes.
- ALL is classified according to the FAB classification, on the basis of cytological appearance, into L1, L2, and L3 types. Immunophenotyping allows the distinction of B-, T-, and null (rare) ALLs.
- Acute myeloid leukaemia has also been classified by the FAB group into M0–M7, depending on the predominant cell type identified by morphology and cytochemistry. Cases of AML may be secondary to Wiskott–Aldrich syndrome, Chediak–Higashi syndrome, and Fanconi anaemia, as well as to the use of cytotoxic drugs such as cyclophosphamide.
- Occasionally, biphenotypic leukaemias may be detected, defined as the presence of at least two markers from each lineage (e.g. lymphoid and myeloid). They account for 5–10% of acute leukaemia and tend to have a poor prognosis. Often they present as AML, but have evidence of clonal rearrangements of immunoglobulin and Tcr genes.

Immunological features

- In ALL the immune system is usually normal, although primary IgM responses to some antigens (viruses) may be poor.
- Secondary immune responses are usually normal.
- Non-neoplastic cells are normally present in normal numbers.
- Leukaemic clones rarely have functional activity, although there have been reports of cytokine production.
- Rare cases may be hypogammaglobulinaemic at presentation.
- Chemotherapy is profoundly immunosuppressive, affecting both T- and B-cell function and rendering patients neutropenic. Careful attention to prevention of infection (isolation, irradiation of food, gut decontamination) is essential.

Immunological diagnosis

- Diagnosis of leukaemia is usually made on the basis of suspicious blood films, supplemented by immunophenotyping of both peripheral blood and bone marrow, to identify the characteristics of the leukaemic clone. This is supplemented by genetic analysis to identify any translocations: probes to the sites of recombination for these translocations give a very sensitive tool for detecting minimal residual disease in bone marrow after treatment.
  ▶Leukaemia phenotyping is best undertaken by haematologists who will have access to supportive evidence from blood films, bone marrow smears, and trephines, as well as cytochemical enzymatic studies. They will also undertake the therapy.
- Monitoring of humoral and cellular function post-treatment, and especially after BMT/HSCT, is essential.

Immunotherapy

- The management of ALL involves intensive chemotherapy and radiotherapy to sanctuary sites such as the nervous system (often with intrathecal methotrexate). For relapse or high-risk patients bone marrow or stem cell transplantation is used, either matched unrelated donors or purged autologous if an HLA-identical donor is not available. There is a high risk of long-term development of non-Hodgkin's lymphoma and acute myeloid leukaemia.

• AML is treated similarly with intensive chemotherapy, with the option for BMT/HSCT when remission is obtained. Acute promyelocytic leukaemia associated with the t(15;17) translocation may be treated with all-*trans* retinoic acid, which allows differentiation of the blocked cells to mature neutrophils, although BMT is still required.

• Certain cytokines may have a role as adjunctive agents, allowing intensification of chemotherapy, but with the increased risk of later myeloid lineage leukaemias.

Bone marrow and stem cell transplantation

• Bone marrow (BMT) or stem cell (HSCT) transplantation is part of the treatment for a variety of inherited diseases (SCID and SCID variants, CGD, HIGM, Wiskott–Aldrich syndrome, osteopetrosis, Gaucher's disease) in addition to its role in the acute leukaemias and CML with blast transformation. The process is discussed in more detail in see also ➔ Chapter 15.

• BMT leads to an immediate severe immunodeficiency, due to the conditioning required to allow 'take'. All blood products must be irradiated to prevent viable lymphocytes engrafting and must be CMV⁻.

• There follows a period of gradually improving immune function while the immune system reconstitutes. This recapitulates immunological ontogeny.

• T-cell function reconstitutes early, but full B-cell function may take up to 2 years to develop. IgG_2 levels may remain depressed and there are frequently poor responses to polysaccharide antigens.

• Degree of reconstitution is affected by the degree of mismatch and by GvHD.

• Return of T-cell function *in vitro* (positive PHA) is usually taken to define the time when release from isolation is safe, but this is usually the last parameter to normalize. Anti-CD3 stimulation responses usually return early.

• Appearance of recent thymic emigrants may be detected by measurement of TRECs (T-cell receptor excision circles) and by the use of CD45RA and CD27 to define naïve and effector CD4⁺ T-cell re-appearance.

• While B-cell function is poor during the acute phase, and for the first year thereafter, IVIg prophylaxis is essential.

• Return of B-cell function can be monitored by IgA/IgM levels and development of isohaemagglutinins. Reappearance of class-switch memory B cells is also valuable, especially in patients transplanted for hyper-IgM syndromes.

- Once off IVIg, a full programme of immunizations should be undertaken, starting with killed vaccines (killed polio, DPT, Hib, and Pneumovax® 23). The response to these can be assessed (pre- and post-levels are required, and remember that antibody from IVIg may persist for up to 6 months or longer).
- Once there is a good response to killed/subunit vaccines, then live vaccines can be administered (MMR).
- Immunological function in chronic GvHD is markedly abnormal, with a persisting risk of invasive infections of all types. The gastrointestinal involvement superimposes a severe nutritional defect, which further reduces immune function.

Extremes of age: prematurity

- At birth, infants are dependent for the first 6 months of life on maternally transferred immunoglobulin (IgG only).
- Immune function gradually develops, although there is usually a physiological trough in IgG levels at around 6 months: if this is prolonged, then transient hypogammaglobulinaemia of infancy results (see ⊃ Chapter 1).
- Additional protection to the neonatal gut is provided by breastfeeding, particularly in the first few days when the IgA-rich colostrum is produced.
- Maternal antibody transfer is an active process in the placenta that begins at around 14 weeks' gestation and accelerates markedly after 22 weeks. The process can take place against a concentration gradient and is selective for some IgG subclasses: IgG_2 is transferred relatively less well.
- Antibody-deficient mothers will also be at risk of producing hypogammaglobulinaemic infants, who will require IVIg for the first 6 months of life. Good replacement therapy during pregnancy will obviate the need for this.
- Premature delivery interrupts the placental transfer and leaves the infant deficient in immunoglobulins and with a relatively less mature humoral and cellular immune system. Breastfeeding is rarely possible, but oral administration of colostrum is desirable to prevent necrotizing enterocolitis. Infections are often problematic, although other factors, such as ITU nursing, venous and arterial lines, and lung immaturity, all contribute. Group B streptococcal infections are particularly troublesome.

Immunological features and diagnosis

- All immunoglobulins will be low, as will be IgG subclasses. However, the 'normal' ranges are calculated from full-term delivery.
- Provided that there are no major complications, the immune system rapidly catches up after delivery and there are rarely long-term sequelae.
- Responses to standard immunization schedules may be poor—consider additional boosters.

Immunotherapy

- The role of IVIg replacement as routine for premature infants has been investigated extensively, with conflicting results, and a consensus as to the value is difficult to obtain.
  - Differences in products and batches may relate to highly variable levels of anti-group B streptococcal antibodies.
  - Better products, enriched for specific antibodies to the problem pathogens, may be required.
  - Oral, IgA-rich products have also been used to reduce the risk of enterocolitis.
- Immunization of the premature may cause problems in timing, as there may be very poor responses if routine immunizations are given at intervals calculated from date of delivery uncorrected for gestational age.

Extremes of age: the elderly

Immunological changes in the elderly are multifactorial, relating to the decline in normal immunoregulatory processes, the increased incidence of disease, and the increased use of drugs. Nutritional status is also important. There is no relationship to chronological age.

Immunological features

- There is no significant change in lymphocyte numbers or subsets in the healthy elderly, although lymphoid organs show a reduction of germinal centres.
- Thymic function declines, but not as much as previously assumed!
- NK-cell numbers increase in the long-lived elderly.
- Mucosal immunity seems to be reasonably intact, although the non-specific inflammatory response is reduced.
- Aged lymphocytes have metabolic abnormalities such as reduced 5'-nucleotidase activity (also associated with CVID), and there are changes in the expression of surface antigens.
- Immunoglobulin levels change with age: IgG and IgA tend to rise while IgM and IgE fall. Primary humoral responses are reduced and secondary responses give lower peak titres and a more rapid fall with time. Antibody affinity may also be poorer. Some studies have shown that vaccine responses in the elderly may be as good as in younger people.
- CVID may present for the first time post retirement, but this diagnosis should only be entertained when other secondary causes have been eliminated.
- With increasing age there is an increasing incidence of small monoclonal bands on electrophoresis (MGUS), such that 20% of 95-year-olds will have bands. These are present at low levels and are rarely of great significance. They may however predispose to myeloma over the very long term.
- There is a parallel increase in autoantibodies of all types. These are usually present at low titres and are not associated with disease. Normal ranges for antibody titres should be adjusted to take account of these changes.

- Cell-mediated immunity, as tested by mitogen responses and by DTH testing, is reduced in the elderly. Thymic function is probably better than previously thought and new thymic emigrants can be detected in the blood of the elderly.
- Biologically, the healthy very elderly (> 85 years old) represent a special group. There may be combinations of MHC genes that can be associated with survival (in Japan, a high frequency of DR1 and low frequency of DR9), but this might be due to selection out of those individuals with less favourable MHC types associated with autoimmune disease.
- Coexisting disease imposes additional strains on the immune system, for example, chronic lung disease from smoking, cardiac failure with pulmonary oedema, and malnutrition. These often tip the balance away from the immune system in favour of invading pathogens.
- Diseases such as influenza have a disproportionate effect on the elderly through the risks of secondary bacterial infection and exacerbating pre-existing underlying diseases. Infections common in early childhood, such as meningitis, are also more common in the elderly.
- CMV has been suggested as an important risk factor for immunological decay.

Immunological diagnosis
- The investigation of the elderly for immunodeficiency should be symptom driven.

Immunotherapy
- Preventative vaccination of at-risk groups is thought to be helpful, for instance, with influenza vaccine and Pneumovax® 23. Risk groups are those with underlying significant disease, particularly chronic lung disease.
  - Protection may be poor because of the underlying decay of immune function!
- Consideration should also be given to ensuring that other vaccines such as tetanus are kept up to date (this tends to be forgotten in the elderly) as tetanus antibodies may fall below protective levels. Keen gardeners are at most risk.
- Immunoglobulin therapy may be required for those with significant symptomatic hypogammaglobulinaemia.
- Other approaches being studied include:
  - nutrition;
  - low-dose sirolimus (improves response to influenza vaccine);
  - adjuvants with vaccines and/or increased doses;
  - IL-7, keratinocyte growth factor.

Transfusion therapy
- In addition to immediate reactions to blood products due to transfused white cells, pre-formed antibodies (to HLA or IgA), etc., there is evidence for an immunosuppressive effect. This is most noticeable in the effect on renal allograft survival (see ➥ Chapter 14).

- IVIg has complex immunoregulatory properties when used in high doses (see ➲ Chapter 16).
- Crude factor VIII (FVIII) concentrates were immunosuppressive, although this may relate as much to chronic hepatitis due to hepatitis C. High-purity FVIII is much less immunosuppressive.
- Other infections transmissible by blood, such as HIV and CMV, can have major immunosuppressive effects.
- The use of unirradiated blood in the immunocompromised (with poor/absent cell-mediated immunity (CMI)) may lead to engraftment of viable lymphocytes and the development of GvHD.
  - Lymphocytes may be viable for up to 2 weeks in bank blood.

Chronic renal disease (nephrotic syndrome and uraemia)

Nephrotic syndrome

- Renal protein loss should always be considered when investigating hypogammaglobulinaemia.
- Investigation of humoral function is essential if there is significant proteinuria.
- In the nephrotic syndrome there is an increased susceptibility to Pneumococcus and other streptococci.
- Typical pattern is loss of immunoglobulins in order of ascending molecular weight, depending on the selectivity of the proteinuria, with preferential loss of IgG, then IgA, and preservation of IgM until gross nephrosis ensues.
- The IgG synthetic rate is normal or increased and the IgM catabolic rate is normal.
- Responses to Pneumovax® 23 are poor but responses to influenza are normal.
- Poor neutrophil chemotaxis and opsonization are also described.
- Loss of complement proteins such as C3 and factor B may also contribute to poor bacterial handling through decreased opsonization.

Uraemia

- Chronic uraemia is immunosuppressive with poor humoral and cellular immune responses. The molecules responsible for this are uncertain.
- Lymphopenia is common, affecting $CD4^+$ and $CD8^+$ T cells; DTH and mitogen responses are reduced.
- Immunoglobulins and specific antibody responses to pneumococcal and hepatitis B vaccines may be low. Double-strength HBV vaccines (40 µg) are advised.
- Lymph nodes show a loss of secondary follicles.
- Neutrophil function shows defective chemotaxis and phagocytosis, with impaired oxidative metabolism, leading to poor bacterial killing.
- Certain types of dialysis membrane (cellophane, now no longer used) activated the alternate pathway of complement, with release of

anaphylotoxins and neutrophil activation leading to severe circulatory and respiratory problems.
- Dialysis patients often have a CD4$^+$ T-cell lymphopenia; increased expression of CD11b/CD18 is seen on neutrophils. Increased T-cell apoptosis may occur.

Renal transplantation
- Renal transplant recipients will be on long-term immunosuppressive therapy.
- Increased risk of papillomavirus-induced skin tumours, EBV-induced lymphomas, and B-lymphoproliferative disease.
- Poor humoral and cellular immune function.
- Monitoring is required, especially if irreversible lymphocytoxic agents such as azathioprine are used long term.

Protein-losing enteropathy and liver disease (cirrhosis)

Protein-losing enteropathy

Causes
- Secondary hypogammaglobulinaemia may be due to protein-losing enteropathy, for which there are many causes:
  - Ménétrier's disease (giant rugal hypertrophy).
  - Coeliac disease and other types of sprue.
  - Inflammatory bowel disease (Crohn's disease).
  - Infections—hookworm, TB.
  - Fistulae; post-gastrectomy syndrome.
  - Neoplasms.
  - Allergic gut disease (eosinophilic enteritis).
  - Secondary to constrictive pericarditis and gross right heart failure.
  - Whipple's disease.
  - Chylous effusions.
  - Genetic causes, e.g. mutations in plasmalemma vesical associated protein (*PLVAP*) and *TTC7A*.
  - Intestinal lymphangiectasia (dilated lymphatics), including CD55 deficiency, CHAPLE syndrome (see ➲ Chapter 1).

Immunological features
- Immunoglobulins are low, with a short half-life, but the synthetic rate may be increased.
- Specific antibody responses may be normal, although they may decline rapidly.
- Lymphopenia is associated with dilated or blocked lymphatics (intestinal lymphangiectasia, constrictive pericarditis, right heart failure). This may lead to poor mitogen responses and DTH reactions.

Diagnosis
- Proof that the bowel is the source of immunoglobulin and cellular loss is difficult as most laboratories are singularly unkeen on trying to measure

faecal immunoglobulin excretion! Whole bowel perfusion studies may make this more tolerable.
- Radiolabelled albumin excretion in the faeces will quantitate the loss.
- Full studies of humoral and cellular function are required, together with investigation for the underlying cause (radiology, endoscopy, and biopsy).

Liver disease (cirrhosis)
- Increased infections are seen (especially with alcohol which directly impairs macrophage function) with bacteria and mycobacteria.
- Complement components are reduced (decreased synthesis).
- Neutrophil phagocytosis and chemotaxis occur.
- T-cell function is poor.

Metabolic disorders

A number of metabolic diseases are associated with concomitant immunological impairment.
- Glycogenosis type Ib: neutropenia and neutrophil migration defect. Recurrent infections a problem: septicaemia, wound infections, osteomyelitis, and sinusitis.
- Mannosidosis: recurrent severe infections; impaired neutrophil chemotaxis. Poor T-cell responses to PHA and concanavalin A (ConA).
- Galactosaemia: increased risk of Gram-negative septicaemia due to abnormalities of neutrophil motility and phagocytosis.
- Myotonic dystrophy: hypercatabolism of IgG but not albumin, IgA, or IgM may occur, although infections are not usually a major problem.
- Sickle-cell disease: increased susceptibility to meningitis and septicaemia. There is an acquired splenic dysfunction, due to infarction. Tissue hypoxia also contributes to bacterial infection. Serum immunoglobulins and vaccine responses are usually normal, even to polysaccharide antigens. It is recommended that all patients should be treated as other asplenic or hyposplenic patients and should receive Pneumovax® 23 and Hib vaccines, and be considered for prophylactic antibiotics.
- Coeliac disease: this may be accompanied by splenic atrophy and these patients should be investigated and treated as other asplenic patients.
- Prolidase deficiency: rare autosomal disorder with rashes, skin ulceration, dysmorphic features, splenomegaly, and recurrent infections. It also appears to be associated with a risk of developing SLE. It is diagnosed by the presence of iminopeptiduria.

Diabetes mellitus

Immunological mechanisms
- There is an underlying genetic susceptibility to type I diabetes (the MHC type is shared with CVID) and consequent immune dysregulation. As a result of the association with the A1, B8, DR3, C4Q0 haplotype, there is an increased incidence of C4 deficiency in diabetes.

- In established disease, the raised glucose itself interferes with both innate and specific immune functions. Most of the research has been done on chemically induced or genetic diabetes in mice; much less work has been done on human diabetes.
- Humoral function is impaired: IgG levels may be reduced, while IgA may be increased. Specific antibody responses may show poor primary immune responses and the non-enzymatic glycation of immunoglobulin may interfere with function. Both T-dependent and T-independent antigens are affected.
- Lymphoid organs are essentially normal but peripheral blood lymphocytes may show variable abnormalities. CMI may be depressed with poor DTH responses and abnormal mitogen responses and poor cytokine production (IL-2).
- Macrophage and neutrophil function is also reduced.
- Type I diabetes is strongly associated with coeliac disease: hyposplenia may occur.
- Infections with *Candida* and other fungi, TB, and pneumococci are more common in diabetes. Staphylococcal colonization of the skin is higher in diabetics than in normal individuals.
- Abnormalities of immune function are more marked in type I diabetes but correlate poorly with blood glucose levels. It is possible that immune dysfunction relates to glycation of surface antigens on immunologically important cells.

Diagnosis and treatment
- Recurrent infections in diabetics should be investigated in the normal way and not merely accepted, particularly if diabetic control is not bad. This should include humoral and neutrophil function.
- In the USA, regular pneumococcal vaccination is recommended, but this policy has not been adopted in the UK.
- Treat hyposplenia as for other causes of asplenia/hyposplenia (see ➲ 'Asplenia', p. 120).

Iron deficiency and nutritional status

Iron deficiency
- Induced sideropenia due to sequestration is part of the body's response to chronic infection, as iron is essential to bacteria. However, it is also essential to host defences.
- Iron deficiency due to loss or inadequate intake impairs neutrophil bactericidal activity, as it is essential for the activity of myeloperoxidase. There is often a T lymphopenia. Immunoglobulins are usually normal but specific antibody production is reduced. All the changes are reversible with iron.

Nutritional status
- The immunodeficiency of malnutrition is difficult to disentangle because it is usually accompanied by multiple other health problems, which make identification of cause and effect impossible.

- Marasmus is total nutritional deficiency, while kwashiorkor is protein deficiency in a high-calorie diet.
- Both are usually accompanied by vitamin deficiency.
- Increased susceptibility to infection seems to be the rule.
- Non-specific barriers are impaired (especially in vitamin A deficiency).
- There may be variable abnormalities of neutrophil bactericidal activity, but these may well be secondary to infection.
- Immunoglobulins are often normal or high, even if the albumin is low. IgE levels may be elevated, even in the absence of significant parasitic infections, suggesting dysregulation of the Th1:Th2 axis.
- Mitogen responsiveness is reduced in kwashiorkor. Lymph nodes show germinal centre depletion and there is thymic atrophy, although the latter is also a feature of infection.

Asplenia

- Congenital (see ⊙ Chapter 1) or acquired asplenia (surgery, trauma) or hyposplenia (sickle-cell disease, coeliac disease) is associated with an increased susceptibility to overwhelming infection with capsulated organisms, *Capnocytophaga canimorsus* (dog bites), and problems in handling malaria, *Babesia*, and *Bartonella* (all intra-erythrocytic organisms).
- Risk appears to be lifelong, and is not limited to the first 2–3 years after splenectomy, as was previously thought. However, BSH guidelines still refer to the risk being of limited duration. Late overwhelming post-splenectomy sepsis (OPSS) is well documented.
- Degree of compromise also depends on the reason for splenectomy. For example, individuals splenectomized for lymphomas often have a more severe defect than those splenectomized for trauma.
- Ideally, all patients undergoing elective splenectomy should be immunized with Pneumovax® 23 and Hib vaccine and with the quadrivalent meningococcal conjugate vaccine preoperatively. If this is not possible, then immunization prior to discharge may be adequate, although responses immediately post-surgery will be reduced.
- The value of conjugated pneumococcal vaccines as routine first-line vaccines in asplenic/hyposplenic patients is uncertain.
- All asplenic patients should be on prophylactic antibiotics (phenoxymethylpenicillin, 500 mg twice a day, for choice); erythromycin can be used for penicillin-allergic patients. Where there is a high level of penicillin-resistant pneumococci (Mediterranean countries), amoxicillin 500 mg daily can be used.
- Patients should have their antibodies to Pneumovax® 23 and Hib measured annually. Those with suboptimal levels should be (re)-immunized and the levels rechecked.
- Those with poor responses to Pneumovax® 23 should receive the conjugated pneumococcal vaccine Prevenar 13®.
- Repeated doses of Pneumovax® 23 close together should be avoided as this may induce tolerance rather than boost immunity.

- Annual influenza immunization is essential to reduce risks of secondary bacterial sepsis.
- Asplenic patients may also not maintain adequate levels following vaccination for more than 3–5 years and regular checks should be carried out to ensure that protection is adequate. Note that the licence for Pneumovax® 23 does not indicate that it can be given this frequently. However, provided steps are taken to avoid immunizing patients with high antibody levels, the risk of adverse events appears to be low.
- Dog bites are dangerous and patients must seek immediate assistance: antibiotic treatment is essential.
- Specific advice is required for foreign travel to malarial areas (increased risk of cerebral malaria and massive haemolysis (Blackwater fever))— refer to Infectious Disease Team for advice.

Drugs and toxins

Drugs

In addition to the drugs discussed in Chapter 16, the major therapeutic action of which is immunosuppression, other drugs have also been reported to cause immunodeficiency. In many cases the evidence is poor, because pre-existent immunodeficiency has not been excluded. However, anticonvulsants, especially phenytoin and carbamazepine, both have strong associations with humoral immune deficiency, which may or may not resolve on withdrawal of the drugs. Newer anticonvulsants may also be associated with immunodeficiency. Lamotrigine has been associated with a combined immunodeficiency and opportunist infection.

Toxins

- Smoking suppresses mucosal immune responses, improving some allergic diseases such allergic alveolitis.
- Illegal drugs have considerable immunosuppressive potential, in part due to contaminants. Cannabis is particularly dangerous to severely immunocompromised patients as it may contain fungal spores.
- Alcohol in excess suppresses macrophage function, and as result increases the risk of tuberculosis.

Burns

- Burns cause a highly significant acquired T- and B-cell immunodeficiency.
- Disruption of the integrity of the normal cutaneous barriers and associated non-specific defences is a serious problem. Complement levels will be reduced by loss.
- In severe burns, neutrophil function is impaired and there is a lymphopenia, with depletion of lymphoid organs.
- DTH, mitogen, and allogeneic responses are reduced.
- These changes may be stress-related, due to excessive endogenous steroid production (Curling's ulcer is also associated) or to the release at the burned site of bacterial products.

- Immunoglobulin levels fall, often dramatically, due to reduced synthesis and increased loss through exudation. However, there is no benefit from IVIg replacement therapy.
- The best treatment is good intensive care and rapid grafting to re-establish normal barrier function.

Thoracic duct drainage

- This used to be used as an immunosuppressive technique for the treatment of rheumatoid arthritis.
- It usually occurs now as an unintended consequence of radical oesophageal surgery; chylothorax results, usually draining through the surgical drains.
- Loss of the circulating lymphocyte pool occurs within 48–72 hours and leads to severe prolonged lymphopenia, followed by severe panhypogammaglobulinaemia.
- Opportunist infections (PCP, *Candida*) occur.
- Chylothorax should be drained to the abdominal cavity, if possible, to allow conservation of lymphocytes. IVIg will be required, together with prophylactic co-trimoxazole, antivirals, and antifungals.
- Reconstitution of the immune system is dependent on thymic function and may take up to 2 years. Once normal lymphocyte numbers are achieved, a programme of re-immunization is required, commencing with killed/subunit vaccines.

Cardiac surgery in children

- Cardiac surgery in children < 2 years old is frequently associated with secondary immunodeficiency (?due to thymic disruption).
- Poor development of humoral immune responses.
- Test immunization may be required.
- Poor antibody function and history of infections are indications for the use of IVIg therapy.
- IVIg has also been used in adult cardiac transplant patients with hypogammaglobulinaemia and infections.

Physical and environmental factors

Radiotherapy and ionizing radiation

- Specific immune responses are affected (T and B cells); neutrophil and macrophage function is usually spared unless there is radiation damage to bone marrow.
- T-cell proliferative responses to mitogens and antigens remain depressed after irradiation for years.
- Lymphopenia, particularly of $CD4^+$ T cells, is common; humoral immune function is reduced.

Ultraviolet light
- Photoimmunosuppression occurs even with low levels of UV light exposure.
- Apoptosis may be increased.
- NF-κB in T cells is activated by UV light.

Chronic hypoxia (altitude)
- Increased infections are noted at high altitude.
- Hypoxic therapy has been used as an adjunct to sports conditioning: this is associated with measurable alterations in circulating lymphocyte profiles, although the patterns are not consistent.

Trauma and surgery
- Systemic inflammatory response syndrome (SIRS) is recognized in trauma and major surgery. It is caused by cytokine release (TNFα, IL-1β, IL-6) and may lead to multi-organ failure.
- A Th1 to Th2 switch and reduced T-cell proliferation have been noted but this is in part mediated by prostaglandin release from macrophages.
- Antibody production is inhibited by β-endorphin (reversible by naloxone).
- Prolonged administration of anaesthetic agents in ITU may contribute to worse immune function.
- Preventing tissue hypoxia is crucial (supplemental oxygen).

Lymphoedema syndromes

A number of familial syndromes have been identified that are associated with lymphoedema. These include:
- Milroy syndrome. Mutations in *VEGFR3* and *VEGFC*. Associated with congenital lower limb oedema, hydrocele, upslanting toenails, papillomatosis, and urethral abnormalities in males. Paucity of lymphatics.
- Lymphoedema-distichiasis syndrome. Mutations in *FOXC2* causes lymphoedema syndromes, with marked heterogeneity. Lower limb lymphoedema, aberrant extra eyelashes, cleft palate. Congenital heart disease.
- Emberger syndrome. Autosomal dominant mutations in *GATA2*, causing bilateral early-onset lower limb and genital lymphoedema and predisposition to develop myelodysplasia, acute myeloid leukaemia, and immune dysfunction.
- Meige syndrome. Autosomal dominant but no identified mutations. Presents with lower limb lymphoedema in adolescence or adulthood.
- *GJC2*-related lymphoedema. Autosomal dominant, presenting in first two decades with four-limb lymphoedema and varicose veins.
- Hennekam syndrome. Autosomal recessive with mutations in *CCBE1* and *FAT4* genes. Congenital or antenatal onset with generalized severe lymphoedema, lymphangiectasia, learning difficulties, epilepsy, microcephaly, and short stature.

- *PIEZO1*-related hydrops. Autosomal recessive, similar to Hennekam syndrome but with normal intelligence. Generalized lymphatic dysplasia. Pulmonary manifestations (effusions, chylothorax, pulmonary lymphangiectasia, and pericardial effusions).
- Others include: Turner's syndrome, Noonan syndrome, *EPHB4*-related lymphatic-related hydrops, and *PIK3CA*-related overgrowth spectrum.

Proteus syndrome

- A hamartomatous condition with partial gigantism of hands and feet, with pigmentary lesions, cerebriform connective tissue naevi, bony abnormalities (hyperostosis and skeletal abnormalities), multiple benign tumours (lipoma, haemangioma) and malignant tumours, capillary and lymphatic vascular malformations, venous thrombosis with pulmonary embolism, and developmental delay.
- Mild hypogammaglobulinaemia, with T- & B-cell lymphopenia has been reported.
- Mosaic activating mutation in the *AKT1* gene has been identified. This gene is involved in control of cell proliferation and apoptosis.
- A drug, ARQ092, which is a pan-AKT inhibitor, is being investigated as a treatment.

Yellow nail syndrome

- Rare syndrome of pleural effusions, lymphoedema, and yellow dystrophic nails.
- Cause uncertain: most cases appear to be acquired.
- Associated with bronchiectasis in 40% of cases.
- May have history of previous malignancy.
- Hypogammaglobulinaemia reported.
- Treatment should target underlying chest disease.
- May respond to high dose vitamin E ± biotin.

Cilial dyskinesia (Kartagener's syndrome)

- Rare autosomal recessive disease with defective cilia.
- Poor/absent cilial function.
- Genetics complex: 38% of dynein mutations are associated with DNAI1 and DNAH5 (latter associated with situs inversus). Multiple other genes (> 30) have been identified.
- Clinical features include:
  - Sinusitis, otitis media, hearing loss.
  - Bronchitis, recurrent pneumonia, bronchiectasis.
  - Infertility.
  - Situs inversus (partial or complete)—Kartagener's syndrome.
  - Asplenia/hyposplenia.
- Other related ciliopathies*.

- Infections are typically with *Staphylococcus aureus, Haemophilus influenzae, Streptococcus pneumoniae*, and *Moraxella catarrhalis*.
- Diagnosis is confirmed by EM of biopsies to assess cilial structure; video of cell cultures to assess ciliary movement and genetic studies.
- Treatment includes aggressive anti-infective treatment to prevent infection-related lung damage.
- Manage asplenia as previously described (see ➡ 'Asplenia', p. 120).

* ℛ http://ciliopathyalliance.org.uk
  ℛ http://www.pcdsupport.org.uk

Young's syndrome

- Rare syndrome of rhinosinusitis, recurrent chest infections, and bronchiectasis, associated with azoospermia.
- Possibly secondary to contact with mercury.
- Cilial function is normal.

Cystic fibrosis (CF)

- Autosomal recessive disease causing respiratory and pancreatic damage.
- Clinical features include:
  - Chronic sinusitis.
  - Bronchitis, bronchiectasis.
  - Recurrent pulmonary staphylococcal infections.
  - Malabsorption.
  - Failure to thrive.
  - Infertility.
- Disease is caused by mutations in the CF transmembrane conductance regulator (CFTR; chromosome 7q31.2). Heterozygosity for the mutated gene is common in Caucasian populations.
- Many mutations described: some are compatible with longevity and late presentation.
- Genetics should be checked in all patients presenting as adults with bronchiectasis/recurrent chest infections, where there is no other explanation, particularly if there are recurrent staphylococcal chest infections.
- Coexistent MBL deficiency is associated with worse prognosis.
- *Aspergillus* colonization may occur; development of IgE to *Aspergillus* is a poor prognostic sign.
- Chronic carriage of *Pseudomonas* and *Burkholderia* tend to be late events and are poor prognostic indicators. These patients need to be segregated to avoid infecting other patients.
- Aggressive antibiotic therapy is required; malabsorption and secondary diabetes are managed normally.
- Lung transplantation is successful.
- Drugs to improve CTFR function are undergoing trials (ivacaftor, a CFTR potentiator, and lumacaftor, a CFTR corrector).

- Gene replacement therapy is being studied. Early studies using viral vectors were only transiently successful. Newer administration modes (nanoparticles and biodegradable polymers) are being tested.

Pulmonary alveolar proteinosis

- Rare disease characterized by accumulations of surfactant-derived PAS-positive material in the lungs and impaired GM-CSF signalling.
- May occur due to mutations in the *CSF2RA* (autosomal recessive) and *CSF2RB* (X-linked) genes.
- An acquired form, due to neutralizing autoantibodies to GM-CSF, is described.
- Treatment is currently by whole lung lavage.
- Administration of GM-CSF (nebulized or systemic) helps in the autoimmune but not congenital types.
- Gene therapy is effective in a murine model of congenital disease.

α_1-Antitrypsin (α_1-AT) deficiency

- Autosomal co-dominant genetic disorder leading to reduced levels of α_1-AT. Associated with mutations in the *SERPINA1* gene
- Causes neonatal jaundice, cirrhosis, and liver failure. Liver disease is caused by accumulation of unsecreted variant α_1-AT protein.
- Later in life, emphysema (rarely bronchiectasis), especially in smokers, and panniculitis and angioedema. Polymers of Z variant appear chemotactic to neutrophils so increase recruitment of inflammatory cells.
- > 80 genetic variants identified by isoelectric focusing. Main types are shown in Table 2.2.
- Severe cases (very low α_1-AT levels, established lung disease) have been treated with infusions of α_1-AT. This may cause anaphylaxis, the formation of IgE anti-α_1-AT antibodies, and may contain low levels of IgA, causing problems in patients with concomitant IgA deficiency.
- Smoking avoidance is crucial to prevent accelerated lung damage.

Table 2.2 Main genetic variants of α_1-AT deficiency

Phenotype	α_1-AT level
PiMM (normal)	100%
PiMS	80%
PiSS	60%
PiMZ	60%
PiSZ	40%
PiZZ (severe phenotype)	10–15%

Hidradenitis suppurativa (acne inversa)

- A chronic inflammatory condition characterized by recurrent or chronic boils affecting the apocrine glands.
- Sinus and fistula formation is common, leading to deep-seated chronic inflammation. Pain is common.
- May be associated with arthritis, Crohn's disease, and lymphoedema.
- Chronic disease leads to significant psychological morbidity.
- Much commoner than previously thought.
- Link to obesity and smoking.
- Bacteria involved are multiple but include staphylococci, streptococci, and corynebacteria. Mixed infection is common.
- Three genes associated with familial HS (*PSENEN, NCSTN, PSEN*), coding for presenilin and nicastrin; activate Notch signalling and modulate activity of gamma-secretase.
- High copy numbers of beta-defensin gene cluster on chromosome 8p23.1 associated with increased susceptibility.
- Chronic inflammation is a risk factor for amyloidosis. Also increased risk of malignancy.
- Medical therapy is difficult and of variable efficacy. European Guidelines for management exist:
  - Topical and systemic antibiotics (clindamycin (topical/oral), tetracyclines, rifampicin (with clindamycin).
  - Intralesional steroids.
  - Systemic steroids.
  - Dapsone (check G6PD and monitor for haemolysis).
  - Ciclosporin.
  - Biologics (adalimumab, infliximab, etanercept, ustekinumab).
  - Retinoids.
  - Immunoglobulin (IM! not advised in UK).
  - Colchicine.
- Surgical therapy:
  - Excision of lesions and apocrine tissue.
  - Primary closure or grafting.
  - Deroofing of deep abscesses/sinuses.
  - Laser therapy may give fewer complications.

Allergic disease

Introduction

Allergic diseases are common: it has been estimated that 15% of the population will suffer from some sort of allergic reaction during their lifetime. It is clear that there has been an increase in atopic diseases since the Second World War. The precise cause of this change is unknown but undoubtedly reflects changes in lifestyle, in particular 'improvements' in housing, rendering houses more heavily colonized with dust mites. A reduction in breastfeeding may also have contributed, particularly atopic eczema. The evidence for air pollution, particularly car exhaust fumes, contributing to the increase is conflicting. It is also likely that the improvements in public health, leading to elimination in the Western world of parasitic infections, may contribute through a lack of physiological function for the IgE–mast cell axis. This has been formalized in the hygiene hypothesis ('dirt is good for you!').

In the mind of the public, allergy is responsible for all ills but in most cases the blame is wrongly apportioned. This perception has led to a proliferation of alternative practices pandering to these beliefs and using diagnostic techniques and treatments that have little to do with allergy as understood by immunologists and more to do with the gullibility of members of the public. That these practitioners can flourish indicates that we are failing our patients in being unable to cure their perceived illnesses, either through lack of knowledge or through lack of appropriate allergy facilities.

Anaphylaxis

Anaphylaxis represents the most severe type of allergic reaction and is a medical emergency.

Cause

- Sudden massive degranulation of mast cells, releasing histamine.
- Mast cells are stimulated to produce leukotrienes (cause of late reaction).
- Degranulation can be mediated by bound IgE-allergen cross-linking on the surface or direct, IgE-independent, mast cell degranulation (anaphylactoid reaction) responses. Mechanism is calcium dependent.
- Reaction is an example of type I hypersensitivity, dependent on the presence of specific IgE. Other reactions may mimic the clinical symptoms but without the involvement of IgE (see ➔ 'Anaphylactoid reactions', p. 137).
- Repeated challenge at short intervals may lead to progressively more severe reactions, but otherwise the severity of a reaction does *not* predict the severity of subsequent reactions.

Presentation

- Usual features are:
  - generalized giant urticaria;
  - angioedema, often involving face, lips, tongue, and larynx, causing stridor;
  - bronchospasm;

- hypotension with loss of consciousness;
- gastrointestinal symptoms (nausea, vomiting, abdominal cramps, diarrhoea).
- Not all symptoms will be present during an attack and only 50% of patients will have a rash.
- Onset is rapid after exposure, usually within minutes, although some agents (foods and latex) may lead to a slower onset. Agents that are injected (drugs, venoms) give the fastest reactions.

Substances causing anaphylaxis

Any substance may cause anaphylaxis, but the most common causes are:
- venoms: bee and wasp venoms;
- legumes: peanuts (and related legumes, soya, and other beans/peas);
- true nuts (walnut, almond, cashew, hazelnut, etc.);
- shellfish (crustacea, prawns, shrimps, crab, lobster) and fish;
- latex (and related foods: banana, avocado, kiwi, chestnut, potato, tomato);
- egg, milk;
- antibiotics: penicillin, cephalosporins, other antibiotics;
- anaesthetic drugs: neuromuscular blocking agents (e.g. suxamethonium, vecuronium);
- peptide hormones (ACTH, insulin);
- heterologous antisera (antivenins, antilymphocyte globulins, monoclonal antibodies);
- antiseptics: on the increase especially chlorhexidine, octenidine. polyhexamide; povidone iodine (very rare).

In some cases a cofactor is required for the reaction, such as concomitant aspirin ingestion with the food, or exercise. It is probable that these cofactors alter the amount of allergen entering the circulation.

Immunological features

- Involvement of IgE requires prior exposure to sensitize the patient. In childhood, sensitization to peanut may occur via formula milk, which may contain peanut oil. Following sensitization, only tiny amounts may be required to trigger subsequent reactions.
- Reaction is triggered by cross-linking of mast-cell cytophilic IgE by the allergen, leading to degranulation and activation of the mast cell.
- Symptoms occur as a result of mast-cell release of histamine, which is responsible for bronchoconstriction, increased airway mucus secretion, stimulation of gut smooth muscle, hypotension due to increased vascular permeability, and vasodilatation and urticaria/angioedema.
- Other mediators include mast cell tryptase and chemotactic factors for eosinophils. Activated mast cells also synthesize prostaglandins and leukotrienes, which reinforce the effects on smooth muscle. Tosyl-L-arginine methyl ester (TAME) has a similar effect. Platelet-activating factor (PAF) causes the activation of platelets, leading to the release of histamine and serotonin and augmenting the effects on vascular tone and permeability.

- Mast-cell numbers at sites of allergen exposure are critical. It is speculative that there are variations in the output of mast cells from bone marrow that influence the possibility of developing reactions.
- Complement and kinin systems are activated (basophils release kallikrein when activated). Bradykinin, C3a, and C5a all act as smooth muscle constrictors and increase vascular permeability.
- Reactions may recur after 2–6 hours, despite successful initial treatment, due to the continuing synthetic activity of mast cells and the release of leukotrienes.
- Those with underlying atopic disease are said to be more at risk of developing serious allergic responses.

Immunological diagnosis

- History is all-important, particularly the timing of reaction in relation to the suspected trigger. If the trigger is not clear, a detailed review of all exposures over the preceding 24 hours is required.
- Reaction should be graded.
  - Mild: a feeling of generalized warmth, with sensation of fullness in throat, some localized angioedema and urticaria, but no significant impairment of breathing or features of hypotension.
  - Moderate: as for mild, but with more widespread angioedema and urticaria, some bronchospasm, and mild gastrointestinal symptoms.
  - Severe: intense bronchospasm, laryngeal oedema, with severe shortness of breath, cyanosis, respiratory arrest, hypotension, cardiac arrhythmias, shock, and gross gastrointestinal symptoms.
- Attention must be paid to other conditions that may appear similar clinically:
  - pulmonary embolus;
  - myocardial infarction (but this may follow anaphylaxis in those with pre-existing ischaemic heart disease);
  - hyperventilation;
  - hypoglycaemia;
  - vasovagal reactions;
  - phaeochromocytoma;
  - carcinoid syndrome;
  - systemic mastocytosis;
  - rarely the symptoms may be factitious (typically occur in those who also have true anaphylaxis).
- Confirmation of the nature of the reaction may be obtained by taking blood for mast cell tryptase (levels will be elevated for up to 12 hours and it is stable). This is valuable where there is doubt about the nature of the reaction.
- Urinary methyl histamine and prostaglandins may be useful adjuncts (see ➲ Chapter 19 for further information).
- Evidence should also be sought for activation of the complement system (measurement of C3, C4, and C3 breakdown products). Measurement of C3a and C5a is possible but requires a special tube, which is unlikely to be available in time.
- Total IgE measurements are of no value.

- Tests for specific IgE (RAST, etc.) may give false-negative results in the immediate phase, even when it is quite clear what has caused the reaction, due to consumption of the IgE. Repeating tests 3–4 weeks later may be helpful.
- Skin-prick testing may be sufficient to trigger a further systemic reaction and should be undertaken with great caution and only in a situation in which full facilities for cardiopulmonary resuscitation are immediately available.
- Where no cause is obvious the use of multi-allergen chip-based tests (ISAC) may be of assistance, but its sensitivity is lower than standard ImmunoCAP® allergen-specific IgE tests.

Management of anaphylaxis

- ❶Immediate management comprises adrenaline (epinephrine) *given intramuscularly* in a dose of 0.5–1 mg (0.5–1 ml of 1 in 1000) for an adult. The dose can be repeated if required.
- If the reaction is severe, the adrenaline may be given intravenously, using 10 ml or 1 in 10 000 adrenaline diluted in 100 ml N-saline, via an infusion pump. This should only be given with continuous cardiac monitoring by an experienced ITU specialist.

❶Never give IV bolus adrenaline to a conscious patient with anaphylaxis under any circumstances.

- Give high-flow oxygen by mask.
- Antihistamine should be given intravenously (chlorphenamine 10 mg).
- A bolus of hydrocortisone (100–200 mg) should be given. The latter has no effect on the immediate reaction but reduces the possibility of a late reaction. Use hydrocortisone sodium succinate; do not use hydrocortisone phosphate as this is frequently associated with severe burning genital pain, which makes a sick patient feel much worse.
  - Cochrane reviews of antihistamines and steroids in the treatment of anaphylaxis conclude that evidence is lacking for both, but custom and practice recommend continued use.
- Support blood pressure with IV fluids (colloid or crystalloid): persisting hypotension may require further vasopressor agents.
- Tracheotomy may be required if there is major laryngeal oedema.
- Admission for observation is required (risk of late reactions); a period of 8 hours is usually adequate
- Great care must be taken with latex-allergic patients, as hospital staff with latex gloves and resuscitation with latex-containing equipment (masks, catheters, etc.) may make the reaction paradoxically worse during resuscitation.
- Patients who have had severe reactions should be trained to self-administer adrenaline using a self-injection aid and should carry a Medic-Alert bracelet or equivalent. See later in this topic for indications.
- Regular annual follow-up by a practice nurse should be undertaken to ensure that patients remain competent in using the adrenaline injector.
- Carrying a supply of antihistamines may also be helpful (used prophylactically if entering a situation of unknown risk, e.g. eating out).

- ❶Patients deemed to be at risk of further anaphylaxis should preferably not receive treatment with β-blockers, as these agents will interfere with the action of adrenaline if required.
  - ❶For venom-allergic patients with ischaemic heart disease, there may be advantages of continuing with β-blockers.
- ❶ACE-inhibitors should be avoided, as bradykinin-mediated effects will be worse during reactions (increased severity).
- Patients should receive detailed counselling on how to avoid the triggering allergen; if a food is involved this should be undertaken by a dietician experienced in dealing with food allergy. Many foods may be 'hidden', so that the consumer is unaware of the contents. This applies particularly to pre-prepared foods and restaurant meals.
- For bee/wasp anaphylaxis, patients should be warned to avoid wearing brightly coloured clothes and perfumes as these attract the insects. They should also stay away from fallen fruit and dustbins. Desensitization is possible (see ➲ Chapter 16). This is a process that requires considerable dedication on the part of the patient (and the hospital staff!). It should be reserved for those who have had a systemic reaction and where the risk of further stings is considered to be high.
- Latex-allergic patients need to be warned about possible reactions to foods (banana, avocado, kiwi fruit, chestnut, potato, and tomato) and be given advice on avoidance. It is important that they tell doctors and dentists as reactions may be triggered during operations by surgical gloves or anaesthetic equipment and by investigations such as barium enema (rubber cuff on tubing) and dental treatment.
- The Anaphylaxis Campaign can provide support and advice to patients and families: ✎ https://www.anaphylaxis.org.uk/

Testing
- See Table 3.1.

Indications for prescription of adrenaline for self-injection (EpiPen®, Emerade®, Jext®)
- Adrenaline for self-injection should be given when:
  - patient has had a severe allergic reaction;
  - there is a risk of re-exposure or the allergen cannot easily be avoided;
  - patient has had a moderate reaction, but access to rapid medical assistance is impossible;
  - patient has asthma—reactions are likely to be more severe;

Table 3.1 Testing for anaphylaxis

Immediate tests	Later tests
Mast cell tryptase (clotted blood)	Specific IgE/skin prick/testing/challenges
Complement C3, C4 (if angioedema is prominent without urticaria)	
Consider other tests in light of differential above	

- pregnancy is not a contraindication, as the risk to the fetus from hypoxia due to anaphylaxis is greater than the risk of adrenaline.
- Adrenaline should *not* be given when:
  - reaction is mild (urticaria or urticaria with minimal angioedema not involving throat);
  - allergen is avoidable;
  - patient is unable to use injection device;
  - patient has or is at risk of ischaemic heart disease; this may include the elderly;
  - patient is on β-blockers. This is a relative contraindication and there is some evidence that the effect is not significant. However, it is recommended that the dose of adrenaline be halved in patients on β-blockers, to avoid paradoxical hypertension due to unopposed α-adrenergic activity. Whether this is required is debated;
  - β-blockade can be reversed with glucagon (but this effect is short-lived);
  - patients are on tricyclic antidepressants or abuse cocaine (increased risk of cardiac arrhythmias).

Problems with adrenaline self-injection devices

- All adrenaline autoinjectors in the UK operate in a similar fashion, but with minor differences. To avoid confusion, patients should receive only one type of injector and should be trained on that injector.
- Alternative devices are available in other parts of the world.
- Jext® and EpiPen® contain 0.3 mg and 1–2 doses are usually sufficient to provide relief. Paediatric doses of 0.15 µg are available.
- Emerade® is also available in a 0.5 mg strength. It also has a slightly longer needle, which means it may be suitable for those with high BMI.
- Studies have shown that much of the adrenaline is not injected intramuscularly, but subcutaneously with the current needle lengths.
- Adrenaline degrades faster in the heat, so patients with adrenaline autoinjectors should aim to travel with them in a cool bag if visiting a hot country.
- The agreed advice is that it is better to use an expired adrenaline autoinjector, than not use anything. At worst it will not have a full dose but will not do harm.
- Accidental injection into fingers occurs: there is a risk of digital ischaemia and patients should be advised to go to casualty (intravenous α-blocker may be required).

Idiopathic anaphylaxis

This refers to anaphylaxis, often recurrent, where the trigger cannot be ascertained. It is suggested that this may be up to 30–60% of all cases of anaphylaxis in adults and 10% in children. It is commoner in women and in those with atopic disease. Careful investigation may identify potential triggers.

Causes

Potential causes include:
- Unsuspected food allergens.
- Latex.
- Alpha-gal allergy (red meat allergy triggered by tick bites).
- Mast cell disorder.

Differential diagnosis

- As for anaphylaxis.
- Consider factitious anaphylaxis.

Investigation

- Skin-prick testing to common foods, including fresh food skin-prick tests with 'as eaten' foods.
- Specific IgE testing to latex, alpha-gal.
- Baseline tryptase and measurement during attacks.
- Urinary methylhistamine/prostaglandins.
- Bone marrow examination and c-kit mutation.

Treatment

- Standard anaphylaxis rescue medication package (as previously noted).
- Continuous high-dose antihistamines.
- Consider ketotifen (said to be advantageous).
- Where attacks are frequent, consider prolonged oral prednisolone, starting at 40–60 mg/day and tapering to eventual withdrawal. Some patients may end up on long-term steroids.
- Omalizumab has been used (unlicensed indication).

Kounis syndrome

This refers to an acute coronary syndrome (coronary artery spasm, myocardial infarction, stent thrombosis) occurring in the setting of anaphylaxis. Cerebral and mesenteric arteries may also be affected.

Causes

- The syndrome is caused by pro-inflammatory and procoagulant mediators released during anaphylaxis (histamine, prostanoids, platelet activating factor, cytokines).
- Any allergic trigger can trigger the syndrome.

Diagnosis

- Clinical symptoms and signs supported by ECG abnormalities and angiography.
- Elevated mast cell tryptase (be aware that myocardial infarction in the absence of anaphylaxis may also elevate tryptase!).

Treatment

- Difficult!

- Adrenaline may worsen ischaemia and trigger arrhythmias. Methoxamine, an α-blocker, may be better.
- Treat coronary artery spasm appropriately with nitrates, calcium-channel blockers, and follow myocardial infarction protocols.
- Use morphine with care as it may increase histamine release and worsen symptoms. Fentanyl has less histamine-releasing effect and may be better.

Anaphylactoid reactions

These may be every bit as severe as IgE-mediated reactions. In most cases they are due to activation of mast cells directly or via other mechanisms that will indirectly activate mast cells.

Causes

The most common causes are:
- direct mast-cell stimulation: drugs (opiates, thiamine, vancomycin, radiocontrast media, some anaesthetic agents, especially those dissolved in cremophor, tubocurarine), foods (strawberries), physical stimuli (exercise, cold, trauma), venoms;
- immune complex reactions (types II and III), with release of anaphylotoxins C3a, C5a: reactions to IVIg, other blood products, heterologous antisera;
- cyclo-oxygenase inhibitors: non-steroidal anti-inflammatory drugs (may also stimulate mast cells directly);
- massive histamine ingestion: eating mackerel and other related oily fish that are 'off' (scombroid poisoning due to breakdown of muscle histidine to histamine caused by bacterial spoilage).

Immunological diagnosis
- History usually gives the clue. No tests are entirely specific. Challenge is very risky, except in the case of scombroid poisoning.
- Tryptase will be elevated.
- Specific IgE will not be detectable.

Management
- Acute management is the same as for anaphylaxis.
- For patients who require IV radiocontrast media and are known or suspected to react, then pre-treatment with oral corticosteroids (40 mg prednisolone, 13, 7, and 1 hour prior to examination), together with an antihistamine (cetirizine 10–20 mg or fexofenadine 120–180 mg orally 1 hour before) and an H_2-blocker (cimetidine, 400 mg orally 1 hour before) should be used. Low-osmolality dyes should be used as these have a lower incidence of reactions.
- Current Royal College of Radiologists' guidelines advise the radiologist to refer patients with severe reactions to a specialist allergy unit for further advice and comment that there is no strongly supporting evidence for the use of prophylaxis as previously described: ℘ https://www.rcr.ac.uk/sites/default/files/Intravasc_contrast_web.pdf

Angioedema

Angioedema is a deep-tissue swelling that must be distinguished from urticaria. It is rarely itchy, and tends to give discomfort from pressure. In hereditary angioedema and sometimes in idiopathic angioedema, there is often a premonitory tingling before the swelling occurs. Any part of the body (including gut) may be involved.

Causes

- Allergic (accompanied by other features such as urticaria, anaphylaxis, etc.).
- Hereditary C1-esterase inhibitor or C4BP deficiency (see ➲ Chapter 1).
- ACE deficiency.
- Acquired C1-esterase inhibitor deficiency (autoantibody-mediated, SLE, lymphoma). Lymphoma-associated acquired C1-esterase inhibitor deficiency is usually due to splenic villous lymphomas.
- Physical (pressure, vibration, water—often with urticaria).
- Drugs ACE inhibitors, angiotensin-II receptor blockers (ARBs), NSAIDs, statins, proton-pump inhibitors are the commonest drugs).
- Idiopathic (rarely involves larynx)—other causes excluded.

Immunological features

- Mechanism is thought to involve activation of the kinin system with bradykinin production, leading to tissue oedema.
- ACE inhibitors inhibit bradykinin breakdown (also cause cough due to excess bradykinin).
- ARBs have now been shown to reduce bradykinin breakdown and may therefore not be a suitable alternative to ACE inhibitors.
- Histamine is not involved (unless there is accompanying urticaria).
- C1-esterase inhibitor is a control protein for the kinin cascade in addition to its role in the complement and clotting systems.
- There are polymorphisms of ACE but it is not known whether they correlate with the tendency to develop angioedema.
- Congenital ACE deficiency has also been associated with angioedema.

Diagnosis

- History will give useful clues: family history, connective tissue disease, lymphoma (may be occult), drug exposure, association with physical stimuli.
- Differential is wide (see Table 3.2).
- Angioedema with urticaria will not be due to hereditary angioedema.
- In angioedema without urticaria, C1-esterase inhibitor deficiency should be excluded.
  - C4 will usually be low, even between attacks; a normal C4 does NOT however exclude HAE.
  - C1-inhibitor will be low in type I but high in type II (see ➲ Chapter 1); functional C1-inhibitor test will distinguish type II.
  - Consider type III HAE (FXII and plasminogen mutations) if family history and normal C1-inhibitor.

Table 3.2 Differential diagnosis of facial swelling

Condition	Features
Contact dermatitis	Includes facial and periorbital oedema followed by peeling; usually secondary to cosmetics (patch testing appropriate); also consider plant allergy (poison ivy)—blistering may occur, usually worse in spring
Cellulitis/erysipelas	Erythema and warmth of skin; fever; inflammatory markers and WCC raised; peeling may occur after resolution
Facial lymphoedema	May occur with rosacea (morbus morbihan); accompanied by flushing (alcohol, spicy foods, temperature); slow onset
Blepharochalasis	Recurrent eyelid oedema causing atrophy and bronze discoloration (mainly children & young adults); IgA deposits seen—?immune pathogenesis
Hypothyroidism	Facial puffiness/myxoedema
SVC obstruction	Generalized oedema of head and neck, with venous engorgement
Orofacial granulomatosis	See ➜ Chapter 14
Idiopathic oedema	Often associated with facial oedema. See ➜ Chapter 14
Dermatomyositis (acute)	Periorbital swelling associated with heliotrope rash and Gottron's papules
Hypocomplementaemic urticarial vasculitis (HUVS)	Facial angioedema may occur in the early stages. See ➜ Chapter 13
Gleich's syndrome	Episodic angioedema with eosinophilia. See text
Clarkson's syndrome	Capillary leak syndrome, causing episodes of sudden hypovolaemic shock accompanied by generalized tissue swelling due to oedema. See text

- Levels of C2 are said to distinguish acquired from inherited C1-esterase inhibitor deficiency (low in inherited deficiency) but this test is not reliable.
- If acquired C1 esterase inhibitor deficiency is suspected, check:
  - for lymphadenopathy and splenomegaly clinically;
  - serum immunoglobulins;
  - serum and urine electrophoresis;
  - serum free light chains;
  - consider chest/abdominal CT scan.
- Check ACE level to exclude ACE deficiency.
- Connective tissue disease will usually be obvious, but detection of autoantibodies (antinuclear antibody (ANA), dsDNA, and extractable nuclear antigen (ENA) antibodies) may be necessary.

Acute treatment
- Treatment is dependent on the cause.
- The management of C1-esterase inhibitor deficiency (HAE) is discussed in Chapter 1.
- Acquired C1-esterase inhibitor deficiency (AAE) due to lymphoma will be improved by effective treatment of the underlying disease, as will the autoimmune-associated angioedema.
  - Purified C1-esterase inhibitor may be required in acquired C1-esterase inhibitor deficiency.
  - Frequent doses may be required, due to the presence of inhibitory antibodies: in severe cases, plasmapheresis and immunosuppression may be required.
  - FFP is less effective and may actually make the angioedema worse by providing extra substrate.
- There is **NO** role for C1-esterase inhibitor concentrate in idiopathic angioedema without evidence of deficiency.
- Icatibant (bradykinin B2 receptor antagonist) may have a role in the management of severe recurrent angioedema (limited clinical trial data and not licensed for this indication); it can be self-administered by SC injection.
- In acute attacks of HAE and AAE attacks, adrenaline, antihistamines, and steroids are less effective than in anaphylaxis. Laryngeal involvement is less common in the non-hereditary forms.
- For other types of recurrent angioedema without systemic features, prednisolone 20 mg plus cetirizine 20 mg (chewed—tastes horrible!) is appropriate immediate treatment. Prolonged courses of steroid are unhelpful.

Prophylactic treatment
- Control may be helped with antifibrinolytics (tranexamic acid, 2–4 g/day), or modified androgens (stanozolol, 2.5–10 mg/day; danazol, 200–800 mg/day). If stanozolol is not available, oxandrolone may be used as an alternative.
  - Monitor LFTs every 4–6 months.
  - Regular ultrasound of the liver (every 1–3 years).
- Idiopathic form (other causes excluded) responds best to tranexamic acid and less well to modified androgens.
- Management of allergic angioedema requires avoidance of triggers and prophylaxis with long-acting non-sedating antihistamines.

Tests
- See Table 3.3.
- ❶Patients with a history of angioedema for any reason should never be given ACE inhibitors, as these drugs may precipitate life-threatening events.

Episodic angioedema with eosinophilia (Gleich's syndrome)
- Recurrent angioedema associated with cyclic weight gain (up to 15%), fever, urticaria, and eosinophilia. Cycles every 28–32 days.
- Some patients have a clonal CD3⁻CD4⁺ population but the disease is most probably multilineage.

Table 3.3 Testing for angioedema

Immediate tests	Later tests
C3, C4, C1 esterase inhibitor	Consider immunoglobulins, electrophoresis (serum, urine), β_2-microglobulin (immunochemical and functional)—urticaria not present
Tryptase (if urticaria present)	ANA, ds-DNA, ENA (suspected CTD)
ACE	CT scan chest/abdomen if lymphoma suspected

- Cause unknown but IL-5 and IL-6 may be elevated.
- Serum IgM is typically elevated.
- Attacks will respond to corticosteroids.

Systemic capillary leak syndrome (Clarkson's syndrome)
- Recurrent episodes of life-threatening hypovolaemic shock, accompanied by generalized swelling (not localized) due to leakage of plasma into tissues.
- Blood tests show reduced albumin, and haemoconcentration.
- Cause is unknown.
- Treatment is supportive: corticosteroids have been used and IVIg has been tried with benefit in some cases (not an approved indication in England).

Urticaria 1

Urticaria is common, affecting 10–20% of individuals at some time. Urticaria is dependent on mast cells and histamine is the principal mediator. The reaction may be due to IgE on mast cells or stimuli that directly activate mast cells (see ➷ 'Anaphylactoid reactions', p. 137). Urticaria may occur alone or be accompanied by more systemic symptoms, including angioedema, although (as noted earlier) histamine is not involved in the latter.

Causes
- Urticaria may be acute or chronic (more than 1 month's duration). Chronic urticaria is often idiopathic (75% of cases) and rarely associated with allergy. 5% of the population may develop a physical urticaria. Idiopathic urticaria may disappear spontaneously after 1–2 years.
- Commonest causes include:
  - stress;
  - infections: in association with common viral infections (concomitant drug therapy usually gets the blame!); *Helicobacter*; prodrome of hepatitis B, Lyme disease, cat-scratch disease; acute or chronic bacterial infections; parasitic infections;
  - also consider sites of chronic infection/inflammation (teeth, sinuses, gall bladder);
  - allergic (ingested allergens, injected allergens, e.g. cat scratch);

- autoimmune: autoantibodies to IgE and to FcεRI (probably rare); also in association with connective-tissue diseases (antibodies to C1q): SLE;
- physical: sunlight (also think of porphyria), vibration, pressure (immediate and delayed, dermographism), aquagenic, heat;
- cold: familial (FCAS, autosomal dominant—*C1AS1* gene mutations— see ➔ Chapter 13); acquired (cryoglobulins, cryofibrinogen, mycoplasma infections);
- cholinergic (much smaller wheals, often triggered by emotion, heat, and sweating);
- adrenergic: provoked by stress;
- contact (e.g. urticaria from lying on grass, wearing latex gloves, occasionally from aeroallergens);
- urticaria pigmentosa: rare disease with reddish-brown macules in skin (accumulations of mast cells);
- vasculitis: usually a leucocytoclastic vasculitis, painful not itchy; also serum sickness (immune complex)—see also ➔ 'Urticarial vasculitis', p. 145;
- hormonal: autoimmune progesterone-induced urticaria, related to menstrual cycle; occasionally other steroids may cause the same reaction; hypothyroidism;
- papular urticaria: related to insect bites (may last several days);
- rare syndromes: Muckle–Wells and related syndromes (see ➔ Chapter 14); mastocytosis (see ➔ 'Mastocytosis', p. 145); PUPP (pruritic urticaria and plaques of pregnancy);
- urticaria may occur with vitamin D, iron, vitamin B$_{12}$, and folate deficiency.

Immunological features

- Mast-cell activation is the cause, with local release of mediators and activation of other pathways, complement, and kinin.
- Autoantibodies against IgE and the IgE receptor (FcεRI) have been proposed as a mechanism in some patients with chronic urticaria. These lead to activation of mast cells by cross-linking surface IgE or receptors. How generally applicable this mechanism is remains to be determined. Assays are dubious.
- Mast cells can be stimulated through other pathways, either directly by drugs, etc. (as previously described) or by the anaphylotoxins C3a, C5a (type II) and by immune complexes (type III). In cholinergic urticaria, mast cells are unusually sensitive to stimulation by acetylcholine released by local cholinergic nerves.

Diagnosis

- See Table 3.4.
- The history is everything! The appearances of the lesions may give clues (distinctive lesions in cholinergic urticaria).
- Dermographism should be sought.
- Physical causes can usually be replicated in the clinic to confirm the diagnosis: pressure tests; ice cube test (wrap ice cube in plastic bag to ensure that it is cold not water that causes the problem).

Table 3.4 Testing for urticaria

Immediate tests	Later tests
Full blood count—check for haematinic deficiency—MCV; ferritin	Drug monitoring as required Anti-C1q antibodies Skin biopsy
Thyroid function	
Liver function Inflammatory marker (ESR/CRP)	
Infection screen—*Helicobacter*	
Tryptase Consider autoimmune serology Cryoglobulins & cold agglutinins (cold induced) Genetic studies if FCAS suspected	

- Other diagnostic tests should depend on likely cause.
- Allergy testing is rarely justified in chronic urticaria as the yield is low.
- Check thyroid function, acute-phase response, full blood count, and think of infective causes.
- For acute urticarias, foods may play a role, exclusion diets may help but only if there is a strong suspicion on clinical grounds. The role of natural dietary salicylates and/or preservatives in chronic urticaria is controversial.
- In cold urticaria, seek family history and check for cryoglobulins and causes thereof (electrophoresis of serum, search for underlying diseases, infections, connective tissue disease, lymphoproliferation).
- Autoantibodies (ANA, ENA, dsDNA, RhF) and complement studies (C3, C4) may be relevant in some instances. In SLE with urticarial or suspected urticarial vasculitis, think of autoantibodies to C1q.
- Tryptase is helpful when mast-cell disorders are suspected.
- Skin biopsy should be considered if there are atypical features (if urticarial vasculitis suspected).

Urticaria 2: treatment

- Urticaria may be difficult to manage, especially cold urticaria. Commonest failing is inadequate dosage of antihistamines. The new antihistamines are safe in doses well above the recommended doses and do not interfere with cardiac potassium channels to cause prolonged QT interval.
- Acute urticaria should be treated with potent non-sedating antihistamines. Short-acting ones such as acrivastine may be appropriate for intermittent attacks. Potent long-acting non-sedating ones, such as fexofenadine, levocetirizine, and cetirizine (also said to have mast-cell stabilizing activity, of uncertain clinical significance), are

useful for prophylaxis against frequent attacks. A few patients may still be sedated by these drugs.
- Loratadine and desloratadine have been reported by the EMEA to be associated with a small increase in minor malformations if taken in pregnancy.
- Doses up to four times the normal dose may be required in difficult cases.
- If these are unsuccessful alone, then the addition of an H_2-blocker may be helpful, although the evidence is weak. There is no evidence to suggest whether ranitidine or cimetidine is preferable.
- Montelukast or zafirlukast are alternatives to H_2-blockers.
- Other therapeutic options include:
  - doxepin, an antidepressant with potent H_1- and H_2-blocking activity;
  - ketotifen, which has mast-cell stabilizing activity in addition to anti-H_1 activity (it increases appetite and is sedating);
  - mirtazapine is also a valuable third-line agent and has anti-histaminic properties;
  - calcium channel blockers may have some beneficial effect as they stabilize mast cells (nimodipine is said to be better than nifedipine);
  - β_2-agonists (terbutaline) and phosphodiesterase inhibitors (theophylline) may help in rare cases;
  - oxypentifylline has been reported to reduce cytokine synthesis by macrophages and may be helpful;
  - colchicine is helpful in delayed pressure urticaria but is poorly tolerated;
  - resistant urticaria may respond to low-dose warfarin (mechanism unknown);
  - modified androgens (stanozolol, danazol)—require monitoring of LFTs;
  - methotrexate—reduces neutrophil accumulation and decreases leukotriene synthesis.
- Non-familial cold urticaria may respond to cyproheptadine, calcium-channel blockers, β_2-agonists, and phosphodiesterase inhibitors, although responses tend to be poor. Omalizumab and reslizumab have also been used.
- Familial cold urticaria does not respond to antihistamines, but may respond to NSAIDs. Anakinra is effective.
- Steroids may be effective but should be used as a last resort as chronic therapy is not justified by the side-effects. Short courses may be helpful for acute disease. Withdrawal of steroid is often marked by worse flares of rash.
- Ciclosporin or tacrolimus may also be helpful, but the disease relapses once the drug is withdrawn. The side-effects (hypertension, nephrotoxicity, increased risk of malignancy) make them undesirable drugs for urticaria, unless symptoms are severe. Mycophenolate has also been used.
- High-dose IVIg has been used in resistant cases but the benefits are variable. It is not endorsed by the current UK guidance.
- NICE guidelines recommend omalizumab for resistant urticaria and persistently high UAS7 scores. This is given as a fixed dose of 300 mg

monthly for six injections. Not all patients respond and those that do frequently relapse when the course is complete, requiring retreatment.
- Whenever chronic therapy is started, it is important to withdraw it at intervals to see whether it is still required in the light of possible spontaneous remission.
- Consider stress management training.

Urticarial vasculitis

- Urticarial vasculitis is distinguished from ordinary urticaria by the persistence of the lesions for > 24 hours. Lesions usually fade to leave brown staining, due to erythrocyte extravasation.
- Biopsies show evidence of cutaneous vasculitis.
- Antihistamines are ineffective.
- The condition is discussed in more detail in Chapter 13.

Mastocytosis

Mastocytosis includes a range of related disorders, characterized by excessive accumulations of mast cells in tissues.

Classification
- Cutaneous mastocytosis:
  - urticaria pigmentosa;
  - solitary mastocytoma;
  - diffuse cutaneous mastocytosis (rare);
  - telangiectasia macularis eruptiva perstans.
- Systemic mastocytosis:
  - involvement of gut, bone marrow, bone. This may be indolent or aggressive.
- Mastocytosis in association with haematological disorders:
  - leukaemia, lymphoma, myelodysplastic syndrome.
- Lymphadenopathic mastocytosis with eosinophilia.
- Mast cell leukaemia (very rare!).
- Secondary: mast cell hyperplasia related to chronic infection, malignancy, or autoimmune disease.

Presentation
- Cutaneous involvement with itchy brown macules; Darier's sign = urticaria on rubbing or scratching cutaneous lesions. Dermographism.
- Systemic symptoms include nausea, vomiting, diarrhoea, headache, shortness of breath, flushing, palpitations, loss of consciousness, malaise, and lethargy.
- Systemic attacks triggered by heat, emotion, aspirin, opiates.
- Evidence of associated haematological malignancy.
- Symptoms may be confused with carcinoid and phaeochromocytoma.

Diagnosis

- Biopsy of skin, bowel; endoscopy will be required for gut involvement.
- Patients with persistently elevated mast cell tryptase should have a bone marrow examination, at least to provide a baseline against which to monitor for progressive disease.
- Mast cell tryptase (serial measurements may be required); urinary methylhistamine can be helpful, but is not readily available.
- Exclude carcinoid by measurement of 5-HIAA, phaeochromocytoma by urinary catecholamines/serum metanephrines.
- Serum immunoglobulins and electrophoresis; serum free light chains.
- Blood film.
- Bone scan/MRI skeletal survey for infiltrations.

Treatment

- High-dose antihistamines (H_1 and H_2).
- Aspirin may reduce prostaglandin production causing flushing, but should be used with caution as it can directly activate mast cells; leukotriene antagonists (montelukast) will prevent leukotriene-related symptoms.
- Oral sodium cromoglicate may help bowel symptoms.
- Caution with drug use: avoid opiates and other drugs directly activating mast cells (radiocontrast dyes, dextrans); anaesthesia needs to be approached carefully.
- Wasp/bee stings may lead to severe reactions.
- Interferon alfa (disappointing in most cases) and c-*kit* inhibitors (mast cells express increased c-*kit*) are being used experimentally. PUVA may help in skin lesions.
- Stem cell transplantation can be considered for severe systemic mastocytosis or mast cell leukaemia in the young.
- For those not suitable for transplantation midostaurin may be an alternative

Mast cell activation syndrome (MCAS)

- This is a concept used to account for a variety of non-specific symptoms which strongly overlap with chronic fatigue syndrome and fibromyalgia.
- It has been particularly associated with Ehlers–Danlos syndrome type III.
- Conventional markers of mastocytosis (mast cell tryptase) are not elevated. Bone marrow examination is normal and excess mast cells are not seen in tissues. Other conditions need to be excluded.
- Management is symptomatic.

Histamine intolerance

- Histamine intolerance may be caused by impairment of the activity of the enzyme diamine oxidase, responsible for the metabolism of histamine. Reduced activity may be due to genetic defects.
- Low DAO activity may predispose to severe reactions, and recurrent anaphylaxis.

- Reduced DAO may be seen in association with drugs (Table 3.5) and with chronic renal and liver failure, and in chronic urticaria.
- A trial of a low-histamine diet may be beneficial.
- Supplementation with vitamins C and B_6 is said to help by increasing DAO activity.
- Some patients may try buying DAO as a dietary supplement over the internet. This approach has not been validated.

Table 3.5 Drugs associated with reduced DAO activity (not exhaustive)

Contrast media	Antibiotics (cefuroxime, clavulanic acid)
Muscle relaxants	
Morphine	Aminophylline
	Cimetidine
Aspirin	Cyclophosphamide
Metoclopramide	Amitriptyline

Pruritus (itch)

Pruritus (itch without rash) is a common problem and is frequently referred to immunology/allergy services for 'allergy diagnosis', whereas in fact allergy is rarely the cause. There are many conditions which cause chronic/intractable itch. Management is difficult.

Causes
- Primary skin diseases:
  - Atopic eczema.
  - Urticaria.
  - Xerosis.
  - Psoriasis.
  - Nodular prurigo.
  - Stasis dermatitis/varicose eczema (legs—beware of reactions to topical treatments).
  - Mast cell disorders.
  - Dermatitis herpetiformis.
  - Lichen simplex.
  - Lichen sclerosus; lichen planus.
  - Infestations (scabies).
  - Fungal skin infections.
- Neurological disorders:
  - Brachioradial pruritus.
  - Notalgia paraesthetica.
  - MS.
  - Post-herpetic neuralagia.
  - Small fibre neuropathy (hands and feet).

- Liver disease:
  - PBC (early in disease).
  - Cholestasis (all causes).
- Renal disease:
  - Uraemia.
- Neoplasia and haematological disorders:
  - Lymphoma.
  - Myeloma.
  - Myelofibrosis.
  - Hypereosinophilic syndromes.
  - Iron deficiency.
- Endocrine disorders:
  - Thyroid disease.
  - Diabetes and diabetic neuropathy.
  - Parathyroid disease.
- Drugs:
  - Opioids.
  - ACE inhibitors.
  - Statins.
  - Metformin.
- Pregnancy:
  - PUPPP (persistent urticarial papules and plaques of pregnancy): a self-limiting condition usually seen in third trimester and resolving after delivery.
- Infections:
  - HIV.
- Psychological:
  - Depression/anxiety/stress.
  - Delusional parasitosis.
  - Anorexia nervosa.
  - Obsessive-compulsive disorder.

Investigation

- History and examination are critical.
- Investigations should be based on the differential diagnosis formulated for each patient.

Treatment

- In the allergy clinic this is primarily about explaining that allergy is not the cause and allergy tests will not be helpful.
- Treatment needs to be directed against the most likely cause.
- Some of the diagnoses listed earlier will have specific therapies.
- Treatments may include:
  - Antihistamines: usually not effective but should be tried. Use non-sedating antihistamines during the day and sedating antihistamines (with anticholinergic activity) at night.
  - Topical doxepin.
  - Topical menthol in aqueous cream (TRPM8 agonist).
  - Topical capsaicin (TRPV1 agonist, reduces release of substance P from C-fibres).

- Topical tacrolimus/pimecrolimus.
- Topical lidocaine.
- Mirtazapine (SNRI, SSRI).
- Amitryptiline.
- Carbamazepine.
- Gabapentin/pregabalin.
- Naltrexone (μ-opioid receptor antagonist).
- Butorphanol (κ-opioid receptor antagonist).
- Psychological interventions.
- ❶*Avoid oral and topical steroids!*

Asthma 1

Asthma is one of the atopic diseases and is characterized by broncho-spasm. It is also a chronic inflammatory disease. However, the cause is multifactorial, with a complex interaction of genetic background with environmental factors. There is also a complex interaction at the local level between changes in the airway (reactive airways disease), neurogenic components (particularly involving vasoactive intestinal polypeptide (VIP) and substance P), and the innate and specific immune system.

Causes

Many factors, including occupational exposures, combine to give the clinical pattern of asthma:

- *Genetic background*. There is no doubt that there is a familial tendency, with inheritance more obvious through the maternal line. The loci involved are controversial, with loci on chromosome 5 (mapping to the region containing the genes for IL-4, IL-5, and the β-adrenoreceptor) and on chromosome 11 being proposed.
- *Allergy*. Inhaled allergens (aeroallergens) such as pollens, danders, dust mites, etc. are potent triggers: IgE will be involved. Allergy is less commonly demonstrated in late-onset asthma. Occupational allergens may cause symptoms, with small, reactive molecules such as platinum salts acting by reaction with self-proteins to produce neo-antigens: IgE may be difficult to demonstrate.
- *Th1:Th2 balance*. An intrinsic bias towards Th2-mediated reactions will lead to higher IgE production and levels of Th2 cytokines (IL-4, IL-5) which, in turn, downregulate potentially balancing Th1 responses.
- *Irritants*. Some agents cause asthma without the involvement of IgE, e.g. sulphites (see ➲ 'Sulphite sensitivity', p. 152); in part the effects here may be due to non-specific inflammation with recruitment of eosinophils and an IgE-independent cycle of cytokine and mediator release. Smoking and viral infections may contribute through this mechanism and through direct epithelial damage. Cold air and exercise may also be non-specific triggers to the hyperreactive airway.
- *Smooth muscle abnormalities*. Abnormally low numbers of β-adrenoreceptors have been documented in asthma. This may contribute to the reactivity of airways.

- *Neurogenic*. Local axon loops involving C-type fibres releasing substance P and neurokinin A contribute to smooth muscle constriction. VIPergic neurons antagonize this response, and these neurons may be reduced in asthma.
- *Chronic inflammatory response*. Unchecked acute inflammation in the lung proceeds via cytokine release to chronic inflammation, with damage to bronchial epithelium and increased collagen deposition, leading to end-stage irreversible airways disease.

Immunological features

- Activation of mast cells leads to immediate and delayed mediator release and synthesis of cytokines (IL-3, IL-4, IL-5—chemotactic for and stimulatory to eosinophils).
- Lung eosinophilia may be marked, continuing the inflammatory process through the release of cytokines.
- Lymphocytes are recruited and activated, releasing Th2 cytokines and stimulating further IgE production.
- The chronic phase may be considered to include a type IV reaction.

Diagnosis

- The diagnosis is dependent on history and examination. There is frequently an atopic background and a family history of atopic diseases. Wheeze is less common in children, who tend to cough instead.
- Serial peak flow measurements may show the typical asthmatic pattern. Chronic disease may show loss of reversibility and be difficult to distinguish from chronic obstructive pulmonary disease (COPD). Reactive airways may be demonstrated with challenge tests (methacholine—see ➲ Chapter 19).
- A high total IgE makes asthma more likely but does not correlate well with symptoms. A low IgE only excludes IgE-mediated bronchospasm. Skin-prick tests to common aeroallergens may pick up positives, but the history will indicate whether these are relevant clinically.
- There may be an eosinophilia on full blood count, although this is rarely marked and is only present in about 50% of asthmatics; sputum eosinophilia is much more common.
- Other serum markers have been proposed for assessing the severity of disease and adequacy of therapy. These include soluble CD23 (a cytokine involved in IgE production) and eosinophil cationic protein (ECP), which is said to correlate well with the underlying chronic eosinophilic inflammation. These tests are expensive and their role in monitoring remains to be determined.

Asthma 2: treatment

Standard treatment

- The mainstay of treatment remains inhaled short- and long-acting bronchodilators (β_2-agonists, anticholinergics) together with inhaled corticosteroids (SMART regimens).

- The current view of the inflammatory nature of asthma makes the use of inhaled steroids more important in preventing long-term lung damage. β_2-agonists relieve symptoms but have little/no effect on the underlying inflammation. Long-acting beta-2 agonists (LABA), such as salmeterol, may lead to a false sense of security, as symptoms are suppressed, and should be used with care. They may have some intrinsic anti-inflammatory effect.
- Leukotriene antagonists (montelukast) are valuable.
- Courses of oral corticosteroids may be required.
- Sodium cromoglicate inhibits degranulation of connective tissue mast cells only and inhibits the activation of neutrophils, eosinophils, and monocytes. It is most effective in children and in exercise-induced asthma. Nedocromil sodium is similar but inhibits both mucosal and connective-tissue mast cells and is a more potent inhibitor of neutrophils and eosinophils.
- Phosphodiesterase inhibitors (theophyllines) are decreasing in popularity. Intravenous aminophylline is no longer recommended for acute attacks: intravenous magnesium has superseded it.
- Antihistamines have little effect in acute asthma.
- Experimental immunosuppressive therapy with low-dose methotrexate or ciclosporin has been used with success in severe disease.

Immunotherapies

- Omalizumab, a monoclonal anti-IgE, has been shown to be highly beneficial. Use is limited by the degree of elevation of total IgE, and (in the UK) by financial restraints to those with severe asthma (requiring frequent hospital admissions).
- Sublingual allergen immunotherapy (house dust mite) is effective in mild-moderate asthma, with caution.
- Other immunotherapies under evaluation are shown in Table 3.6.

Environmental control

- Environmental control is important both in the home and in the context of occupational asthma.
  - Attempts should be made to reduce house dust-mite exposure by reducing ambient temperature and avoiding high humidity (fewer house plants).

Table 3.6 Immunotherapies for asthma under evaluation

Target	Biologic	Activity
IL-4 & IL-13	Pitrakinra	Mutant IL-4
	Lebrikizumab; tralokinumab	Anti-IL-13
	Dupilumab	Anti-IL-4Rα
IL-5	Mepolizumab; reslizumab	Anti-IL-5
	Benralizumab	Anti-IL-5Rα
Thymic stromal lymphopoietin	Anti-TSLP mAb	Anti-TSLP

- Avoid thick-pile carpets, heavy curtains, and other dust traps.
- Regular vacuuming with a high-efficiency vacuum cleaner (cyclonic or HEPA filter) is necessary (ones that do not spray dust back into the room may be better, although much more expensive).
- Mattress covers are desirable and all bedclothes should be washable (at high temperatures).
- De-miting mattresses is difficult: liquid nitrogen is effective but needs specialist services. Acaricides such as benzyl benzoate may also be effective but may be irritant.
- If animal danders are a problem, the animal should go, although this news is rarely popular with patients!
- Animal removal remains controversial as there is some evidence that early exposure of children to pets in atopic families may reduce rather than increase the chance of developing allergies.

Sulphite sensitivity

Some individuals are unusually sensitive to sulphites. These agents include sulphur dioxide, sodium and potassium metabisulphite, and sulphite. These agents are used widely in foods and drinks as antioxidants and preservatives.

Presentation
- Reactions include severe wheeze accompanied by flushing, tachycardia, and, if severe, may mimic anaphylaxis.
- Urticaria and angioedema are not usually features.

Cause
- Mechanism is unclear but probably involves direct mast-cell stimulation and cholinergic stimulation.
- IgE antibodies have occasionally been detected.
- There does not appear to be any cross-reactivity with other agents.

Diagnosis
- The history is usually diagnostic, with reactions typically to white wine or beer, soft drinks, pickles, salami and preserved meats, dried fruits, shrimps/prawns, and prepared salads.
- Certain drugs for injection contain sulphites, particularly adrenaline-containing local anaesthetics used by dentists.
- No tests are of particular value except for exclusion followed by re-challenge under controlled conditions (with facilities for resuscitation).

Treatment
- Management is by avoidance and proper dietary advice is required.
- Care must be taken with the prescription of drugs.
- Severe reactors may need to carry adrenaline (without sulphites).

Aspirin sensitivity and nasal polyps

Presentation

- Acute angioedema.
- Aspirin is also associated with a triad of asthma, nasal polyposis, and hyperplastic sinusitis (Samter's triad). Each feature can occur without the others.

Cause

- Effect is due to a sensitivity to cyclo-oxygenase (COX) inhibition, and therefore occurs with other NSAIDs but not usually with choline or sodium salicylate or paracetamol.
  - Paracetamol has weak COX-1 inhibitory function and may rarely cause angioedema.
- There is a loss of bronchodilating prostaglandins and a shunting of substrate to the lipo-oxygenase pathway with the production of bronchoconstrictor leukotrienes.
- Some patients with aspirin intolerance also react to tartrazine and related azo-dyes.

Diagnosis

- Specific IgE tests are of uncertain value. Flow-CAST® assay may show positives in some patients (see ➲ Chapter 19).
- Aspirin challenge is not recommended unless there is doubt about the diagnosis, as reactions may be severe.

Treatment

- Exclusion of natural salicylate from the diet may be helpful if asthmatic symptoms and nasal polyps are troublesome.
- Obstructing polyps need to be removed surgically; oral or topical corticosteroids will lead to shrinkage. Regrowth after surgery may be prevented by diet and drug therapy with topical nasal steroids and oral agents.
- Large polyps may need treatment for short periods with betnesol drops, before nasal steroid sprays will be effective. The combination of oral antihistamines and montelukast can be helpful.
- Aspirin desensitization can be undertaken: incremental doses of aspirin are administered over 2 days; tolerance persists only while aspirin is administered regularly. Risks of triggering severe acute asthma are high, and the treatment should be undertaken with ITU back-up.
- Nasal furosemide drops (50 µg per nostril bd) can be very effective in reducing polyp size, if available. Treatment needs to be continued long term. Extemporaneous preparation of the drops by the pharmacy is required.
- Mepolizumab and reslizumab (anti-IL-5) appear to be helpful in persistent nasal polyps, and reduce the need for surgery. Dupilumab (anti-IL-4/IL-13) also appears helpful for nasal polyps.
- Omalizumab may be considered (unlicensed indication).

Allergic rhinitis

Allergic rhinitis needs to be distinguished from non-allergic causes, such as vasomotor rhinitis, rhinitis medicamentosa, and infectious cause. This is not always easy. Timing of symptoms (seasonal versus perennial) will give useful clues. Perennial rhinitis is often due to dust mite allergy: symptoms often worsen in October when windows are shut and the central heating is switched on, as mite numbers increase with rising humidity and temperature. Guidelines on investigation and management have been published in 2017 by EAACI and BSACI.

Causes of rhinitis
- Allergic.
- Vasomotor (autonomic).
- Non-allergic rhinitis with eosinophilia (NARES): may go on to develop asthma.
- Drug-induced: α-agonist nasal sprays, cocaine abuse (direct); antihypertensives (ACE inhibitors, β-blockers); NSAIDs and aspirin, clomethiazole (indirect).
- Hormonal: pregnancy (last trimester), puberty, OCP, HRT, possibly hypothyroidism.
- Irritant: fumes, solvents; alcohol, spicy foods, pepper, sulphites.
- Infectious: viral, bacterial, leprosy, cilial dyskinesia, cystic fibrosis.
- Vasculitis: Wegener's granulomatosis, Churg–Strauss (EGPA).
- Mechanical: nasal polyps, septal deviation, foreign bodies, tumours (lymphoma, melanoma, carcinoma), sarcoidosis.
- Atrophic: following trauma, surgery, radiation.
- CSF leak.
- Idiopathic aspirin sensitivity.

Immunological mechanisms
- Mechanisms in allergic rhinitis are very similar to those described previously for asthma, although histamine release plays a more significant role and the role of neurogenic mechanisms is less well established.
- Histamine and leukotrienes are thought to be responsible for the itch, sneezing, rhinorrhoea, and nasal obstruction, through swelling and hyperaemia.
- There is a predominant eosinophilia in tissue and secretions.
- Perennial rhinitis may be a manifestation of chronic antigen exposure and, like chronic asthma, may lead, via type IV mechanisms, to chronic tissue damage with connective tissue proliferation.
- Allergens involved are similar to those involved in asthma, i.e. aeroallergens, although larger allergens will tend to be trapped preferentially in the nose.
- Nasal polyps may occur as a result of chronic allergic stimulation.

Diagnosis
- Diagnosis relies heavily on the history and on examination of the nose. Rhinoscopy may be necessary to obtain a good view; use of an otoscope is adequate for most purposes.

- Elevated total IgE may indicate an allergic basis, but a normal IgE does not exclude allergy.
- Skin-prick tests (SPTs) demonstrate sensitization to aeroallergens, but the clinical relevance can be determined only from the history.
- Specific IgE (RASTs) should be limited only to confirming equivocal SPTs, or when drugs such as antihistamines cannot be discontinued. Both RASTs and SPTs may be negative even in the presence of significant local allergy if no specific IgE is free to spill over into the bloodstream.
- Examination of nasal secretions for excess eosinophils may be helpful, although there is a condition of NARES. This is often associated with aspirin sensitivity and asthma; sinusitis is also common.
- Peripheral blood eosinophilia is variable and is a poor diagnostic marker.
- If the suspect allergen is available, then nasal provocation tests may be possible (see Part 2).

Treatment

- Topical or systemic antihistamines provide relief in mild cases.
- More severe cases may require topical steroids or mast-cell blocking agents such as sodium cromoglicate or nedocromil sodium. Combined intranasal antihistamine and steroid may be more effective.
- Ipratropium bromide may be particularly helpful in vasomotor rhinitis.
- Ensure patient understands optimum head position for use of nasal sprays: head forward looking at feet, with nozzle pointed away from the nasal septum.
  - ❶Most therapeutic failures are due to incorrect use of sprays!
- Saline washes may be helpful.
- Carbon dioxide washing may be helpful (available over the counter as Serenz).
- Decongestants should be used with caution (or not at all) because of a rebound increase in symptoms.
- Leukotriene antagonists may be beneficial.
- Very severe cases may require courses of oral corticosteroids. Depot injections of long-acting steroid have been used in the past in seasonal rhinitis: these are *not* recommended (risk of avascular necrosis of joints).

Immunotherapies

- If triple drug therapy fails at maximal levels, then immunotherapy may be appropriate if a single allergen is responsible and there are no contraindications such as severe asthma, pregnancy, β-blockers, or ischaemic heart disease. This should only be undertaken through specialist centres. Results for seasonal (grasses, tree pollens) and perennial allergens (house dust mite) are excellent. Immunotherapy to animal allergens is more variable in effect. Sublingual (tablets or drops) or subcutaneous therapies are both effective. In the UK few products are licensed. Combination allergens are available from some manufacturers. *Ad hoc* extemporaneous mixtures prepared by allergists are not supported, due to difficulties in standardization.
- There is some concern that sublingual therapies could potentially be a trigger for eosinophilic oesophagitis.

- Surgery may be required for sinus involvement and for polyps, if topical steroid therapy fails to reduce them.

Environmental control
- Environmental control may be important as an adjunctive measure. Avoidance of allergens where possible should be tried.
- In the grass-pollen season, avoid opening windows more than necessary during the day (especially in the afternoon and evening when pollen count is high).
- Air filtration systems able to trap pollens are available for cars and for houses, although the latter are expensive to install. Masks are likely to be of little value.
- Cold air, alcohol, and spicy foods may exacerbate symptoms in vasomotor rhinitis.

Allergic conjunctivitis

Allergic conjunctivitis often accompanies rhinitis (the two areas are connected by the lacrimal ducts). The mechanisms are identical.

Presentation
- Typical features include itching and watering of the eye, with redness and swelling.
- More extreme forms include vernal conjunctivitis, in which giant papillae are seen on the tarsal surface of the eyelid. In this condition the allergic component is a trigger. This disease is difficult to treat but may burn out after 5–10 years.

Diagnosis
- As for rhinitis.
- Specific IgE may be detected in tears but it is rarely of value as a diagnostic test.
- Challenge tests may be helpful in very rare circumstances.

Treatment
- Topical antihistamines and mast-cell stabilizing agents (sodium cromoglicate and nedocromil) may help to relieve symptoms. Lodoxamide is another mast-cell stabilizer specifically available for allergic eye problems.
- Oral antihistamines are valuable for more severe symptoms.
- Topical steroids may be very valuable but should only be prescribed under ophthalmological supervision, as long-term use may lead to glaucoma and cataract.
- Short-course oral steroids may be used for severe symptoms unresponsive to topical treatment, and may be used to cover periods of exams, etc.
- Topical ciclosporin and NSAIDs (flurbiprofen and diclofenac) have also been used successfully in vernal conjunctivitis.
- Immunotherapy (either injected or sublingual) is often valuable; vernal conjunctivitis however responds less well.

Sinusitis

Causes
- Allergy, with secondary infection due to allergic swelling closing off the drainage ostia. Usually associated with other allergic features.
- Primary infective: due to mechanical drainage problem; secondary to humoral immune deficiency.
- Aspirin intolerance.
- Ethmoiditis in children may mimic conjunctivitis.
- Inflammatory disease such as Wegener's granulomatosis and midline granuloma.
- Chronic fungal sinusitis is recognized by ENT specialists, even in the absence of immune deficiency.

Presentation
- Usually obvious with pain over sinuses.
- Maxillary sinusitis may also present as dental pain in upper molars.

Diagnosis
- Plain radiographs not recommended; CT scanning is most sensitive.
- Nasal smears will demonstrate eosinophilia if there is an allergic cause, but neutrophilia will be present in infective cases.
- Measurement of humoral immune function (immunoglobulins, IgG subclasses, and specific antibodies) and antineutrophil cytoplasmic antibodies (ANCA) should be considered in chronic sinusitis.

Treatment
- Treat underlying cause.
- Obstructed sinuses can be washed out. This can be done by an endoscopic procedure that allows the sinuses to be inspected.
- Nasal decongestants and topical steroids assist in reducing oedema and promoting free drainage.
- Antibiotics are required for infective problems. *Haemophilus influenzae* and pneumococcus are the most common organisms. Ciprofloxacin, clarithromycin, and azithromycin are appropriate as they penetrate well into sinus fluids.
- If all else fails—try a prolonged course of an oral antifungal such as itraconazole.

Secretory otitis media (glue ear)

It has been suggested that this is related to underlying allergy but there is little evidence for this in children, unless there is allergic disease elsewhere in the respiratory tract. Rarely, it may be related to specific antibody deficiency or a more widespread antibody deficiency. The history will reveal if there are other infective problems that would suggest such a diagnosis.

Atopic eczema (dermatitis)

Atopic eczema is the most common manifestation of atopic disease. It is usually worst in childhood, improving with age in 80%. It affects particularly the cheeks and flexures and is a risk factor for the development of contact dermatitis in later life. Asthma or rhinitis will develop in 50–75% of patients. It is on the increase. Eye involvement may occur, with an atopic keratoconjunctivitis, and in severe cases subcapsular cataract may form.

Causes

- There is a genetic basis, as demonstrated by twin studies, although whether the background is the same as for asthma (chromosome 11 or 5) has not yet been demonstrated.
- In addition to the immunological factors, there are abnormalities of the lipids of the skin and evidence for autonomic nervous abnormalities (white dermographism). There is a reduced threshold for itch, which leads to a vicious cycle of itch and scratch, leading to the lichenification of chronic eczema.
- Non-specific irritants make the disease worse, such as wool, heat, and stress.
- Staphylococcal infection is common, and may play a role in exacerbating the disease: IgE against the bacterium may be detected, although the role is unclear. Staphylococcal superantigens have also been suggested to play a role. Cutaneous fungi may also exacerbate the disease.
- Role of diet is controversial. It has been suggested that maternal diet during pregnancy may contribute, as may a lack of breastfeeding. The contribution of diet to established symptoms is even more controversial, although some children are helped by exclusion diets. It is rare that adults are helped by dietary manoeuvres.

Immunological features

- Precise role of type I responses is unclear. IgE levels are often very high, and specific IgE may be detected against a variety of aero- and food allergens, although most of the IgE is 'junk', with no recognizable specificity.
- Langerhans cells in the skin do have IgE receptors, although their role in atopic eczema is speculative. Keratinocytes release cytokines when damaged, which will excite the immune response (TNFα, IL-1, IL-6, IL-8).
- There is more evidence for a type IV reaction with an infiltrate of CD4$^+$ T cells into the epidermis and dermis; most of these cells are of the Th2 phenotype which will support IgE production. As part of the inflammatory response, eosinophils, mast cells, and basophils are all increased in the affected skin, and mechanisms similar to those found in the chronic phase of asthma probably predominate.

Diagnosis

- Blood eosinophilia is common.
- 80% of cases will have a high IgE, often > 1000 kU/l. Specific IgE may be detected by SPT or RAST, but this rarely helps in management.

- Atypical patterns of eczema with other infections should raise the possibility of hyper-IgE syndrome. Here the IgE is even higher, usually > 50 000 kU/l, and there may be evidence of other humoral abnormalities such as low IgG_2, so a full investigation of humoral immunity is warranted.
- Viral infections such as eczema herpeticum, molluscum contagiosum, and warts are common in atopic eczema and do not indicate a significant generalized immunodeficiency, but are a manifestation of disturbed local immunity.

Treatment
- Reduce itch by the use of emollients and antihistamines, inflammation by the use of topical steroids, and staphylococcal superinfection by the use of appropriate oral antibiotics.
- Ciclosporin is helpful in severe disease as a temporary measure but the disease relapses as soon as the drug is withdrawn. Topical agents, tacrolimus and pimecrolimus, may be effective and do not have the same adverse effects as steroids.
- PUVA.
- Dupilumab, which blocks both IL-4 and IL-13, has been shown to be effective.
- A Cochrane review in 2016 did not find any good-quality evidence to support the use of allergen-specific immunotherapy in atopic eczema.
- High-dose IVIg has also been shown to be beneficial in resistant cases.
- Theoretically, γ-interferon should be helpful, by reducing the Th2 predominance, and this has been borne out in several small trials.
- Where babies, by virtue of a strong family history, are at risk of developing atopic eczema, avoidance of cows' milk for the first 6 months of life and late weaning may be helpful. The additions of γ-linoleic acid and fish oil have been suggested to be helpful; the evidence from controlled trials is less supportive.
- Avoidance of egg, milk, or wheat may help some children. In adults if there is concern over the contribution of food, then a 2-week trial of an elimination diet will identify whether food is contributing.

Contact dermatitis (hypersensitivity)

Presentation
- Contact hypersensitivity is a localized type IV reaction due to contact with a triggering allergen. Reaction is eczematous, often with blistering and weeping. The pattern of rash together with a careful exposure history usually identifies possible allergens.
- It needs to be distinguished from straightforward irritant dermatitis due to a localized toxic effect that does not involve the immune system. Typical irritants are solvents, acids, alkalis, and other chemicals. The skin has a limited number of ways in which it can respond, and the appearance of irritant and allergic dermatitis can be clinically similar.

Causes
- Many topically applied compounds can cause DTH reactions.
  - Nickel allergy often leads to dermatitis affecting the ear lobes, under the back of watches, and where jean studs press on the skin. Those regularly handling coins will get hand eczema. This is the commonest contact dermatitis.
  - Aniline dyes in leather cause dermatitis affecting the feet and where leather belts come in contact with skin.
  - Chromium: hand eczema, usually in those handling cement.
  - Cobalt: used as a stabilizer for the head on beer!
  - Latex and synthetic rubbers: related to chemical accelerators and hardeners (thiurams, mercapto compounds, carbamates); there is no evidence that latex proteins themselves cause type IV reactions.
  - Hair dyes (PPD, henna), formaldehyde (perming lotions).
  - Fragrances and cosmetics (biocides, phenylenediamine, parabens).
  - Topical antibiotics (gentamicin, neomycin, bacitracin, benzocaines).
  - Antiseptics: these may cause both irritant and allergic contact dermatitis.
  - Colophony (rosin) and other resins (adhesives in plasters).
  - Ivy, sumac tree, chrysanthemum, feverfew, primula (gardeners).
- Some allergens require concomitant exposure to sunlight for the effect to develop; rash only develops on sun-exposed areas of contact.
  - Plants: limes, lemons, figs, giant hogweed, pine wood.
  - Drugs, including sulfonamides, tetracylines, and phenothiazines; sunscreens (p-aminobenzoic acid, oil of bergamot).

Immunology
- Types I and IV hypersensitivity may coexist.
- In most cases the allergens are low molecular weight substances that penetrate the skin readily and lead to neoantigen formation. As with all T-lymphocyte-mediated responses, sensitization precedes reactivity.
- Active lesions show a sparse CD4+ T-lymphocytic infiltrate but few eosinophils.

Diagnosis
- The history and examination give the most important information.
- This should be supplemented by patch testing (see ➲ Chapter 19).
- SPT and measurement of total IgE are of little value.

Treatment
- This should be undertaken by a dermatologist.
- Antihistamines may be needed to control itch.
- Wet compresses may be required for weeping eczema.
- Potent topical steroids accompanied by avoidance of the offending agents usually lead to resolution.
- Low-nickel diets may be tried for those with proven type IV sensitivity to nickel and oral symptoms.

Food allergy 1

Food allergy causes more trouble than any other aspect of immunology. Foods are blamed by the general population for a multitude of sins. However, the public perception of food allergy is not reflected by its true incidence when large-scale population studies are undertaken. True food additive intolerance is very rare (< 0.23% of the population) when those claiming to be intolerant are formally tested. Food allergy (in which IgE is involved) must be distinguished from food intolerance, which may have a variety of causes, and from psychogenic causes.

Symptoms of true food allergy are invariably limited to the gut, the skin, and the respiratory tract. Symptoms outside these systems are much less likely to be due to true allergy. There is no convincing association with arthritis. There is no evidence that food allergy is a cause of chronic fatigue syndromes (see ➋ Chapter 14), and thus 'desensitization' therapies have nothing to offer; equally there is no evidence to support *Candida* overgrowth as a cause of CFS.

Causes—true food allergy

- True food allergy is very real and may be severe (see ➋ 'Anaphylaxis', pp. 130–36). It is most common in children (up to 0.5% may be allergic to cows' milk). Almost any food can cause true allergy mediated via IgE.
- Most allergens involved in food allergy are heat stable (resisting cooking) and acid stable (resisting stomach acid). There are exceptions to this, so that a food will be allergenic cooked but not raw or vice versa: these foods are typically fruit and vegetables.
- Cows' milk allergy is common, especially in children under 5 years. The proteins responsible for the allergic response include β-lactoglobulin, α-lactalbumin, casein, bovine serum albumin, and bovine immunoglobulins. Often the response is against more than one antigen. This allergy usually disappears by the age of 5 years. Rarely, gastrointestinal haemorrhage may result (Heiner's syndrome: cows' milk intolerance accompanied by iron-deficiency anaemia and pulmonary haemosiderosis).
- Egg, milk, and wheat allergies are common in the under-fives, and often disappear with age, although anaphylactic responses may occur. The major antigens are ovomucoid and ovalbumin. Cross-reaction with chicken meat is unusual.
- Fish allergy may be severe, such that inhalation of allergens in the vapour from cooking fish or second-hand contact (e.g. kissing someone who has eaten fish) may be enough to trigger reactions. The allergens are species-specific in 50% and cross-reactive with all fish in the remainder. Fish allergy is usually permanent. Similar constraints apply to shellfish, both crustacea (prawns, crabs, and lobster) and molluscs (mussels, scallops, and oysters).
- The legumes, peanuts and soya, are major causes of severe allergic reactions. These agents cause major problems because they are widely used as food 'fillers' and may not be declared on labels. Avoidance may be difficult. Sensitization is often extreme, such that small amounts of residual protein in peanut (groundnut) oil may be enough to trigger

reactions. Sensitization may occur through the use of groundnut oil in formula milks. Arachis oil (groundnut oil) is used as a carrier in certain intramuscular injections. True nuts may be equally troublesome. These reactions are often lifelong, although a proportion of children who develop peanut allergy early in life may grow out of it (oral challenge required).

- Cereals may cause direct allergic responses if ingested or cause symptoms via gluten intolerance (coeliac disease). Flour also causes baker's asthma as an occupational disease. Wheat, barley, and rye are all closely related. Symptoms are less extreme and this is hypothesized to be due to proteolysis reducing the allergenicity, although why this does not apply to other foods is unclear. Rice and maize allergies are rare.
- Oral allergy syndrome (see ➲ 'Oral allergy syndrome', p. 165 for more detailed discussion), where there is allergy to pollens and cross-reactive food allergies (usually non-anaphylactic). Allergens tend to be heat-labile.
  - Birch-pollen allergy with allergy to hazelnut, apple, pear, and carrot.
  - Birch pollen allergy with stone fruits (plums, peaches, cherries, almonds).
  - Ragweed allergy with melon, banana.
  - Grass pollen allergy with tomato, melon.
  - Mugwort pollen allergy with celery, carrots, spices (includes vermouth!).
- Other described associations include latex with banana, avocado, kiwi fruit, chestnut, lettuce, pineapple, and papaya.
- Occasionally trace contaminants may be responsible for allergy, as in the case of antibiotics in meat (used by farmers to improve the animals' weight gain), which may lead to reactions to meat and to therapeutic drugs.
- Concomitant administration of proton-pump inhibitors and H_2-blockers, which reduce stomach acid, may increase allergenicity of foods.

Causes—food intolerance
True food allergy must be distinguished from food intolerance, which takes many forms.
- Pharmacological: caffeine and theobromine (tachycardias in heavy tea/coffee drinkers), tyramine (headaches, hypertension in patients on MAOIs), alcohol (obvious symptoms, plus beer drinkers' diarrhoea), NSAIDs (may include natural salicylates), figs (laxatives).
- Toxic: scombrotoxin (histamine from spoiled mackerel), green potatoes (solanins), flavotoxins (peanuts), lectins (PHA in undercooked kidney beans), food poisoning (*Bacillus cereus* (fried rice), staphylococcal toxins), monosodium glutamate (headaches, nausea, and sweating—Chinese restaurant syndrome).
- Enzyme deficiencies: lactase deficiency (common in Asians; diarrhoea due to laxative effect of lactose), also sucrase and maltase deficiency.
- Fructose intolerance: excess undigested fructose causes diarrhoea, abdominal cramp, and bloating; high levels in dried fruits, onions, peppers, some sports drinks, and fruit juices.

- Other bowel disease: Crohn's disease, coeliac disease, infections (*Giardia*, *Yersinia*), bacterial overgrowth (in association with reduced motility, e.g. systemic sclerosis), 'irritable bowel syndrome' (other causes must be excluded).
- Pancreatic insufficiency: cystic fibrosis, Shwachman's syndrome (see ➲ Chapter 1).
- Psychogenic: 'smells', somatization disorder.

Food allergy 2: immunological mechanisms, diagnosis, and treatment

Immunological mechanisms

- For true allergic reactions pre-sensitization is required. The bowel contains a specific subset of mast cells (MC_T), which are capable of being armed by IgE. Activated T cells are also present. The pattern of reactions is probably very similar to that in mechanisms involving mast cells in other sites, although it is less well studied because of inaccessibility.
- Abnormalities of mucosal immunity may contribute to the generation of IgE antibodies to foods. IgA deficiency may be a predisposing factor to allergic disease in general and also to coeliac disease, although cause-and-effect has not been proven beyond reasonable doubt. Exposure of an immature mucosal immune system may also be a factor; hence the lower rates of food allergy in babies breastfed and weaned late.
- It has been suggested that some of the slower-onset food reactions may involve type III (immune complex reactions): this is difficult to prove as IgG anti-food antibodies are not uncommon in healthy individuals. Publications indicating that irritable bowel disease is associated with IgG anti-food antibodies need to be viewed with caution. Current understanding of IBS suggests that disturbance of the microbiome of the gut plays a significant role.

Diagnosis

- The history may give good clues about particular foods that cause problems.
- Skin-prick tests are helpful for foods causing severe reactions (milk, egg, fish, peanuts, true nuts), while being less useful for other food groups.
- If commercial reagents do not work, then the fresh food should be tried (stab lancet into food then into patient). However, SPT to fresh foods may be dangerous in those who have had severe anaphylactic reactions. Dose is unstandardized.
- RAST tests are less sensitive.
- Total IgE is not especially helpful.
- The allergy practitioner will need to have a good understanding of the biological families in which plants are grouped, as this often helps explain patterns of reactivity: members of the same biological family often share common antigens.

- Dietary manipulation plays an important role in diagnosis, but is time-consuming and should be undertaken only in collaboration with a dietician. Elimination diets (oligoallergenic diets), with gradual reintroduction of foods in an open but controlled manner, may be helpful in identifying troublesome foods. Formal confirmation requires a double-blind placebo-controlled food challenge, in which the suspect food is disguised in opaque gelatine capsules or, if bland, in another tolerated food.
- Differentiation of food intolerance requires careful history-taking. Patients should be investigated for evidence of malabsorption (iron, vitamin B_{12}, folate, clotting, calcium, and alkaline phosphatase) and for coeliac disease (endomysial or tissue transglutaminase antibodies); if there is diarrhoea, do stool microscopy and culture. Acute-phase proteins and faecal calprotectin will indicate likely inflammatory bowel disease.
- Bacterial overgrowth, lactose intolerance, and pancreatic insufficiency can be diagnosed on appropriate radioisotopic tests or by measuring breath hydrogen production. Lactose intolerance can be identified using a modified oral tolerance test similar to a glucose tolerance test but substituting lactose for glucose. In lactase deficiency the normal rise in blood glucose is abolished. Faecal elastase is a useful test of pancreatic exocrine function.
- Radiology of the bowel may be revealing and biopsy should always be considered: enzyme levels can be measured and coeliac disease confirmed rapidly. In early coeliac disease, histology may show only a lymphocytic infiltrate without complete villous atrophy.

Treatment

- Distinguish food allergy from intolerance and non-food-related symptoms.
- Education of the patient about their symptoms and the cause. This may be hard if the patient already has a well-established preconception that he/she has a 'food allergy'.
- Management of food allergy is mainly avoidance, while maintaining a nutritious diet: specialist dietetic support is required.
- Antihistamines (H_1 and H_2) may be of value taken prophylactically when patients with true food allergy are eating in unfamiliar surrounding; routine use is unnecessary.
- Patients who have had anaphylaxis need to have adrenaline for self-injection.
- Oral sodium cromoglicate may help occasional patients.
- Short course of steroids may be necessary for severe disease (eosinophilic gastropathy, enteritis; see ➲ Chapter 7).
- Enzyme-potentiated desensitization (EPD) is not of proven value despite claims by some practitioners to the contrary.
- Management of food intolerance depends on the underlying cause.
- The Anaphylaxis Campaign provides useful information and support. ⌕ https://www.anaphylaxis.org.uk/

Contact allergy to food

Causes

Contact reactions to food may be due to:

- Irritant dermatitis:
  - Citrus juices.
  - Mustard family.
  - Corn (usually farmers and processing workers).
  - Pineapple (bromelin)—proteolytic enzyme.
  - Spices.
  - Chilli peppers—capsaicin.
- Allergic contact dermatitis (common in chefs). Includes (non-exhaustive list):
  - Mango sap (and related foods: cashew).
  - Mustard family.
  - Olive oil.
  - Citrus fruits.
  - Artichoke.
  - Asparagus.
  - Celery family (carrots, parsley, parsnip).
  - Garlic.
  - Spices (cinnamon especially).
- Contact urticaria:
  - Immunological or non-immunological.
- Phototoxic or photo-allergic dermatitis.
- Photoxic reactions mainly due to psoralens, e.g. celery family, citrus family (mixing or drinking Margaritas!).
- Photoallergic reactions are rare—mainly garlic.

Immunology and diagnosis

- History of exposure and type of rash is crucial.
- Patch testing may be useful.
- Photopatch testing may be required.

Oral allergy syndrome

The oral allergy syndrome (OAS) is caused by IgE to heat-labile allergens in fruits. These are highly cross-reactive. Symptoms are *usually* mild and restricted to oropharynx (itching and local swelling).

Immunology and diagnosis

- Standard commercial skin-prick test solutions and *in vitro* specific IgE tests do not reliably identify the allergy, as the antigens are labile.
- The use of recombinant allergens may help.
- May be linked to pollen allergies (Birch, Bet v1, Bet v2).
- Direct skin-prick testing with fresh fruits/vegetables may be helpful.
- Knowledge of the cross-reacting families is helpful (Table 3.7).
- Full details of key allergens can be found at: ℘ http://www.phadia.com/en-GB/allergens.

Table 3.7 Main cross-reacting families and key allergens

Allergen group	Key foods	Key allergens
PR-10 (Bet v1 homologues)—associated with pollen allergies to hazel, alder, birch Allergens are heat labile—symptoms will be typical OAS; commonest cause of reactions to fruit and vegetables in Northern Europe	Hazelnut Rosacea family fruits (apple, almond, apricot, cherry, peach, pear, raspberry, strawberry) Carrot, celery, parsley Peanut Soya bean Asparagus Potato, pepper Mango Melon	Cor a1 Ara h8 Gly m4
Non-specific lipid transfer proteins (nsLTPs). Heat stable. Reactions are more severe and often systemic. Commonest in southern Europe	Hazelnut Rosacea (as for PR-10) Carrot, parsley Asparagus Cabbage, turnip Castor bean Oil seed rape Grape Sunflower, lettuce Wheat, barley, maize, rice Lemon Peanut Tomato Walnut	Cor a8 Ara h9
Profilins (Bet v2). Highly cross-reactive, heat labile allergens	Hazelnut Rosacea (as for PR-10) Asparagus Banana Rice, wheat Potato, tomato, pepper Carrot, celery, parsley Mango Melon Peanut Soya bean Sunflower Sesame Oil seed rape Walnut Pineapple	Cor a2 Ara h5 Gly m3

Allergen group	Key foods	Key allergens
Storage proteins (albumins, vicilins, legumins). Heat stable. Associated with severe reactions. Polysensitization common	Peanut	Ara h1, h2, h3
	Other legumes	
	Lupin	
	Tree nuts (Brazil nut, walnut, pecan, almond, hazelnut)	
	Cashew, pistachio	
	Sesame	
	Sunflower	
	Mustard, turnip	
	Buckwheat	
Cross-reactive carbohydrate determinants (CCDs). IgE may not give rise to clinical symptoms		

Treatment
- Careful dietary review is required: patients need to be made aware of potential cross-reactions.
- For heat labile allergens, cooked fruits are usually not a problem. For fresh fruits (apples) 10–15 seconds in a microwave on full power is usually enough to destroy the allergens (which are concentrated under the skin).
- An estimate of the likelihood of severe reactions needs to be made (requires adrenaline for self-injection).
- Typical OAS patients require only standby antihistamines + prednisolone (cetirizine 20 mg chewed + prednisolone 20 mg as stat dose).

Risk stratification and role of food challenge
An increasing problem for adult allergists is the question of whether young adults with a childhood history of nut/peanut allergy have outgrown their allergy. This may have employment implications (e.g. entry into the Armed Forces).
- The use of recombinant peanut allergens may provide prognostic information:
  - Positivity for rAra h2 is associated with risk of severe systemic reactions.
  - Positivity for rAra h8 is associated with localized OAS symptoms.
- Food challenges with graded exposure may be required to confirm reactivity.

Desensitization to foods
- Desensitization to peanut using peanut flour has been used with success.
- The identification of key allergens will lead to suitable immunotherapeutic vaccines becoming available in the near future.
- Anti-IgE therapy (omalizumab) may be valuable as sole or adjunctive therapy.

Latex allergy

Latex allergy is an increasing problem in hospitals, mainly triggered by the massive increase in latex glove usage during the 1980s when AIDS was identified. Up to 20% of staff in high glove-usage areas (theatres, ITU) may become sensitized to latex.

Presentation

- Type I reactions occur with anaphylaxis, asthma, angioedema, rhinoconjunctivitis, and contact urticaria.
- Typical reactions occur with gloves, condoms, and new elasticated clothing.
- Range of latex-containing domestic and medical products is very large.
- Cross-reaction to foods is frequent: bananas, avocado, kiwi fruit, potato, tomato, chestnut, lettuce, pineapple, papaya.
- Type IV reactions occur due to plasticizers used in the manufacture (not latex), and cause a localized dermatitis.

Cause

- Type I reactions develop against a range of proteins present in the latex.

Immunology and diagnosis

- Current specific IgE tests (RAST) identify only 85% of allergic patients.
- Recombinant allergens are now available (see Box 3.1).
- SPT with commercial latex solutions (preferably from two different manufacturers) identifies 96% of allergic patients.
- A proportion of patients have clear histories of reactions on exposure, but no positive tests. Challenge tests may be required: blind glove challenge (in a box), open glove challenge, and SPT with prick through a glove have all been used.
- Type IV reactions are identified by patch testing.

Management

- For type I reactions avoidance is required. This requires education of patient and employers.
- Occupational issues are difficult, especially in the Health Service.

Box 3.1 Recombinant latex allergens
rHev b1*
rHev b3*
rHev b5*
rHev b6.01*
rHev b6.02*
rHev b8 (latex profilin)
rHev b9
rHev b11

* Associated with high risk of severe reactions.

- Latex is a substance identified in the Control of Substances Hazardous to Health (COSHH) regulations as hazardous to health. Employers are therefore required by law to minimize exposure and carry out risk assessments where latex is used. Employees have successfully sued for large sums of money where this has not been carried out.
- Latex-allergic patients often develop an anxiety-depression related to their inability to avoid latex and subsequent reactions: support from psychologists is required.
- Attendance at A & E is often difficult. Consideration of management of anaphylaxis away from hospital, including self-administration of hydrocortisone, may be desirable.
- The Anaphylaxis Campaign can provide support and advice (℡ https://www.anaphylaxis.org.uk/).
- Pharmacy will advise on latex content of drugs: latex is used in bungs in drug vials.
- Supplies departments should be able to access information on the latex content of hospital products.
- Hospitals should keep identified boxes of latex-free equipment in key areas (theatres, A & E, Medical Admissions).
- All employers are required by the Health and Safety Executive to have policies on latex. The HSE Website contains further advice: ℡ http://www.hse.gov.uk/skin/employ/latex.htm. Hospitals should also have a specific risk management committee to review these policies for staff and patients.

Drug allergy 1: penicillin, other antibiotics, and insulin

Drugs may cause allergic reactions due to all four mechanisms of hypersensitivity, or combinations thereof. For example, penicillin may cause anaphylaxis (type I), a haemolytic anaemia (type II), serum sickness (type III), and interstitial nephritis (type IV). As noted previously, drugs may also cause reactions through other mechanisms, such as direct histamine release (opiates, radiocontrast media), undue sensitivity to the pharmacological effect (NSAIDs), and direct complement activation. Drug fever may be the primary manifestation of an adverse reaction to antibiotics. This may be difficult to detect when the drug is an antibiotic being used to treat an infective condition, where the reappearance of fever may lead to further investigation for an infective focus. The CRP will also be elevated during a drug fever.

Penicillin allergy
- Penicillin allergy is very common, perhaps occurring in up to 8% of treatment courses. Most of the reactions are trivial. Severe reactions are rare and occur mainly after parenteral administration.
- Occasional patients react on apparent first exposure and it has been suggested that sensitization may occur through antibiotics occurring in food.
- All evidence suggests that patients with vague/poor histories of reactions to penicillin in childhood (usually non-specific rashes) have a very low probability of true allergy.

- All four types of Gell and Coombs' hypersensitivity reactions may occur with penicillin, together with reactions of uncertain aetiology such as Stevens–Johnson syndrome.
- There are major antigenic determinants (benzylpenicilloyl nucleus) and minor determinants (benzylpenicillin, benzylpenicilloate, and others), although both are capable of causing severe immediate reactions.
  - Currently available tests (RAST and SPT/IDT) detect only major determinants, although benzylpenicillin may detect some minor-determinant-only reactions if suitably diluted and used for SPT.
- Tests for IgE (i.e. RAST and SPT) have no predictive value for other types of reactions. Up to 3% of SPT-negative patients may subsequently have reactions, although the reaction rate falls if both major and all minor antigens are used for testing. Some recent studies have claimed very few false-negative results with SPT. Conversely, not all SPT-positive patients will react when subsequently challenged.
- There have been difficulties in obtaining skin test reagents containing minor determinants, which makes accurate testing difficult.
- Up to 75% of patients who have had a reaction to penicillin will tolerate the drug subsequently. This probably applies to patients with non-specific reactions of dubious allergic aetiology (nausea, vomiting, diarrhoea) but more care should be taken in patients with a history of angioedema, Stevens–Johnson syndrome, etc. A previous confirmed Stevens–Johnson reaction is a contraindication to challenge testing including IDT.
- There is a high level of cross-reactivity with other semisynthetic penicillins with a β-lactam ring, such as the carbapenems and the monobactams (up to 50% in the case of imipenem), for IgE-mediated reactions.
- Cephalosporins and cephacarbams also cross-react, but at a lower level: up to 5.6% of penicillin-allergic (SPT positive) patients may also react to cephalosporins. Older figures are higher, but may relate to first-generation cephalosporins. Anaphylaxis to cephalosporins is said to be very unlikely if there are no responses to major or minor determinants of penicillin. In some cases the IgE is directed not at the nucleus but at the side-chain, which may be shared between a penicillin and a cephalosporin (e.g. aztreonam and ceftazidime).
- The specific morbilliform rash associated with the administration of amoxicillin to patients with acute EBV infection does not indicate a likelihood of subsequent true penicillin allergy.

Management
- The management of the penicillin-allergic patient depends on obtaining a clear history from the patient.
- For patients with severe reactions, avoidance is the best course, including other semisynthetic β-lactam antibiotics.
- If penicillin or equivalent is essential, rush desensitization schedules may be used, although there is a high risk of reactions, for which supportive therapy will be required. The desensitization must be followed by the treatment course and there is no lasting tolerance. Desensitization should *not* be attempted in those who have had a Stevens–Johnson reaction.

- NICE guidelines recommend testing where there is an absolute requirement for use of a penicillin, where there is a chronic condition requiring frequent courses of antibiotics, and where there are multiple antibiotic allergies/intolerances.

Other antibiotics

- Little is written about true allergy to other antibiotics.
- Patients with AIDS have a very high reaction rate to trimethoprim–sulfamethoxazole (co-trimoxazole). This has been associated with IgE to a derivative of the sulfamethoxazole.
- Abnormal metabolism with generation of toxic intermediates has been proposed as a mechanism for the generation of erythema multiforme and Stevens–Johnson syndrome. Cross-reactivity to sulfonamides may also affect other drugs that are closely related such as furosemide, hydrochlorothiazide, and captopril.
- Skin-prick and intradermal testing can be carried out where reactions are suggestive of a type I reaction (but *not* if the reaction is Stevens–Johnson).

Insulin allergy

- Insulin allergy may occur due to changes in the tertiary structure of insulin engendered in the manufacturing process for human insulin, or previously due to the sequence differences in bovine and porcine insulin, with the production of IgE antibodies. These do not recognize natural human insulin.
- Other components such as protamine and zinc may also cause allergic reactions.
- There is urticaria at the site of injections and frequently induration. Rarely, systemic reactions occur.
- Treatment is difficult: local reaction may be amenable to the prophylactic use of antihistamines or the inclusion of a tiny dose of hydrocortisone (1–5 mg) with the insulin.
- 'Desensitization' regimens have been used where there are major problems and diabetic control has failed.
- Skin testing with a range of insulins may be appropriate: desensitization may be undertaken with the least reactive.

Drug allergy 2: anaesthetic allergy, diagnosis and treatment of drug allergies, and drug-induced Stevens–Johnson syndrome

Anaesthetic allergy

- The major difficulty of the investigation of anaesthetic reactions is that multiple drugs are administered nearly simultaneously.

- Patients suffering an acute reaction to anaesthetics should be referred to a specialist centre for investigation (the Royal College of Anaesthetists has produced guidelines on management for anaesthetists).
- Confirmation of the reaction at the time requires a blood sample for mast cell tryptase, complement C3 and C4, and albumin (for calculation of dilutional effects).
- Complex regimes of serial blood sampling have been recommended: these are impractical and add nothing to the subsequent investigation.
- Measurement of specific IgE at the time of the reaction is unhelpful, as a negative result may be due to consumption.
- Detailed anaesthetic records must be forwarded to the drug allergy testing unit.
- Some of the drugs used (opiate derivatives) are capable of inducing mast-cell degranulation, while solvents such as cremophor, used to dissolve lipophilic drugs, may activate the complement system.
- Problems of severe reactions peroperatively may also arise from synthetic plasma expanders and blood products and in patients with unrecognized (or ignored) sensitivity to latex. Chlorhexidine and other antiseptics (octenidine, polyhexamide) are increasingly recognized as causes of anaphylaxis.
- There is extensive cross-reactivity between the neuromuscular blocking agents; prior exposure is not necessary (possibly cross-reaction with microbial products or prior exposure to the over-the-counter cough suppressant pholcodine).
- RAST tests for specific IgE are currently limited commercially to suxamethonium and thiopental, although research centres may have tests for IgE to other agents.
- SPT and intradermal testing are necessary to identify causative agents and identify safe alternatives.
- Challenge testing should only be carried out with full resuscitation facilities to hand.
- Guidance on testing is detailed in Chapter 19.

Local anaesthetics

- Local anaesthetics may cause both type I and type IV reactions, so a careful history is required to identify the nature of the reaction and guide subsequent testing.
- IgE-mediated allergy to local anaesthetics is exceedingly rare.
- Overdose of local anaesthetic may cause significant adverse reactions; it is essential to exclude this possibility.
- Inadvertent intravenous administration may give rise to non-specific symptoms: these are not due to allergy and do not contraindicate further use.
- Vasovagal reactions need to be identified.
- Local anaesthetics divide into two groups: group I are the benzoic acid esters, including benzocaine and procaine; group II are the amides, including lidocaine, bupivacaine, and prilocaine. There is little cross-reactivity between the two groups, but there is often cross-reactivity within the groups.
- Local anaesthetics may contain sulphites (particularly if adrenaline is present) and other preservatives such as parabens, which may cause adverse reactions in their own right.

- Articaine appears to be the local anaesthetic least likely to cause reactions and is the drug of choice where there is doubt about previous reaction history.

Diagnosis
- Diagnosis of drug reactions requires a good history.
- For tests, see Table 3.8.
- Investigation of an acute reaction requires confirmation of the nature of the reaction.
- Ideally, it should be possible to measure complement breakdown products (C3d, C3a, C5a) and urinary methylhistamine but, due to the withdrawal of appropriate commercial assays and the need for usually unobtainable stabilizers in blood tubes (Futhan–EDTA), these additional tests are not usually done.
- Some authorities recommend complex time schedules for blood sampling post-reaction. These are impractical and never adhered to; if the lab gets one post-reaction clotted sample it has done well!
- Reliable specific IgE tests are available to only a few drugs (thiopental, suxamethonium, major determinants of penicillin).
- Skin-prick testing followed by intradermal testing is required (see ➲ Chapter 19 for suggested protocols).
- Challenge tests are of more value but are time-consuming and potentially dangerous.

Treatment
- Treatment of all drug reactions involves immediate cessation of the drug and, if the reaction is severe, resuscitation as for anaphylaxis (see ➲ 'Anaphylaxis', pp. 130–36).
- Appropriate warnings should be incorporated into the notes.
- Patients must be informed of the cause of their reaction and, if it is thought likely to recur, then they should be advised to wear a Medic-Alert bracelet or equivalent.

Table 3.8 Testing for drug allergies

Immediate tests	Later tests
Mast cell tryptase, C3, C4, as soon after the reaction as possible and at 24 hours	Refer to immunologist/allergist for investigation
Serum albumin	Specific IgE, SPT and intradermal testing: Flow-CAST; drug challenge (DBPC)

Drug-induced Stevens–Johnson syndrome
Drugs, particularly sulfonamides and penicillins, may cause the Stevens–Johnson syndrome. The immunological mechanism is uncertain.
❶Stevens–Johnson syndrome is a contraindication to any form of cutaneous challenge testing or further administration of the drug.
A useful source of information on drug allergy can be found at:
🔊 http://www.phadia.com/PageFiles/27357/Drug-Book-web.pdf

DRESS syndrome

DRESS = drug reaction with eosinophilia and systemic symptoms.

Presentation
- Begins several weeks after starting drug. Drugs involved include:
  - sulfonamides, dapsone, minocycline, carbamazepine, phenytoin, lamotrigine, modafinil, allopurinol.
- Features include rash (generalized), fever (> 38°C), lymphadenopathy, evidence of at least one internal organ involved, and haematological abnormalities.
- Organ involvement:
  - Liver (80%), kidney (40%), lung (33%).
- Haematological abnormalities include: eosinophilia, lymphopenia/ lymphocytosis, thrombocytopenia.
- Mortality up to 10%.

Diagnosis
- Typical features and associated drug therapy.
- No specific immunological tests.

Treatment
- Stop offending drug (and do not reintroduce!).
- Treat with corticosteroids.

Vaccine reactions

Vaccines have been blamed for a multitude of medical problems. Frequent concerns are raised about egg allergy and vaccination, latex allergy, and allergy to antibiotics.

Vaccine composition
- Depends on vaccine.
- May contain egg proteins (viral vaccines grown in eggs), antibiotics (neomycin), and latex components (stoppers, manufacturing plant equipment).
- May contain other preservatives.

Egg allergy
- Data are now published each year of the ovalbumin content of flu vaccines: this is available through the Department of Health's Green Book on Infectious Diseases (now only electronic!): ℘ http://www. dh.gov.uk/en/Publichealth/Immunisation/Greenbook/index.htm
- Advice is available: the BSACI has published a position statement on egg allergy including advice: ℘ http://onlinelibrary.wiley.com/doi/10.1111/ j.1365-2222.2010.03557.x/pdf
- Patients where the history is uncertain should be formally investigated by an allergist/immunologist to confirm or refute the diagnosis of egg allergy.
- Almost all patients will tolerate vaccines with very low ovalbumin content, unless they still have severe reactions to egg.

Latex allergy
- Drug information departments can obtain information on latex content of flu vaccines; information is also available from the Anaphylaxis Campaign.

Antibiotic allergy
- Confirmatory tests may be required (patch testing for neomycin).
- Decision on safety can be taken on a patient-by-patient basis, depending on need.

Adjuvant-induced disease
- Controversial.
- Claimed that adjuvants may trigger an autoimmune process, leading to CFS-like syndrome.
- Immunological evidence is lacking so far.

Venom allergy

Allergy to bee and wasp venom can be associated with severe reactions. It is commonest in those with occupational risk factors (bee keepers, gardeners, forestry workers, pest controllers).

Presentation
- Systemic reactions (anaphylaxis).
- Large local reactions (not usually IgE-mediated).
- Identity of the insect may be in doubt.

Diagnosis
- SPT with graded concentrations of venom is helpful. Bee and wasp should always be tested, unless the history is very clear (e.g. beekeeper stung at hive).
- Double positives may be seen due to cross-reactive carbohydrate determinants—test for specific IgE to recombinant bee allergens to identify primary sensitizer.
- If there is a good history and negative SPTs, consider intradermal testing.

Treatment
- Give avoidance advice: no perfumes, no brightly coloured clothes, no bare feet in gardens, avoid fallen fruit.
- For severe systemic reactions provide emergency treatment kit: adrenaline for self-injection (see p. 133), prednisolone, cetirizine.
- Consider immunotherapy:
  - Large local reactions are not an indication for immunotherapy.
  - Cardiac disease is not a contraindication, as risk of death from wild sting is high—get cardiology opinion first.
  - β-blockers may provide cardio-protection and are not necessarily a contraindication (provide half-strength adrenaline for self-injection—0.15 mg per pen).

- ACE inhibitors must be stopped (ARBs may also impair kinin breakdown) as reactions will be severe (both wild and treatment) and accompanied by more marked swelling and hypotension.
- Risk of severe reactions returns to baseline anyway over 10 years.
- Some authorities advocate sting challenge at the end of immunotherapy (no consensus).
- No consensus on optimum duration of treatment (3–5 years).
- Immunotherapy may be carried out as normal, semi-rush, or rush, depending on urgency.
- It should not be started during flying season for insects (risk of wild sting).
- Other insects may cause specific problems: e.g. bumblebees in commercial fruit growers (vaccine available); hornets, some parts of UK and Europe (use wasp venom immunotherapy); fire ants (USA).

Extrinsic allergic alveolitis (EAA)

Presentation
- Typical features of EAA are fever, shortness of breath, and cough within 4–6 hours of allergen exposure, i.e. much slower than for type I reactions. Rhonchi are present and there is acute hypoxaemia.
- About 10% of patients are also asthmatic and then show both an immediate (type I) and a later (type III) reaction.
- For occupational allergens, features are often most marked on Monday morning (after a weekend free of exposure) and improve somewhat later in the week: this is 'Monday morning fever'.
- Chronic allergen exposure leads to a more insidious deterioration in lung function, often without much in the way of fever, but a steadily progressive shortness of breath.

Cause
- EAA is a hypersensitivity reaction mediated by IgG, mainly through a type III reaction, although there may well be a type IV reaction in addition. The antigens are inhaled and must be of such a size (< 5 mm) to enable them to penetrate to the alveolus.
- Many different antigens have been associated with this type of disease, including animal, fungal, bacterial, plant, and chemical allergens. Many are associated with occupational exposure. In the UK, the most widely recognized diseases are bird-fancier's lung (pigeons, caged birds) and farmer's lung (thermophilic fungi).
- Curiously, smoking appears to have a protective effect against the development of EAA. This may be due to the inhibition of macrophage function.

Immunology
- Total IgG is often raised and precipitating IgG antibodies to the offending allergen may be detected. However, these specific antibodies are a marker of exposure and do not correlate with the presence of disease. Precipitins may also decline with time, so that a negative test does not exclude the diagnosis.

- IgE levels are not usually elevated, and specific IgE is not detected; SPT has no role in the diagnosis of type III reactions.
- In the acute stage, there is a peripheral blood neutrophilia, rather than the eosinophilia seen in type I reactions.
- Bronchoalveolar lavage (BAL) studies typically show a lymphocytosis with a reversal of the normal CD4$^+$:CD8$^+$ T-cell ratio, due to an expansion of the CD8$^+$ T-cell population. The CD8$^+$ T cells show evidence of activation, expressing CD25 and VLA antigens. However, as with precipitins, BAL also shows changes in exposed but asymptomatic individuals, although the most extreme elevations of CD8$^+$ T cells are seen in those with active disease.

Diagnosis

- The diagnosis is based on typical symptoms together with evidence of allergen exposure.
- Precipitin tests provide supportive evidence only.
- The chronic disease, with interstitial changes, may be difficult to diagnose, but BAL may help differentiate EAA from sarcoidosis and idiopathic pulmonary fibrosis.
- In the occupational setting, challenge tests within an environmental chamber may be required as proof positive of the causal link. Pure allergens are required and the process may make the patient seriously unwell.

Treatment

- Avoidance is the mainstay. This may require difficult decisions if the patient's livelihood is affected; hence the need for positive evidence of causation through a challenge. If the disease is identified early and the allergen exposure terminated, no permanent harm will be done. However, in chronic cases, if fibrotic lung damage has occurred, then this will be irreversible.
- Oral corticosteroids may help to deal with acute symptoms.

Allergic bronchopulmonary aspergillosis (ABPA)

Presentation

- ABPA is a specific entity in which there are both type I and type III reactions to *Aspergillus*.
- Presentation is with bouts of wheeze, fever, cough, and haemoptysis.
- Bronchiectasis may develop.
- Chest radiographs show transient infiltrates.
- Symptoms are often most marked in the winter.
- Similar features of a mixed type I and type III response to *Aspergillus* may occur in some patients with cystic fibrosis. This appears to be a poor prognostic sign.

Cause
- The causative fungus, *Aspergillus*, is usually present in the sputum of patient with ABPA, and can be seen on microscopy and often cultured from serial specimens.

Immunology
- Both IgE and IgG precipitins to the relevant strain of *Aspergillus* can be detected.
- SPTs against *Aspergillus* are also strongly positive and give both an immediate and a late response.
- Total IgE is usually very high and there is a marked peripheral blood eosinophilia during acute episodes. Both fall during remission.

Treatment
- Acute flares are treated with high-dose corticosteroids; some patients require continuous low-dose steroids to maintain remission.
- Bronchodilators are also required.
- Immunotherapy with extracts of *Aspergillus* is unhelpful!

Other pulmonary eosinophilic syndromes

- Pulmonary eosinophilia may also be caused by drug reactions, parasitic infestations (*Ascaris, Strongyloides*, filariasis), vasculitis (Churg–Strauss vasculitis, see ➲ Chapter 13), and idiopathic eosinophilic pneumonias, including Löffler's syndrome and hypereosinophilic syndromes.
- Diagnosis can be difficult. Involvement of other organs may occur.
- There are no specific immunological tests of value.
- Idiopathic pulmonary eosinophilia is treated with steroids and is exquisitely sensitive to very small doses.

Allergic renal disease

- A seasonal nephrotic syndrome has been described in atopic patients, corresponding to the pollen season.
- IgE has been documented in the glomeruli.
- This appears to be very rare.

Hypereosinophilic syndromes (HES)

The investigation of hypereosinophilia is difficult. Presentations vary widely and the response to treatment is equally variable. Cardiac involvement may occur.

Causes
- Causes are numerous—see Table 3.9.
- Elevations of IL-5 may be responsible in some cases.

Table 3.9 Causes of hypereosinophilia

Infections	Parasitic infections
	Fungal infections
	HIV
Allergic diseases	Eczema
	Drug reactions—DRESS syndrome
Immunological disease	Hyper-IgE syndrome, DOCK8 deficiency, Omenn's syndrome
	Graft-vs-host syndrome
	Transplant rejection
	IL-2 treatment
Malignant disease	Myeloid leukaemia
	Lymphoma (esp. Hodgkin's)—associated with PDGFRA–FIP1L1 gene rearrangements
	Mastocytosis
	Some adenocarcinomas
Pulmonary disease	Loeffler's syndrome
	ABPA
	Eosinophilic pneumonia
	Sarcoidosis
Gastrointestinal disease	Eosinophilic oesophagitis/enteritis
Skin disease	Bullous diseases
	Eosinophilic cellulitis (Wells syndrome)
	Kimura's disease
	Eosinophilic fasciitis (Shulman's disease)
	Episodic angioedema with eosinophilia (fever and weight gain)
Vasculitis	Churg–Strauss syndrome (EGPA)
	Cholesterol emboli
Miscellaneous	Radiation
	Addison's disease
	Idiopathic
	Familial—autosomal dominant mapped to 5q31–33

Diagnosis
- Low levels of eosinophilia (0.4–3.0 × 10⁹/l) may be associated with atopic disease.
- Investigations depend on the probability of the conditions listed in Table 3.9.
- Bone marrow examination, eosinophil clonality studies, and scanning (CT, PET-CT) for evidence of lymphoma may be required.

- A proportion of patients with Churg–Strauss syndrome (CSS, eosinophilic granulomatosis with polyangiitis) will be ANCA$^+$ (see **➔** Chapter 13).
- Troponin, echocardiography, and ECG should be carried out to check for cardiac involvement.
- IgE levels will be raised significantly in Job's syndrome, atopic eczema, and sometimes in CSS.

Treatment
- Treatment will depend on underlying diagnosis.
- Corticosteroids are the first-line treatment.
- Second-line treatments include hydroxycarbamide, interferon alfa, and tyrosine kinase inhibitors (imatinib).
- Anti-IL-5 mAbs (mepolizumab) may be helpful.
- Some idiopathic HES patients may be exquisitely sensitive to tiny doses of steroid (1–3 mg per day!).
- Cardiac monitoring may be necessary.

Websites

American Academy of Allergy, Asthma and Immunology (AAAAI): *ℛ www.aaaai.org*
American College of Allergy, Asthma and Immunology (ACAAI): *ℛ www.acaai.org*
European Academy for Allergology and Clinical Immunology (EAACI): *ℛ www.eaaci.net*
Health and Safety Executive: *ℛ www.hse.gov.uk/latex*
Joint Council of Allergy, Asthma and Immunology: *ℛ www.jcaai.org*
World Allergy Organization: *ℛ www.worldallergy.org*

Autoimmunity and the endocrine system

Classification of autoimmune thyroid disease

- Autoimmune hyperthyroidism.
- Graves's disease.
- Autoimmune thyroiditis.
- Hashimoto's thyroiditis.
- Postpartum thyroiditis.
- Atrophic thyroiditis.

Graves's disease

Presentation
- Usually presents with thyrotoxicosis and a diffusely enlarged thyroid gland.
- Often accompanied by exophthalmos and occasionally by thyroid acropathy.
- Stress and environmental factors may be triggers.
- It is recorded during the reconstitution phase after HAART treatment for HIV and after alemtuzumab therapy.

Immunogenetics
- Strong female predominance, F:M = 7:1.
- Disease runs in families and it is associated with HLA-A1 B8 DR3, although less strongly than some other autoimmune diseases.
- In Asians the disease has been associated with HLA-Bw35 and Bw46.
- Strong association of exophthalmos with HLA-DR3.
- A weak association exists with polymorphisms of *CTLA-4*, *CD25*, *FCRL3*, *CD226*, and *PTPN22* (a T-cell regulatory gene, lymphocyte-specific tyrosine phosphatase).

Immunopathology
- Disease has been associated with aberrant MHC class II expression on thyrocytes, which is thought to play a role in the induction of the autoimmune response.
- There is predominant CD4$^+$ T-cell infiltration of the thyroid gland.
- Exophthalmos may be due to an autoantibody directed to unknown antigens expressed on retro-orbital connective tissue, probably fibroblasts or fat cells, leading to a localized inflammatory response, with plasma-cell infiltrate, and consequent hypertrophy and hyperplasia.

Autoantibodies
- Patients with Graves's disease have elevated levels of:
  - antibodies to thyroid peroxidase (present in 50–80%) and antibodies to thyroglobulin (20–40%);
  - thyroid-stimulating antibodies, both growth promoting (TGSI, 20–50%) and stimulating (TSI, 50–90%);
  - antibodies that compete with the binding of thyroid-stimulating hormone (TSH) (TBII, 50–80%). These autoantibodies are directly involved in the pathogenic process.

- Graves's goitre has been associated with stimulating autoantibodies to both the TSH receptor (TSH-R) and to the insulin-like growth factor receptor (IGF1-R), which both promote growth of the gland.
- Presence of TSI and TBII correlate with risk of relapse and of neonatal hyperthyroidism if present in pregnancy.
- Exophthalmos may be due to a separate autoantibody directed against yet unknown antigens or due to antibodies to autoantigens that are common to both the thyroid gland and the orbits.

Immunotherapy

- Treatment of the thyrotoxicosis does not involve immunotherapy.
- Eye disease may require treatment with steroids, ciclosporin, or irradiation to control the inflammatory process. Rituximab is now being used. Surgical intervention may be required.
- ^{125}I ablation of the thyroid to control the thyrotoxicosis may be associated with a flare-up of the eye disease, and pre-treatment with steroids may be helpful.

Hashimoto's thyroiditis

Presentation

- Patients are usually hyperthyroid initially and then progress to hypothyroidism as fibrosis of the gland occurs.
- There is usually a goitre.
- It is the most common cause for hypothyroidism.
- Hashimoto's thyroiditis also tends to occur in families with other thyroid disease or autoimmune disease, and has a predilection for older females.

Immunogenetics

- Association of DR5 with goitrous Hashimoto's disease.
- DR3 and DR4 are also associated.

Immunopathology

- There is an acute inflammatory thyroiditis, accompanied by a lymphocytic infiltrate of the gland, of unknown aetiology.
- Lymphocytic infiltrate comprises all types of cells and may result in germinal centre formation within the gland. These may play a key role in the production of autoantibodies and cytokines.
- Increased HLA class II antigen expression on infiltrating lymphocytes and thyrocytes in affected glands.
- An increased number of helper and cytotoxic T cells are found with decreased suppressor T-cell numbers.

Autoantibodies

- Anti-thyroid peroxidase antibodies will be present in 80–95% of patients, usually at extremely high titres (higher than in Graves's disease).
- Autoantibodies to multiple other thyroid antigens, including thyroglobulin, can be detected.

- Up to 20% of patients may have antibodies (stimulatory or blocking) directed at the TSH receptor.
- Anti-TPO assays should be incorporated in main biochemistry analysers as part of thyroid profiles.

Immunotherapy
- No immunotherapeutic manoeuvres are used.

Subacute thyroiditis syndromes

- These include transient thyroiditis syndromes such as granulomatous thyroiditis (de Quervain's syndrome) and postpartum thyroiditis.
- Patients are initially hyperthyroid but may become transiently hypothyroid in recovery before the euthyroid state is restored.

Immunopathology
- De Quervain's thyroiditis may be caused by viral infections (mumps, measles, adenovirus, Epstein–Barr virus, coxsackievirus, and echovirus), which lead to an acute, painful thyroiditis.
  - No single agent has been unequivocally linked to the disease.
  - Antithyroid antibodies, against thyroglobulin and thyroid peroxidase, are present (usually in low titres), in 10–50% of patients with de Quervain's thyroiditis.
- Postpartum thyroiditis usually occurs within 3 months of delivery and is usually painless:
  - it appears to be common (1–11% of pregnant women);
  - it is associated with HLA-DR5;
  - complement-fixing anti-TPO antibodies are present in the majority of patients and the titre correlates with disease severity;
  - presence of such antibodies during or after pregnancy in otherwise well women has a predictive value of subsequent thyroid dysfunction.

Testing
- See Table 4.1.

Table 4.1 Testing for subacute thyroiditis syndromes

Tests for diagnosis	Tests for monitoring
Thyroid function	Thyroid function
Anti-TPO antibodies	Thyroglobulin (thyroid carcinoma)
Other thyroid antibodies	Vitamin B_{12} status
Thyroglobulin (thyroid carcinoma)	
Antibodies to gastric parietal cells and intrinsic factor (consider PA)	
Vitamin B_{12} status	
Consider other endocrinopathies (diabetes, Addison's disease)	

Immunotherapy
- No immunotherapeutic manoeuvres are used.

Primary hypothyroidism and sporadic goitre

Primary hypothyroidism
- This may well be caused by previous occult thyroiditis, leading eventually to presentation with overt hypothyroidism years later.
- There may be a lymphocytic infiltrate of the gland, with marked fibrosis.

Autoantibodies
- 80% of patients will have antibodies to thyroid peroxidase, and a lower proportion will have antibodies to thyroglobulin.
- Some cases may have antibodies that block the TSH-R, preventing normal function.

Immunotherapy
- No immunological treatments are used.

Sporadic goitre
- This has been associated with stimulating autoantibodies to the IGF1-R, in the absence of other antibodies, leading to glandular growth.

Thyroid disease and other symptoms

Arthropathy
- Both hypo- and hyperthyroidism can be a cause of significant joint pain.
- Detection of thyroid antibodies in a patient with joint pain may therefore be significant and should not be ignored.

Urticaria
- Occult hypo- or hyperthyroidism has also been associated with the development of urticaria, although the reasons are unclear.
- Unfortunately, the urticaria does not always settle when the thyroid abnormality is treated.
- The association appears to be with thyroid peroxidase antibodies.

Anti-thyroid antibodies in euthyroid patients
- The wider use of autoantibody testing has led to the detection of anti-thyroid antibodies in fit euthyroid patients.
- The Wickham community survey has demonstrated that a significant number of these patients go on to develop overt thyroid disease subsequently.
- The detection of such antibodies in asymptomatic patients should therefore lead to a high index of suspicion for thyroid disease and a low threshold for requesting thyroid function tests when the patient re-presents with symptoms.
- It may be worth screening the thyroid function annually.

Association with other autoimmune disease
- Autoimmune thyroid disease is strongly associated with pernicious anaemia and vice versa.
- Gastric parietal cell antibodies may therefore be detected in patients with thyroid disease.
- Such patients should be monitored for the subsequent development of vitamin B$_{12}$ deficiency.
- Thyroid disease may be accompanied by Addison's disease, in addition to pernicious anaemia (Schmidt's syndrome/type II autoimmune polyglandular syndrome (APS)).
- Generally, patients and family members of a patient with Graves's disease are more likely to have other autoimmune disease, e.g. type I diabetes, lupus erythematosus, chronic active hepatitis, coeliac disease, dermatitis herpetiformis, and Sjögren's syndrome, than the general population.

Autoantibodies to thyroxine
- May be seen in paraproteinaemic states (Waldenström's macroglobulinaemia).
- Cause hypothyroidism.
- Interfere with assays for FT4.

Amiodarone and thyroid function
- Amiodarone-induced thyroid disease is more common in women and in individuals who are positive for antibodies to TPO.

Classification of diabetes mellitus
- There are four types of diabetes:
  - type Ia (immune-mediated) or insulin-dependent diabetes mellitus (IDDM);
  - type Ib as type Ia but without evidence of immune involvement;
  - type II or non-insulin-dependent diabetes mellitus (NIDDM);
  - type III: due to other genetic defects, insulin resistance syndromes, other endocrinopathies, etc.
- There is considerable clinical overlap, although type II does not have an immunological basis.

Type I diabetes (insulin-dependent)

Presentation
Patients may present with symptoms related to an elevated blood sugar, or a raised fasting blood sugar level may be an isolated finding.

Immunogenetics
- Males and females are almost equally affected, unlike other autoimmune diseases.
- Twin concordance for IDDM is only 30–70%.

- Major susceptibility gene is in HLA region, accounting for 40–60% of risk.
- Genotyping has shown that DQA1*0301, DQB1*0302, DQA1*0501, and DQB1*0201 are strongly associated with type Ia.
- DQA1*0102, DQB1*0602 protect against the development of diabetes.
- CTLA-4 and PTPN22, the IL-2 receptor (CD25), interferon-induced helicase, and a number of other genes (including some of unidentified function) are also associated with increased susceptibility to type I diabetes.
- Other specific loci have been associated with the shared risk of developing coeliac disease with diabetes, although the effects are small. The greatest risk appears to be with CCR5.
- At least 17 other genetic loci contribute to susceptibility including polymorphisms in the promoter of the insulin gene.
- Tenfold increased risk of developing diabetes in family members.

Immunopathology

- A disease characterized by immunological destruction of the islets of Langerhans in the pancreas, with subsequent insulinopenia.
- There is a seasonal fluctuation in the presentation.
- It has been postulated that there is an initial viral infection, leading to subsequent autoimmune damage in a genetically susceptible host.
- Viruses that have been proposed include coxsackievirus, reovirus, mumps, influenza, rubella, and cytomegalovirus.
- In the early stages of the disease there is a lymphocytic infiltrate, predominantly of $CD8^+$ T cells, but with small numbers of other types too.
- Islet beta cells are particularly susceptible to damage by $TNF\alpha$.
- As diabetes has been described in a patient with X-linked agammaglobulinaemia, T cells are more important than autoantibodies in causing diabetes.

Autoantibodies

- GAD autoantibodies:
  - β-cell-specific antibodies have been detected that recognize glutamic acid decarboxylase (GAD).
  - This antigen occurs in both nerve and pancreas in two isoforms (65 kDa and 67 kDa), encoded by separate genes.
  - Autoantibodies against this antigen have also been described in the stiff-person syndrome (see → Chapter 5).
  - Primary target in type Ia diabetes appears to be the 65kDa protein, and antibodies to this are found in up to 80% of newly presenting IDDM.
  - Antibodies to GAD-67 are also found.
  - There is sequence homology between GAD and a coxsackievirus antigen.
  - GAD autoantibodies may be found in first-degree relatives.
- Insulinoma-associated protein 2 autoantibodies (IA2)
  - IA2 antibodies are found in 58% of type 1 diabetics at first diagnosis.
  - They appear later than GAD and insulin antibodies but strongly predict progression to diabetes.

- Zinc transporter (ZnT8) autoantibodies.
  - 60–80% of newly diagnosed type I diabetics have antibodies to ZnT8.
  - They may be the only autoantibody detectable in patients negative for GAD, IA-2, and insulin antibodies.
  - They appear early in the process and are lost quickly after the onset of diabetes.
  - Polymorphisms of the gene for ZnT8 are associated with type II diabetes.
- Insulin autoantibodies (IAA).
  - Insulin antibodies appear first in children developing diabetes.
  - As insulin antibodies develop in patients treated with insulin, they cannot be used as diagnostic markers once insulin has been commenced.
- Islet cell autoantibodies (ICA).
  - ICA also recognize cell types in the islets other than the insulin-producing β-cells.
  - ICA are not involved in the autoimmune destruction, but are merely a marker of the disease process (secondary autoantibodies).
  - With the identification of more specific markers, the role of ICA in diagnosis is uncertain.
  - Antibodies are present in 65–85% of newly presenting IDDM, but disappear within 1–2 years.
  - They also occur in the first-degree relatives of patients with IDDM, who have a high risk of developing the disease.
  - Studies in healthy children have shown that large numbers have ICA but do not progress to diabetes.
- Autoantibodies have also been described to a number of other putative target antigens although the relevance of these is yet to be determined, including:
  - insulin (30–50% IDDM positive for insulin antibodies by radio-immunoassay, RIA), more common in children developing IDDM;
  - gangliosides, GT3, GM2, and others, antigens shared between β-cells and neuronal tissue;
  - an autoantigen that cross-reacts with a rubella capsid antigen;
  - a glucose transporter (GLUT-2, not β-cell specific);
  - ICA p69, which has sequence homology with bovine serum albumin;
  - ICA-512, a protein whose intracellular sequence has some homology to other protein tyrosine phosphatases;
  - heat-shock protein 65 (Hsp-65);
  - insulin receptor;
  - carboxypeptidase H.
- Presence of autoantibodies is helpful in distinguishing type I and type II diabetes.
- Screening of first-degree relatives for GAD and insulin antibodies may be valuable in identifying those at risk of developing diabetes.
- The optimal screening profile for autoimmunity in Type I diabetes has not been defined. It is likely that ICA will be replaced by an automated screen of GAD, IA-2, insulin antibodies, and possibly ZnT8.
- The more autoantibodies that are present, the higher the risk of developing diabetes.

- For patients thought to have type II diabetes, the presence of autoantibodies is predictive of the need for insulin therapy.

Immunotherapy

- Identification of patients in the pre-diabetic phase may well become more important, as trials of immunoregulatory therapies become more widespread.
- Aim is to prevent damage to the islets, as the presentation with overt diabetes clearly represents the end-stage of the disease when insufficient islet tissue remains.
- Studies of immunotherapy are aided by the existence of a mouse model (NOD mouse).
- Aggressive therapy with corticosteroids, azathioprine, ciclosporin, tacrolimus (FK506), and anti-thymocyte globulin (ATG) has been tried with some success in newly presenting patients and has staved off the requirement for insulin for some time.
- Many monoclonal antibodies and polyclonal antibodies, including Campath®-1, anti-CD4, anti-CD8, and anti-CD45, that are directed against the T cell are immunosuppressive and have been shown to prevent the onset of diabetes in pre-diabetic NOD mice.
- Anti-CD3 mAbs are able to reverse diabetes in new-onset diabetic NOD.
- Initial clinical trials in humans are promising with moderate loss of β-cell function during and after therapy.
- Tolerance induction using parenterally administered GAD and Hsp p277 peptide has been successfully used in mice. The oral route has also been used.
- Clinical trials are underway, using Hsp p277, GAD, and insulin in newly diagnosed patients.
- Cytokine-based immunotherapy has been tried.
  - In particular IL-4 has been targeted as a possible treatment although the feasibility of treatment with this remains to be confirmed.
  - The alternative cytokine-based approach consists of blocking IL-12 or γ-IFN.
- Early insulin treatment may also assist by β-cell rest, and perhaps by decreasing MHC class II expression, although the role of this in diabetes is controversial.
- Other potential therapies include MHC class II blockade with peptides and stem cell therapy.
- Pancreatic islet cell transplantation is now being undertaken.

Association with other autoimmune disease

- There is a clinical association of type I diabetes with coeliac disease and thyroid disease.
- In children, there is strong association with coeliac disease: all children with type Ia diabetes need regular endomysial/tTG antibodies checking (recommended annually).

Testing

- See Table 4.2.

Table 4.2 Testing for type I diabetes

Tests for diagnosis	Tests for monitoring
Blood glucose and glucose tolerance test; urinalysis	Glucose and glycated Hb; urinalysis
IA-2 & ZnT8 antibodies	Endomysial/tTG antibodies
Anti-GAD antibodies	
Endomysial/tTG antibodies	

Immunological complications of insulin therapy

Allergic reactions

- As noted in Chapter 3, reactions may occur to administered insulin: these are rare now that diabetics are treated with human insulin, rather than that from pigs or cattle, but they still occur.
- The manufacturing process for the human insulin is capable of altering the tertiary structure of the molecule in a way that can render it immunogenic.
- Other agents such as zinc and protamine, used to alter the pharmacokinetics of the drug, may also contribute.
- Reactions may include local or generalized urticaria and, very rarely, severe systemic reactions.
- Both immediate and late reactions may occur.
- Insulin oedema is non-immunological.
- Oral antihistamines and the inclusion of 1–5 mg of hydrocortisone in the syringe with the insulin may be helpful.
- Desensitization may be possible, but should only be attempted where severe reactions are occurring that compromise diabetic control.
- Development of antibodies to protamine in diabetics may lead to major systemic reactions if intravenous protamine is used to reverse anticoagulation with heparin (e.g. after cardiac bypass surgery).
- IgE antibodies have been documented.

Insulin resistance

- Insulin resistance may occur due to IgG anti-insulin antibodies.
  - May arise spontaneously or as a result of attempted desensitization where reactions have occurred.
  - Resistance to insulin action may occur as a result of abnormalities of the peripheral insulin receptor (type A, severe insulin resistance, hirsutism, and acanthosis nigricans) or due to IgG insulin-receptor-blocking antibodies (type B, often associated with other autoimmune diseases).
- Insulin resistance due to anti-insulin antibodies has also been reported in ataxia telangiectasia.

Autoimmune insulin syndrome
- Autoantibodies against insulin may occur leading to complex formation. The complexes dissociate some hours after a meal, releasing free insulin and causing hypoglycaemia.
- Seen in Japan (possible genetic basis) and in association with myeloma (paraprotein with specificity for insulin).

Crow–Fukase syndrome (POEMS syndrome; Takatsuki syndrome)
- Characterized by:
  - Polyneuropathy
  - Organomegaly
  - Endocrinopathy
  - Monoclonal proteins
  - Skin changes
  - = POEMS.
- Clinical features include:
  - Papilloedema.
  - Symmetrical distal polyneuropathy (motor and sensory); may cause erectile dysfunction.
  - Lung disease with pulmonary hypertension.
  - Hepatosplenomegaly, lymphadenopathy.
  - Peripheral and pulmonary oedema, pleural effusions, ascites.
  - Hyperprolactinaemia causing amenorrhoea (women), gynaecomastia (men), testicular atrophy, type II diabetes, hypothyroidism, adrenal insufficiency.
  - Skin changes include thickening, hypertrichosis, hyperpigmentation, clubbing, or sclerodermatous changes.
  - Thrombophilia, cardiomyopathy, thrombocytosis, and polycythaemia may also occur.
- Plasma cell dyscrasia (IgG or IgA); invariably λ light chain.
  - Osteosclerotic myeloma.
  - Castleman's disease (non-clonal lymphoid proliferation due to IL-6 hypersecretion).
- May be due to elevated IL-6 and IL-1 levels.
- Elevated VGEF.
- Check serum immunoglobulins, electrophoresis, and immunofixation.
- Treatment is with steroids and alkylating agents (cyclophosphamide).
- Bone marrow transplantation has been used successfully.
- Anti-VGEF mAb, bevacizumab may be beneficial in some cases but can cause severe capillary leak syndrome.

Classification of adrenal insufficiency
- Autoimmune Addison's disease (commonest cause in Western countries).
- Tuberculosis (commonest worldwide).

- Malignancy.
- Sarcoidosis.
- Haemochromatosis.
- Haemorrhage (post-partum).
- Thrombosis (anti-phospholipid syndrome (APS)).
- Infections (fungi, viruses).
- Genetic causes include X-linked adrenoleucodystrophy, congenital adrenal hypoplasia, familial glucocorticoid deficiency, triple A syndrome, and Kearns–Sayre syndrome.

Addison's disease

Presentation
- Includes collapse, faintness, nausea, weight loss, and anorexia.
- Findings include pigmentation, postural hypotension, hyponatraemia, and an absent response to ACTH stimulation test (Synacthen test).
- There is a strong association with autoimmune ovarian disease and therefore females with Addison's should also be checked for the presence of ovarian antibodies and other features of the autoimmune polyglandular syndrome (APS; see ➋ sections on types I, II, and III APS, p. 193).

Immunogenetics
- In DR4-positive patients DRB1*0404 is the most frequently carried allele.
- The MICA-5.1 allele is an additional major independent determinant of Addison's disease.
- Polymorphisms in *CTLA4* and the class II transactivator (*CIITA*) have been associated with autoimmune Addison's disease.

Immunopathology
- Lymphocytic infiltrate in the adrenal gland is confined to the cortex and comprises mainly activated CD4+ T cells, with some B cells and CD8+ T cells.
- It has been suggested that Addison's disease is a Th2 disease.

Autoantibodies
- Adrenocortical autoantibodies are found in two-thirds of patients.
- Autoantibodies are rarely found in normal individuals or in first-degree relatives. They may be found in small numbers of patients with other autoimmune endocrine diseases (1.7% type I diabetics).
- 21 hydroxylase (21OH; CYP21A2) has been identified as the major autoantigen, which is localized to the endoplasmic reticulum of zona glomerulosa cells.
- 17 α-hydroxylase (CYP17, expressed in adrenal gland and gonads) and P450scc (CYP11A1, expressed in adrenals, gonads, and placenta) can also be the target of autoantibodies in autoimmune Addison's disease.
- Autoantibodies are normally detected by indirect immunofluorescence on adrenal sections: this detects mainly antibodies to CYP21A and CYP17.

Testing
- See Table 4.3.

Table 4.3 Testing for Addison's disease

Tests for diagnosis	Tests for monitoring
Endocrine function tests (basal cortisol, short and long Synacthen tests)	Endocrine function tests
Antibodies to adrenal, steroid-producing cells, TPO, GPC	Monitor for development of associated endocrinopathies and vitamin B_{12} deficiency

Treatment
- Patients should be on long-term steroid replacement therapy and the dose increased if the patient is unwell, undergoing surgery, etc.
- Medic-Alert bracelet is essential.

Classification of autoimmune polyglandular syndromes (APS/APGS)
- See Table 4.4.

Table 4.4 Classification of autoimmune polyglandular syndromes

Syndrome	Major criteria	Minor criteria
Type I	Candidiasis Adrenal failure Hypo-parathyroidism	Gonadal failure Alopecia Malabsorption Chronic hepatitis
Type II (Schmidt's syndrome)	Adrenal failure Thyroid disease IDDM	Gonadal failure Vitiligo Non-endocrine autoimmunity (myasthenia)
Type III	Thyroid disease	*Either* IDDM *or* Pernicious anaemia *or* Non-endocrine autoimmunity (myasthenia)

Type 1 APS (autoimmune polyendocrinopathy candidiasis ectodermal dysplasia; APECED)

Presentation

- Presentation is usually during teenage years.
- First sign is often chronic *Candida* infection.
- This is generally followed by autoimmune hypoparathyroidism and Addison's disease.
- At least two of these three features should be present for diagnosis.
- Other autoimmune disease may be present:
  - Alopecia, vitiligo, chronic active hepatitis, hypogonadism, type I diabetes, hypothyroidism, pernicious anaemia, intestinal malabsorption, and autoimmune gastritis.
- It forms part of the spectrum of chronic mucocutaneous candidiasis (see ➲ Chapter 1).

Immunopathogenesis and immunogenetics

- Type 1 APS is thought to be a Th2-type disease.
- There is no strong HLA linkage, although several reports have suggested a link to HLA-A28.
- APS type 1 is the result of mutations of the recessive autosomal autoimmune regulator element (*AIRE*) gene localized on chromosome 21q22.3: autosomal recessive.
- Equal male and female incidence.
- Autoantibodies to 21OH, 17OH, and/or P450scc are found.
- Antibodies to NALP5 (NACHT leucine-rich repeat pyrin domain-containing protein 5), expressed in the parathyroid and the ovaries, BPI fold containing family member B (BPIFB1), potassium channel regulator KCNRG (lung), and transglutaminase 4 (prostate) appear to be fairly specific to APS1.
- Antibodies to tryptophan hydroxylase (an endogenous intestinal antigen) have been described in patients with gastrointestinal complications.
- Autoantibodies to interferon (particularly interferon-omega) have been described.
- Other disease specific autoantibodies will be found.
- *AIRE* gene:
  - AIRE protein localizes in the nucleus and contains several motifs found on proteins involved in transcriptional regulation.
  - At least 50 different mutations of the *AIRE* gene have been identified, with many of the APECED-causing mutations clustered within the putative DNA binding and transactivation domains.
  - AIRE is involved in the expression of a variety of peripheral tissue antigens in the medullary thymus, a function that seems to be required for purging the immune system of autoreactive T cells and therefore the development of tolerance.
  - Exact mechanism by which AIRE exerts its effect is yet to be identified.

Types II (Schmidt's syndrome) and III APS

Type II APS (Schmidt's syndrome)

Presentation
- This comprises Addison's disease + autoimmune thyroid disease (Graves's disease) ± IDDM.
- Pernicious anaemia, chronic active hepatitis, vitiligo, and hypogonadism may also occur.
- Peak age of onset is 20–30 years of age.
- Females are more commonly affected than males (2:1).

Immunopathogenesis and immunogenetics
- It may be a Th1-type disease.
- Abnormal cellular immune function may occur.
- Autosomal dominant and recessive patterns of inheritance have been identified, with multiple genes.
- There is an association with HLA-B8, DR3, and with certain subtypes including DQA1*0501, DRB1*0301, and DQB1*0201.
- This syndrome is also associated with polymorphism of the MHC class I chain-related A (*MICA*) gene.

Autoantibodies
The presence of antibodies to 17OH and P450scc is strongly associated with a primary gonadic failure that often evolves into early menopause.

Type III APS
- This comprises autoimmune thyroid disease with either IDDM or pernicious anaemia.
- Non-endocrine autoimmune disease may also occur, for example, myasthenia gravis.
- Vitiligo and alopecia may also be present.
- There is a very strong female predominance and an association with HLA-DR3.

IPEX syndrome

- IPEX syndrome (immune dysregulation, polyendocrinopathy, enteropathy, X-linked)—see **➲** Chapter 1.
- Presentation is in infancy with enteropathy, IDDM, and thyroiditis.
- It is an X-linked condition.
- Gene defect (*FOXP3*) has been localized to Xp11.23–13.3.
- Antibodies to GAD65, harmonin, and villin (proteins of the intestinal brush border and villi) are detectable.
- BMT/HSCT has been used as a treatment.

Cushing's syndrome

In Cushing's syndrome due to pigmented nodular dysplasia, stimulating IgG antibodies have been described, which are thought possibly to bind to the ACTH receptor, analogous to thyroid-stimulating antibodies.

Pernicious anaemia

Pernicious anaemia (PA) is the end-stage of autoimmune gastritis that typic-ally affects persons > 60 years.

Presentation
- Patients develop vitamin B_{12} deficiency and hence megaloblastic anaemia and, in severe cases, subacute combined degeneration of the spinal cord.
- Patients often have prematurely grey hair and blue eyes.
- Increased risk of both gastric carcinoma and carcinoid tumours.
- Females are more commonly affected than males.
- More common in people with blood group A.

Immunogenetics
- No strong HLA association has been identified.
- Increased incidence in family members.
- Strong association with other endocrine autoimmune disease such as autoimmune thyroiditis, IDDM, and adrenalitis.

Immunopathology
- Megaloblastic anaemia is the direct result of the vitamin B_{12} deficiency.
- Vitamin B_{12} deficiency is a consequence of the loss of intrinsic factor producing gastric parietal cells in the corpus of the stomach afflicted by autoimmune gastritis.
- Pathological lesion of autoimmune gastritis, also known as type A chronic atrophic gastritis, is restricted to the parietal-cell-containing corpus of the stomach with sparing of the gastric antrum.
- Gastric lesion is characterized by chronic inflammatory (mainly lymphocytic) infiltrate in the submucosa.
- Advanced lesions are characterized by intestinal metaplasia with replacement of resident parietal and zymogenic cells of gastric glands by mucus-secreting cells.
- Intrinsic factor antibody (IgA isotype) secreted on to the gastric lumen by local lymphoid cells is likely to contribute to the deficiency of intrinsic factor by complexing with intrinsic factor and preventing the absorption of the intrinsic factor–vitamin B_{12} in the terminal ileum.
- Progression to overt pernicious anaemia may span 20–30 years.

Autoantibodies

- Gastric parietal cell (GPC) antibodies:
  - GPC antibodies, directed against the gastric H^+/K^+ ATPase are diagnostic of the underlying pathological lesion of autoimmune gastritis.
  - Not diagnostic of pernicious anaemia as the gastric lesion may not yet have progressed to this end-stage condition.
  - GPC antibodies are found in up to 85% of patients with PA.
  - Also present on some patients with other autoimmune endocrinopathies and in 3–10% healthy individuals (increasing incidence with age).
  - Antibodies to parietal cells directed towards the gastric ATPase have been reported in about 20–30% of patients with *H. pylori* associated gastritis.
  - It is hypothesized that *H. pylori* may be the environmental trigger for autoimmune gastritis.
  - GPC antibodies may also arise, with the appearance of thyroid antibodies, during treatment of hepatitis C infection with α-interferon.
- Intrinsic factor antibodies:
  - Intrinsic factor antibodies have a much higher disease specificity, but lower sensitivity, than GPC antibodies.
  - Intrinsic factor antibodies are found in approximately 60% of patients with PA.
  - Two types of intrinsic factor antibodies have been described.
  - Type 1 antibodies bind to the vitamin B_{12} binding site of intrinsic factor while type 2 bind to a site remote from this and block uptake in the terminal ileum.
  - IF antibodies are unreliable if the patient has been started on parenteral vitamin B_{12} injections.
  - Serum vitamin B_{12} levels may be reduced in patients on the oral contraceptive.

Treatment

- No immunotherapeutic manoeuvres are used.
- Patients who have vitamin B_{12} deficiency due to pernicious anaemia should be given replacement intramuscular vitamin B_{12} (given initially in high doses with supplemental potassium, having checked that other haematinics, especially iron, are adequate and then 3-monthly).
- Erroneous treatment of patients with folic acid may not only mask the anaemia caused by vitamin B_{12} deficiency but can permit the development of irreversible neurological damage.
- Asymptomatic GPC antibody positive patients with normal MCV and vitamin B_{12} should be monitored annually for development of vitamin B_{12} deficiency, especially if other family members have PA.
- GPC antibody positive patients should be screened for autoimmune thyroid disease.

Testing
- See Table 4.5.

Table 4.5 Testing for pernicious anaemia

Tests for diagnosis	Tests for monitoring
FBC and MCV	FBC and MCV
Thyroid function	Thyroid function
Vitamin B_{12}	Vitamin B_{12}
GPC and TPO antibodies	
Intrinsic factor antibodies	
Schilling test—due to manufacturing and clinical issues, the Schilling test has now been withdrawn	

Premature ovarian failure, gonadal autoimmunity, and immunological infertility

Premature ovarian failure

Presentation
- Affects 1% of women (defined as a menopause < 40 years of age).
- 20% of these are associated with Addison's, but the remainder are not associated with APS.

Autoantibodies
- Ovarian, adrenal, and steroid cell antibodies may be detected in patients.
- Steroid cell antibodies are directed at 17α-hydroxylase and P450 side-chain-cleavage enzyme.
- Another target enzyme appears to be 3β-hydroxysteroid dehydrogenase, which may be a more sensitive and specific marker of premature ovarian failure.
- Antibodies have been described against the follicle-stimulating hormone (FSH) receptor and other unidentified surface receptors in premature ovarian failure, although this appears still to be controversial.
- Screening of patients with premature ovarian failure should include a search for ovarian-, adrenal-, and steroid-cell antibodies by indirect immunofluorescence.

Gonadal autoantibodies
- Found in patients with Addison's and hypogonadism.
- React with steroid-producing cells of the adrenal cortex, syncytiotrophoblasts, Leydig cells of the testis, and the theca interna/granulosa cell layer of the ovary.

- Associated with type I APS.
- The target antigens are 17α-hydroxylase (CYP17) and P450 side-chain-cleavage enzyme (CYP11A1).
- Steroid-cell antibodies are found in 15% of Addison's without hypogonadism, but in > 80% with hypogonadism.
- They rarely disappear and infertility is usually lifelong.

Immunological infertility

- Infertile women may have anti-oocyte antibodies (approximately 9% of patients) that inhibit adherence and penetration of spermatozoa through the zona pellucida.
- ZP3, the primary sperm receptor, has been identified as a target antigen in an experimental mouse system.
- Antibodies have also been described against spermatozoa, causing agglutination or immobilization.
- It is not now thought that these antibodies play a major role in the genesis of the infertility, as they may also be detected in 12% of fertile women.

Pituitary autoimmunity

Autoimmune hypophysitis (lymphocytic hypophysitis) is very rare and is characterized by a lymphocytic infiltration. Both anterior and posterior pituitary may be involved leading to endocrine dysfunction and diabetes insipidus. The gland and stalk may appear swollen on MRI.

- Anterior hypophysitis may be associated with type I APS.
- Target antigens are unknown at present but a possible target is the prolactin-secreting cell.
- Antibodies may also be detected against vasopressin-producing cells, associated with autoimmune diabetes insipidus.
- A lymphocytic hypophysitis associated with pituitary failure has been found in young women during or after pregnancy; this may be associated with pituitary-reactive autoantibodies.
- Care needs to be taken to exclude a rare presentation of Wegener's granulomatosis.
- Pituitary antibodies may also be found in some patients with Sheehan's syndrome (pituitary infarction).
- Treatment with immunosuppressive drugs (corticosteroids, azathioprine) has been used.

Parathyroid autoimmunity

- Antibodies may be detected that recognize parathyroid gland surface membrane antigens and that may inhibit parathyroid hormone (PTH) secretion *in vitro*.
- They recognize the external domain of the calcium-sensing receptor and are associated with CMC and APS.

- Antibodies to mitochondria of parathyroid chief cells have been described.
- Blocking antibodies to the parathyroid hormone receptor have been described in secondary hyperparathyroidism of renal failure.
- Detection is by immunofluorescence on parathyroid sections, but normal mitochondrial and antinuclear antibodies must be excluded first, using a standard multiblock slide, as these will interfere with the detection of parathyroid antibodies.

Vitiligo and alopecia

Vitiligo
- Vitiligo is due to melanocyte loss and occurs in isolation or in association with other autoimmune diseases, typically thyrogastric autoimmunity and type II APS.
- It can also occur in association with inflammatory diseases.
- Multiple susceptibility gene loci have been identified, including *PTPN22* (generalized vitiligo), IL-2RA, and MHC class I and class II (DRB1, DQA1). Mutations (SNPs) have been identified in the *NALP1* gene.
- High levels of IL-1β expression are found.
- Target antigen of the immune response is tyrosinase and antibodies are present in most patients.
- This enzyme is an important target antigen in melanoma and patients with vitiligo and melanoma who have detectable antibodies do better than those without.
- Anti-tyrosinase antibodies are only found in patients with type II but not type I APS or sporadic vitiligo.
- Specific treatment is rarely successful: topical tacrolimus and UVA or UVB therapy may be tried.

Alopecia
- Alopecia frequently accompanies autoimmune diseases, especially thyroid, vitiligo, and SLE.
- There is no conclusive evidence for autoantibodies to the hair follicles, although this would not preclude a T-cell-mediated disease process.

Turner's syndrome

People with Turner's syndrome (45XO, or mosaics of 45XO/46XX) are infertile with multiple medical problems, including autoimmune hypothyroidism, cardiac disease, hypertension, and recurrent infections (chest, ears, sinuses). Specific antibody responses are reduced, with poor immunization responses. Antibiotic prophylaxis may be required in some cases.

Autoimmunity affecting the nervous system

Myasthenia gravis (MG)

Presentation

- Patients complain of double vision, muscle weakness, and fatigue (worse later in the day).
- Ptosis and diplopia are typical signs.
- Examination reveals generalized fatiguable muscle weakness.
- It is a heterogeneous condition with varying ages of presentation.
- Diagnosis of a neuromuscular junction defect can be confirmed by electrophysiological tests and the Tensilon test.

Immunogenetics

- In younger patients there is an association with HLA-A1, B8, and DR3, and with a strong female predominance.
- Disease may also be induced by penicillamine, and is mostly found in those who are HLA-Bw35/DR1 positive.
- Congenital myasthenic syndromes are described due to gene mutations in the AChR and associated molecules.

Immunopathology

- Muscle weakness is due to impaired action of acetylcholine (ACh) at the muscle endplate.
- Cause is unknown but the disease is strongly associated with thymomas (benign and malignant), thymic hyperplasia, and other autoimmune diseases such as SLE, polymyositis, haemolytic anaemia, and thyroid disease (especially in those < 40 years old).
- Prevalence is 2–10/100 000.
- Patients with thymoma are usually older and both sexes are affected equally; about 10% have thymomas, but removal of the tumour does not always affect the course of the disease.

Autoantibodies

- IgG anti-ACh-receptor (AChRAb) are detected in 75–95% of patients.
- 15% are seronegative for AChRAb.
- 50% with pure ocular myasthenia are seronegative for AChRAb, but may have other antibodies.
- Disease is caused by direct receptor blockade by AChRAb, complement-mediated endplate damage, and enhanced recycling of the receptor off of the endplate surface membrane.
- AChRAb levels are variable, but high titres are found in those less than 40 years old with thymic hyperplasia.
- Antibodies are IgG isotype (IgG$_1$ and IgG$_3$) and therefore can be transmitted across the placenta, causing neonatal myasthenia.
- The presence of striated muscle antibodies is a marker for the presence of a thymoma. These include antibodies to the ryanodine receptor and titin antibodies.
- Cardiac arrythmias may occur in the presence of anti-cardiac muscle antibodies.
- Other antibodies associated with seronegative MG include antibodies to low-density lipoprotein receptor-related protein (LRP4) and contactin.

- Antibodies to MuSK (muscle-specific tyrosine kinase) have been shown in up to 40% of patients with AChRAb-negative MG.
  - MuSK is a receptor tyrosine kinase that is restricted to the neuromuscular junction.
  - Patients with these antibodies are typically female with bulbar disease who may be difficult to treat with immunosuppression.
  - Antibodies to MuSK interfere with agrin-triggered stimulation of MuSK.
  - Antibodies are usually IgG_4.

Treatment
- Treatment is with oral anti-cholinesterases.
- Immunosuppressive therapy may be required: prednisolone (1–1.5 mg/kg) alone or with azathioprine is the treatment of choice.
- Mycophenolate mofetil, cyclophosphamide, methotrexate, and ciclosporin have all been used.
- Thymectomy may be required to prevent local extension and to exclude malignancy.
- Plasma exchange may be helpful in myasthenic crisis, but must be coupled with other immunosuppressive therapy.
- High-dose IVIg (hdIVIg) has also been demonstrated to be helpful in acute crises.

Testing
- See Table 5.1.

Table 5.1 Testing for myasthenia gravis

Tests for diagnosis	Test for monitoring
Edrophonium (Tensilon®) test	AchRAb
AChRAb	
Striated muscle antibodies	
MuSK antibodies	

Lambert–Eaton myasthenic syndrome (LEMS)

Presentation
- LEMS is an idiopathic or paraneoplastic syndrome.
- It is associated with small cell lung cancer as a paraneoplastic phenomenon (1–3% of cases of SCLC); 50–70% of cases of LEMS will have a malignancy.
- Some cases occur without cancer (especially in children) and are associated with HLA-B8, DR3.
- Proximal muscle weakness is marked but bulbar and ocular muscles are spared.
- Associated with other autoimmune diseases, especially thyroid and vitiligo.

Immunopathology
- There is a decrease of voltage-gated calcium channels (VGCC) on presynaptic nerve terminals, caused by an autoantibody reactive with the channels, particularly P/Q-type.
- Some patients have antibodies to synaptotagmin.
- Anti-glial nuclear antibody (AGNA), recognizing SOX1, is a specific marker for LEMS associated with SCLC.
- Patients with LEMS may also have antibodies to AChR.

Treatment
- Treatment of the tumour with chemotherapy may give temporary benefit.
- 3,4-diaminopyridine (blocks potassium channels) or guanidine may be needed to control the weakness.
- Plasma exchange or hdIVIg may be of significant (but temporary) benefit.
- In both non- and paraneoplastic forms, prednisolone is an option combined with azathioprine in non-paraneoplastic LEMS.

Acquired neuromyotonia (Isaac's disease) and stiff person syndrome (SPS)

Acquired neuromyotonia (Isaac's disease)

Presentation
- This syndrome is marked by acquired spontaneous and continuous muscle contraction.
- Patients develop stiffness, twitching, cramps, sweating, and other autonomic problems.

Immunopathology
- Some cases are due to autoantibodies against voltage-gated potassium channels (VGKC) at presynaptic nerve terminals.

Treatment
- Treated with phenytoin, carbamazepine, or immunosuppression.

Stiff person syndrome (SPS)
Presentation
- It causes a fluctuating and progressive muscular rigidity, which is painful.
- Men are more commonly affected than women.
- Up to a third of patients will develop diabetes and there may be features of autoimmune glandular disease.
- In approximately 10% of patients, SPS develops as a paraneoplastic disorder, associated with breast cancer.

Immunopathology
- This rare neurological syndrome is associated with anti-GAD antibodies.
- The finding of the autoantibody ties in with the neurological conclusion that GABAergic neurons, which regulate muscle tone, are involved.

Autoantibodies
- Anti-GAD antibodies are found in > 60% of patients with stiff person syndrome. See ➲ Chapter 18.
- Anti-amphiphysin antibodies are sometimes elevated in blood and CSF of patients with paraneoplastic SPS and, rarely, in non-neoplastic SPS.
- Anti-GlyR antibodies may be seen in paraneoplastic SPS.
- There is evidence that the autoantibodies are pathogenic in some cases of paraneoplastic SPS.

Treatment
- Muscle relaxants such as diazepam, baclofen, vigabatrin, and valproate are used.
- HdIVIg has been shown to be effective in a single trial in non-paraneoplastic SPS.
- Immunosuppression is frequently attempted.
- Case reports of complete remission with rituximab (anti-CD20).

Morvan's syndrome
- Rare syndrome of neuromyotonia, hyperhidrosis, insomnia, and delirium.
- Autoimmune aetiology; may be associated with thymoma (and solid tumours).+
- Associated with antibodies to VGKC and to CASPR2.
- May respond to corticosteroids, plasmapheresis, hdIVIg, and thymectomy.

Rasmussen encephalitis
- This rare syndrome usually presents in children with hemiparesis and intractable focal epilepsy, dementia, and cerebral atrophy.
- Associated with autoantibodies in some cases to glutamate R3 receptors and the synaptic protein munc-18. A subset is associated with antibodies to the NMDA receptor.
- It may respond to hdIVIg.

PANDAS (paediatric autoimmune neuropsychiatric disorders associated with *Streptococcus*)
- Syndrome with dramatic onset of symptoms including motor and vocal tics. Possibly similar to Sydenham's chorea, but no evidence of cardiac involvement. Basal ganglia affected.
- May be a genetic susceptibility to this syndrome after group A streptococcal infection, linked to expression of B-cell antigen D8/17.
- May respond to hdIVIg.

Paraneoplastic autoimmune neurological syndromes

Paraneoplastic cerebellar degeneration

- Associated with carcinoma of the breast and carcinoma of the ovary.
  - Anti-Yo antibodies, directed against the cytoplasm of cerebellar Purkinje cells and recognizing two antigens of molecular weights 34 and 62 kDa, are found.
- Associated with Hodgkin's lymphoma.
  - Anti-Tr antibodies.
  - Anti-mGluR1.
- Associated with small cell lung cancer, without LEMS.
  - Antibodies to P/Q VGCC.
  - Anti-PCA2 (also causes encephalomyelitis).
  - Zic4 (often in association with anti-Hu and anti-CV2/CRMP5).
- Associated with germ cell tumours, and breast and colon cancer.
  - Antibodies to Ma (Ma1, Ma2, Ma3).
- May be treated with immunosuppression, tumour removal, and hdIVIg.

Paraneoplastic neurological syndrome of ataxia and myoclonus (opsoclonus–myoclonus (OM))

- This has been described in patients with carcinoma of the breast, gynaecological cancer, and small cell carcinoma of lung.
- 50% of children with neuroblastoma develop OM.
- Patients may have anti-Yo or an anti-neuronal nuclear antibody, anti-Ri.
- May be treated with immunosuppression, tumour removal, plasma exchange, and hdIVIg.

Paraneoplastic ataxic sensory neuropathy or paraneoplastic encephalomyelitis

- This can occur in patients with small cell carcinoma of the lung, although less commonly patients may have anaplastic, bronchial, or squamous carcinoma of the lung, or reticuloendothelial neoplasms.
- Anti-Hu is an anti-neuronal nuclear antibody (ANNA), recognizing a group of proteins of molecular weight 35–40 kDa.
- Anti-Hu is one of the autoantibodies now known to penetrate intact cells containing the Hu antigen in their nucleus, indicating that it may have a primary pathogenic role.
- Other antibodies associated with paraneoplastic encephalomyelitis include anti-Zic4 and anti-Ma (brainstem encephalitis).
- Paraneoplastic tranverse myelitis with SCLC is associated with anti-Hu, anti-CV$_2$/CRMP5, or anti-amphiphysin antibodies.
- Paraneoplastic autonomic neuropathy is associated with anti-Hu, anti-CV$_2$/CRMP5, and antibodies to ganglionic AChR.
- Multiple other target antigens have been identified, but they occur extremely rarely.

Limbic encephalomyelitis

- This may occur alone or in association with malignancy.
- Encephalitis associated with antibodies to N-methyl-D-aspartate receptor (NMDAR) can affect any age or sex.
- Prodrome appears viral followed by psychiatric symptoms, memory loss, seizures, reduced consciousness, abnormal movements and autonomic instability. Diagnosis is often delayed.
- May be associated with teratomas, as well as lung, breast, or ovarian cancer.
- Other variants include:
  - Morvan's syndrome (see ➲ 'Morvan's syndrome', p. 205).
  - Encephalitis with antibodies to GABA$_{B1}$ receptor. Symptoms may include seizures, cerebellar symptoms, and opsoclonus. 50% will have SCLC.
  - Encephalitis with antibodies to GABA$_A$ receptor, presents with status epilepticus. May be associated with thymoma.
  - Encephalitis with AMPA (alpha-amino-3-hydroxyl-5-methyl-4-isoxazolepropionic acid) receptor antibodies, typically affects middle-aged women. 70% associated with tumours of breast, lung, and thymus.
  - Progressive encephalomyelitis with rigidity and myoclonus (PERM) is seen with antibodies to glycine receptor (GlyR). Mostly occurs in the absence of cancer but can be associated with lung cancer, thymoma, and Hodgkin's disease.
  - Encephalitis with antibodies to dpeptidyl peptidase-like protein 6 (DPPX) causes a syndrome with agitation, hallucinations, delusions, tremor, myoclonus, nystagmus, and seizures. GI symptoms may occur. Usually no tumour association.
  - Encephalitis with Parkinsonian features, dystonia, and chorea has been associated with dopamine-2 receptor antibodies (D2R antibodies).
  - Encephalitis with antibodies to glial fibrillary acidic protein (astrocytopathy).

Demyelinating diseases 1: multiple sclerosis (MS) and acute demyelinating encephalomyelitis (ADEM)

Multiple sclerosis (MS)

Clinical presentation

- Pattern of illness is difficult to predict and may be chronic and progressive, or relapsing and remitting.
- Progressive form of disease leads to disability.
- It affects any age, but predominantly the young and with a 2:1 female predominance.
- Clinical presentations are highly variable and include visual disturbance (optic neuritis), ataxia, weakness, and sensory signs, which usually, at least in initial attacks, resolve completely over a few days.

Immunogenetics
- MHC susceptibility loci have been identified, although these differ in different racial groups.
- DR2, DQ1, and DQ6 seem to be particularly important; DRB1*1501 is the strongest HLA association.
- Other genetic susceptibility loci are located on chromosomal regions 19q35 and 17q13.
- Monozygotic twin concordance is only 25–30%.

Immunopathology
- Cause of MS is unknown, although there are strong indications that it is triggered by infection.
- Disease seems to involve abnormal T cells reactive to myelin basic protein.
- Th 17 cells (and IL-17) are increased in lesions.
- Macrophages and microglia are involved, with local release of inflammatory cytokines and upregulation of MHC class II antigens.
- Plasma cells also localize to lesions, increasing local synthesis of IgG.
- There is selective destruction of myelin sheath and demyelination.
- Animal studies show that the disease can be transferred with CD4$^+$ T cells.
- CSF may contain membrane attack complexes of complement.
- Cytokines may be involved (TNF, IFNs, and IL-2).
- A high salt diet may activate autoreactive T cells.
- There may be a link to EBV infection.

Autoantibodies
- Autoantibodies to myelin oligodendrocyte glycoprotein (MOG) may occur.
- Some patients with a typical MS pattern of demyelination may demonstrate anti-nuclear antibodies and antibodies to dsDNA, without other features of SLE.
- Conversely, some patients who clearly have SLE develop MS-like symptoms and signs.

Investigations
- There are no specific diagnostic immunological tests.
- Examination of serum and CSF demonstrates increased intrathecal immunoglobulin synthesis, with a CSF IgG/albumin ratio of > 22%.
- Isoelectric focusing and immunoblotting demonstrate the presence of oligoclonal IgG bands, but these are not specific for MS, being also found in neurosarcoid, neurosyphilis, acute viral infections of the CNS, SLE, and Sjögren's syndrome.
- Other helpful tests include evoked potentials (visual, auditory, peripheral).
- MRI scanning shows typically placed demyelinating lesions.
- Rarely, patients with MS develop a uveitis as well as an optic neuritis: this may be associated with autoantibodies to the retinal S-antigen.

Treatment

- Acute attacks may respond to high-dose steroids, but chronic steroid therapy does not prevent relapses.
- Cytotoxic agents mitoxantrone, cladribine, azathioprine, and cyclophosphamide have also shown some benefit.
- Interferon beta (1a and 1b) (8 mU/alternate days subcutaneously) has shown considerable promise in decreasing the relapse rate in the relapsing–remitting form. Utility of therapy may be limited by anti-interferon antibodies.
  - Drugs have significant immunomodulatory effects, including reducing T-cell proliferation, decreasing induced MHC class II antigen expression, and reducing the production of inflammatory cytokines (TNFα and γ-IFN).
  - Effect may be monitored by measuring production of myxoma resistance protein A (MxA).
- Natalizumab is a mAb against α4-integrin; shown to be useful in MS. Concerns raised about possible association with progressive multifocal leukoencephalopathy (PML) and it should only be used in JC-virus negative patients.
- Other biologicals in trial include daclizumab (anti-IL-2R), rituximab (anti-CD20), and alemtuzumab (anti-CD52). Daclizumab has been suspended due to reports of serious/fatal encephalitis thought to be due to the drug.
- Glatiramer acetate is an immunomodulatory drug comprising synthetic polypeptides and also reduces attack rate in relapsing–remitting disease.
- Fingolimod is a sphingosine analogue that modulates the sphingosine-1-phosphate receptor and alters lymphocyte migration. Benefit identified, possibly best for newly diagnosed patients.
- Dimethyl fumarate (Tecfidera®, also used in skin disease) has been shown to reduce new lesions. This causes marked T-cell lymphopenia, so regular monitoring is advised.
- Teriflunomide inhibits the mitochondrial enzyme dihydro-orotate dehydrogenase and is the active metabolite of leflunomide. Pyrimidine synthesis is blocked. It is teratogenic and can remain in the circulation for up to 2 years, but the use of colestyramine or activated charcoal will accelerate removal.
- Evidence for the use of hdIVIg is sparse.
- TNFα blockade is not helpful.

Acute demyelinating encephalomyelitis (ADEM)

- A monophasic demyelinating disease usually associated with a preceding infection, typically childhood viral infections (measles, varicella) and rarely with vaccination to measles.
- Other associated infections include EBV, HHV6, HIV, rubella, mumps, influenza, mycoplasma.
- Children affected most frequently but may occur in adults.
- May present as acute haemorrhagic leukoencephalitis.
- MRI changes can be distinguished from MS.

- Associated with cross-reactive autoimmune response, leading to demyelination. Antibodies to myelin basic protein may be found.
- Oligoclonal bands in CSF occur less frequently than in MS and are usually transient.
- Some patients progress on to an MS-like illness.

Demyelinating diseases 2: Guillain–Barré syndrome and variants

Clinical presentation
- An inflammatory demyelinating peripheral neuropathy that frequently follows 1–3 weeks after infection, particularly with *Campylobacter jejuni*.
- Begins with ascending weakness, which may progress with alarming rapidity and involve bulbar and respiratory muscles, including the diaphragm, leading to respiratory failure.
- Sensory symptoms are mild.
- There may be marked autonomic instability.
- Demyelination may progress for up to 4 weeks before remyelination begins.
- Recovery may be very prolonged.
- There are a number of variants to this classical presentation and progression, including acute motor axonal neuropathy, acute motor sensory axonal neuropathy, and the Miller–Fisher variant, with ophthalmoplegia, ataxia, and areflexia.

Immunopathology and autoantibodies
- Antibodies to membrane gangliosides (glycolipids including GM1, LM1, and GD1b) are detected in sera from up to 40% of patients with GBS.
- These antibodies interfere with nerve conduction and have been shown to activate phagocytes via IgG receptors.
- Antibodies to GQ1b are present in 90–100% of cases of the Miller–Fisher variant and seem to be specific for this condition, related possibly to the very high expression of this antigen in the third cranial nerve.
- Antibodies to GT1a are associated with acute pharyngeal cervicobrachial neuropathy (APCBN).
- Antibodies to GD1a, GM1, GM1b, and GalNAc-GD1a are associated with acute motor axonal neuropathy.
- Anti-GM1 antibodies are known to cross-react with lipopolysaccharides from *C. jejuni*.
- CSF will contain increased levels of cytokines (IL-6, TNFα, γ-IFN).

Treatment
- Treatment is best undertaken with plasmapheresis or hdIVIg, which appear to be equally effective if begun early.
- There is a suggestion that the relapse rate may be higher with hdIVIg.
- Steroids are of no benefit, and may make symptoms worse.
- Miller–Fisher variant appears to be relatively benign and resolves without treatment.

Demyelinating diseases 3: chronic inflammatory demyelinating polyneuropathy (CIDP), related conditions, and Devic's syndrome (neuromyelitis optica)

Chronic inflammatory demyelinating polyneuropathy (CIDP)

Clinical features

- CIDP resembles a chronic form of GBS.
- Characterized by mainly distal weakness and areflexia as well as marked sensory signs.
- There is usually no history of antecedent infection.

Investigations

- The diagnosis is confirmed by the course, exclusion of other diseases, and by typical electrophysiological studies, compatible with demyelination.
- Complement-fixing IgG and IgM antibodies may be demonstrated in affected nerves.
- Autoantibodies to the gangliosides GM1, LM1, and GD1b can be found in some patients. Other antibodies have been detected to P0, myelin P2 protein, PMP22, or neurofascin.
- 25% of cases with features of CIPD have a monoclonal gammopathy of uncertain significance (MGUS), usually IgG or IgA. POEMS syndrome should be excluded.
- Patients with predominantly sensory symptoms and an IgM paraprotein may have antibodies against myelin-associated glycoprotein (MAG). The IgM antibodies are incorporated into the myelin, giving a distinctive pattern on EM. This condition is often refractory to treatment.

Treatment

- Steroids, cytotoxic agents, plasmapheresis, and hdIVIg have all been used successfully.
- If hdIVIg is to be given, current practice is to give three courses at monthly intervals and a further three courses if there is benefit.
- Treatment is then discontinued, to see whether patients maintain a remission.
- Some patients require long-term hdIVIg therapy.
- Refractory patients may respond to rituximab.

Related conditions

- Other related conditions that may have an autoimmune basis include amyotrophic lateral sclerosis and multifocal motor neuropathy with conduction block.
  - Multifocal motor neuropathy with conduction block is associated with high-titre polyclonal antibodies to GM1. Plasma exchange and steroids

may not be effective, but hdIVIg is usually helpful. Rituximab and cyclophosphamide have been used for resistant cases.
- Chronic sensory ataxic neuropathy is associated with antibodies to GD1b and GQ1b.
- Treatment is the same as for CIDP.

Devic's syndrome (neuromyelitis optica)

- Comprises attacks of optic neuritis and myelitis but, unlike MS, there is no brainstem, cerebellar, or cognitve involvement. It is an aggressive disease with 60% of patients blind after 8 years.
- Seen mainly in Asian and African people but not Caucasian people.
- May be associated with other autoimmune conditions: SLE, Sjögren's syndrome, P-ANCA+ vasculitis, mixed connective tissue disease, myasthenia gravis, Hashimoto's thyroiditis.
- Can be triggered by varicella, EBV, TB, or HIV infection.
- May rarely be paraneoplastic (breast, lung, and other cancers).
- Autoantibodies to aquaporin 4 (channel for water transport in astrocytes) are frequently found and are diagnostic. Seropositive patients have high rate of relapse.
- Oligoclonal bands are seen in < 30% of cases.
- Demyelination is complement-mediated and thus distinct from MS.
- Treatments include high-dose steroids and plasma exchange for acute attacks. Rituximab, mycophenolate and azathioprine are used to reduce the risk of relapses. Interferon beta is not effective and may increase the risk of relapses.

Demyelinating diseases 4: paraproteinaemic neuropathy and paraproteinaemic myopathy

Paraproteinaemic neuropathy

- Demyelinating polyneuropathies may be associated with paraproteins of all classes.
- Anti-MAG neuropathy is particularly associated with IgM paraproteins directed against MAG, a 100 kDa glycoprotein of central and peripheral nerves.
  - The light chain of the monoclonal protein is invariably lambda.

Paraproteinaemic neuropathies may be associated with:
- Waldenstrom's macroglobulinaemia.
- Amyloidosis (see ➲ Chapter 14).
- Type II cryoglobulinaemia.
- POEMS syndrome (polyneuropathy, organomegaly, endocrinopathy, monoclonal gammopathy, and skin changes; see also ➲ Chapter 4).
  - Skin changes tend to be a sclerodermatous thickening.
  - Endocrine diseases include diabetes, thyroid disease, gonadal failure, and hyperprolactinaemia.

- Lymph nodes may show the changes of Castleman's syndrome, or angiofollicular lymph node hyperplasia (with 'onion-skin' lesions), which is of itself also associated with a polyneuropathy; the lesion is not thought to be malignant.
  - IL-6 levels are said to be raised, explaining the plasma-cell abnormalities.
- CIDP associated with MGUS: a MGUS will be found in approximately 10% of patients for whom no diagnosis has been identified.
- A severe motor and sensory polyneuropathy is seen in up to 50% of patients with osteosclerotic myeloma and can be the presenting feature of the illness.

Treatment
- Treatment of paraproteinaemic neuropathies should include treatment of the underlying plasma-cell clone with steroids, melphalan, or chlorambucil.
- Plasmapheresis and hdIVIg are useful as for CIDP.

Paraproteinaemic myopathy: anti-decorin (BJ) antibodies have been associated with myopathy associated with Waldenström's macroglobulinaemia (specificity of the paraprotein).

Vasculitic neuropathy and Degos's disease

Vasculitic neuropathy

Systemic causes
- Behçet's disease.
- Giant cell arteritis (GCA).
- Takayasu's arteritis.
- Wegener's granulomatosis (granulomatous polyangiitis).
- Churg–Strauss syndrome (eosinophilic granulomatous polyangiitis).
- Cogan's syndrome.
- Kawasaki's disease.
- Henoch–Schönlein purpura in children.
- Polyarteritis nodosa.
- Systemic lupus erythematosus.
- Rheumatoid arthritis.

Clinical features
- Clinical deficits arise from nerve ischaemia or infarction.
- Patients may present with a variety of symptoms including mononeuritis multiplex, asymmetric neuropathy, and a distal polyneuropathy.

Investigations
- Nerve biopsy shows a vasculitis of the epineurial arterioles, focal or multifocal fibre loss, and areas of segmental demyelination and remyelination.
- Investigation should follow the guidance in Chapter 13.

Treatment
- Steroids are the mainstay of treatment with or without the addition of cytotoxics.
- Cyclophosphamide appears to be the most effective treatment.

Degos's disease
- See ➲ Chapter 13.
- A vasculitic syndrome, in which cerebral infarction is a major feature.
- Associated with the presence of anti-cardiolipin antibodies and a lupus anticoagulant.
- Activated T cells (virally triggered) may be the pathogenic mechanism.

Neuropathy associated with Sjögren's syndrome (SS)

Clinical features
Patients may present with a number of neurological conditions:
- Chronic and slowly progressive sensorimotor neuropathy.
- Sensory neuropathy.
- Neuronopathy.
- Mononeuritis multiplex.
- Multiple recurrent cranial neuropathies.
- Subacute demyelinating polyradiculopathy.

Autoantibodies
- An IgG antibody can be detected against Ro and La in approximately 50% of patients.
- See ➲ Chapter 12 for details of investigation of suspected SS.

Treatment
- Response to treatments has generally been disappointing.
- Steroids, immunosuppression, plasma exchange, and hdIVIg have all been used.

Autoimmune encephalopathies

Encephalopathies have been associated with the following.
- Sjögren's syndrome: this is not well established.
- Hashimoto's thyroiditis with high levels of anti-thyroid antibodies.
  - α-Enolase has been identified as an autoantigen in this syndrome.
  - Treatment is with corticosteroids and hdIVIg.
- Coeliac disease in association with occipital lobe epilepsy and intracranial calcification has been described. Seizure control may improve with a strict gluten-free diet
- Coeliac disease may also be associated with a cerebellar syndrome which may respond to gluten withdrawal.

- Claims have been made that this syndrome is associated with IgG anti-gliadin rather than endomysial or tTG antibodies. Evidence is weak.
- Synapsin I has been identified as a possible target of cross-reactive anti-gliadin antibodies.

Primary angiitis of the central nervous system (PACNS)

- See ➔ Chapter 13.

Autoimmunity in other neurological diseases

Research suggests that some diseases not previously considered to have an immunological basis may in fact be immune (autoimmune) mediated. Further research is clearly needed. These include:

- Schizophrenia.
  - Autoimmune mechanism has been proposed.
- Sporadic Parkinson's disease.
  - Autoreactive T cells identified against pluripotent stem cells.
- Chronic fatigue syndrome (ME).
  - Autoantibodies to CNS adrenoreceptors have been described.
  - Rituximab and plasmapheresis have been used with success in some (but not all) patients.

Autoimmunity associated with cardiac, respiratory, and renal disease

Cardiac diseases 1: myocarditis and cardiomyopathy

Myocarditis

- This is associated with infections (coxsackievirus, HIV, trypanosomes, spirochaetes, rickettsia), connective tissue diseases, especially SLE, and vasculitis, particularly Churg–Strauss syndrome, sarcoidosis, and giant cell myocarditis.
- May present with congestive heart failure, arrhythmias, and chest pain.
- There appears to be an association with anti-ribonucleoprotein (RNP) antibodies.
- After viral myocarditis, autoantibodies to β-adrenergic receptors, troponin, and Na^+/K^+ ATPase have been reported—significance is uncertain.
- Endomyocardial biopsy may be helpful
- There is usually a good response to steroids.

Cardiomyopathy

- Anti-cardiac antibodies are associated with dilated cardiomyopathy, which may also have features of myocarditis on biopsy.
- Anti-cardiac antibodies are also found in 20% of cases of type II autoimmune polyglandular syndrome, but in this syndrome are not associated with cardiomyopathy, but with an increase in blood pressure.
- Antibodies are directed against cardiac atrial cells producing atrial natriuretic peptide.
- Dilated cardiomyopathy is associated with M7 anti-mitochondrial antibodies recognizing mitochondrial flavoproteins, including riboflavin.
- Cardiomyopathy may be associated with amyloidosis (light chain; transthyretin, senile).

Cardiac diseases 2: eosinophilic syndromes

- Rare eosinophilic syndromes may affect the myocardium, leading eventually to endomyocardial fibrosis.
- Churg–Strauss (eosinophilic granulomatosis with polyangiitis, EGPA) syndrome frequently involves the myocardium—check ANCA and IgE.
- Idiopathic eosinophilic syndromes may affect the heart.
- Echocardiography is required.

Cardiac diseases 3: recurrent pericarditis and Dressler's syndrome

Recurrent pericarditis

- May occur as a disease in its own right, although it is a common feature of connective tissue diseases including:
  - SLE and rheumatoid arthritis (RhA);
  - auto-inflammatory diseases e.g. familial Mediterranean fever (see ➲ 'Familial Mediterranean fever', see ➲ Chapter 14).
- Pericardium is thickened, with an infiltrate of inflammatory cells.
- No specific immunological tests.
- NSAIDs are the first line of treatment. Steroids may be required, and colchicine has been suggested as a useful agent.
- Pericardectomy may be required.

Dressler's syndrome

- This is (myo-)pericarditis following 2–3 weeks after a myocardial infarction and presenting with typical pericarditic pain.
- It is very rare since thrombolytic therapy has been introduced.
- Antibodies to cardiac muscle are often present.
- Post-pericardotomy syndrome is similar but follows cardiac surgery.
- NSAIDs and steroids may be required but the syndromes settle spontaneously.

Cardiac diseases 4: rheumatic fever

Clinical features

- Incidence is now increasing.
- Mainly affects children but can be seen in adults.
- Clinical features include carditis, polyarthritis, chorea, cutaneous nodules, erythema marginatum, prolonged PR interval on ECG, and raised CRP/ESR, together with evidence of previous streptococcal infection with group A streptococci.

Immunopathology

- Appears to be due to an aberrant immunological response to the streptococcal M-proteins (M-proteins 5, 14, 24), some of which generate antibodies that are cross-reactive with human sarcolemmal proteins and with myosin.
- Other streptococcal M-proteins cause cross-reactive antibodies reacting with the vimentin of glomerular mesangial cells, and are therefore associated with glomerulonephritis.
- M-protein types 1, 5, and 18 cross-react with cartilage epitopes, thus potentially leading to arthritis.
- In addition, the M-proteins may act as bacterial superantigens, enhancing the autodestructive immune response.
- Genetic studies have identified that polymorphisms in MBL2, Ficolin 32, TLR2, TNF, TGFβ1, and CTLA4 can increase susceptibility. HLA-B5 is also associated.

Diagnosis
- There are no specific immunological tests.
- Diagnosis is clinical, supported by ECG, elevated acute-phase proteins, and raised antistreptolysin O titre (ASOT).

Treatment
- Antibiotics are prescribed to eliminate the organism.
- NSAIDs for arthralgia.
- Corticosteroids for carditis.
- Long-term penicillin prophylaxis is required as the syndrome will recur on subsequent group A streptococcal infection.

Respiratory disease 1: idiopathic pulmonary fibrosis (cryptogenic fibrosing alveolitis)

Clinical features
- Patients present with severe progressive breathlessness; a fulminant presentation, often with fever and cough, is referred to as the Hamman–Rich syndrome.
- Inflammatory lung fibrosis may occur in association with connective tissue diseases (SLE, Sjögren's syndrome, antisynthetase syndrome—see ➜ Chapter 12) and as a consequence of drug exposure, especially nitrofurantoin.
- Many cases have no obvious trigger or association.

Immunopathogenesis
- Biopsies show activated macrophages and a neutrophil infiltrate.
- In the early stages there is a lymphoid infiltrate (before fibrosis develops), and excess local cytokine production can be demonstrated (TNFα, IL-2, γ-IFN, TGFβ, IL-8).

Investigations
- Lung function shows a reduced forced vital capacity (FVC) and diffusion capacity, with desaturation on exercise.
- BAL may be helpful as part of the diagnostic work-up (see ➜ Chapter 20), particularly where there is a lymphocytosis.
- Biopsy (transbronchial or transthoracic) may be required.
- Chest X-ray (CXR) and lung CT demonstrate the typical interstitial fibrosis.
- Most patients show an acute-phase response with a polyclonal hypergammaglobulinaemia.
- RhF is found in 50% and ANA in 20%.

Treatment
- Treatment is with steroids, with either azathioprine or cyclophosphamide, but the response is often poor and the disease is progressive.

Respiratory disease 2: pulmonary alveolar proteinosis (PAP)

Clinical features
- May be congenital (see ➲ Chapter 1) or acquired (silicosis, immunodeficiency, malignancy).
- Gradual onset of exertional dyspnoea, fever, fatigue, and weight loss.

Immunopathogenesis
- Congenital PAP is an autosomal recessive disease caused by mutations in the surfactant protein B (SP-B) gene.

Investigations
- Associated with polyclonal hypergammaglobulinaemia (unless secondary to immune deficiency).

Treatment
- Whole lung lavage may be helpful.

Respiratory disease 3: lymphoid interstitial pneumonitis and sarcoidosis

Lymphoid interstitial pneumonitis

Clinical features
- Patients present with chronic cough, shortness of breath, and chest pain.
- May occur alone, but is more usually found in autoimmune diseases such as Sjögren's syndrome, SLE, dermatomyositis, polymyositis, and in association with drugs.
- Also associated with viral infection (particularly HIV, EBV), and common variable immunodeficiency.

Investigations
- Biopsy and BAL are the most helpful tests.
- There is a lymphocytic alveolitis (CD8$^+$ T cells in HIV and CD4$^+$ T cells in Sjögren's syndrome).
- Hypergammaglobulinaemia is usually found, but is anyway associated with the primary disorders (with the exception of CVID).

Treatment
- Corticosteroids and immunosuppressive drugs (rituximab, cyclophosphamide, and azathioprine) may be used.
- Treatment of underlying infection, where present.

Sarcoidosis
- See ➲ Chapter 14.
- Although not normally considered an autoimmune disease, some patients with histologically proven sarcoidosis have anti-nuclear and dsDNA antibodies.

Respiratory disease 4: eosinophilic lung syndromes

The lung is affected by a variety of hypereosinophilic syndromes:
- Löeffler's syndrome (a hypersensitivity reaction to drugs, parasites, or idiopathic).
- Chronic eosinophilic pneumonia.
- Tropical pulmonary eosinophilia (due to filariasis).
- Churg–Strauss syndrome (eosinophilic granulomatosis with polyangiitis, EGPA—often associated with neuropathy), see ➔ Chapter 13.
- Eosinophilia–myalgia syndrome (contaminated L-tryptophan).
- Bronchopulmonary aspergillosis.
- Eosinophilic granuloma (Langerhans cell histiocytosis).

Investigations
- Investigations that may help distinguish the cause, other than standard respiratory investigations (CXR, respiratory function tests, CT), include:
  - BAL, with lymphocyte subpopulation analysis; if Langerhans cell histiocytosis is suspected, then antibodies to the S-100 antigen should be included in the panel;
  - biopsy;
  - ANCA (including MPO and PR3 antibodies);
  - IgE and specific IgE (*Aspergillus*);
  - *Aspergillus* precipitins;
  - identification of parasitic infection (direct identification, serology).
- Eosinophil cationic protein (ECP).
  - The role of serum ECP levels is uncertain, as it is likely to be raised whatever the cause of eosinophil activation.
  - It may, however, have a role in monitoring the response to treatment and be a more sensitive marker of damaging activity than eosinophil number in the peripheral blood.

Treatment
- Treatment is usually with steroids, once an underlying infective trigger has been excluded.
- Churg–Strauss syndrome (EGPA) usually requires additional cytotoxic therapy.

Respiratory disease 5: other respiratory diseases

Various aspects of respiratory disease are covered in other chapters (Chapter 3, ➔ 'Allergic disease'; Chapter 13, ➔ 'Vasculitis'; and Chapter 14, ➔ 'Miscellaneous syndromes'). Goodpasture's syndrome is covered in this chapter under ➔ 'Renal disease 5', p. 226.

A useful website
British Thoracic Society: ℘ www.brit-thoracic.org.uk

Renal disease 1: glomerulonephritis—an overview

The diagnosis of glomerulonephritis is complex and specialized. It relies upon the synthesis of multiple diagnostic strands, including routine histology, immunofluorescence on biopsies, electron microscopy, and serological tests. All the histology should be done in the same laboratory and reported by the same person: it is inappropriate for immunology laboratories to do the direct immunofluorescence while not seeing the H & E sections, special stains, and EM.

Renal disease 2: necrotizing crescentic glomerulonephritis

Clinical features
- Presentation is usually fulminant.
- Associated with systemic vasculitis (Wegener's granulomatosis (granulomatosis with polyangiitis (GPA)), microscopic polyarteritis), or with renal-limited disease.
- See ⤷ Chapter 13.

Investigations
- ANCA and anti-GBM antibody are required.
- Positive ANCA by immunofluorescence should be titred (so that the reduction by plasmapheresis can be checked) and should be typed as proteinase 3 (Pr3)- or myeloperoxidase (MPO)-positive.
- Quantitative anti-GBM is also helpful when patients are plasmaphoresed.
- A small number of patients will have both ANCA and GBM antibodies.
- Routine serology for ANA, dsDNA, C3, C4, and acute-phase reactants should also be taken as a baseline.
- Renal biopsy: examination should include direct immunofluorescence and EM as well as normal histological stains.
- Monitoring of patients subsequently should include ANCA titre and CRP/ESR—a rising titre of ANCA may herald relapse, but the numeric value has no relation to disease activity.

Treatment
- Patients should be plasmaphoresed acutely, starting immunosuppressive therapy at the same time
- Treatment should not be delayed waiting for antibody results.
  - 5% of patients will be ANCA negative.
  - Out-of-hours ANCA are therefore not required.
- Immunosuppression is with high-dose steroids with cyclophosphamide.
- Initial treatment is given as pulsed intravenous therapy: the merits of continuous oral cyclophosphamide therapy versus pulsed intravenous or oral are still debated.
- Azathioprine and mycophenolate mofetil have been suggested as possible alternatives to cyclophosphamide after the initial phase.
- Rituximab may be used.

Testing
- See Table 6.1.

Table 6.1 Testing for necrotizing crescentic glomerulonephritis

Tests for diagnosis	Tests for monitoring
Urinalysis (sediment for casts)	Urinalysis (sediment for casts)
Cr & E	Cr & E
FBC	FBC
ESR and CRP	ESR and CRP
ANCA and titre	ANCA and titre
Anti-GBM (quantitate if positive)	Quantitative GBM (if being plasmapheresed or considered for transplant)
ANA, dsDNA, C3, C4	

Renal disease 3: immune complex glomerulonephritis

- Immune complex glomerulonephritis may be triggered by a host of antigenic stimuli including:
  - bacteria: nephritogenic streptococci; staphylococci (SBE); treponemes; mycoplasma; salmonella;
  - viruses: EBV, CMV, HIV, hepatitis B, hepatitis C;
  - fungi: *Candida* (systemic infection);
  - parasites: *Plasmodium* species, *Schistosoma*, *Toxoplasma*;
  - drugs: xeno-antisera (serum sickness);
  - connective tissue diseases: SLE, mixed connective tissue disease (MCTD; rarer);
  - tumours: lymphoma, carcinoma.
- Also associated with complement deficiency.
  - Any component.
  - C3-nephritic factor (secondary consumption).

Diagnosis
- The circumstances under which the glomerulonephritis develops gives useful clues as to the diagnosis.
- Activity of the renal disease is marked by the presence of casts (especially red cell) in the urinary sediment.
- The type of immune deposits in the biopsy also gives important clues as to the underlying aetiology.

Testing
- See Table 6.2.

Table 6.2 Testing for immune complex glomerulonephritis

Tests for diagnosis	Tests for monitoring
Urinalysis for casts	Urinalysis for casts
Cr & E	Cr & E
FBC	FBC
ESR & CRP	ESR & CRP
ANA, dsDNA, ENA	Other tests, depending on underlying diagnosis
C3, C4, complement breakdown products	
C3-nephritic factor (persistent low C3 > 6 weeks)	
Cryoglobulins (low C4, no ANA, dsDNA, check for HCV)	
RhF	
Serum immunoglobulins and electrophoresis (monoclonal component in type II cryoglobulins, HCV; raised IgA in HSP)	
Infectious serology (ASOT)	

Renal disease 4: post-streptococcal glomerulonephritis, mixed essential cryoglobulinaemia, and IgA nephropathy

Post-streptococcal glomerulonephritis

- This is accompanied by a reduced C3, normal C4, and elevated complement breakdown products (C3d).
- ASOT will be high, although the rise may take at least a week.
- Normally, the C3 level will return to normal within 8 weeks.
- Persistently low C3 with normal C4 beyond this time, in the presence of renal disease, suggests the presence of a C3-nephritic factor (see ➲ 'Renal disease 8: C3-nephritic factors and C4-nephritic factors', p. 230).

Mixed essential cryoglobulinaemia

- Caused by hepatitis C, which explains the high incidence of mixed essential cryoglobulinaemia in northern Italy.
- Type II cryoglobulin with rheumatoid-factor activity.

- Paraprotein component is usually IgMκ, and the bone marrow often shows a monoclonal expansion of B cells.
- Features of the disease, other than immune complex glomerulonephritis and hepatitis, include arthralgia, skin rashes, and neuropathy.

Treatment
- Treatment of the underlying HCV infection (with α-IFN ± ribavirin) often improves the paraproteinaemia and cryoglobulinaemia.
- Treatment of the abnormal plasma cell clone may require cytotoxics.
- Plasmapheresis may be necessary to reduce the cryoglobulin level. Rituximab may be useful.
- Type II or type III cryoglobulins may also be detected in other chronic infections that cause glomerulonephritis, such as SBE.

IgA nephropathy
- The renal lesion is characterized by deposition of IgA immune complexes in the glomerulus, as also seen in the renal lesions associated with Henoch–Schönlein purpura (HSP).
- Both this and HSP may be associated with HLA-Bw35.
- Serum IgA levels are variable but may be significantly elevated. However, this is not a specific test, as liver disease and infections may also lead to persistent elevation of IgA.
- Some types of IgA nephropathy may be associated with IgA class ANCA, although this is not fully substantiated.
- Rituximab has been used for treatment.

Renal disease 5: anti-GBM disease (Goodpasture's syndrome)

Clinical features
- Characterized by glomerulonephritis and sometimes pulmonary haemorrhage, which may lead to secondary pulmonary haemosiderosis.
- Lung involvement without renal disease is rare.
- Onset is usually sudden and may be preceded by flu-like symptoms and arthralgia.
- Disease may be triggered by toxin exposure (hydrocarbon solvents) or infections.
- Smokers are more likely to develop lung haemorrhage than non-smokers.
- May also be caused by penicillamine therapy.
- Associated with other autoimmune diseases, including Wegener's granulomatosis (GPA), M-PAN, thyroid disease, Behçet's disease, coeliac disease, inflammatory bowel disease, thymoma, lymphoma, and other malignancies.

Immunopathology

- Characterized by the presence in almost all cases of an autoantibody directed against the non-collagenous region of the α3-chain of type IV collagen (anti-GBM antibodies).
- This antigen is missing in patients with Alport's syndrome (hereditary deafness and glomerulonephritis), and these patients make a nephritogenic antibody if transplanted with a normal kidney.
- Type IV collagen forms the basement membrane in both the glomerulus and lung, but is also found in the cochlear basement membrane, eye, choroid of the brain, and in liver, adrenal, pituitary, and thyroid.
- Eye and brain disease may occasionally be found in anti-GBM disease.

Immunogenetics

- Disease is strongly MHC-associated (DRw15(DR2)/DQw6, DR4/ DQw7).
- Male:female ratio 6:1.

Investigations

- Renal biopsy shows the typical appearance of basement membrane deposition of IgG (rarely IgA or IgM) and a C3 (linear staining) which is best seen in the glomeruli. This can also be seen on good bronchial biopsies.
- Serum invariably contains high levels of circulating anti-GBM antibodies (> 90% of patients positive), which should be quantitated to allow monitoring of therapy.
- Patient should be screened for coincident ANCA-positive vasculitis.
- Disease can recur in a transplanted kidney: if antibodies are still present, transplantation should be deferred for a minimum of 6 months and preferably 12 months after the antibody has disappeared from the circulation.
- Serial monitoring over long periods is therefore justified where transplantation is considered or has been undertaken.

Treatment

- Acute treatment involves plasmapheresis (although the controlled trial data to support this are sparse) or immunoadsorption with protein G columns (experimental).
- Longer-term therapy involves steroids and cyclophosphamide (intravenous pulsed therapy), although the optimal regimen has not been defined.
- Rituximab may be used.
- Aggressive therapy should be continued until the antibody level drops significantly.

Testing

- See Table 6.3.

Table 6.3 Testing for anti-GBM disease

Tests for diagnosis	Tests for monitoring
Urinalysis for casts	Urinalysis for casts
Cr & E	Cr & E
FBC	FBC
ESR and CRP	ESR and CRP
Renal biopsy	Anti-GBM (quantitate)
ANCA	Pulmonary function tests including diffusing capacity
Anti-GBM (quantitate)	
Pulmonary function tests including diffusing capacity	

Renal disease 6: typical and atypical haemolytic–uraemic syndrome (HUS)

Clinical features

- Characterized by acute severe illness with haemolytic anaemia, thrombocytopenia, and acute kidney injury. Diarrhoea, peripheral ischaemic vasculopathy, myocardial infarction, and liver involvement are all described.
- Most cases occur in children but can be seen in adults. 90% are due to Shiga toxin-producing E. coli (STEC).
- In 10%, no association with STEC (atypical)—associated with abnormalities of the complement system.
- May need to be distinguished from thrombotic thrombocytopenic purpura (TTP) due to acquired or congenital ADAMTS13 deficiency.
- May occur secondary to other diseases:
  - SLE, scleroderma, antiphospholipid syndrome.
  - Malignant hypertension.
  - Deficiency in cobalamin metabolism (methylmalonic aciduria).
  - Malignancy.
  - Associated with pregnancy (pre-eclampsia, HELLP syndrome).
  - GvHD after BMT.
  - *DGKE* mutation (diacylglycerol kinase epsilon)—aHUS before age of 1.

Immunopathology

- Characterized by the presence on renal biopsy of thrombotic microangiopathy.
- Autoantibodies to factor H have been documented.

- C3 will be reduced; haemolytic complement will be reduced.
- May recur in renal transplants.
- *DGKE* mutations increase endothelial ICAM-1 expression producing a pro-inflammatory and pro-thrombotic endothelium.

Immunogenetics

- Disease is strongly associated with complement gene abnormalities:
  - Complement factors H & I.
  - MCP.
  - Thrombomodulin.
  - Gain-of-function mutations in C3 and factor B.
  - Some factor H mutations are protective.

Investigations

- Rapid recognition is required.
- Cr & E.
- Full blood count; film will help (fragmented red cells).
- Clotting studies, including fibrinogen and degradation products.
- Haptoglobin & LDH for haemolysis.
- Complement studies (C3, C4, factor B, haemolytic complement, C5a–C9).
- MCP expression by flow cytometry.
- Factor H autoantibodies.
- Faecal sample for STEC detection.
- Tests to exclude secondary causes (other infections, autoimmune diseases).
- Genetic studies for complement mutations.
- Exclude TTP with ADAMTS13 assays.
- Exclude methylmalonic aciduria.
- Consider renal biopsy.

Treatment

- Discuss with Specialist HUS Centre.
- Plasma exchange. Especially beneficial if factor H autoantibodies are present.
- Eculizumab: blocks conversion of C5 to C5a and C5b, preventing generation of terminal lytic sequence.
- Other drugs are being developed—see ➡ Chapter 16.
- Renal replacement therapy.
- Renal transplantation if end-stage renal disease—note risk of recurrence.
- Consider risks of invasive meningococcal infection (immunize and consider prophylactic antibiotics).

Testing

- See Table 6.4.

Table 6.4 Testing for HUS disease

Tests for diagnosis	Tests for monitoring
Urinalysis for casts	Urinalysis for casts
Cr & E	Cr & E
LFTs	LFTs
FBC & blood film	FBC
ESR and CRP	ESR and CRP
Renal biopsy	Haptoglobin, LDH
Haptoglobin & LDH (haemolysis)	Complement studies
Clotting studies	
Complement studies (C3, C4, factor B, CH50/APCH50, C5b-C9)	
ADAMTS13	
Autoantibodies to factor H	
MCP by flow cytometry	
Genetic testing	

Renal disease 7: idiopathic membranous nephropathy

Idiopathic membranous nephropathy is a common cause of nephrotic syndrome in adults.

- May be associated with autoantibody against phospholipase A_2 receptor (PLA2R1) in the majority of cases.
- 10% of anti-PLA2R1-negative patients have antibodies to thrombospondin type-1 domain-containing 7A (THSD7A).
- Autoantibody may be IgG_4.
- Levels of anti-PLA2R1 correlate with disease activity and disease progression.
- There is linkage to HLA (DRB1*1501 & DRB3*00202).

Renal disease 8: C3-nephritic factors and C4-nephritic factors

C3-nephritic factors (C3nef) are autoantibodies which bind to and stabilize the alternate pathway C3-convertase (C3bBb). C4nef, much rarer, stabilize the classical pathways C3-convertase (C4bC2b). Both lead to uncontrolled complement activation.

- May occur in some healthy individuals.
- Seen in patients with post-streptococcal glomerulonephritis (see
  ➔ 'Renal disease 4: post-streptococcal glomerulonephritis, mixed essential cryoglobulinaemia, and IgA nephropathy', p. 225).

- Most common in membranoproliferative glomerulonephritis:
  - 80% of patients with dense-deposit disease.
  - 40% of patients with C3 glomerulonephritis.
  - Cause proteinuria, haematuria, nephrotic or nephritic syndromes.
  - Disease will recur in 80% of patients receiving renal transplant for end-stage renal disease.
- Found in patients presenting with acquired partial lipodystrophy (which may precede kidney disease by many years).
  - Mediated by alternate-pathway complement destruction of adipocytes through factor D.
- Macular degeneration occurs in patients with C3nef. Regular eye checks are therefore required.
- Treatment includes conventional immunosuppression, plasmapheresis, rituximab, and eculizumab (to prevent activation of the final lytic sequence of complement).

Autoimmunity in gastrointestinal disease

Autoimmune enteropathy

Autoantibodies against gut enterocytes and goblet cells have been associated with the following.
- Coeliac-like enteropathy (DQ2 positive), unresponsive to gluten-free diet, with villous atrophy.
- IPEX syndrome (see ➲ Chapters 1 and 4).
- Post-stem cell transplantation.
- Olmesartan-triggered enteropathy.
- Other cases not associated with the above-mentioned factors.
- Presentation with diarrhea and malabsorption.
- May be complicated by bowel lymphoma.

Achalasia

Clinical features
- Patients develop dysphagia for both liquid and solids.
- Eventual massive dilatation of the oesophagus occurs.
- Occurs in early to middle adult life.
- Marked increase in the risk of subsequent oesophageal carcinoma.
- Similar features occurs in the trypanosomal infection, Chagas' disease.

Immunopathology
- Achalasia results from damage to the myenteric inhibitory neurons of the lower oesophagus.
- Autoantibodies have been described that recognize the neurons of Auerbach's plexus in the oesophageal wall in the idiopathic form of the disease (anti-myenteric plexus). Also may be positive for anti-Ma2/Ta).
- 25% of patients with achalasia have autoimmune thyroid disease.
- Strong association with HSV-1 infection
- Genetic association includes MHC class II (DQA1*0103 & DQB1*0603) and other genes (*ALADIN* (Allgrove (4A) syndrome: alacrimia, achalasia, autonomic dysfunction, and ACTH insensitivity), *VIPR1*, *IL-23*).

Treatment
- The lower oesophageal sphincter is dilated endoscopically or the muscle divided surgically (Heller's myotomy).
- Drugs to relax smooth muscle are also used (calcium-channel blockers and nitrates).
- Botulinum toxin injections may give temporary relief.

Eosinophilic gastroenteritis (including oesophagitis)

Presentation

- Non-specific GI symptoms: abdominal pain, nausea, vomiting, weight loss, distension, reflux-like disease, dysphagia (oesophagus).
- Associated with cholangitis, appendicitis, pancreatitis, giant duodenal ulcer, and eosinophilic infiltration of spleen.
- Incidence increased with associated atopic disease and urticaria, and coeliac disease.
- Any age/race/sex; higher incidence in later life. Incidence appears to be increasing.
- May be seasonal variation in presentation (higher in summer).
- Has been seen as a complication of sublingual immunotherapy with pollens.

Immunopathology

- Possible association with food allergy (increased IgE to foods).
- Association with hypereosinophilic syndromes (see ➲ Chapter 3).
- Increased IL-5, IL-13, IL-15, fibroblast growth factor 9, and eotaxin increased.

Diagnosis

- Confirm by biopsy: > 15 eosinophils per high power field.
- Bowel wall may be thickened on scans.
- Exclude other systemic and local diseases where bowel eosinophilia may be seen (Crohn's disease, polyarteritis nodosa, Churg–Strauss syndrome, malignancy, parasites).

Treatment

- Corticosteroids; may be used as swallowed steroid from inhaler for oesophagitis; oral budesonide for eosinophilic enteritis.
- Trial of elimination diet if specific IgE to foods identified (only 45% long-term benefit):
  - Six-food elimination (wheat, milk, soya, nuts, eggs, seafood).
  - Four-food elimination.
  - Elemental diet.
- Sodium cromoglicate, ketotifen, and montelukast may be tried.
- Omalizumab, anti-IL5, and anti-IL13 mAb have been tried successfully in a small number of cases.

Crohn's disease

Presentation

- Crohn's disease is an inflammatory disease affecting any part of the bowel, which may also be accompanied by disease distant from the bowel (skin, muscle).

- Presents with diarrhoea and abdominal pain, or with evidence of the extra-gastrointestinal complications.
- Inflammation is transmural and granulomata are present.
- There is superficial ulceration and crypt abscesses.
- Skin lesions are common, and the deep penetrating ulceration frequently gives rise to fistulas.
- Associated with seronegative arthritis, uveitis, and sclerosing cholangitis.
- Malabsorption (especially of vitamin B_{12}, as the terminal ileum is frequently affected) may occur.

Immunogenetics

- Associated with DR5, DQ1 haplotype, or DRB*0301 allele.
- Strong association with NOD-2 (*CARD15*) gene on chromosome 16 that senses bacterial peptidoglycan and regulates NF-κB expression. This gene is also involved in Blau syndrome (see ➔ Chapter 14) and juvenile sarcoidosis.
- Over 30 genes have been identified which contribute directly or indirectly including:
  - X-box binding protein 1 (*XBP1*) is a transcription factor regulating immune system genes in response to stress (endoplasmic reticulum and unfolded protein response).
  - Autophagy-related protein 16-1 (*ATG16L1*).
  - Genome wide screening (GWAS) has identified four genes/genetic areas associated with worse prognosis: *FOXO3, XACT*, a region linked to *IGFBP1*, and the ancestral MHC 8.1 haplotype.
  - *IL10* or *IL10RA* and *IL10RB* mutations all cause severe inflammatory bowel disease within the first year of life, presenting with severe enterocolitis. There may be folliculitis, recurrent fever, and chronic large joint arthritis. HSCT may be considered.

Immunopathology

- It has long been suspected that the disease is related to an infection and current attention has focused on *Mycobacterium paratuberculosis*, which causes Johne's disease in cattle.
- Measles has also been suggested as a possible trigger.
- There is evidence of both a cell-mediated response and defective T-cell suppressor function.
- Excess Th17 cells are critical to disease development.
- Increased B-cell activity with immunoglobulin and complement deposition in damaged bowel.
- Activated macrophages are present and mast-cell numbers are increased.
- Excessive inflammatory cytokines are present (TNFα).
- Crohn's disease should be considered a form of host defence disease with impairment of the ability to handle intestinal bacteria correctly.

Diagnosis

- Crohn's disease is associated with specific autoantibodies.
  - Non-MPO P-ANCA (up to 25% of patients).
  - P-ANCA in Crohn's is associated with colonic disease.
  - Anti-*Saccharomyces cerevisiae* antibodies (ASCA; present in 60–70% of patients).
  - Combination of ANCA with ASCA is said have a 97% specificity for Crohn's (49% sensitivity).
- Other antibodies found in Crohn's disease include:
  - anti-cardiolipin;
  - anti-mycobacterial heat-shock protein;
  - rheumatoid factors;
  - anti-goblet cell;
  - outer membrane porin C (OMPC, bacterial antigen);
  - pancreatic autoantibodies;
  - antibodies against tropomyosin isoform 5;
  - antibodies against red cell membrane antigens that cross-react with *Campylobacter*: associated with haemolysis in Crohn's;
  - antibodies to a range of glycans (laminanbioside, chitobioside, mannobioside, laminarin, chitin);
  - none of these antibodies has realistic diagnostic value.
- Monitoring is best done with acute-phase markers ESR/CRP.
- Faecal calprotectin will be elevated and provides a useful monitoring tool, although the assays have poor reproducibility and EQA performance.
- α1-acid glycoprotein (orosomucoid) was said to be more sensitive as an acute-phase marker for inflammatory bowel disease, but it really adds nothing clinically over CRP.

Treatment

- Treatment is with steroids, azathioprine, 6-mercaptopurine, methotrexate, ciclosporin, mycophenolate mofetil, and 5-aminosalicyclic acid derivatives.
  - Patients on immunosuppression need monitoring for side-effects and need prophylaxis against opportunist infections.
- Thalidomide is also used for its anti-TNF effect.
- Resistant disease is treated with anti-TNF agents, infliximab (5 mg/kg), etanercept or adalimumab, certolizumab (pegylated Fab' fragment of humanized anti-TNF).
  - Complications include development of TB, lymphoma, and autoimmune disease.
- Natalizumab, a humanized mAb against the α4 integrin, has been licensed in the USA for remission induction and maintenance of severe Crohn's. Major risk is development of progressive multifocal leukoencephalopathy (PML).
- Vedolizumab, an antibody to α4β7 integrins is also effective.
- Ustekinumab (anti-IL-12/IL-23) is effective.

Testing

- See Table 7.1.

Table 7.1 Testing for Crohn's disease

Tests for diagnosis	Tests for monitoring
ESR and CRP	ESR and CRP
FBC	FBC
LFTs	LFTs
Faecal calprotectin	Faecal calprotectin
ANCA	Radiography (including labelled white cell scans)
ASCA	
Radiography (including labelled white cell scans)	
Biopsy	

Ulcerative colitis (UC)

Presentation

- An inflammatory disease limited to the colon.
- Presentation is usually with bloody diarrhoea.
- Extra-intestinal manifestations include:
  - seronegative arthritis (sacroiliitis);
  - uveitis;
  - pyoderma gangrenosum;
  - erythema nodosum;
  - sclerosing cholangitis.
- Pancolitis may cause a toxic megacolon, a medical/surgical emergency.

Immunogenetics

- Pancolitis is associated with HLA-DRB1*0103—this is also associated with an increase in extra-intestinal complications.
- Also associated with allele 2 of the IL-1 receptor antagonist.
- Multiple genetic loci associated with UC.

Immunopathology

- Unlike Crohn's disease, the disease is continuous and does not include the presence of granulomata. Otherwise the histology is similar.
- Activated T cells (CD4+, DR+, CD45RO+) and also of inflammatory cells, including neutrophils.

Autoantibodies

- Autoantibodies to colonic epithelial cells have been described (which are cytotoxic): these are not diagnostically valuable.
- Atypical P-ANCA (non-MPO) are also seen; a number of candidate antigens have been suggested as the target for this atypical P-ANCA, including lactoferrin and cathepsin G (? related to reactions to enteric bacteria).
- 50–70% of UC patients will be atypical P-ANCA+.

- P-ANCA positivity is associated with pancolitis and primary sclerosing cholangitis.
- 10–15% may have anti-*Saccharomyces cerevisiae* antibodies (ASCA)—diagnostic utility is low.

Diagnosis

- Is made on colonoscopic appearance and biopsy.
- Inflammatory markers (ESR/CRP) are elevated and provide a useful way of monitoring disease.
- Faecal calprotectin will be elevated.

Treatment

- Treatment is with topical or systemic steroids, azathioprine, and 5-aminosalicyclic acid derivatives.
- Anti-TNF agents appear to be less effective in UC compared to Crohn's disease. Infliximab, adalimumab, and golimumab are all used.
- Tofacitinib, a JAK1/JAK3 inhibitor, blocks signalling via the common-gamma-chain cytokines and is effective in moderate-to-severe UC.
- Significantly increased risk of carcinoma of the colon, so those with pancolitis will usually have a total colectomy, which is curative. For milder disease regular surveillance by colonoscopy may be sufficient.

Whipple's disease

Presentation

- Multisystem disease with diarrhoea, steatorrhoea, fever, weight loss, abdominal pain, migratory arthritis, and eye and CNS involvement.
- Features of a significant protein-losing enteropathy may occur.
- Dementia occurs as late complication.
- More common in men.

Aetiology

- Now known to be caused by infection with an unusual bacterium called *Tropheryma whipplei*.
- This is a common mouth commensal, and therefore rarely causes disease, suggesting a subtle immunodeficiency in those that develop disease. Deficiency of IRF4 may contribute to increased susceptibility.

Immunopathology

- There is a secondary hypogammaglobulinaemia, and also gut loss of T cells, leading to a secondary combined immunodeficiency.
- Biopsies show typical Schiff-positive macrophages abundant in the bowel wall.

Diagnosis

- There are no routinely available serological tests, but PCR-based tests are available.

Treatment
- Prolonged courses (> 1 year) of antibiotics (ampicillin, doxycycline (with hydroxychloroquine), co-trimoxazole if there is neurological involvement).
- Treatment courses < 1 year associated with 40% relapse rate.

Coeliac disease

Presentation
- Common inflammatory disease of the small intestine, triggered by wheat gliadin (gluten).
- Particularly common in western Ireland (prevalence 1 in 300).
- In the UK occurs in 1 in 1500 people.
- The symptoms can come on at any age.
- In childhood there is failure to thrive, while in adults it often comes to light during the investigation of unexplained anaemia (usually iron deficient).
- Malabsorption may be obvious, but many patients do not have significant steatorrhoea.
- Many adult patients may have a normal or increased weight (due to compensatory hyperphagia).
- Strong associations with the blistering skin rash, dermatitis herpetiformis (see ◑ Chapter 10), and with autoimmune diseases particularly diabetes, thyroid disease, Addison's disease, and SLE.
- Gluten sensitivity has been associated with an encephalopathy and a cerebellar syndrome, which respond to gluten withdrawal.

Immunogenetics
- It is associated with HLA-B8, DR3, DQ2.
- 95% of patients with coeliac disease are DQ2 positive (and 5% DQ8 positive), but only a minority of people with DQ2 develop coeliac disease.
- 10% of patients will have selective IgA deficiency.

Immunopathology
- Typical histological features are of total villous atrophy.
- Sub-total villous atrophy, and in the early stages an increase in intra-epithelial lymphocytes are also compatible with the diagnosis.
- Total villous atrophy is *not* required to make the diagnosis.
- Amount of gluten being consumed by the patient at the time of biopsy will have a significant bearing on the biopsy findings.

Autoantibodies
- The standard serological tests for coeliac disease are IgA endomysial antibodies (EMA, monkey oesophagus sections, or human umbilical vein) or ELISA assays for antibodies against recombinant human tTG.
  - IgA tTG assays have been recommended by NICE for screening but are too sensitive (increased false-positive rate); IgA EMA are better for screening.

- IgA tTG are better for monitoring response to gluten-free diet (quantitative).
- NICE recommends the annual screening of children with type I diabetes for the development of IgA EMA/tTG antibodies.
- As IgA deficiency may occur, testing for IgA deficiency as part of screening has been recommended, although some centres have dropped this.
- In IgA deficiency IgG anti-EMA or tTG have the same significance.
- There is no place for the use of R1 reticulin antibodies or IgA and IgG anti-gliadin antibodies, which have low sensitivity and specificity.

Diagnosis

- Differential diagnosis for coeliac disease is wide, and includes inflammatory bowel disease, true food allergy (excess eosinophils on biopsy), infections (*Giardia*), and connective tissue diseases (scleroderma).
- Gold standard for diagnosis is still biopsy of the jejunum, although endoscopic biopsy of the duodenum usually gives satisfactory and equivalent results.
- Serological tests are now recognized to have high sensitivity and specificity, and many patients, particularly children, will not be biopsied, although best practice indicates that patients should still be biopsied if possible.
- Positive antibodies with normal biopsy may represent a prodromal state.
- Absence of DQ2/DQ8 has a > 99% negative predictive value: testing is appropriate where other tests are equivocal and where biopsy is not possible.
- Children with type I diabetes should be screened annually for coeliac disease.

Treatment

- Treatment is lifelong gluten avoidance.
- Abnormal bowel returns to normal when gluten is withdrawn from the diet.
- Antibodies gradually disappear with gluten avoidance and reappear on gluten challenge.
  - IgA/IgG EMA/tTG can be used as a tool to monitor compliance with the diet.
- Compliance is important, as continued exposure to gluten increases the risk of intestinal lymphoma (T cell).
- Secondary splenic atrophy may occur (Howell–Jolly bodies on blood film).
  - Such patients should be treated in the same way as fully asplenic patients, with prophylactic antibiotics and regular checks on pneumococcal and Hib antibodies, with appropriate booster immunizations as required to maintain antibody levels (see ➔ Chapter 2).
- Dermatitis herpetiformis usually responds to gluten withdrawal, but may require treatment with dapsone (care in G6PD-deficient patients).

Testing
- See Table 7.2.

Table 7.2 Testing for coeliac disease

Tests for diagnosis	Tests for monitoring
FBC	FBC
Markers of malabsorption (Fe, vitamin B_{12}, folate, Ca^{2+}, clotting)	Markers of malabsorption (Fe, vitamin B_{12}, folate, Ca^{2+}, clotting)
IgA endomysial antibody/tTG antibody DQ2/DQ8 testing	IgA endomysial antibody/tTG antibody (compliance); if IgA deficient monitor IgG EMA/tTG
Small bowel biopsy	Asplenic follow-up antibodies (pneumococcal, Hib)
Other organ-specific autoantibodies (TPO, GPC, islet/GAD)	Markers of lymphoma (immunoglobulins, electrophoresis, β_2-microglobulin)
Blood film ± USS abdomen for hyposplenism	
IgA (if deficient, check IgG EMA/tTG)	

Sclerosing mesenteritis

- Uncommon condition, presenting with abdominal pain, nausea, vomiting, anorexia.
- May overlap with IgG_4 disease.
- CRP may be elevated; CT scans may be helpful.
- May include mesenteric panniculitis.
- Biopsy will be required for confirmation.
- May be associated with other autoimmune conditions (thyroid, sclerosing cholangitis, SLE) and autoimmune pancreatitis (see next topic).
- Treatment may include corticosteroids, tamoxifen (to reduce production of TGFβ), colchicines, cyclophosphamide, and thalidomide.

Autoimmune pancreatitis (AIP)

- Rare disorder, presenting with abdominal pain, pancreatic masses, pancreatic duct strictures, obstructive jaundice (and obstructive LFTs).
- AIP1 characterized by IgG_4 plasma cell infiltrate in pancreas.
- Raised serum IgG_4.
- Considered to be part of the spectrum of IgG_4 Disease and other features may be present.
- Autoantibodies to plasminogen-binding protein (PBP) may be a marker, but can be found also in patients with pancreatic cancer.

- Other autoantibodies may be found (ANA, AMA, ASMA, ANCA).
- Responds to corticosteroids; steroid-sparing agents may be required (mycophenolate mofetil, cyclophosphamide, ciclosporin, rituximab).
- AIP2 shows granulocytic infiltration without IgG_4+ cells and without systemic features.

Irritable bowel syndrome (IBS)

- Common condition of unknown aetiology. Theories include:
  - disturbance of brain–gut axis;
  - infection;
  - disturbance of the microbiome.
- Evidence supporting the role of IgG antibodies to foods is weak.
  - Such antibodies can be found in healthy normal individuals.
  - There is insufficient evidence to justify the use of extensive IgG antibody testing to direct dietary modification.
- NICE-BDA Guidelines advise the avoidance of 'resistant starches' (starchy foods that have been cooked or reprocessed more than once).
- A low FODMAP diet, under supervision by a dietician, may help some patients. FODMAP = fermentable oligosaccharides, disaccharides, monosaccharides, and polyols.
- All patients claiming that wheat exacerbates symptoms must have coeliac disease excluded (as previously described).
- There is a strong association with CFS/ME, fibromyalgia, depression, and anxiety; stress invariably exacerbates symptoms.
- Treatments, apart from diet, include stool bulking agents, anti-spasmodics, tricyclic antidepressants, $5HT_4$ antagonists (tegaserod (due to side effects, use restricted by FDA)), chloride channel activators (lubiprostone), and guanylate cyclase-C agonists (linaclotide).

NICE-BDA Diet sheet
🔗 https://www.nhs.uk/conditions/incontinence-bowel/documents/NICE%20guidelines%20IBS.pdf

Low FODMAP Diet
🔗 http://fodmapliving.com/wp-content/uploads/2013/02/Stanford-University-Low-FODMAP-Diet-Handout.pdf

Autoimmunity in liver disease

Primary biliary cirrhosis (PBC)

Presentation
- PBC is a disease of older women (90% of patients are female).
- Clinical features include initially:
  - profound fatigue starting in the prodrome;
  - intense itch;
  - severe fatigue and pruritus at presentation tend to be associated with more aggressive disease;
  - arthralgia.
- With disease progression:
  - hepatosplenomegaly;
  - xanthelasma;
  - skin pigmentation;
  - eventually hepatic decompensation with jaundice.
- Disease is strongly associated with other autoimmune diseases, including Sjögren's syndrome, thyroid disease, cryptogenic fibrosing alveolitis, CREST (calcinosis, Raynaud's, oesophageal dysmotility, sclerodactyly, and telangiectasia), and renal tubular acidosis.
- Other autoimmune diseases (any type) occur more rarely.

Immunogenetics
- Multiple genes have been identified: GWAS has identified at least 27 non-HLA risk loci.
- Epidemiology suggests a possible infectious aetiology.
- It is particularly common in the north-east of England.

Immunopathology
- Not strictly a cirrhotic disease, as the primary pathology is inflammation around the portal triads (intrahepatic bile ducts), leading eventually to fibrosis.
- 10% will have overlap feature with autoimmune hepatitis, and show typical interface hepatitis.
- Increased HLA-DR expression on the biliary epithelium and an infiltrate of CD4$^+$ T cells specific for biliary epithelial antigens.
- An excess of IgM-producing B cells is seen around the biliary ducts.

Diagnosis
- Liver function tests show elevated alkaline phosphatase. Caeruloplasmin, lipoproteins, and cholesterol are also raised.
- Biopsy shows typical features.
- Total IgM levels are polyclonally raised, often significantly (20–30 g/l), although the reason for this is not known.
- Occasionally small monoclonal IgM bands will be seen on electrophoresis.
- Autoantibodies are diagnostic.

Autoantibodies

- Typical immunological features are the presence of mitochondrial antibodies, found in 96% of cases.
- A variety of different mitochondrial antibody patterns are identifiable (with difficulty!) by immunofluorescence (see ➲ Chapter 18 for descriptions).
- The M2 pattern is most commonly associated with PBC.
- M2 autoantigens have now been identified as trypsin-sensitive molecules on the inner mitochondrial membrane.
- Primary antigen is the large multimeric 2-oxo-acid dehydrogenase complex, pyruvate dehydrogenase complex (PDC).
  - M2a recognizes the E2 subcomponent (dihydrolipoamide acyltransferase) of PDC (95% of PBC).
  - M2c recognizes the E2 antigen of oxoglutarate dehydrogenase (OGDC) (39–88% of PBC) and branch-chain 2-oxo-acid dehydrogenase (BCOADC) (54%), and the protein X component of PDC (95%).
  - M2d and M2e antigens are E1-α and E1-β components of PDC (41–66% and 2–7%, respectively).
- Solid-phase assays are available for M2 antigens and should be used to confirm the specificity of antibodies identified by immunofluorescence.
- Antibodies recognize conserved epitopes on related proteins found in fungi and bacteria.
- Antibodies, which are mainly IgM and IgG$_3$, are known to inhibit enzyme function and may penetrate viable cells.
- Other antibodies have been thought to identify subgroups of PBC.
  - M9 antibody (anti-glycogen phosphorylase) may be marker for early PBC with a benign prognosis (also found in low titres in healthy individuals).
  - M4 antibody may be a marker of aggressive disease (anti-sulphite oxidase).
  - Non-M2 anti-mitochondrial antibodies (AMAs) are found in myocarditis, SLE, syphilis, and in some drug reactions.
- Antinuclear antibodies are also found in PBC and are associated with more severe disease: HEp-2 cells may show multiple nuclear dots (MND) and perinuclear staining.
  - MND-ANA (Nsp-1, Nsp-2) are found in 10–44% of PBC patients, especially associated with Sjögren's syndrome. The Nsp-1 antigen is p80-coilin. Nsp-2 antigen is Sp100 (pseudocentromere). Both may occur in the absence of AMA, but it is not clear whether this subgroup is clinically different.
  - As CREST may also be associated with PBC, true centromere antibodies may be found (very confusing!). The presence of true anti-centromere antibodies in PBC is prognostic for portal hypertension.
  - Punctate perinuclear staining is due to autoantibody to the major glycoprotein of nuclear pores (gp210, found in up to 27%) and laminin B receptor. Both may occur in AMA-negative PBC. Antibodies to gp210 are associated with higher mortality and poorer outcome.

- Antibodies to p62 (nucleoporin) are more frequent in stage IV disease and are associated with more severe disease.
- Antibodies to carbonic anhydrase II have been identified in mitochondrial antibody negative and positive PBC.
- Multiple other antibodies have been described in PBC, including antibodies to GW bodies, PML (promyelocyte leukaemia antigen), GRASP-1, and VCP (valosin-containing protein), among others.
- Attempts have been made to correlate antibody patterns with risks of hepatic decompensation and response to ursodeoxycholic acid.
- See: ℘ https://www.ncbi.nlm.nih.gov/pmc/articles/PMC2915421/pdf/WJG-16-3616.pdf for a listing of associated antibodies.

Treatment

- Treatment with immunosuppressive drugs is thought to be unhelpful; the response to rituximab has not been encouraging.
- Colchicine and penicillamine have both been tried with limited benefit.
- Ursodeoxycholic acid may improve symptoms but does not alter the prognosis. Methotrexate may be used in combination.
- Obeticholic acid (farnesoid X receptor agonist) and fenofibrate/bezafibrate have all shown promise in early trials.
- Colestyramine and naltrexone are used to relieve itch.
- Transplantation is used for end-stage disease.

Table 8.1 Testing for primary biliary cirrhosis

Tests for diagnosis	Tests for monitoring
FBC	FBC
LFTs	LFTs
Caeruloplasmin	Caeruloplasmin
Cholesterol and lipoproteins	Cholesterol and lipoproteins
CRP/ESR	CRP/ESR
Anti-mitochondrial antibodies (also check for other organ-specific autoantibodies, TPO, GPC, true centromere)	Serum immunoglobulins and electrophoresis
M2 antibodies	
HEp-2 cell screen (Nsp-1, Nsp-2, gp210, laminin B receptor)	
Serum immunoglobulins and electrophoresis	

Testing
- See Table 8.1.

Autoimmune hepatitis

Presentation

- Before a diagnosis of autoimmune hepatitis can be made, it is important to exclude other causes:
  - toxic (alcohol, drugs);
  - metabolic diseases (Wilson's disease, haemochromatosis, α_1-antitrypsin deficiency);
  - viral causes, although there is a complex link between autoimmune hepatitis and HCV.
- Predominantly a disease of younger women (90% of patients are female).
- May present with acute hepatitis, jaundice, profound malaise and fatigue, and amenorrhoea in women (?autoimmune).
- May be marked extrahepatic features: vitiligo and alopecia, thyroid disease, pernicious anaemia, type I diabetes mellitus, autoimmune haemolytic anaemia and ITP, rheumatoid arthritis, ulcerative colitis, glomerulonephritis, cryptogenic fibrosing alveolitis, and coeliac disease.

Immunogenetics

- There is a strong association with HLA-B1, B8, DR3, DR4.

Immunopathology

- Major features are piecemeal necrosis of hepatocytes in the periportal region.
- There is an infiltrate of $CD4^+$ T cells and B cells.
- Later stages of the disease show typical cirrhosis.

Diagnosis

- Liver function tests show markedly elevated transaminases.
- Prothrombin time may be prolonged in late disease.
- Markers of hepatitis virus infection are absent.
- Polyclonal hypergammaglobulinaemia (mainly IgG and IgA).

Autoantibodies

- Antibodies to HCV or HCV PCR^+ = exclusion criteria for autoimmune hepatitis!
  - Type 2b hepatitis is associated with antibodies to hepatitis C in addition to the LKM antibodies.
- Autoantibodies to nuclear components, dsDNA, smooth muscle (anti-actin), LKM antibodies, and liver membranes can be detected.
- Low-titre AMA may also be detected.

The pattern of antibodies present has led to a classification scheme for autoimmune hepatitis.

- Autoimmune hepatitis type 1 (AIH-1) is ANA^+, smooth muscle antibody $(SMA)^+$, $P\text{-}ANCA^+$, and soluble liver antigen (SLA) $antibody^+$.
  - In AIH-1, 50% are ANA^+/SMA^+, 15% are ANA^+ only, and 35% are SMA^+ only.
  - 8% of AIH-1 are SLA^+ only.
  - Typically occurs in adults and has a better prognosis and responds well to therapy; 90% female.

- High frequency of extrahepatic features.
- Previously known as lupoid hepatitis.
- Autoimmune hepatitis type 2a (AIH-2a) is typically liver–kidney microsomal (LKM-1, LKM-3) antibody+ and liver cytosol (LC-1) antibody+.
  - 43% of AIH-2 are LC-1+ only.
  - AIH-2a is seen in children (50% of cases) and has a worse prognosis with poor response to therapy.
  - Associated with thyroid and gastric parietal cell autoimmunity.
  - Hypergammaglobulinaemia is less marked; IgA is usually low.
- Autoimmune hepatitis type 2b (AIH-2b).
  - HCV-associated; HCV-RNA positive, antibodies to HCV positive.
  - No female predominance; occurs in over 40s; milder disease.
  - No extrahepatic features.
  - LKM-1 positive (NB HCV antigen cross-reactive with P450 (IID6) cytochrome).
- Autoimmune hepatitis type 3 (AIH-3) is ANA⁻, LKM⁻, SLA⁺. SMA and AMA are seen less commonly.
  - Most patients are women (90%) and have a similar presentation to that of type 1.
- Autoimmune hepatitis type 4 (AIH-4).
  - Overlap syndrome of autoimmune hepatitis and PBC; AMA positive with antibodies to M2 antigen.
- There are cases of biopsy-proven but serologically negative hepatitis.
- Tests for both SLA and LC-1 should be performed.
- LKM-1 antibodies recognize the cytochrome P450IID6 and are associated with types 2a and 2b autoimmune chronic active hepatitis.

Other autoantibodies in hepatitis

- Liver–kidney microsomal antibodies may be found in autoimmune hepatitis and recognize different hepatic cytochrome enzymes:
  - LKM-1: cytochrome P450 (IID6): associated with types 2a and 2b autoimmune hepatitis. Antibodies to LKM-1 may be triggered by HCV and HSV as both have proteins sharing homology with P450 (IID6).
  - LKM-2: cytochrome P450 (IIC9). Drug-induced, tienilic acid, in France only.
  - LKM-3: UDP glucuronosyl transferase. Hepatitis delta infection. These antibodies are specific to human liver.
  - LKM-4: P450 (IA2) and P450 (IIA6) is seen in autoimmune hepatitis associated with APECED (see ⊃ Chapter 1).
  - Liver microsome antibodies (LM): cytochrome P450 IA2. Drug-induced hepatitis, dihydralazine.
- SLA (liver-pancreas) antibodies recognize liver cytokeratins 8 and 18.
- LC-1 antibodies recognize formiminotransferase cyclo-deaminase.

Treatment

- Prognosis is dependent on type and early diagnosis.
- Treatment depends on the underlying cause.
- Treat any viral trigger (HCV) with interferon alfa ± ribavirin.

- Immunosuppressive therapy with corticosteroids (high dose) is used and a good initial response defines a good prognosis.
- Azathioprine/mycophenolate are useful for maintaining remission.
- Ciclosporin, tacrolimus, and sirolimus have been used.
- Rituximab is also valuable.
- Liver transplantation may be required for end-stage disease in young patients.

Testing
- See Table 8.2.

Table 8.2 Testing for autoimmune hepatitis

Tests for diagnosis	Tests for monitoring
FBC	FBC
LFTs + GGT	LFTs + GGT
Autoantibody screen (ANA, SMA, AMA, GPC, TPO)	Clotting studies
SLA, LC-1	Serum immunoglobulins and electrophoresis
Liver biopsy	
Clotting studies	
Serum immunoglobulins and electrophoresis	

Primary sclerosing cholangitis

- An inflammatory disease of intra- and extrahepatic bile ducts, leading to fibrosis.
- More common in men than in women and can occur at any age.
- Associated with HLA-A1, B8, DR3.
- May lead to cholangiocarcinoma.
- Strongly associated with inflammatory bowel disease (see ➲ Chapter 7). It is thought that PSC occurring as a primary condition and PSC occurring with other conditions are different.
- May occur with autoimmune pancreatitis as part of IgG_4 disease: IgG_4 may be raised.
- May be associated with immune deficiencies, Langerhans cell histiocytosis, cystic fibrosis, sickle cell anaemia.
- Liver function tests are similar to those for PBC.
- IgG may be raised in children and neutrophil ANA positive.
- Anti-mitochondrial antibodies are absent, the IgM is not raised, and atypical P-ANCA may be found. P-ANCA is present in about 80% of cases.

- Anti-nuclear and anti-smooth muscle antibodies may be present in 25–50% of cases.
- Diagnosis is made by endoscopic retrograde cholangiopancreatography (ERCP) or magnetic resonance cholangiopancreatography (MRCP).
- Immunosuppressive treatment is unhelpful. Simtuzumab (IgG$_4$ anti-LOXL2) may be beneficial. Liver transplantation may be required.

Autoimmune haematological disorders

Immune thrombocytopenia (ITP)

Presentation
- ITP can occur at any age and is characterized by thrombocytopenia, with increased marrow megakaryocytes, and shortened platelet survival.
- Presentation is usually with sudden onset of petechiae, particularly around the feet, and bleeding (nose, gums, bowel, urinary tract).
- Can occur with:
  - infection (including HIV);
  - drugs (the list is very long!);
  - malignancy (lymphoma, adenocarcinoma);
  - common variable immunodeficiency;
  - other autoimmune diseases (SLE, thyroid disease, autoimmune hepatitis).
- Neonatal alloimmune thrombocytopenia may occur in mothers who are negative for the platelet antigen PLA1, who become sensitized in prior pregnancies where infants are PLA1 positive, or by blood transfusion; other platelet antigen systems have also been involved.
- Evans syndrome refers to the occurrence of ITP with autoimmune haemolytic anaemia. It may occur with congenital immune deficiencies and with common variable immunodeficiency (see ➲ Chapter 1).

Immunopathology
- Antibody-coated platelets are destroyed by the phagocytic cells in the peripheral blood.
- Many platelet antigens have been shown to be targets for the autoimmune response, including GPIIb/IIIA, GPIb/IX, and GP V (after chickenpox).
- Detection of anti-platelet antibodies is difficult and few centres offer this routinely.
- A wide variety of tests are used.

Diagnosis
- Diagnosis can usually be made clinically, with the assistance of a bone marrow examination.
- Investigations are needed to rule out associated autoimmune disease (SLE), immunodeficiency, and malignancy.
- Drug history should be reviewed.

Testing
- See Table 9.1.

Treatment
- Treatment is complex and should be undertaken by a haematologist.
- Any underlying cause should be treated or removed (drugs).
- Therapy is determined by the severity of the thrombocytopenia: counts of $< 20 \times 10^9/l$ usually lead to bleeding problems.
- First-line therapy is either steroids or hdIVIg. Advised dosage of IVIg has been reduced to 1 g/kg. Anti-D immunoglobulin can be used in RhD$^+$ patient who have not undergone splenectomy.

Table 9.1 Testing for immune thrombocytopaenia

Tests for diagnosis	Tests for monitoring
FBC, platelet count and film review	FBC, platelet count
Viral serology	
Serum immunoglobulins	
Autoantibodies (ANA, dsDNA, ENA, TPO)	
Anti-platelet antibodies	
Bone marrow biopsy	

- Thrombopoetin receptor antagonists (romiplostim = fusion protein analogue of thrombopoetin and eltrombopag) are replacing hdIVIg and have been approved by NICE. Romiplostim is administered weekly as a subcutaneous injection.
- Second-line therapies include cytotoxics, danazol, dapsone, and splenectomy.
- Rituximab may be valuable in resistant cases (unlicensed indication).
- If splenectomy is undertaken, the usual precautions should be taken (see ➋ Chapters 2 and 7 under ➋ 'Coeliac disease').

Autoimmune haemolytic anaemia

Classification

Immune haemolytic anaemia is divided into two categories dependent on the temperature at which haemolysis takes place.

- Warm haemolytic anaemia:
  - idiopathic autoimmune (AIHA);
  - secondary to other diseases: SLE, CVID, lymphoid malignancy, sarcoidosis, PBC, ulcerative colitis;
  - infections: hepatitis C, HIV, CMV, VZV, pneumococcus (and rarely pneumococcal vaccine), leishmaniasis, TB.
- Cold haemolytic anaemia:
  - idiopathic cold agglutinin disease;
  - cold agglutinins secondary to infection (*Mycoplasma pneumoniae*, EBV);
  - cold antibody disease (Donath–Landsteiner antibody, occurs in childhood or secondary to syphilis): paroxysmal cold haemoglobinuria;
  - cold antibody disease secondary to lymphoma (CHAD).
- Other causes of haemolytic anaemia include:
  - drug-induced (which may be due to bystander immune-complex-mediated damage or due to direct binding of antigen, e.g. penicillin, to the red cell membrane causing the formation of an immunoreactive neo-antigen);

- massive haemolysis may occur following mismatched blood transfusions (ABO incompatibility, pre-formed isoagglutinins);
- as a result of rhesus incompatibility (rhesus haemolytic disease of the newborn);
- in association with ITP (Evans syndrome).

Presentation
- Depends on the underlying cause.
- Signs of anaemia ± jaundice will usually be the presentation.

Diagnosis
- Immunological process is identified by the Coombs' test (direct anti-globulin test, DAT), which identifies the presence of immunoglobulin and C3 on the red cell membrane.
- Assays are done at different temperatures to identify warm or cold antibodies.
- Panels of typed red cells may be used to identify the specificity of the antibody.
- In the direct test, an anti-human IgG is used to demonstrate pre-bound IgG on the patient's red cells.
- In the indirect test, the patient's serum is incubated with normal erythrocytes to demonstrate the presence of anti-red cell antibodies in the serum.
- Pre-bound antibody can be eluted from the red cell for further studies.
- Serum haptoglobins are decreased during active haemolysis and serum LDH is increased.
- Check autoantibody screen for ANA (dsDNA, ENA) if appropriate.

Autoantibodies
- Antigenic specificities vary according the cause of the anaemia.
  - Most warm antibodies are against the rhesus system antigens or against the band 3 anion transporter.
  - Cold antibodies due to *Mycoplasma* recognize the I-antigen.
  - Those induced by EBV recognize I-antigen.
  - Lymphoma-associated cold agglutinin disease is characterized by a monoclonal IgM (usually κ not λ) with anti-I specificity.
  - Donath–Landsteiner antibody recognizes the P antigen (receptor for parvovirus B19).
- Three classes of drug-induced antibodies to red cells are recognized.
  - Antibodies binding to the drug itself on the red cell, where red cell damage is 'accidental': these antibodies are usually warm.
  - Drugs binding to a complex of drug and red cell membrane antigen (but binding only weakly or not at all to red cells without the drug): these may be cold antibodies.
  - Antibodies induced by the drug but binding to the red cell in the absence of the drug and recognizing rhesus antigens: these antibodies are usually warm.

Testing
- See Table 9.2.

Table 9.2 Testing for autoimmune haemolytic anaemia

Tests for diagnosis	Tests for monitoring
FBC and film	FBC and film
LFTs including bilirubin and LDH	LFTs including bilirubin and LDH
Direct and indirect Coombs' test	Direct and indirect Coombs' test
Cold agglutinins	Cold agglutinins
Bone marrow	Haptoglobin & LDH
Viral serology	
Serum immunoglobulins and electrophoresis	
Cryoglobulins	
Haptoglobin & LDH	
Autoantibodies (ANA, dsDNA, ENA, TPO)	
Splenic imaging (USS)	

Treatment
- Treatment is complex and should be undertaken by a haematologist.
- Treatment of any underlying disorder is required (lymphoma, infection).
- Any suspect drug should be stopped.
- Treatment is similar to that for ITP: high dose steroids are first-line therapy.
- Rituximab is second-line therapy.
- Azathioprine, mycophenolate, ciclosporin, and danazol are used as third line.
- Splenectomy may be required.
- Cold haemagglutinin disease is treated with rituximab or fludarabine if there is evidence of clonal disease.
- Cold avoidance is required where there is cold-associated haemolysis. Special precautions required during surgery to prevent cold-induced haemolysis.
- Folic acid supplementation is required.
- hdIVIg is much less effective than in ITP.

Autoimmune neutropenia

Presentation
- Usually with bacterial and fungal infections.
- Distinguish in children from congenital neutropenias (isoimmune neonatal neutropenia, similar to neonatal haemolytic anaemia).
- May occur alone or in conjunction with:
  - autoimmune diseases, such as SLE, rheumatoid arthritis (Felty's syndrome, especially if DR4+), Sjögren's syndrome, PBC, autoimmune hepatitis;

- malignancy such as lymphoma or large granular lymphocyte (LGL) leukaemia;
- infection (CMV, EBV, HIV, parvovirus B19); overwhelming sepsis;
- drug exposure (penicillins and cephalosporins), due to immune mechanisms. Agranulocytosis may occur after exposure to a number of drugs, of which the most important is carbimazole. Other drugs include carbamazepine, sodium valproate, sulfonamides, clozapine, and olanzapine.

Diagnosis

- All patients will require a bone marrow examination if neutropenia is severe and persistent.
- Screen for associated autoimmune disease (ANA, dsDNA, ENA, TPO, GPC).
- Attempts to detect anti-neutrophil specific antibodies are hampered by the non-specific binding of immunoglobulins via neutrophil Fc receptors.
  - Two surface antigens (HNA1a and HNA1b, previously known as NA1 and NA2, recognizing isoforms of CD16, FcγRIII) have been identified in primary autoimmune neutropenia of childhood.
  - In adults some patients have had antibodies against the complement receptor CD11b/CD18; also CD35 and CD177 (neutrophil glycoprotein, previously known as NB1).
  - Patients with Felty's syndrome may have antibodies to an elongation factor eEFIA-1.

Treatment

- Treatment is not usually required until the neutrophil count falls below 0.5×10^9/l.
- Co-trimoxazole and antifungal prophylaxis may be required.
- G-CSF may be valuable in shortening the period of agranulocytosis, and may be given as a test in patients who are chronically neutropenic in order to assess the response: responders can then be given treatment if they develop infection.
- Treatments with immunosuppressive drugs (steroids, interferon alfa and cladribine) have been used.
- Splenectomy may be required with the usual precautions (see Chapter 2).
- hdlVIg has been used in primary autoimmune neutropenia, but is much less effective than in ITP.

Paroxysmal nocturnal haemoglobinuria (PNH)

- Disease is due to an acquired (clonal) deficiency of complement control proteins on the red-cell surface.
- Caused by a failure to synthesize glucosylphosphatidylinositol (GPI) membrane anchors (common to a number of important surface molecules), due to somatic mutation in the *PIGA* gene on the X-chromosome.

- Affected molecules of red cells include CD55 (decay accelerating factor), CD59 (homologous restriction factor-20, HRF20), and homologous restriction factor (HRF65, C8-binding protein), all of which prevent accidental lysis of red cells by complement.
- Red cells tend to lyse at night when the pH of serum drops (hence the name), and the diagnostic test is flow cytometric demonstration of the absence of the relevant surface molecules (CD55, CD59).
- Flow cytometry using the FLAER reagent (fluorescent aerolysin, derived from bacterial aerolysin) which binds to GPI anchors, can be used in addition.
- Ham's acidification test is no longer used.
- Haptoglobin will be reduced; haemoglobin–haptoglobin multimers may be seen on protein electrophoresis; LDH & bilirubin will be increased.
- Free haemoglobin scavenges nitric oxide and this inhibits smooth muscle relaxation causing abdominal pain, oesophageal spasm, erectile dysfunction, and pulmonary hyperternsion.
- There is often an associated iron deficiency and leucopenia and an increased risk of haematological malignancy. Bone marrow examination is required.
- Androgen therapy may be helpful; steroids are not.
- Anticoagulation may be required due to increased thrombotic risk, especially in pregnancy.
- Eculizumab (Soliris®, a monoclonal antibody that binds to C5 and prevents cleavage by the C5 convertase) blocks complement activation and prevents haemolysis. In the UK, it is available through designated supra-regional specialist PNH centres. It can be used in pregnancy and is associated with improved maternal and fetal outcomes.
- The sudden rise in nitric oxide when eculizumab is administered will cause headache.
- It is advisable that all patients receiving eculizumab receive quadrivalent meningococcal, Hib, and pneumococcal vaccines within 2 weeks of starting, to prevent overwhelming infection.
- New therapies include a subcutaneous C5 inhibitor coversin, and a long-acting version of eculizumab (ALXN1210). C3 inhibitors such as pegylated compstatin has been given orphan status for PNH, although there is concern over the risks of invasive infection and autoimmunity, based on the profile of inherited C3 deficiency.
- Stem cell transplantation may be required.

Aplastic anaemia (AA) and pure red cell aplasia

Aplastic anaemia (AA)

- Aplastic anaemia, affecting all bone marrow lineages, may arise from the following:
  - infections (hepatitis B, hepatitis C);
  - exposure to toxins: benzene;
  - drugs: chloramphenicol, carbamazepine, phenytoin, quinine;

- idiopathic;
- congenital (Fanconi anaemia, dyskeratosis congenita).
- In idiopathic forms, a cellular immune response inhibiting erythropoiesis is present.
- About 50% of patients with idiopathic AA respond to treatment with anti-thymocyte globulin (ATG).
- Alemtuzumab is also used but not as first-line therapy.
- Androgenic steroids may help, but corticosteroids do not.
- Growth factors are not recommended.
- Ciclosporin is of benefit, combined with ATG. Other immunosuppressive agents are not recommended.
- Vaccines should be avoided as they may trigger relapse unless the patient has received HSCT.
- Infection is a major cause of death: prophylactic antibiotic and anti-fungals are used.
- Blood transfusion support is required (all cellular products should be irradiated to prevent GvHD if receiving ATG or alemtuzumab) and stem cell transplantation is the definitive procedure.
- 10–33% may develop PNH.

Pure red cell aplasia

- Causes are similar to those of aplastic anaemia but limited to red cell lineage.
- Other causes include HIV and herpesvirus infections, T-cell LGL leukaemia and thymoma.
- Parvovirus B19 can cause prolonged red cell aplasia in the immunosuppressed (PID and HIV)—may respond to hdIVIg.
- Autoantibodies to red cell precursors can be detected.
- T-cell responses and inhibitory NK cells have also been demonstrated.
- It may respond to treatment with rituximab.

Anti-factor VIII antibodies (acquired haemophilia)

- Acquired FVIII inhibitory autoantibodies may occur in association with:
  - SLE and other autoimmune diseases;
  - drug therapy (phenytoin, penicillin, chloramphenicol, and sulfonamides);
  - as an idiopathic autoimmune disease.
- Antibodies may occur in patients with congenital haemophilia receiving exogenous FVIII.
- Autoantibodies can cause a severe clotting disorder.
- Two types of patient are identified:
  - Type I—high-titre antibodies with a high response to further FVIII challenge. Avoid further FVIII.
  - Type II—low-titre antibodies with a low/absent response to FVIII challenge. Treat with high-dose FVIII.

- Plasmapheresis or specific immunoadsorption with protein A columns (antibodies are usually IgG_1 or IgG_4) may be required acutely.
- hdIVIg may also be beneficial.
- Rituximab may reduce autoantibody production.
- Steroids and cyclophosphamide may also be used in conjunction with other measures.
- Tolerance induction using regular FVIII treatment has been tried with variable success, but is only recommended if nothing else works!
- Desmopressin mobilizes FVIII from storage and may be a useful adjunct to treatment when inhibitor levels are low.
- Clotting can be controlled using partially activated complexes that bypass the level of inhibition.
  - Prothrombin complex concentrate.
  - Recombinant FVIIa (directly activates FX, bypassing need for FVIII) or recombinant activated FVII (rFVIIa).

Heparin-induced thrombocytopenia (HIT)

- Type I HIT is caused by direct heparin-induced platelet aggregation.
- Type II HIT is caused by an IgG autoantibody recognizing neoepitopes on the complex of heparin and platelet factor 4. The resulting complex binds to platelet and monocyte Fc receptors and activates platelets. Thrombin generation is increased.
- Assays for anti-heparin-PF4 complex antibodies are available.
  - 90% of these antibodies cross-react with low molecular weight heparins.
  - Low molecular weight heparins have a reduced risk of inducing autoantibodies.
  - Anticoagulation is achieved with non-heparin anticoagulants such as thrombin inhibitors (argatroban) or danaparoid/fondaparinux/bivalirudin (FXa inhibitors).
  - Danaparoid disrupts the heparin-PF4 complexes so reducing the target for the autoantibody.

Thrombotic thrombocytopenic purpura and haemolytic–uraemic syndrome

Thrombotic thrombocytopenic purpura

- A fulminant acquired syndrome triggered by:
  - pregnancy;
  - metastatic cancer;
  - bone marrow transplantation;
  - viral infections (HIV);
  - drugs (ticlopidine, clopidogrel, ciclosporin, tacrolimus, interferon alfa).
- Clinical features include fever, transient focal neurological symptoms, severe thrombocytopenia, microangiopathic haemolytic anaemia, and renal impairment.

- The disorder needs to be distinguished from haemolytic–uraemic syndrome.
- Diagnostic tests include the full blood count, platelet count, absent haptoglobin, raised LDH, and typical blood film. Screening for ADAMTS13 activity and the presence of an autoantibody to ADAMTS13 is required.
- The autoantibody inhibits metalloproteinase ADAMTS13 involved in breakdown of high molecular weight von Willebrand factor (vWF), causing platelet activation.
- Recurrent TTP is associated with genetic deficiency of ADAMTS13 (Upshaw–Schulman syndrome).
  - Phenotype is usually mild.
  - TTP develops when vWF levels are elevated (infections).
- Treatment involves plasmapheresis and replacement with fresh frozen plasma on a daily basis ± immunosuppressive therapy (high-dose steroids, rituximab). Recombinant ADAMTS13 is undergoing clinical trials. Caplacizumab inhibitor of vWF glycoprotein 1b also shows promise.
- Prophylactic fresh frozen plasma has been used in ADAMTS13 deficiency.

Haemolytic–uraemic syndrome

- Major cause (90% of cases) is infection with a strain of *E. coli* expressing a Shiga-like toxin (STEC; O157).
- The toxin inactivates the endothelial metalloproteinase ADAMTS13 and allows formation of multimers of von Willebrand factor which initiates platelet activation and microthrombus formation.
- See ➜ Chapter 6 for more details.

Anti-phospholipid syndrome (Hughes' syndrome)

- See ➜ Chapter 12.

Autoimmune skin disorders

Overview

- The skin is a very easy organ in which to investigate autoimmune disease, due to its accessibility for biopsy.
- Autoantibodies may be detected either by direct immunofluorescence (DIF) of snap-frozen biopsies or by indirect immunofluorescence (IIF) using the patient's serum.
- Use of hypertonic saline prior to staining of biopsies splits the epidermis away from the dermis, between the lamina lucida and the lamina densa, and allows the site of autoantibody binding to be more clearly identified: this is important in distinguishing epidermolysis bullosa acquisita from bullous pemphigoid.
- Significant disease may be present with little or no circulating antibody and therefore DIF plays a major role in diagnosis.
- Reliable results require an experienced laboratory!
- For testing, see Table 10.1.

Table 10.1 Testing for autoimmune skin disorders

Tests for diagnosis	Tests for monitoring
Skin biopsy (H&E, DIF, split skin, EM) Indirect IF (monkey oesophagus)	IgA EMA/tTG (compliance with gluten-free diet in dermatitis herpetiformis)
IgA EMA/tTG	
Other associated autoantibodies (by EIA)	

Bullous pemphigoid

Presentation

- Disease of the elderly characterized by the presence of tense, itchy blisters over limbs and trunk.
- Blistering stage may be preceded by papules or urticaria.
- Mucous membranes may be involved in up to one-third of patients.

Immunogenetics

- Increased prevalence of HLA-DQB1*0301.

Immunopathology and diagnosis

- Blister is subepidermal on histology.
- DIF and IIF show mainly linear IgG and C3 at the dermo-epidermal junction, binding to the epithelial side of the basement membrane (on a saline-split preparation).
- On immunoelectron microscopy the IgG is located on the lamina lucida.
- Rate of positivity in DIF is up to 90% and for IIF up to 70%.
- Other immunoglobulin classes may be detected.
- Drug reactions may cause similar bullous lesions but with negative immunofluorescence.
- IgE and eosinophil counts may be raised, although these are not diagnostically useful.

Autoantibodies
- Two autoantigens have been identified:
  - BPAg1, 230 kDa (chromosome 6);
  - BPAg2, 180kDa (chromosome 10).
- BPAg1 is similar to desmoplakin I and is likely to form part of the hemi-desmosome, which provides the major site of attachment between the internal cytoskeletal proteins and the external matrix.
- Antibodies to BPAg1 are only found in bullous pemphigoid.
- BPAg2 is also a hemi-desmosomal protein, but antibodies are also found in herpes gestationis.

Treatment
- Mild disease can be treated with topical steroids.
- Severe disease requires high-dose oral steroids, which can be tapered once remission is obtained.
- Remission may be sustained once steroids are withdrawn.
- Additional immunosuppressive therapy is rarely required, but azathioprine, cyclophosphamide, ciclosporin, mycophenolate mofetil, and dapsone have all been used.
- Plasmapheresis has been found not to be of benefit. Rituximab has not been very successful either.
- hdlVIg may be of benefit.
- Small studies have shown benefit from omalizumab.
- Tetracycline and niacinamide have also been proposed as treatment, although this is controversial: the mechanism of action is obscure.

Herpes gestationis and cicatricial pemphigoid

Herpes gestationis
Presentation
- Rare itchy and blistering rash associated with pregnancy. < 1 in 50 000 pregnancies.
- Onset is in the second or third trimester or occasionally in the immediate postpartum period.
- Infant may also be affected due to transplacental passage of the IgG antibody; this usually resolves spontaneously as maternal antibody decays.
- The umbilicus is involved, in contrast to another rare disease: pruritic urticaria and plaques of pregnancy (PUPP).
- May recur in subsequent pregnancies and in response to hormonal changes during the menstrual cycle or in response to the oral contraceptive pill.

Immunogenetics
- Associated with HLA-DR3 and DR4.
- C4 null alleles are increased.

Immunopathology
- Pathology shows the presence of eosinophils, which may be accompanied by a peripheral blood eosinophilia.
- Staining on immuno-EM is localized to the epithelial lamina lucida.
- IIF is positive in only 30% of patients, with C3 and IgG at dermo-epidermal junction. Occasionally other isotypes are present. The antibodies bind to the epidermal side of a saline split skin.
- Biopsy with DIF is therefore the diagnostic test of choice.

Autoantibodies
- Autoantigen is the 180 kDa BPAg2 antigen (see ⊃ 'Bullous pemphigoid', p. 264) and DIF shows linear deposits of C3 at the dermo-epidermal junction in almost all cases, with IgG in up to 50%.
- Serum autoantibodies to epidermal basement membrane only positive in 30%.

Treatment
- Treatment is with steroids (20–60 mg/day) together with antihistamines to control itch.
- This may pose problems for the pregnancy (increased incidence of 'small for dates') and careful monitoring is required.

Cicatricial pemphigoid
- See ⊃ Chapter 11.

Pemphigus vulgaris

Presentation
- Serious blistering disease that, if unrecognized and untreated, is invariably fatal.
- Blisters are flaccid and tend to rupture, with the split occurring in the epidermis itself.
- Causes the characteristic sign (Nikolsky's sign), where gentle lateral pressure leads to sloughing of the skin both in affected areas and in apparently normal areas.
- Blisters typically occur on the head and trunk and in the groins, although no part of the skin is spared.
- Mucosal lesions are common and the disease often presents with oral involvement.

Immunogenetics
- Disease is more common in middle age and particularly in persons of Jewish or Mediterranean extraction.
- Rarely, it may occur as a familial disease.
- Associated with HLA-A10 and also HLA-DR4/DQw3 (DRB1*0402) or DR6/DQw1 (DQB1*0503).

Immunopathology
- Histology shows acantholysis or separation of the keratinocytes.
- DIF on skin biopsies shows the deposition of IgG and C3 in the intercellular spaces of the epidermis, giving a chicken-wire appearance, in almost all cases.

- IIF on monkey oesophagus gives a similar pattern in over 90% of patients.
- Diagnosis requires both DIF on a suitable biopsy, together with IIF on serum.
- Low titres of serum antibodies giving a similar staining pattern have been reported in SLE, myasthenia gravis with thymoma, burns, and some cutaneous infections (leprosy).

Autoantibodies

- Autoantigen is now known to be a 130 kDa protein identified as a cadherin (Dsg3), which is homologous to desmoglein and occurs complexed to plakoglobin.
- Some patients have antibodies to desmoglein-1 (Dsg-1) in addition.
- Immune complex occurs at sites of adherence between neighbouring keratinocytes.
- Complement plays a key role in the immune process and complement breakdown products can be detected in blister fluid.
- Local plasmin formation is also important in separation of the cells.
- A rare form of pemphigus, with a characteristic neutrophilic infiltrate, has been described in which the antibody is IgA and the autoantigens are desmocollin I and II components of the desmosome (intraepidermal neutrophilic IgA dermatosis).
- The DIF shows a chicken-wire staining pattern, located in the basal layers only with anti-IgA antiserum.

Treatment

- Treatment is with corticosteroids in high dose (1–2 mg/kg/day).
- Azathioprine is the preferred second-line agent, although cyclophosphamide, ciclosporin, mycophenolate mofetil, and methotrexate have all been used successfully.
- In the neutrophilic variant, dapsone is helpful because of its effects on neutrophil activity.
- Plasmapheresis may be of benefit when combined with other therapies in refractory disease.
- hdIVIg and rituximab are valuable in resistant cases; early use of rituximab may prevent the development of resistant disease.

Pemphigus foliaceus

- Rare variant of pemphigus vulgaris that rarely involves the mucosal surfaces.
- Blistering is more superficial than in pemphigus vulgaris, giving a better prognosis.
- Endemic form in Brazil (fogo selvagem) may be triggered by an infectious agent, perhaps transmitted by an insect vector—this is characterized unusually by an IgG_4 autoantibody.
- May also be seen as a reaction to certain drugs (penicillamine, captopril, and other ACE inhibitors). Drugs containing thio groups more likely to act as triggers.

- Increased incidence of HLA-DQ1, DR4; DR7 may confer resistance.
- DIF may show that the immunofluorescence is more superficial than in pemphigus vulgaris.
- Autoantigen is different from that in pemphigus vulgaris (PV) and is a 160 kDa component of the desmosome, desmoglein-1 (a cadherin).
- Treatment is the same as for PV: antimalarials and oral gold may also be useful.

Paraneoplastic pemphigus

- A severe variant of pemphigus, accompanied by erythema multiforme, may occur in association with lymphomas, chronic lymphocytic leukaemia, and thymoma.
- Pathology shows acantholysis with necrosis of the keratinocytes and basement membrane damage.
- Involvement of the trachea and bronchi may occur with bronchiolitis and respiratory failure.
- DIF shows IgG and C3 deposition, both in the intercellular substance and along the basement membrane.
- Autoantigens are desmosomal proteins, desmoplakin I and II, desmogleins 1 and 3, and possibly other antigens (230 kDa BPAg1, envoplakin, plectin, and periplakin).
- No effective treatment is known. Complete excision of tumour may lead to slow recovery.
- Death occurs from respiratory failure and sepsis.

Epidermolysis bullosa acquisita

- A blistering disease accompanied by marked skin fragility affecting particularly sites of trauma such as hands and feet.
- Associated with inflammatory bowel disease, especially Crohn's disease, and bullous SLE.
- Disease can often be difficult to distinguish from other blistering diseases.
- Increased prevalence of HLA-DR2.
- DIF shows linear staining with IgG and C3 of the basement membrane, but this is not diagnostic. These are localized below the lamina lucida.
- On split-skin preparations the antibody is seen to localize to the dermal side. This test is more sensitive.
- IIF may also be positive.
- Autoantibody appears to react with type VII procollagen, reacting with epitopes in the NC1 non-collagenous domain.
- Treatment is difficult and the response to steroids and cytotoxics is poor.
- Plasmapheresis, photophoresis, rituximab, and hdIVIg may be more effective.
- Hsp-90 inhibitors are being studied.

Dermatitis herpetiformis (DH) and linear IgA disease

Dermatitis herpetiformis (DH)

- DH is an intensely itchy blistering rash that is associated with gluten intolerance.
- Typical sites for the rash include the elbows, buttocks, and thighs.
- As with coeliac disease, associated with increased risk of lymphoma (NHL).
- Also associated with achlorhydria and gastric atrophy and other organ-specific autoimmune diseases and connective tissue diseases.
- Increased incidence of HLA-A1/B8/DR3/DQw2 and associated organ-specific autoimmune disease.
- DIF on the skin biopsy shows typical granular IgA deposits on the dermal papillae.
- IgA endomysial or tissue transglutaminase antibodies will be positive.
- Jejunal/duodenal biopsies will often show features of coeliac disease even in the absence of clinical symptoms.
- Gluten-free diet will eventually lead to resolution of the rash.
- Resistant cases may require treatment with dapsone, having first excluded G6PD deficiency (monitor all patients for haemolysis and methaemoglobinaemia—see ➜ Chapter 16).
- Other drugs that may be used if dapsone is not tolerated include tetracycline, colchicine, and nicotinamide.

Linear IgA disease

- A group of rare blistering disorders, also associated with IgA deposition in the skin on DIF, that are not associated with gluten intolerance.
- May be induced by vancomycin (antigen is type VII collagen).
- Rash is often similar to that of DH.
- DIF shows linear (rather than granular) IgA deposition along the basement membrane and a 97 kDa antigen (LAD-1) has been identified in most cases.
  - Antigen appears to be a domain of the BPAg2 antigen (180 kDa).
- Treatment is with dapsone (with the caveats noted earlier), or low-dose corticosteroids.

Erythema multiforme (EM)

- Presents with rash (target lesions); usually self-limiting but may be chronic.
- Can be triggered by infections.
  - HSV, EBV, HIV, influenza.
  - Prophylaxis with aciclovir may be useful if this is the cause.
  - Mycoplasma, typhoid, streptococci.
  - Fungal and protozoal infection.

- Can be triggered by drugs:
  - Sulfonamides
  - Penicillins
  - Allopurinol
  - Phenytoin
  - Tetracyclines
  - Barbiturates.
- Possible link to dietary benzoates.
  - Trial of benzoate-free diet may be helpful.
- Role of corticosteroids is uncertain.

Stevens–Johnson syndrome (SJS)/toxic epidermal necrolysis (TEN)

- SJS = milder form of TEN.
- Associated with fever, sore throat, mucosal ulceration, and conjunctivitis.
- Triggered by drugs:
  - Allopurinol
  - Carbamazepine, phenytoin, valproate, lamotrigine
  - Nevirapine, abacavir
  - Imidazole antifungals
  - Trimethoprim, sulfonamides
  - Salicylates, NSAIDs
  - Sertraline
  - Bupropion.
- Triggered by infections:
  - HSV, EBV, HIV, enterovirus, influenza, hepatitis viruses, mumps, coxsackieviruses
  - Group A beta-haemolytic streptococci, diphtheria, brucella, mycoplasma, mycobacteria
  - Fungi
  - Malaria, trichomoniasis
  - Immunization (measles, hepatitis B).
- May be associated with lymphoma and GvHD.
- Drug-induced SJS more likely in patients with HIV, SLE, RhA, and Still's disease.
- Immunopathology: massive death of keratinocytes, excess CD8+ T cells, and possible involvement of FasL.
- MHC link in some cases, mainly in East Asian but not Caucasian populations (HLA-B15 (B75) with phenytoin or carbamazepine, or B58 with allopurinol).
- Short-course high-dose steroids may have survival benefit.
- Meta-analysis suggests hdIVIg and all other therapies were not beneficial with the possible exception of ciclosporin.
- Mortality is significant.
- Where drugs are suspected, allergy testing is contraindicated, as re-exposure even to minuscule amounts may retrigger the disease.

Sweet's syndrome (acute febrile neutrophilic dermatosis)

- Acute-onset tender plaques associated with fever, arthritis, conjunctivitis, and oral ulcers.
- Associated with autoimmune diseases (RhA), inflammatory bowel disease, and acute myeloid leukaemia (AML), especially if G-CSF used in treatment.
- May precede diagnosis of AML.
- 50% of cases associated with underlying systemic disease.
- Neutrophilia, increased ESR, and increased alkaline phosphatase; skin biopsy shows mixed infiltrate of neutrophils and histiocytes and evidence of vasculitis.
- Treat with corticosteroids, colchicine, or potassium iodide. Alternatives include dapsone (check G6PD status), doxycycline, clofazimine, and ciclosporin.

Lichen planus (LP)

- Chronic inflammatory condition that may also affect the oral mucosa.
- Associated with non-scaly papules and Whickam's striae; other variants exist. Usually itchy.
- Cause unknown.
- Associated with:
  - other autoimmune conditions (alopecia, vitiligo, ulcerative colitis);
  - hepatitis B, hepatitis C;
  - drugs (gold, penicillamine, β-blockers, thiazides, NSAIDs, and anti-TNF agents).
- Treat with topical corticosteroids, tacrolimus; for severe disease systemic steroids, ciclosporin, retinoids, and UV-B are used.
- Oral LP increases risk of squamous cell carcinoma.
- For oral LP, worth patch testing for type IV reactions to metals (nickel) and oral flavourings (cinnamon): trial of low-nickel diet and avoiding cinnamon is worthwhile.

Alopecia areata

- Loss of hair that may be localized or generalized.
- T-cell mediated, with circulating IgG autoantibodies to anagen hair follicles.
- May be triggered by stress.
- Strongly associated with autoimmune thyroid disease and other endocrine autoimmune diseases. Often accompanied by vitiligo.
- Needs to be differentiated from telogen effluvium, tinea capitis, trichotillomania, drug-induced hair loss, SLE, and syphilis.
- Treated with intra-lesional corticosteroids, topical steroids, and ciclosporin or tacrolimus: results of treatment are variable.
- Pan-JAK inhibitor tofacitinib and JAK 1/2 inhibitors ruxolitinib and baricitinib have shown significant benefit.

- Combination treatment with simvastatin/ezetimibe has also shown benefit in a small trial.
- Ustekinumab (anti-IL-12/IL-23) has been reported to be beneficial in a handful of patients.
- Support for wigs etc. is essential, if alopecia is extensive.

Vitiligo

- Presents with patchy pigmentary loss, often starting in childhood or early adulthood and progressive.
- Inflammatory destruction of melanocytes.
- Strongly associated with other autoimmune diseases.
  - Autoimmune endocrinopathies; pernicious anaemia, autoimmune hepatitis, alopecia, psoriasis, lichen planus, SLE, rheumatoid arthritis, myasthenia gravis.
- Multiple susceptibility genes (at least 10, similar to other autoimmune diseases), but especially alleles of the *TYR* gene.
- Strong family history.
- Treatment is difficult: topical tacrolimus and PUVA or UVB may be helpful.
- JAK inhibitors as for alopecia (as previously described).
- Melanocyte transplants have been used successfully.
- Teaching patients camouflage techniques is essential.

Psoriasis

- Chronic inflammatory skin disease presenting with scaly plaques, caused by hyperproliferation of keratinocytes.
- Complex immunopathology.
  - Infiltrate of CD4+ and CD8+ T cells and increased cytokine production by keratinocytes (γ-IFN, IL-2, IL-12, TNFα). IL-22 and IL-23 also increased, stimulating Th17 cells.
- Associated with at least nine gene loci (*PSOR1-9*).
- Other genes involved include IL-36R antagonist deficiency (*IL36RN*, generalized pustular psoriasis), *CARD14* mutations, APIS3 deficiency (*APIS3*, pustular psoriasis).
  - Strong family history (at least 30% have affected family members.
  - HLA-Cw6 associated with early-onset disease.
  - Shared genes with Crohn's disease (increased incidence of Crohn's in psoriasis).
- Treated with PUVA, vitamin D_3 analogues, oral retinoids, methotrexate, ciclosporin, fumaric acid esters (monitor CD4+ T cells as lymphopenia can be severe), hydroxycarbamide, leflunomide, anti-TNFs, JAK 1/3 inhibitors (tofacitinib, ruxolitinib), and ustekinumab (anti-IL-12/IL-23). Newer drugs, recently licensed, include risankizumab (anti-IL-23 p19 subunit) and tildrakizumab (anti-IL-23).

Website

British Association of Dermatologists: ✆ www.bad.org.uk

Autoimmune eye disease

Overview

The eye has a number of interesting immunological properties that alter the propensity for immune-mediated disease, including the curious feature that antigen injected into the anterior chamber induces tolerance rather than immunity. In addition, the eye has no true lymphatics, relatively poor vascularity, and, as the retina is an extension of the CNS, there is a blood–retinal barrier that limits passage of molecules in either direction. Ocular involvement is a common feature of many connective tissue and vasculitic diseases.

Sicca symptoms are common in connective tissue diseases (see ➲ Chapter 12). Where there is no evidence of a CTD, and fatigue is prominent, consider the dry eyes and mouth syndrome (DEMS—see ➲ Chapter 14).

Uveitis

Causes

Uveitis occurs as a consequence of a wide range of systemic diseases. The site of inflammation gives some clues as to the cause.

- Anterior uveitis:
  - seronegative arthritis (ankylosing spondylitis, Reiter's disease, psoriatic arthropathy);
  - juvenile chronic arthritis (see ➲ Chapter 12);
  - infections (herpes simplex, herpes zoster, TB);
  - idiopathic;
  - vasculitis (Behçet's syndrome).
- Posterior uveitis:
  - infections—mainly in immunocompromised (HIV, CMV, *Candida*, other fungi, syphilis, *Toxoplasma*, TB);
  - vasculitis (Behçet's, polyarteritis);
  - sarcoidosis;
  - rare eye diseases (Eales disease, VKH, birdshot retinopathy).
- Pan-uveitis:
  - connective tissue diseases (polychondritis, SLE);
  - infections (*Brucella, Toxoplasma*, TB, viruses);
  - vasculitis (Behçet's, Wegener's);
  - sympathetic ophthalmitis;
  - sarcoidosis.
- Intermediate uveitis:
  - Fuchs heterochromic iridocyclitis (abnormal pigmentation of the iris);
  - pars planitis (may be associated with MS);
  - juvenile rheumatoid arthritis.

Investigation

- Investigations should therefore be aimed at most likely causes.
- Infection needs to be excluded, as the appropriate treatment for non-infectious uveitis is immunosuppression.
- Presentation with acute anterior uveitis may be a first presentation of a spondyloarthropathy.

- MS may cause intermediate uveitis and bilateral granulomatous anterior uveitis (worse prognosis for the neurological disease). Associated with HLA-DR2.

Treatment
- Aggressive therapy is justified if vision is to be preserved.
- Treatment is with steroids and steroid-sparing agents (ciclosporin, tacrolimus, mycophenolate mofetil, cyclophosphamide, azathioprine, low-dose weekly methotrexate).
- Anti-TNF agents are being used in Behçet's uveitis.
- Patients require regular monitoring of therapy (see ➲ Chapter 16).

Testing
- See Table 11.1.

Table 11.1 Testing for uveitis

Tests for diagnosis	Tests for monitoring
FBC	FBC
Cr & E	Cr & E
Glucose	LFTs (azathioprine, mycophenolate mofetil, tacrolimus)
CRP/ESR	CRP/ESR
ACE	Glucose (steroids)
Serology (viral, *Toxoplasma*, *Brucella*)	Drug levels (ciclosporin, tacrolimus)
TPMT level (azathioprine—see ➲ Chapter 16)	
ANCA	
ANA (dsDNA, ENA, C3, C4)	
Chest radiograph	
Mantoux test	
Fluorescein angiogram	
Ultrasound of retina	

Tubulointerstitial nephritis and uveitis (TINU)

- Rare syndrome of nephritis with uveitis.
- Thought to be caused by autoantibodies against a modified CRP (m-CRP).
- Cellular response (T cells) also involved.
- May be associated with other autoimmune diseases.
- Treated with steroids and second-line agents (mycophenolate mofetil).

Vogt–Koyanagi–Harada disease (VKH)

- Rare bilateral granulomatous pan-uveitis occurring in adults and leading to visual failure.
- More common in Japan and South America.
- Similar to sympathetic ophthalmitis.
- Associated with vitiligo, alopecia, and poliosis.
- Strong HLA association with DR53.
- High titres of anti-retinal antibodies can be detected, against the retinal S-antigen.
- High levels of circulating γ-IFN have been noted.
- Corticosteroids and ciclosporin are the recommended treatments.

Cancer-associated retinopathy and uveitis

- Very rare paraneoplastic syndrome associated with small cell carcinoma of the lung; also with melanoma.
- Associated with destruction of the photoreceptors.
- SCLC-associated retinopathy (CAR) presents with alterations of visual acuity, scotomata, alterations in colour vision, progressive visual dimming, and night blindness.
- Melanoma-associated retinopathy (MAR) presents usually with sudden-onset shimmering, flickering, or pulsating photopsia, night blindness; may be unilateral.
- Autoantibodies against the retina are detectable:
  - Anti-recoverin (CAR, with SCLC).
  - Anti-bipolar cells (MAR, with melanoma)—putative antigens include arrestin and transducin.
  - Anti-enolase antibodies associated with less severe retinopathy, affecting cones.
  - At least 20 other autoantigens identified.
  - Diagnostic significance is debated.
- Cancer-associated uveitis and optic neuritis may occur—associated with antibodies to CV2/CRMP5.
- Associated with SCLC, breast, renal, and thyroid cancer, thymoma.
- Optimal treatment is not defined.

Birdshot retinopathy

- Rare primary uveitis, with a retinal vasculitis.
- Affects predominantly middle-aged Caucasian females.
- Strongly associated with HLA-A29 and the *ERAP2* gene on chromosome 5 and possibly *TECPR2* (in Dutch and Spanish but not British patients).
- Treatment is with immunosuppressive agents, including steroids, ciclosporin, azathioprine, and hdIVIg.

Scleritis

Presentation

- Painful red eye.
- Evidence of scleral thinning (perforation in severe cases = necrotizing scleritis/scleromalacia perforans).
- Posterior scleritis may be difficult to identify (orbital ultrasound may help).
- Must be distinguished from episcleritis, a mild and self-limiting condition (see Table 11.2).

Immunopathology

- Vasculitis of scleral vessels.
- Associated with a range of autoimmune diseases:
  - Rheumatoid arthritis
  - SLE
  - Wegener's granulomatosis
  - Ankylosing spondylitis
  - Inflammatory bowel disease
  - Polychondritis
  - Inflammatory bowel disease
  - Giant cell arteritis/temporal arteritis.

Treatment

- Treatment should be supervised by an ophthalmologist.
- NSAIDs, topical and systemic.
- Topical and systemic corticosteroids.
- Steroid-sparing immunosuppressive drugs (rituximab, anti-TNFs).

Table 11.2 Differentiation of scleritis and episcleritis

Scleritis	Episcleritis
Usually associated with systemic disease	Rarely associated with systemic disease
Chronic persistent	Recurrent short-lived attacks
Usually painful	Pain is minimal
May be necrotizing and lead to perforation if not treated	

Keratitis

- Inflammation/ulceration of the cornea.
- Peripheral ulcerative keratitis, usually associated with RhA, also SLE, Wegener's/PAN—can lead to corneal melt syndrome. Requires aggressive immunosuppression (steroids, rituximab).
- Mooren ulcer: not associated with systemic disease. Antibody to calgranulin may be present (expressed in cornea, neutrophils and filaria).
- Cogan's syndrome (see ➲ Chapter 13).

Ocular cicatricial pemphigoid (mucous membrane pemphigoid)

Presentation
- Causes subepithelial fibrosis of conjunctivae and, if untreated, can cause blindness, through damage to the corneal surface.
- Mouth is also involved, giving a gingivitis and ulceration. This may rarely also spread to involve the larynx and oesophagus.
- Rarely, there is also skin disease.

Immunogenetics
- There is an association with HLA-DQ7 (DQB1*0301) and B11.

Autoantibodies
- Autoantibodies to a 120 kDa basement membrane antigen can be detected.
- On direct immunofluorescence antibodies are found as continuous linear staining at the epithelial basement membrane, located on immuno-EM to the lamina lucida.
- IgG, IgA, and complement are deposited.
- Circulating epithelial antibodies are rarely present: studies claiming to detect them have used neat serum, which is likely to give meaningless results.
- Putative antigens include epiligrin (laminin 5, a ligand for keratinocyte integrins): this antibody is associated with laryngeal involvement.
- Where the skin is involved, antibodies to BPAg1 and BPAg2 have been detected (see **→** 'Bullous pemphigoid', p. 264).

Treatment
- Topical therapy is rarely effective and oral steroids, cyclophosphamide, azathioprine, mycophenolate mofetil, or dapsone will be required.
- Rituximab and hdIVIg may be effective in patients with progressive ocular disease.
- Tetracyclines combined with nicotinamide may be used.
- Drug-induced pemphigoid has been associated with pilocarpine, ephedrine, and idoxuridine.

Corneal transplantation
- Commonly carried out for keratoconus.
- Immunological rejection can occur despite the eye being immunologically privileged. Usually occurs as late event, CD4+ T cell mediated.
- HLA-typing does not reduce risk of rejection.
- Pre-transplant corneal neovascularization is a risk factor and prophylactic immunosuppression may be required.
- Treatment is with immunosuppressive agents, including steroids and steroid-sparing drugs.

Sympathetic ophthalmitis

- Syndrome occurs following penetrating trauma to one eye, which is then followed by a progressive granulomatous pan-uveitis in the uninjured eye after a variable interval.
- It is thought that damage to the uveal tract triggers an autoimmune response: autoantibodies to retinal photoreceptors and Müller cells (normally responsible for nutritional support for the photoreceptor) may be detected.
- One of the major autoantigens is the retinal S-antigen (arrestin).
- It may also be associated with lens-associated uveitis, although the latter may occur alone and may be cured by lens removal.
- Vitiligo, alopecia, and whitening of the eyelashes (poliosis) may occur.
- Early removal of the traumatized eye and aggressive immunosuppressive therapy may be required.

Idiopathic orbital inflammation (orbital pseudotumour)

- Rare disease of the orbit; no clear aetiology.
- Said to be 'benign', but may cause serious visual problems. 10% associated with other autoimmune disease—may be associated with:
  - Crohn's disease;
  - SLE;
  - Rheumatoid arthritis;
  - myasthenia gravis;
  - diabetes mellitus.
- Causes chemosis, ptosis, and optic neuropathy.
- Responds to corticosteroids; cyclophosphamide, ciclosporin, and methotrexate may also be required as steroid-sparing agents.
- Relapse may occur after successful treatment.

Connective tissue disease

Rheumatoid arthritis: aetiology, clinical features, and immunopathology

Aetiology

- RhA is a multisystem disease in which arthritis is a major component.
- Smoking and female gender in association with a genetic background susceptibility are risk factors.
- An infectious trigger has been sought for many years, without success.
- The best candidate pathogens include:
  - EBV;
  - *Mycobacterium tuberculosis*;
  - *Proteus mirabilis*;
  - *Porphyromonas gingivalis* (able to citrullinate proteins).
- The genetic background includes:
  - DR4 (DRβ1*0401), DR1 (DRβ1*0101) in Caucasians;
  - DR10 (DRβ1*1001) in Spanish and Italian patients;
  - DR9 (DRβ1*0901) in Chileans; DR3 (DRB1*0301) in Arabs;
  - Tcr, TNFα, IL-10, and IgG polymorphisms.
  - *PTPN22* (strongest non-HLA gene).

Clinical features

- Early clinical signs include:
  - morning stiffness;
  - fatigue.
- There may be low-grade fever.
- Joint pain and swelling follow and the arthritis is often deforming. Hand joints are typically affected. Radiographic changes are typical.
- Non-articular features include:
  - Sjögren's syndrome;
  - lymphadenopathy;
  - scleritis;
  - cutaneous vasculitis and ulceration;
  - nodules both of skin and lung;
  - pleurisy, alveolitis;
  - pericarditis, endocarditis (with valvular involvement);
  - splenomegaly (with ulceration and neutropenia = Felty's syndrome, see Table 12.1);
  - myositis, mononeuritis multiplex, and cord compression from spinal involvement.
- Amyloid is a long-term complication from chronic inflammation.

Immunopathology

- Most of the pathology is located in the joint.
  - Activation of T cells, macrophages, and endothelial cells.
  - Increased synovial vascularity.
  - Both CD4⁺ and CD8⁺ T cells are found in the joint tissues.
  - 'Memory' T cells (CD45RO⁺, CD29⁺) predominate.
  - Restriction of Tcr Vβ usage suggestive of a superantigenic effect.

Table 12.1 Features of Felty's syndrome

Triad of chronic arthritis, spemomegaly, and granulocytopenia	Associated with HLA-DR4
33% have clonal expansion of large granular lymphocytes	CD3$^+$CD8$^+$CD16$^+$CD57$^+$
Complications	Rheumatoid nodules, weight loss, Sjogren's syndrome, lymphadenopathy
	Leg ulcers, pleuritis, neuropathy, skin pigmentation, episcleritis
	Increased risk of lymphoma (NHL)
	Increased risk of bacterial infections
Immunological abnormalities	98% RhF$^+$
	60–80% ANA$^+$
	77% ANCA$^+$ (mostly anti-lactoferrin)
	Reduced complement
	Increased immunoglobulins
Treatment	As for RA
	Splenectomy may be required
	C-CSF for severe neutropenia

- Large quantities of cytokines can be detected in the joint fluids and contribute to bone destruction.
- Endothelial cell activation/production of chemokines is responsible for influx of inflammatory cells including:
  - interleukin-8 (IL-8);
  - RANTES;
  - MCP-1;
  - Gro-α;
  - ENA-78 (epithelial neutrophil activating peptide).
- Autoantibodies are produced, including:
  - rheumatoid factors;
  - anti-nuclear antibodies; including anti-neutrophil nuclear antibodies;
  - anti-keratin;
  - anti-cyclic citrullinated peptide (CCP); citrullinated vimentin (MCV);
  - anti-calpastatin;
  - anti-Sa (unknown antigen);
  - anti-filaggrin.
  - Other target antigens include fibrin, fibrinogen, enolase, collagen II, aggrecan, HnRNPA2, HCgp39, G6P isomerase.
- Pathogenic role of these autoantibodies is uncertain.
- IgG molecules in RhA have been shown to have markedly reduced glycosylation, although the significance of this is uncertain.
- Complement activation takes place, releasing anaphylotoxins, C3a, C5a.

Rheumatoid arthritis: immunological tests, treatment, and childhood RhA

Immunological tests

- Rheumatoid factors (RhF) are found in 67–85% of patients, depending on the type of assay used.
  - Most detected RhF are IgM class.
  - RhF⁻ patients may have RhF of other immunoglobulin classes, not detected by standard assays.
  - RhF are not diagnostic tests for RhA (see Part 2).
  - Highest titres of RhF are found in patients with extra-articular disease.
  - There is no correlation of disease activity with antibody titres.
  - Detection of RhF is of most value when the diagnosis of RhA has been made.
- Anti-CCP antibodies are valuable, as a more specific marker, in identification of early disease. Anti-citrullinated vimentin may be an alternative, but may be less sensitive.
- Antibodies to filaggrin and keratin have also been said to be more specific for RhA: assays are not widely available.
- Cryoglobulins may be found and these are usually type II or type III (i.e. with RhF activity), often in association with Felty's syndrome.
- Hypergammaglobulinaemia is usually present, due to chronic inflammation, and this is invariably polyclonal, although small monoclonal bands may be present.
- Urine may contain an excess of free polyclonal and sometimes monoclonal light chains.
- Complement C3/C4 are usually elevated, as are acute-phase proteins, although patients with Felty's may have reduced levels.
- Anti-nuclear antibodies may be found, both on rat liver and on HEp-2 cells. ANAs are most commonly found in Felty's syndrome. These include antibodies against:
  - nuclear antigen RA-33, a ribonucleoprotein of the spliceosome;
  - rheumatoid-associated nuclear antibodies (RANA), against an antigen which is present in high levels in EBV-transformed cell lines. This antibody is also found in SLE and MCTD patients.
- Antibodies are also detected against granulocyte nuclei (GS-ANA), which may be difficult to distinguish from P-ANCA when testing is done by fluorescence; these are also associated most strongly with Felty's syndrome.
- True P-ANCA may be found in RhA vasculitis.
- Associated Sjögren's syndrome will be accompanied by the presence of antibodies to Ro and/or La.
- In active disease, both CRP and ESR will be elevated.
- CRP is the most sensitive marker of activity, due to its wide dynamic range, and is the most useful marker to monitor response to treatment.
- Other markers of disease activity that have been studied include cytidine deaminase, calprotectin, and serum hyaluronate. None of these are used routinely yet.
- Monitoring of cytokines is not used routinely.
- Anaemia of chronic disease is often present and there may be lymphopenia (both CD4⁺ and CD8⁺ cells).

Treatment

- Proper supportive care (physiotherapy, occupational therapy) is essential.
- Drug therapy includes NSAIDs, usually with gastric protection, and analgesics as first line.
- Low-dose corticosteroids are now back in favour to slow the progression of erosive disease (prednisolone 5–7.5 mg/day).
- Disease-modifying drugs (DMARDs; see ⊃ Chapter 16) include:
  - sulfasalazine;
  - gold salts;
  - penicillamine;
  - methotrexate (low dose weekly);
  - hydroxychloroquine;
  - azathioprine;
  - leflunomide;
  - gold and hydroxychloroquine both interfere with TNF production;
  - ciclosporin and tacrolimus have been used to reduce the activation of $CD4^+$ T cells.
- Immunotherapies with biological agents include:
  - anti-CD4 monoclonal antibodies (mAbs);
  - anti-CD52 mAbs;
  - anti-TNF agents (adalimumab, infliximab, etanercept, certolizumab, golimumab) are highly effective;
  - IL-1 receptor antagonist (anakinra) seems less effective and has not been endorsed by NICE;
  - rituximab (anti-CD20);
  - humanized anti-IL-6 receptor (tocilizumab/atlizumab).
- Other agents undergoing trials include:
  - oral anti-TNF drugs;
  - CTLA4-Ig (abatacept);
  - anti-CD2;
  - anti-IL-15;
  - anti-IL-12;
  - anti-B-lymphocyte stimulator protein (BLys) (belimumab).
- Problems with all mAb-based therapies have included:
  - high levels of reactions to xenogeneic proteins, even if attempts have been made to humanize the antibodies;
  - severe and persistent T-cell lymphopenia in some trials, raising concerns over risks of opportunist infections;
  - anti-mAb antibodies that block effects.
- Surgical replacement of damaged joints may restore function and relieve pain.

Childhood rheumatoid arthritis

- Childhood-onset seropositive RhA is rare and usually presents with general malaise and polyarthritis of the small joints of the hands and feet.
- Because of the frequent appearance of RhF following infection, European guidance suggests that three positive tests over a 3-month period are required to confirm the diagnosis, although, bearing in mind the half-life of the antibodies, this is probably too short an interval.

- This disease is associated with DR4.
- Diagnosis and management are as for the adult disease.
- An RhF-negative polyarthritis is also seen in children; this may be severe. It is associated with DR5 and DR8.

Tests
- See Table 12.2.

Table 12.2 Testing for childhood rheumatoid arthritis

Tests used for diagnosis	Tests used for monitoring
CRP/ESR	CRP/ESR
FBC	FBC (drug toxicity, anaemia of chronic disease)
LFTs	LFTs (drug toxicity)
Immunoglobulins	ENA (development of Sjögren's)
ANA	ANA, dsDNA (monitoring of anti-TNFs)
	Anti-biological antibodies
ENA	
RhF	
Anti-CCP	
Granulocyte-specific ANA (Felty's syndrome)	
ANCA (RhA vasculitis)	

Juvenile chronic arthritis (JCA) and Still's disease

Clinically JCA is divided into two types: pauci-articular and systemic forms. The latter is usually referred to as Still's disease.

Aetiology and immunopathology
- As with many connective tissue diseases (CTDs), aetiology is not well understood.
- Immunogenetics of pauci-articular disease is complex: DR8 and DR5 show the strongest correlation with pauci-articular disease. Other genes include DPB1 and A2. Multiple genes have been implicated.
- Rubella virus has been implicated as a possible trigger.
- Systemic disease is also associated most strongly with DR5 and DR8, but also with DR4.
- Juvenile Still's disease (systemic juvenile idiopathic arthritis) may be associated with DRB1*11. It may also occur as an autosomal recessive monogenic disease with mutations in the *LACC1* gene, coding for a copper oxidoreductase.

Clinical features

- Clinical diagnosis of pauci-articular disease is one of exclusions.
  - Usual age of onset is 1–3 years, with a 4:1 female predominance.
  - Systemic features are an exclusion, and the usual features are those of painful or painless swelling of one or two joints.
- Uveitis may develop and regular screening is required when ANAs are detected.
- A macrophage activation syndrome resembling familial haemphagocytic lymphohistiocytosis may occur.
- Still's disease typically has a high spiking fever, accompanied by malaise and rigors.
  - A pale, salmon-pink rash that comes and goes is usual, in parallel with the spikes of fever.
  - Hepatosplenomegaly and generalized lymphadenopathy are usually present.
  - There is polyarthralgia and polyarthritis.
  - Pericarditis and pleurisy are also common.
  - A rare macrophage-activation syndrome has been described, with encephalopathy, hepatitis, disseminated intravascular coagulation (DIC), and haemophagocytosis.
  - Amyloid may be a long-term complication.

Immunological tests

- Rhf is rare (< 5%) in pauci-articular disease and, when present, suggests that the course will be that of juvenile RhA with polyarticular disease.
- ANAs are frequently present, and it is important to ensure that the normal range for significance is appropriately adjusted for the paediatric population.
  - In small children, titres of 1/10 and 1/20 are highly significant, whereas such titres would not be considered important in adults.
- High incidence of uveitis in female patients with arthritis and positive ANA, especially if also anti-Ro$^+$.
- Antibodies to histones H1 and H3 are also associated with uveitis.
- Antibodies to retinal S-antigen may also be found (in 30%).
- Other antibodies detected include anti-histone antibodies (often in those without uveitis).
- Detection of anti-dsDNA antibodies should lead to consideration of childhood lupus.
- Frequent evidence of complement consumption with raised C3d, even when C3 levels are within the normal range.
- Acute-phase proteins are minimally elevated.
- High ESR should prompt a search for other causes, including leukaemia and infection.

❶It is important to realize that the development of diagnostically helpful antibodies often follows rather than precedes the development of clinical disease. Repeating antibody measurements at 3-monthly intervals is therefore advised if there is strong clinical suspicion of disease.

- In Still's disease, there are no specific tests. ESR and CRP are very high, with anaemia, leucocytosis, and thrombocytosis.
  - There is a polyclonal hypergammaglobulinaemia, although the incidence of IgA deficiency is increased.
  - A small proportion of patients may have RhF and a larger proportion may have ANA (37%).
  - Complement activation may be present.
  - IL-6 and TNFα levels may be elevated.

Treatment

- NSAIDs form the mainstay of therapy for pauci-articular disease, notwithstanding the risks of Reye's syndrome.
- DMARDs may be required for more severe cases.
- Uveitis may be treated with etanercept, methotrexate, or mycophenolate mofetil.
- Biological agents including anti-TNFs, anti-CTLA4 (abatacept), anti-IL-1 (anakinra, canakinumab), anti-IL-6 (tocilizumab), rituximab, anti-IL-12/23 (ustekinumab) and anti-IL-17A (secukinumab) are all used.
- In Still's disease, NSAIDs are used initially, with steroids reserved for failure of response. Methotrexate is the most effective steroid-sparing agent; gold and sulfasalazine are contraindicated.
- Bone marrow and stem cell transplantation are now being used successfully for severe cases.

Testing

- See Table 12.3.

Table 12.3 Testing for JCA and Still's disease

Tests used for diagnosis	Tests used for monitoring
CRP/ESR	CRP/ESR
FBC	FBC
LFTS	LFTs
ANA	ENA, anti-histone antibodies (uveitis risk)
dsDNA	ANA, dsDNA (monitoring of anti-TNFs)
	Anti-biological antibodies
ENA	
Anti-histone antibodies	
RhF	
C3, C4	
Immunoglobulins	

Adult Still's disease

- Clinical features are very similar to those of childhood Still's, but occurring in young adults.
  - There is the typical fever (for more than 1 week) and rash (evanescent salmon-pink), often accompanied by sore throat.
  - Hepatosplenomegaly and lymphadenopathy are common.
  - Polyserositis occurs frequently.
  - Polyarthralgia or polyarthritis lasting more than 2 weeks.
- Exclusion of lymphoma may be difficult.
- May be complicated by haemophagocytosis (macrophage activation syndrome).
- There are no diagnostic tests other than non-specific inflammatory markers.
  - Neutrophilia is common.
- RhF and ANA will be negative.
- Ferritin levels may be exceptionally high and disproportionately elevated when compared to other acute-phase markers.
  - Ferritin levels are controlled by IL-18 and a polymorphism in the IL-18 gene has been identified in adult Still's patients that may explain the high ferritin.
  - Hyperferritinaemia may be seen if haemophagocytosis is present and may also be found in other haemophagocytic syndromes.
- NSAIDs, corticosteroids, and DMARDS are all required.
- ❶NSAIDs have a risk of inducing hepatitis and possibly of triggering haemophagocytosis.
  - Regular monitoring of LFTs is required.
- Good response to anti-IL-1 therapies; methotrexate is also valuable.
- Role of anti-TNF therapies is unclear: some may benefit.
- Ciclosporin may be beneficial if there is macrophage activation syndrome.
- Disease may run a chronic progressive course, a relapsing–remitting course, or resolve completely.

Ankylosing spondylitis (AS) and related spondyloarthropathies

These are a group of seronegative (RhF-negative) disorders, strongly associated with HLA-B27. The group includes ankylosing spondylitis, reactive arthritis, enteropathic arthritis, psoriatic arthritis, and undifferentiated spondyloarthritis.

Clinical features

- Typical clinical features of AS include spinal pain and restriction in movement, especially in the lumbar and thoracic regions, accompanied by demonstrable sacroiliitis on radiographs.
- Commoner in men than women.
- May be associated with inflammatory bowel disease.

- Complications include:
  - anterior uveitis;
  - cardiac lesions involving the proximal aorta and aortic valve;
  - pericarditis and conduction block;
  - upper-lobe lung fibrosis;
  - amyloidosis;
  - sponylodiscitis and spinal fractures;
  - chronic fatigue.

Immunopathology

- TNFα appears to play a key role: levels are high in affected joints, which are infiltrated with CD4$^+$ and CD8$^+$ T cells.
- IL-6 levels are also elevated.
- HLA-B27 is critical for the development of disease: B27 transgenic mice develop spontaneous spondylitis.
- GWAS have identified up to 70 susceptibility genes.
- Bacterial infections (especially bowel bacteria) are strongly associated.
- Autoantibodies have been identified to aggrecan (a proteoglycan in cartilage) and heat shock proteins—these are not diagnostically valuable.

Diagnosis

- By definition, this is an RhF-seronegative arthritis and there are no defining antibodies.
- Acute-phase proteins may be normal or elevated.
- IgA is often elevated.
- Alkaline phosphatase and creatinine kinase (CK) may also be elevated.
- More than 90% of all cases will be HLA-B27 positive but, as this is a common antigen in the Caucasian population (8%), the diagnostic value of testing for HLA-B27 is limited.
- Of B27-positive persons, 5–10% will develop AS, while 20% go on to develop a reactive arthropathy after infection with agents such as *Salmonella* or *Chlamydia*.
- DR4 is associated with peripheral joint involvement.

Treatment

- Previously the mainstay of treatment has been NSAIDs (with exercise and physiotherapy), sulfasalazine (only effective in peripheral joint not axial disease), and methotrexate.
- AS responds dramatically well to anti-TNF drugs (etanercept, infliximab, adalimumab, golimumab), although the associated uveitis responds less well and may need other immunosupressive agents.
- Tocilizumab (anti-IL-6) and rituximab (anti-CD20) are also useful.
- Anti-IL-17A (secukinumab) appears valuable.
- Other beneficial therapies include bisphosphonates and thalidomide.

Complications

- Amyloid may develop and there is a recognized association with IgA nephropathy.

SAPHO syndrome

- A syndrome of synovitis, acne, palmoplantar pustulosis, hyperostosis, and osteitis (with granulomata).
- Acne is severe.
- Hidradenitis suppurativa is also seen.
- Hyperostosis of especially sternoclavicular joint and spine.
- Peripheral arthritis is seen in 92% of cases.
- ESR is high.
- There is a weak association with HLA-B27.
- May respond to anti-TNF treatment and antibiotics (as used for acne on the basis that *Propionobacterium acnes* has been isolated from bone biopsies).
- Bisphosphonates have also been used successfully.

Psoriatic arthritis

Clinical features

- Usually develops in patients with clinical psoriasis, although, if skin lesions are not present, diagnosis may be difficult.
- Arthritis is frequently asymmetrical and spinal involvement is common, in contrast to RhA, which it most resembles.

Immunopathology

- Disease is associated with HLA-B7 and B27.
- DR4 is linked with a peripheral arthritis.
- A gene has also been identified on chromosome 17.
- GWAS have identified up to 60 susceptibility genes.
- Retroviral-like particles have been described in psoriasis.
- There is a direct association of guttate psoriasis with streptococcal infections.
- Major pathological process is overgrowth of keratinocytes, driven primarily by activated CD4+ T cells and the resultant release of cytokines and growth factors.
- Psoriasis is associated with HLA-Cw6 (also DR7, DQ3, and B57); B27 is associated with spondylitis.

Diagnosis

- There are no specific immunological tests for psoriatic arthropathy.
- Up to 10% of patients will be RhF positive (low titre) and may also have low-titre ANA and autoantibodies against skin antigens.
- There is polyclonal hypergammaglobulinaemia.
- Acute-phase proteins are elevated.
- Anaemia is common and may be both due to chronic disease and also due to folate deficiency from increased cell proliferation.
- Increased cell turnover may cause hyperuricaemia and gout.

Treatment

- The realization of the central role of T lymphocytes in psoriasis has led to a change in the approach to treatment towards immunomodulation.
- Biologicals used for skin psoriasis may also be effective.
- Anti-TNF agents are extremely effective.
- Apremilast, a phosphodiesterase 4 inhibitor, is effective.
- ❶Care must be taken as some NSAIDs and antimalarials may exacerbate psoriasis.
- Gold, penicillamine, hydroxychloroquine, methotrexate, sulfasalazine, azathioprine, ciclosporin, PUVA, and retinoids have all been shown to be useful.

Reactive arthritis (including Reiter's syndrome)

Clinical features

This group of diseases presents with a pauci-articular large-joint arthritis, accompanied by back pain (sacroiliitis) and non-articular symptoms, such as:
- balanitis, urethritis, and cervicitis;
- keratoderma blennorrhagicum;
- pericarditis (with a long PR interval and non-specific T-wave changes);
- conjunctivitis.

Immunopathology

- Symptoms can be triggered by a variety of urogenital and intestinal infections, including *Shigella, Salmonella, Campylobacter, Yersinia, Klebsiella, Proteus, Escherichia coli, Chlamydia, Mycoplasma*, and *Ureaplasma*.
- Also associated with inflammatory bowel disease and HIV infection.
- 55% of cases will be HLA-B27+, but mostly these will be patients with spinal involvement.

Diagnosis

- ESR/CRP will be elevated and there is anaemia and leucocytosis.
- RhF and ANA will be absent. Atypical P-ANCA may be seen where there is inflammatory bowel disease.

Treatment

- Standard treatment is with NSAIDs, together with treatment of the underlying infection or bowel disease.
- Variable response to anti-TNF agents.

Bowel disease and arthritis

Other bowel diseases that are associated with arthritis include:
- coeliac disease (check IgA endomysial antibodies/tTG antibodies), which responds promptly to a gluten-free diet;
- intestinal bypass surgery/bacterial overgrowth (cryoglobulins may be present, and there may be cutaneous vasculitic lesions);
- Whipple's disease due to infection with *Tropheryma whipplei* (malabsorption with migratory arthritis; no specific tests apart from PCR-based detection of organism but hypogammaglobulinaemia may occur—see ➋ Chapter 7).

Systemic lupus erythematosus (SLE) and variants

SLE has taken over from syphilis as being the great mimic. Clinical criteria have been defined by the ARA: 4 out of 11 criteria are sufficient to confirm the diagnosis (within a window of observation, not necessarily concurrently). However, many patients clearly have the disease even though they do not fit the criteria. SLE is strongly associated with other autoimmune diseases through a shared immunogenetic background.

Aetiology and immunopathology

- There is a strong multigenic background to SLE: the main contributing factors being:
  - homozygous complement deficiency (especially C1qrs, C2, C4 deficiency);
  - TREX1 deficiency (X-linked gene): endothelial function gene;
  - HLA-A1, B8, DR3, other HLA genes associated with specific features and/or autoantibodies (DQw1, DQw2 with anti-Ro; DR2, anti-Sm; DQw6, 7, 8 with anti-phospholipid antibodies);
  - multiple immune genes (STAT4, ITF5, IRAK1, PTPN22, OX40L among others);
  - racial background (especially West Indian);
  - female sex (M:F = 1:10–20);
  - men with Klinefelter's syndrome are at increased risk of SLE;
  - mothers of boys with X-linked chronic granulomatous disease are at increased risk of lupus.
- Precise cause of lupus is unknown, although a mouse model is known to be deficient of mechanisms for controlling lymphocyte apoptosis (*fas*).
- Drugs may also trigger lupus, although the association for some of these is weak.
  - Likelihood of a drug causing problems is associated with acetylator status (slow acetylator status increasing the risk).
- SLE is the prototype immune complex disease, with evidence for incorrectly sized immune complexes being formed that are cleared inefficiently, in part due to an acquired reduction in the CR1 receptor on erythrocytes.
- Many antibodies thought to be non-pathogenic are now known to be able to penetrate viable cells and interfere with an intracellular target enzyme. These include:
  - anti-dsDNA;
  - anti-RNP;
  - anti-ribosomal P antibodies;
  - process is trypsin-sensitive.
- Surface DNA-binding proteins and proteins with a similar structure to DNA will also bind anti-DNA antibodies and this may lead to alterations in cell function.
- There is evidence of complement consumption, the level of which corresponds to disease activity.

- FcγRIIA polymorphisms that reduce immune complex binding are associated with lupus nephritis.
- Environmental factors, e.g. UV-induced Ro antigen expression on keratinocytes, smoking, EBV exposure, silica exposure, all contribute.

Clinical features

- There is no typical presentation and the disease may present to any organ specialist (see Table 12.4).
- Any age group may be affected, but younger women are most commonly affected.
- Fatigue, malaise, and weight loss are often marked in the prodrome.
- Lymphadenopathy and splenomegaly are common.
- Presentations with skin disease alone are of a more limited disease (which may progress), discoid lupus, and subacute cutaneous lupus.
- C2-deficient lupus tends to give a very florid disease with marked cutaneous vasculitic symptoms and is invariably anti-Ro positive.
- Arthritis with recurrent polyserositis is a common presentation.
- A high index of suspicion for the disease is required.

Table 12.4 Clinical features of SLE, and associated antibodies

Clinical features	Associated autoantibodies and immunological features
Arthritis (non-deforming)	
Serositis (pericarditis, pleurisy, peritonitis)	
Rashes; photosensitivity; malar (butterfly) rash	Anti-Ro; anti-La
Cutaneous lupus	Deficiency of C2, C4, C1q
Urticaria	
Angioedema	Anti-C1 esterase inhibitor; anti-C1q
Alopecia (scarring); vitiligo	Anti-melanocyte
Mouth ulcers	
Sicca syndrome	Anti-Ro; anti-La
Glomerulonephritis; nephrotic syndrome	Anti-dsDNA; anti-C1q
Neurological disorder (psychosis, seizures)	Anti-ribosomal P; anti-neuronal
Peripheral neuropathy; mononeuritis	
Transverse myelitis; optic neuritis (MS-like)	ANA
Myasthenia gravis	Anti-acetylcholine receptor (AchRAb)
Haemolytic anaemia	Anti-erythrocyte; Coombs' test[+]
Thrombocytopenia	Anti-platelet; anti-phospholipid

Table 12.4 (*Contd.*)

Clinical features	Associated autoantibodies and immunological features
Lymphopenia	Lymphocytotoxic antibodies (anti-MHC)
Neutropenia	Anti-neutrophil antibodies
Venous thrombosis; pulmonary emboli	Anti-phospholipid antibodies
Recurrent miscarriage; livedo reticularis	Anti-phospholipid antibodies
Endocarditis	Anti-phospholipid antibodies
Raynaud's phenomenon	Anti-phospholipid antibodies; cryoglobulins (type II or III)
Shrinking lung	
Hepatitis	Anti-smooth muscle; anti-dsDNA
Mesenteric vasculitis	
Intestinal pseudo-obstruction	
Pancreatitis	
Organ-specific autoimmune disease	Organ-specific autoantibodies (thyroid peroxidase, etc.)
Neonatal lupus; congenital complete heart block	Anti-Ro; anti-La
Drug-induced lupus	Anti-histone; anti-ssDNA

- Disease may be triggered by stress and by UV light (in patients who are photosensitive). The latter not only causes worsening of skin disease but also sets off systemic manifestations.
- Infection may also trigger flares, but the role of immunization is more controversial.
- As the disease often affects young women, pregnancy is a frequent problem.
  - Effect of SLE on pregnancy is unpredictable.
  - Conception is unlikely with severe active disease.
  - Disease may flare or remit during pregnancy.
  - Disease frequently flares postpartum (due to sudden hormonal changes).
- As autoantibodies are invariably IgG, they cross the placenta. Anti-Ro and possibly anti-La have been associated with:
  - congenital complete heart block due to damage to the fetal conducting system;
  - neonatal lupus that disappears as maternal antibody is removed from the circulation;
  - complete heart block occurs in the children of 1 in 20 women positive for the antibodies but, if there has been a previously affected baby, the risk rises to 1 in 4.

SLE: immunological testing

- Detection of autoantibodies and complement abnormalities form the mainstay of diagnosis.
- Full diagnostic screen must include:
  - ANA, dsDNA, ENA, HEp-2 cells (for proliferating cell nuclear antigen (PCNA) and staining pattern);
  - anti-cardiolipin ± anti-β2GP-I, lupus anticoagulant (dRVVT);
  - organ-specific autoantibodies (thyroid, gastric parietal cells, DCT, others as clinically indicated);
  - C3/C4;
  - C2, C1q particularly if atypical skin disease;
  - serum immunoglobulins and electrophoresis;
  - cryoglobulins if Raynaud's is present.

Autoantibody testing

- Antibodies to histones if drug-induced lupus erythematosus suspected.
- Other antibodies may be sought, depending on clinical features (see Table 12.4).
- Pattern of ANAs detected (on HEp2 cells) may give a clue as to other antibodies present (e.g. coarse speckled = anti-RNP), and should always be reported. Homogeneous ANAs are usually associated with antibodies to dsDNA and histones.
- Multiple specificities may be present in a single patient.
- A proportion of SLE patients have always been noted to be ANA-negative: these patients are usually anti-Ro positive.
  - Rodent liver, widely used as a substrate for detecting ANA, has low levels of Ro antigen, which may be leached out during the test procedure.
  - HEp-2 cells have much higher levels, so the proportion of ANA-negative lupus falls when this substrate is used for screening.
  - HEp-2 cells also allow the detection of PCNA (see Part 2), another SLE-specific antibody.
  - Anti-Ku antibodies may be seen (but also seen in other CTDs).
- Antibodies to dsDNA should be checked regardless of the ANA result if SLE is suspected.
  - Certain subsets of dsDNA antibodies (not routinely measurable) appear to be specifically associated with glomerulonephritis.
- Additional antibodies detected on ENA screening give further useful information.
  - Anti-Sm is a rare antibody that is highly specific for SLE and is found mostly in West Indians.
  - Anti-RNP may be found in SLE, but always with dsDNA (if anti-RNP is the only specificity, then MCTD/UCTD is more likely; see ➋ 'Mixed connective tissue disease (MCTD)', p. 306).
  - Anti-Ro and anti-La are associated with features of secondary sicca syndrome, as well as with congenital complete heart block, neonatal lupus, and photosensitivity.
  - Ribosomal antibodies will be detected when a multiblock section is used.

- Anti-C1q antibodies appear to be associated with lupus nephritis, as well as urticarial vasculitis.
- ANCA may also be found in SLE, although it is difficult to identify these accurately in the presence of high-titre ANA: solid-phase assays with specific antigens (PR3 and MPO) help here.
- Antibodies to lipoprotein lipase have been associated with the pathogenesis of lupus nephritis (in association with antibodies to dsDNA, and ribosomal P antigen).
- Rheumatoid factors are usually present but contribute little to the diagnostic process.
- For investigation of anti-phospholipid antibodies, see ➲ 'Anti-phospholipid syndrome (APS)', p. 319.

❶Severe difficulties in diagnosis may occur as ANAs may frequently be found in chronic infection, including bacterial endocarditis and particularly infection with enteric organisms, and in association with drugs (phenothiazines, ACE inhibitors, minocycline—see ➲ 'Drug-induced lupus (DRL)', p. 302).

Complement studies
- Complement studies are essential.
- C4 reductions are common and do not reliably relate to disease activity, as C4 null alleles are common.
- When disease is quiescent, the following rule of thumb applies:
  - complete C4 deficiency: no detectable C4;
  - one functioning allele: C4 is half the lower limit of normal;
  - two functioning alleles: C4 is at or just below the lower limit of normal;
  - three functioning alleles: C4 is midway into the normal range.
- C3 levels are reduced in active disease, although, because of an acute-phase response with increased synthesis, the level may not drop below the lower end of the normal range.
- A measure of C3 breakdown is required (C3d), but suitable assays for routine diagnostic laboratories are limited. C5–C9 assays may be helpful.
- Measuring haemolytic complement as a monitor of disease activity is too crude and not recommended.
- Measurement of haemolytic complement essential when SLE is thought to be due to a complete deficiency, and this testing should always be followed up with measurement of individual components.
- Genetic testing for deficiency may be required.
- Assays of immune complexes are difficult (impossible?) to standardize and add little to the management.
- Activation assays such C5a–C9 may be valuable.
- Rare patients with acquired angioedema may have antibodies to C1q or C1 inhibitor.

Biopsies ('lupus band test')
- Skin biopsies show typical deposits of IgG and C3/C4 along the dermo-epidermal junction in a 'lumpy-bumpy' distribution. There may also be deposits around cutaneous blood vessels. Both normal and affected skin show similar findings (this is used to form the so-called lupus band test).
- Renal biopsy may be helpful in view of the wide range of histopathological abnormalities that may be identified.

Immunoglobulin abnormalities

- Serum immunoglobulins are normally increased polyclonally; small monoclonal bands on a polyclonal background may be seen on electrophoresis.
- Electrophoresis of serum may show a reduction in the β-region due to low C3 and a reduced albumin and raised α2-band will be seen if there is a nephrotic syndrome.
- IgA deficiency is common in SLE, and rare patients may be pan-hypogammaglobulinaemic (distinct from hypogammaglobulinaemia secondary to aggressive immunotherapy).
- Cryoglobulins, if present, will be type II or type III.

Acute-phase response

- ESR is raised in active disease but, paradoxically, CRP is either normal or only trivially raised.
- High CRPs in patients with SLE suggest intercurrent infection (which may be hard to distinguish from a flare).

Other tests

- FBC should be scanned for evidence of haemolysis (reduced Hb, increased MCV, confirmed by low/absent haptoglobin and positive DCT), thrombocytopenia, and other cytopenias.
- Regular monitoring of creatinine and electrolytes, liver and thyroid function tests, and urine (casts, red cells, protein) are all essential.
- Imaging is essential to confirm organ-specific problems and MRI is particularly valuable.

Monitoring of established disease

- Monitoring of lupus patients must include:
  - regular FBC;
  - Cr & E;
  - LFTs;
  - TFTs;
  - urine (protein, albumin/creatinine ratio, blood, casts);
  - CRP/ESR;
  - C3/C4; low C3 indicates active disease;
  - anti-dsDNA: a rising titre of dsDNA often heralds relapse.
- Complement studies and acute-phase markers give an indicator of current activity, although this must always be interpreted in the light of clinical symptoms.
- There is no value in monitoring ANA titres.
- Frequency of monitoring is dependent on disease activity and the type of drugs being used (i.e. more frequent when cytotoxics are being used).
- It is worth rechecking full serology every so often (every 6–12 months), as antibodies may come and go and the clinical disease pattern may evolve or change in parallel. More frequent checking of ENA antibody specificities is unhelpful.
- As the half-life of antibodies is about 3 weeks, measurements of autoantibodies are rarely of value more frequently than monthly (unless a patient is being plasmapheresed).

SLE: treatment and paediatric SLE

❶Treatment protocols change regularly as new drugs are introduced: readers are recommended to check up-to-date literature.

Treatment

- Mild disease can usually be managed with NSAIDs, although there are reports that patients with SLE are more prone to develop hepatic abnormalities and aseptic meningitis.
- Rashes can be treated with topical steroids.
- Sunblocks are essential in sunny climes.
- Fatigue, arthralgia, and skin disease respond well to antimalarials: hydroxychloroquine is the safest. Mepacrine is an alternative (beware skin discoloration). Hydroxychloroquine interferes with TLR7 and TLR9 signalling.
- Dapsone may be useful for cutaneous lupus.
- Systemic disease usually responds to low-dose steroids (20–30 mg/day). Azathioprine (2–4 mg/kg per day—check TPMT level first) can be used as a steroid-sparing agent.
- Mycophenolate mofetil (MMF) is an alternative to azathioprine (and is valuable where there is renal disease). Counsel regarding pregnancy (and effects on male recipients).
- Methotrexate (weekly oral or SC) is now being used for arthritis.
- More serious organ involvement, e.g. glomerulonephritis, haemolytic anaemia, requires aggressive therapy with pulsed intravenous steroid with intravenous 5–10 mg/kg/pulse or oral (2–4 mg/kg/day) cyclophosphamide.
  - ❶High dose cyclophosphamide requires the concomitant use of mesna to prevent haemorrhagic cystitis. Long-term risk of bladder cancer.
- Neurological involvement is difficult to treat and there is no consensus: high-dose steroids can be tried but may be more likely to trigger a steroid psychosis. The role of cytotoxics is uncertain.
- Plasmapheresis may be an adjunct in severe disease while waiting for a clinical effect from cytotoxics, but should not be used alone because of potential rebound worsening of the disease.
- In pregnancy, if possible avoid drugs other than prednisolone (metabolized by placenta).
  - Dexamethasone may be used to treat fetal complications (heart block) in utero as it is not metabolized by the placenta.
  - Hydroxychloroquine may improve pregnancy outcomes.
- IVIg should be used only with care as it may make the immune complex component of the disease worse (contraindicated if there is a high-titre RhF, renal impairment (high dose)).
- Aim should always be for the lowest dose of treatment compatible with maintaining remission.
- Immune ablation with stem cell transplantation has been used for severe disease in adults and children.

Use of biological agents
- Many biological agents have been tried and have failed in SLE!
- Large numbers of drugs are currently undergoing clinical trials.
  - Nelfinavir (HIV protease inhibitor): reduced dsDNA antibody levels.
  - Bortezomib: proteasome inhibitor.
  - Anti-IL-10.
  - Anti-CD40 ligand (dapirolizumab pegol).
  - Ubiquitin ligase modulator (iberdomide).
  - NF-κB inhibitor (iguratimod).
  - Forigerimod.
  - Voclosporin.
- Belimumab (humanized mAb that inhibits B-lymphocyte stimulator BLys) approved by FDA in SLE.
- Rituximab (anti-CD20), in combination with corticosteroids and cyclophosphamide, has been used in refractory disease.
  - Progressive multifocal leukoencephalopathy (PML) may be a risk.
  - Rituximab alone seems to be disappointing.
- Other anti-B-cell agents are undergoing trials.
  - Atacicept: fusion protein of TACI and IgG (appears to significantly increase risk of infection if given with MMF).
  - Epratuzumab: anti-CD22 mAb—disappointing.
- Anti-T-cell treatments undergoing trials.
  - Abatacept (CTLA4 fusion protein)—not successful!
  - JAK (baricitinib, filgotinib) and SYK (GS 9876) inhibitors are being trialled.
- Anti-interferons.
  - Anifrolumab may be of benefit in lupus nephritis and neuropsychiatric lupus.

Other important treatment features
- Chronic steroid therapy requires bone protection therapy (bisphosphonate, calcium, and vitamin D).
- Oral contraceptives are not contraindicated, but low-oestrogen or progesterone-only pills should be used.
- Splenectomy may be required for thrombocytopenia where this is antibody mediated and resistant to immunosuppressive therapy: great care needs to be taken with these patients in view of the increased infective risk.
- Patients on any form of immunosuppressive therapy need to have their humoral and cellular immune status monitored, and preventive measures, such as low-dose co-trimoxazole and antifungals, may be required.
- APS requires anticoagulation (see ⊃ 'Anti-phospholipid syndrome', p. 319).

Testing
- See Table 12.5.

Paediatric SLE
- The disease in children is very similar to that in adults.
- Difficulties arise because the marker antibodies are frequently not present until the child has been ill for some time, making diagnosis

Table 12.5 Testing for SLE

Tests for diagnosis	Tests for monitoring
FBC	FBC
Cr & E	Cr & E
LFTs	LFTs
TFTs	TFTs
Urine (RBCs, casts, protein, creatinine clearance)	Urine (RBCs, casts, protein, creatinine clearance)
ANA	dsDNA
dsDNA	Anti-C1q antibodies (renal disease)?
ENA	C3, C4 (C3d)
HEp-2 screen	ESR, CRP
Histone antibodies (drug-induced only)	
Ribosomal antibodies, neuronal antibodies (CNS only)	
Anti-C1q antibodies (renal disease)?	
Organ-specific autoantibodies	
Anti-phospholipid antibodies	
DCT	
C3, C4 (C3d)	
Haemolytic complement (complement deficiency)	
Immunoglobulins	
Cryoglobulins	
ESR, CRP	

difficult. There is often also overlap of symptoms with childhood connective tissue diseases.
- Before puberty, the male to female ratio is increased compared to that in adults (1:5).
- The use of diagnostic tests should be applied just as in adult disease; however, where there is a high suspicion of disease, but no antibodies, tests should be repeated at regular intervals (every 2–3 months), as antibodies may appear later.
- ▶Remember that significant titres of autoantibodies will be lower in children compared to adults.
- Management follows the same lines as in adults, although greater care needs to be taken over the use of steroids, to avoid stunting growth.

Drug-related lupus (DRL)

A large number of drugs have been associated with DRL.
- Key drugs include:
  - hydralazine;
  - procainamide;
  - methyldopa;
  - quinidine;
  - chlorpromazine;
  - minocycline (particularly associated with autoimmune hepatitis);
  - isoniazid;
  - penicillamine;
  - phenytoin;
  - anti-TNF agents (infliximab, etanercept, etc.);
  - ACE-inhibitors.
- Chemical features of drugs associated with DRL include the presence of:
  - arylamine or hydrazine groups;
  - sulphydryl groups.
- Patient factors include:
  - acetylator status;
  - polymorphisms of P450 cytochrome enzymes.
- Specificity of ANA is usually but not exclusively anti-histone (> 95%).
  - Antibodies recognize complex of histone dimer H2A-H2B + dsDNA.
  - With hydralazine DRL the specificity is H1 and H3/H4 complex.
  - Anti-dsDNA antibodies are usually *absent*.
- The presence of ANCA has also been associated with hydralazine-induced lupus (with glomerulonephritis).
- It is important to take a clear drug history when patients are identified with ANAs in order to exclude the possibility of drug-induced lupus.
- Symptoms tend to be mild.
- ▶Drug-induced ANAs may occur without symptoms.
- Disease often remits once the offending drugs are withdrawn.
- Patients with persistent symptoms should be treated in the normal way.

Sjögren's syndrome

Sjögren's syndrome may occur as both a primary disorder in its own right, or it may accompany other connective tissue diseases. There is a strong association with other autoimmune diseases, particularly thyroid disease and primary biliary cirrhosis (PBC). The primary pathology is a lymphocytic infiltrate into the exocrine glands, affecting salivary and lacrimal glands, but also glands of the genital and respiratory tracts.

HCV infection may give rise to similar symptoms and must be excluded at the outset.

Aetiology and immunopathology

- Cause is unknown, although there is some evidence to suggest that viral infections may contribute substantially, including EBV, HCV, and retroviruses.
- There is an immunogenetic background, shared with other autoimmune diseases, including B8 and DR3. There is a strong association, independent of ethnic background, with DQA1*0501.
- STAT4 and IRF5 are both associated with SS.
- B-cell activating factor (BAFF) elevated, especially in patients with hypergammaglobulinaemia. Possibly produced by glandular epithelial cell in response type I interferons.
- CD40⁺ B cells more resistant to apoptosis.
- Proto-oncogenes are also expressed and the disease is frequently accompanied by monoclonal expansion of B cells within the glands, accompanied by IgMκ paraprotein production and the development of type II cryoglobulins.
- Disease may terminate in frank lymphoma, usually extra-nodal low-grade B-cell lymphomas.
- Antibodies to α-fodrin may be associated with the disease.

Clinical features

- Dry gritty eyes, dry mouth, difficulty swallowing, recurrent parotitis and gingivitis, recurrent chest infections (bronchiectasis), and dyspareunia are the main sicca symptoms.
- There may be subclinical pancreatitis.
- Fatigue and malaise are marked and early features.
  - Increased IL-1RA is found in CSF, suggesting that IL-1 may mediate fatigue.
  - Autonomic dysfunction may be present (orthostatic hypotension, gastroparesis, urinary frequency, etc.).
- Arthralgia and arthritis and fibromyalgic pain are common.
- Interstitial lung disease may be found on CT scanning.
- Fanconi syndrome may occur.
- Both CNS and peripheral nerve involvement have been reported.
  - Hemiparesis, transverse myelopathy, seizures, movement disorders, and aseptic meningitis. MS may occur.
- Features of other autoimmune diseases will be present.
- Raynaud's may be present if there are cryoglobulins.
- Hypergammaglobulinaemia purpura (vasculitis).
- Salivary glands may be enlarged. Lymphadenopathy should always be taken seriously if it does not settle once local infection has been dealt with (risk of lymphoma/maltoma). Consider CT of salivary glands ± biopsy.
- Biopsy of minor salivary glands may be diagnostically useful.
- Secondary Sjögren's appears to be more limited (sicca symptoms).
- Clinical diagnosis may be made by Schirmer's test (normal > 15 mm wetting in 5 minutes; < 5 mm is abnormal); Rose Bengal staining of the cornea may demonstrate corneal damage.

Immunological testing

- Diagnostic testing should include ANA, dsDNA, ENA, RhF, thyroid and mitochondrial antibodies, C3/C4, serum immunoglobulins and electrophoresis, cryoglobulins, β_2-microglobulin, CRP/ESR, and IgG subclasses.
- Typically associated with anti-Ro antibodies (both Ro52 and Ro60) and anti-La antibodies.
- If the ANA is negative and primary Sjögren's is suspected, then salivary gland antibodies may be helpful.
- HEp-2 screening may also pick up other specificities known to be associated, such as antibodies to the Golgi body and the nuclear mitotic apparatus.
- RhF will be found in 90% of patients developing arthritis, 70% will be positive for anti-Ro, and 40% for anti-La. ANA will usually show a fine speckled appearance. DsDNA will be negative.
- Thyroid antibodies are common (30%) and mitochondrial antibodies will be found in those going on to develop PBC.
- Complements will usually be normal or elevated (this is not a complement-consuming disorder). Low levels should raise questions about the primary underlying diagnosis.
- There is invariably a marked restricted-clonality hypergammaglobulinaemia, often with IgMκ paraproteins on immunofixation.
- Increase in IgG is restricted to IgG_1, with reductions seen in IgG_2, IgG_3, and IgG_4: hence the electrophoretic appearances. Measurement of IgG subclasses is therefore a helpful adjunctive test, as no other conditions give this pattern, other than myeloma.
- Cryoglobulins should always be sought, particularly if there is any cutaneous involvement.
- β_2-Microglobulin should be monitored as a marker of lymphoproliferation.
- ESR and CRP are high, with anaemia of chronic disease.
- Raised alkaline phosphatase of liver origin may indicate PBC.
- Thyroid function must be checked at baseline and regularly thereafter.
- Long-term monitoring of patients should be undertaken at the clinical level. Regular checks for paraproteins and evidence of lymphoproliferation are essential.
- Clinical checks should include thyroid and liver, in view of the strong association with Sjögren's syndrome.
- There is no value in monitoring the autoantibodies, unless there is a clinical change.

Treatment

- Symptomatic treatment with lubricants forms the mainstay of treatment.
  - Spectacles help reduce the drying effect of the air.
  - Meticulous attention to oral hygiene reduces the oral infective problems.
  - Pilocarpine has also been used to increase saliva flow.

- Hydroxychloroquine is valuable for the arthralgia and fatigue.
- Topical ocular ciclosporin has been approved by the FDA.
- The role of steroids and cytotoxics is less clear, and often have little benefit for the sicca symptoms. It has been suggested that these may increase the rate of progression to lymphoma. However, they are necessary if there is extraglandular involvement and/or vasculitis.
- Methotrexate (*weekly* PO or SC) may be used.
- Anti-TNF drugs do not appear helpful.
- Other biological agents (rituximab, epratuzumab, belimumab) are undergoing trials, but haven't been very promising.
- Long-term follow-up needs to be instituted for early identification of malignancy.
- Refer all suspicious persistent swellings for CT/MRI and biopsy.

Testing

- See Table 12.6.

Table 12.6 Testing for Sjögren's syndrome

Tests for diagnosis	Tests for monitoring
FBC	FBC
Cr & E	Cr & E
LFTs	LFTs
TFTs	TFTs
Urine (glucose, amino acids; Fanconi syndrome)	Urine (glucose, amino acids; Fanconi syndrome)
ANA	Immunoglobulins, electrophoresis
dsDNA	β_2 MG
ENA	ESR/CRP
HEp-2 screen	CT/MRI scan (lungs, salivary glands, lymph nodes) ± biopsy
Organ-specific autoantibodies	
Immunoglobulins, electrophoresis	
β_2 MG	
Cryoglobulins	
ESR, CRP	
Schirmer's test	
Labial gland biopsy	
CT/MRI scan salivary glands ± biopsy	

IgG₄-related chronic sclerosing dacryoadenitis

- Rare disease mimicking Sjögren's syndrome. Other complications of IgG₄ disease may include:
  - autoimmune pancreatitis;
  - sclerosing cholangitis;
  - non-infectious aortitis.
- Inflammatory sclerosing masses with plasma cell infiltrates in submandibular and lacrimal glands.
- IgG₄ significantly raised without changes in other IgG subclasses (unique abnormality that is diagnostic).
- Responds to corticosteroids.

Undifferentiated connective tissue disease

- This usually comprises a clinical syndrome that does not fulfil the criteria for any one connective tissue disease, either clinically or serologically.
- Typical features include:
  - Raynaud's syndrome;
  - polyarthritis;
  - rash;
  - interstitial lung disease;
  - myalgia.
- Such patients need to be treated symptomatically while being followed clinically and serologically (testing as for lupus, see ➔ 'SLE: immunological testing', p. 296).
- Capillaroscopy may identify abnormalities.
- Some patients with chronic fatigue may have positive ANA and/or low C4: these need to be followed to exclude the possibility of a prodromal CTD.
- Interval measurement of ENA antibodies is helpful (every 6–12 months).
- Some will resolve spontaneously and others will progress to a more clearly defined disease.
- Early intervention with DMARDs may alter the natural history.

Mixed connective tissue disease (MCTD/UCTD)

Whether MCTD/UCTD is truly a distinct entity has been questioned by some experts, on the basis that it may evolve into SLE or other typical connective tissue disease, or that these diseases may evolve into MCTD/UCTD. Even if it forms part of the spectrum of SLE, it is distinct enough to be considered separately.

Aetiology and pathogenesis
• It is associated with DR4 and DQ3.

Clinical features
• Clinical features include: arthralgia (96%), swollen hands (88%), Raynaud's (84%), abnormal oesophageal motility (77%), myositis (72%), and lymphadenopathy (68%).
• Other clinical features that may occur include serositis, leucopenia, thrombocytopenia, sclerodactyly, pulmonary fibrosis (with reduced gas transfer, 70%), pulmonary hypertension (major cause of death), and aseptic meningitis.
• Trigeminal neuropathy may occur in 10%.
• Fatigue and malaise are common in the prodrome.
• Up to 50% of patients develop nephritis.

Diagnosis
• There is polyclonal hypergammaglobulinaemia.
• Cryoglobulins may be detected.
• C3/C4 may be reduced.
• Autoantibodies show a coarse speckled ANA, absent or low level of anti-dsDNA antibodies, and strongly positive anti-U1 RNP (90–100% of true MCTD/UCTD patients).
  • Antibodies to U1 RNP 68kD and A protein are associated with increased severity of symptoms.
• Presence of high levels of anti-dsDNA suggests SLE not MCTD/UCTD.
• RhF is positive in 40–60%.
• Anti-phospholipid antibodies may be associated with pulmonary hypertension.
• ESR/CRP are elevated and there is anaemia of chronic disease.
• Thrombocytopenia may be due to anti-platelet antibodies or the presence of anti-phospholipid antibodies.
• CK may be elevated from muscle involvement but also in aseptic meningitis and trigeminal neuropathy.

Treatment
• Treatment is with NSAIDs and/or hydroxychloroquine for fatigue, myalgia, and polyarthritis.
• Steroids plus cytotoxic agents (azathioprine, cyclophosphamide) are used for severe organ involvement. Methotrexate is used where there is evidence of erosive joint disease.
• Anticoagulation is used for the anti-phospholipid antibodies (see ➲ 'Anti-phospholipid syndrome', p. 319).
• Raynaud's phenomenon (see ➲ 'Raynaud's phenomenon', p. 322).
• Other organ-based symptoms are managed appropriately.

Testing
• See Table 12.7.

Table 12.7 Testing for MCTD

Tests for diagnosis	Tests for monitoring
FBC	FBC
Cr & E	Cr & E
LFTs CK	LFTs CK
TFTs	TFTs
Urine (RBCs, casts, protein, Cr. clearance)	Urine (RBCs, casts, protein, Cr. clearance)
ANA	Immunoglobulins, electrophoresis
dsDNA	C3, C4
ENA (U1-RNP)	Diffusing capacity and lung function
HEp-2 screen	Echocardiogram annually (for PA pressure and development of pulmonary hypertension)
RhF	
Anti-phospholipid antibodies	
Immunoglobulins, electrophoresis	
C3, C4	
Cryoglobulins	
ESR, CRP	
Diffusing capacity and lung function	
Echocardiogram (baseline PA pressure)	

Polymyositis (PM), inclusion body myositis (IBM), and dermatomyositis (DM)

Polymyositis and dermatomyositis may be idiopathic (no known accompanying disease) or they may be associated with malignancy. Juvenile forms also exist. Rare forms of myositis include inclusion-body myositis, eosinophilic myositis, granulomatous myositis, and orbital myositis (orbital pseudotumour).

Aetiology and immunopathology

- These diseases tend to be common in patients of African origin compared to Caucasians (4:1) and also in females (2:1).
- PM and IVBM are associated with HLA-DR3 (DRB1*0301 and DQB1*0201) and DRw52 (75% of cases).
- Juvenile DM associated with DQA1*0501.

- Older patients tend to be more affected, but the diseases can occur at any age.
- In adult patients there is a strong association with underlying malignancy.
  - Carcinoma.
  - More rarely, lymphoma.
  - Muscle disease often appears at a time when the tumour is still occult and it is debated how intensively one should investigate to identify the tumour.
  - Muscle disease will often remit when the tumour is treated.
- Seasonal variations have been noted in onset.
  - Anti-Jo-1 disease occurs mainly in the spring.
  - Anti-SRP myositis in the autumn.
  - Indicates possible association with separate infectious agents, as yet unidentified.
- Muscle infiltrate with both CD4⁺ and CD8⁺ T cells.
  - Restriction Vβ gene usage suggests that the recruitment is specific to muscle antigens.
  - Muscle fibres express MHC class II antigens and there is an increase in local expression of adhesion molecules (ICAM-1).
- B cells seem to play little role, and the pathogenicity of the autoantibodies known to occur is uncertain.
- Complement is involved in the muscle-fibre destruction.
  - Role of hdIVIg in PM/DM is to interfere with complement activation.
- A very wide range of autoantibodies have been identified, although many are not routinely available through diagnostic laboratories. The PM/DM-associated antibodies comprise one of the most complex sets of any autoimmune disease.
  - Most important subgroup of PM/DM is associated with transfer-RNA synthetases, which accounts for about 30% of cases.
- The most important antibody is anti-Jo-1. This antibody, together with the rarer antibodies (see Table 12.8), identifies the anti-synthetase syndrome, characterized by:

Table 12.8 PM/DM-associated anti-synthetase antibodies and corresponding target antigens

Anti-synthetase syndrome antibodies	Target antigen
Anti-Jo-1 (25%)	Histidyl-tRNA synthetase
Anti-PL-7 (rare)	Threonyl-tRNA synthetase
Anti-PL12 (rare)	Alanyl-tRNA synthetase
Anti-OJ (rare)	Isoleucyl-tRNA synthetase
Anti-EJ (rare)	Glycyl-tRNA synthetases
Anti-KS (rare)	Asparaginyl-tRNA synthetase
Anti-Zo (rare)	Phenylalanyl-tRNA synthetase

- Aggressive myositis, prone to relapse, accompanied by a high incidence of interstitial lung disease, mechanic's hands, Raynaud's syndrome, inflammatory polyarthritis, sclerodactyly, and sicca syndrome.
- Response of this subgroup to treatment is much poorer, but it is less likely to be associated with malignancy.
- Anti-Jo-1 antibodies frequently rise before the onset of overt muscle damage, indicating a possible pathogenic role, especially as it is now known that autoantibodies may enter selected viable cells.
- Other antibodies, recognizing other nuclear antigens, have been identified.
  - Anti-signal recognition particle (SRP) in adult PM (lung disease uncommon); disease is associated with severe and aggressive (necrotizing) myopathy.
  - Anti-Mi-2 in dermatomyositis (recognizes helicase). Responds well to therapy.
  - Anti-KS in PM with Raynaud's and lung disease.
  - Anti-Zo in PM and lung disease.
  - Anti-annexin XI in juvenile dermatomyositis (60%).
  - Anti-hPMS-1 (DNA mismatch repair enzyme) in 7.5% of cases of myositis.
  - Anti-MDA5 in amyopathic DM with rapidly progressive lung disease, cutaneous ulcers, and palmar papules.
  - Anti-TIF1-γ in juvenile DM and cancer-associated DM.
  - Anti-SAE with severe skin and oesophageal involvement.
  - Anti-NXP-2 associated with calcinosis and muscle contractures in children.
  - Anti-HMGCR in necrotizing myopathy and very high CK. May be triggered by prior statin use.
- Polymyositis may occur as part of overlap syndromes, such as:
  - MCTD/UCTD (anti-U1 RNP);
  - polymyositis–scleroderma overlap (anti-PM–Scl);
  - SLE–myositis overlap (anti-Ku).
- Amyopathic DM may be associated with antibodies to CDM-140.

Clinical features

- Major clinical feature is proximal muscle weakness with pain. Onset may be acute with fever. Distal muscle involvement is rare, and should raise other diagnostic possibilities (infection (viral, bacterial, parasitic), inclusion-body myositis, and metabolic problems).
- Gottren's papules are often seen on the knuckles, and the typical heliotrope rash around the eyes and a generalized erythematous rash (may be photosensitive) mark out DM.
- Signs of inflammatory arthritis and scleroderma; 'mechanic's hands' (thickened, cracked skin) identify the anti-synthetase syndrome.
- Dyspnoea from lung involvement (interstitial lung disease); with accompanying pain pulmonary embolus may be suspected.
- Although the heart is rarely involved, presentations with atypical chest pain used to be diagnostically difficult due to raised CK. This is now less of a problem since the introduction of cardiac-specific troponins as a diagnostic test for myocardial damage.

- Diaphragmatic involvement typically leads to dyspnoea when lying flat.
- Gastrointestinal disease may occur (slowed transit, reflux).
- Renal disease is rare, but high serum myoglobin levels may trigger renal impairment if there is very active myositis.

PM/DM: diagnosis and treatment

Diagnosis

- Muscle biopsy and electromyogram (EMG) should be considered. As the disease may be patchy within a muscle, a normal biopsy does not categorically exclude disease.
  - Biopsy will exclude IBM.
- MRI is excellent at identifying affected muscles non-invasively. Biopsy may not be necessary in a typical presentation associated with typical autoantibodies.
- Lung function tests, including gas transfer, mouth pressures, and CT of lungs, are essential.
- Anti-Jo-1 recognizes primarily a cytoplasmic antigen: this will not be recognized on rodent liver. If PM/DM are suspected, then screening on HEp-2 cells is most revealing as many of the cytoplasmic and nuclear antigens associated with myositis can be identified from the patterns of staining. Antibodies to Jo-1 should be specifically requested. Confirmatory line blots, EIA, or multiplex assays are required.
- Mi-2 antibodies are preferentially associated with DM rather than PM.
- Nucleolar ANA may also be seen, although these may also be found in patients with scleroderma.
- Antibodies to Ku, SRP, Mi-2, PM–Scl, TIF1γ, MDA5, and other synthetases may be available from certain specialist centres.

Treatment

- Management is with high-dose steroids.
- Failure to control disease with acceptable levels of steroids is an indication for second-line therapy:
  - weekly methotrexate (where there is no lung disease);
  - azathioprine;
  - mycophenolate mofetil;
  - cyclophosphamide;
  - possibly ciclosporin or tacrolimus; tacrolimus may work where ciclosporin has failed.
- Both steroids and cyclophosphamide can be given as intravenous pulse therapy, particularly if there is progressive lung disease.
- Intolerance of, contraindications to, or failure of first- and second-line agents should lead to consideration of the use of hdIVIg.
- Patients with malignancy-associated PM/DM respond poorly to immunosuppressive therapy, as do those with the anti-synthetase syndrome and IBM.
- Rituximab has been used in resistant disease.
- Hydroxychloroquine may help in resistant skin disease.
- Infliximab and etanercept have both been used in small series.

Testing
• See Table 12.9.

Table **12.9** Testing for PM/DM

Tests for diagnosis	Tests for monitoring
FBC	FBC
Cr & E	Cr & E
CK	CK
Serum myoglobin	CRP, ESR
Urinalysis (myoglobinuria)	Lung function, diffusing capacity
HEp-2 screen	MRI (muscle)
ENA (Jo-1, RNP, others)	
CRP, ESR	
Lung function, diffusing capacity	
CT scan (malignancy, interstitial lung disease)	
MRI (muscle)	
EMG	

Overlap syndromes

Patients often exhibit features of more than one connective tissue disease. Moreover, clinical features may change over a period of time, and this may be accompanied by changes in the serological profile. It is therefore wise not to be too dogmatic in pigeon-holing patients.

Recognized overlap syndromes include the following.
• Mixed connective tissue disease: see ➲ 'Mixed connective tissue disease (MCTD/UCTD)', p. 306.
  • Marker antibody profile is anti-U1 RNP in the absence of anti-dsDNA.
• 'Rhupus': a form of lupus with more aggressive destructive arthritis more typical of rheumatoid arthritis, but with other typical lupus features.
  • There are no specific serological markers, as many patients with SLE have rheumatoid factors anyway, without developing overt features of RhA.
  • Whether this is a true overlap syndrome is debatable.
• Polymyositis–scleroderma overlap: features of polymyositis and scleroderma, although the myositis may be mild.
  • Serologically defined by detection of anti-PM–Scl.
  • Calcinosis may be severe.
  • Treatment of calcinosis is difficult: calcium-channel blockers, low-dose warfarin, and anti-TNF agents may all be beneficial.
• SLE–myositis overlap: features of SLE with prominent myositis.
  • Serologically defined by detection of anti-Ku.

Systemic sclerosis (SSc): CREST and limited variants

There are many variants of scleroderma, including localized and systemic forms. There is also considerable overlap with other connective tissue diseases (SLE, MCTD, PM/DM). The pathological process is very similar to that of chronic graft-versus-host disease. The CREST syndrome (calcinosis, Raynaud's, oesophageal dysmotility, sclerodactyly, and telangiectasia) forms an entirely clinically and serologically distinct subgroup: this is now referred to as limited scleroderma, but the acronym reminds one of the expected features. See ➲ 'Scleroderma mimics', p. 317 for mimics of scleroderma. Localized scleroderma includes morphoea and linear scleroderma.

Aetiology and immunopathogenesis

- There is a female preponderance (M:F = 1:4).
- Childhood onset is rare.
- A wide range of MHC antigens have been associated with scleroderma variants, including DR1, DR3, DRw52, DR5, although there is significant racial variation.
- Chocktaw Indians in Oklahoma have a very high incidence of SSc, associated with abnormalities in the fibrillin-1 gene *FBN1*.
  - Autoantibodies have been detected against fibrillin 1.
  - A mouse model of SSc, *tight-skin*, is also associated with a duplication of the *FBN1* gene.
- Chromosomal abnormalities (ring chromosomes, chromatid breaks, etc.) are common in SSc—significance is uncertain.
- Parvovirus B19 has been associated with SSc development.
- Strong association of scleroderma-like conditions with environmental factors including:
  - dust exposures;
  - organic solvents such as vinyl chloride, resins, 'toxic oil' contaminated with aniline;
  - drugs such as cocaine, pentazocine, bleomycin, fenfluramine;
  - contribution of silicone breast implants to scleroderma is uncertain.
- Precise immunological involvement is unclear, but targets include endothelial cells and fibroblasts, with cytokine production leading to increased collagen synthesis.
- Obvious vascular changes, such as vasomotor instability (Raynaud's), but also direct damage to blood vessels, such as can be seen in nailfold capillaries.
- Unlike other connective tissue diseases, there is very little in the way of a systemic inflammatory response, and CRP/ESR may be low or normal.
- A variety of autoantibodies have been identified, although the significance of some of them has not been fully elucidated (see Part 2).
  - ANAs are common (see Table 12.10).
  - Anti-endothelial cell antibodies (AECA) have been reported and may lead to apoptosis of endothelial cells, triggering a cascade of tissue damage.

Table 12.10 Anti-nucleolar antibodies in SSc

Nuclear target antigen	Nucleolar target antigens
Centromere (CENP-A, CENP-B, CENP-C)—80% CREST patients	RNA polymerases I, II, III: 23% systemic disease (speckled nucleolar staining on HEp-2)
Scl-70 (topoisomerase I), 30% SSc, 10% limited scleroderma	Fibrillarin (clumpy nucleolar staining) PM-Scl (homogeneous nucleolar staining)—scleroderma–myositis overlap
	To/Th (homogeneous nucleolar staining)—rare, limited scleroderma, lung and kidney involvement

- Anti-centromere antibodies and anti-Scl-70 antibodies are mutually exclusive: only two cases of the presence of both antibodies together have ever been reported.
- Antibodies to RNA Pol III are found in patients with diffuse cutaneous scleroderma and are a marker for increased risk of renal crisis.
- Antibodies to U3-RNP (fibrillarin) are associated with an increased risk of pulmonary hypertension and skeletal muscle involvement.
- Antibodies to PM-Scl are associated with severe calcinosis.
- Antibodies to beta-2-glycoprotein I (seen in anti-phospholipid syndrome) are associated in addition with macrovascular disease and are a risk factor for digitial ischaemia and pulmonary hypertension.
- Antibodies to Th/To are markers for pulmonary hypertension and renal crisis, with a poor prognosis.
- Antibodies to NOR90 are associated with milder disease and a better prognosis.
- Increased TGFβ and platelet-derived growth factor (PDGF) may play a role in the fibrosis.
- Scleroderma-like disease is seen in chronic GvHD. In SSc, microchimerism due to persistence of fetal cells in the mother or maternal cells in the child is common, and may be the triggering event (i.e. SSc is a naturally occurring chronic GvHD).

Clinical features

- Localized forms include linear morphoea ('coup de sabre') and limited scleroderma where the changes are limited to the extremities, without systemic manifestations.
- Raynaud's phenomenon is severe.
- CREST syndrome has a more generalized involvement, and may give rise to late pulmonary hypertension, but less often to renal involvement.
- SSc, on the other hand, leads to major renal and lung involvement. Involvement of the kidney may lead to rapid onset of severe hypertension and renal failure, due to obliteration of the glomeruli (scleroderma kidney).
- Lung disease includes interstitial fibrosis, an increased risk of carcinoma, bronchiectasis, and pulmonary hypertension.

- Gastrointestinal involvement leads to severe oesophageal reflux, malabsorption due to poor small bowel motility, and bacterial overgrowth. Secondary problems may arise from a deficiency of key vitamins and minerals. Poor colonic motility may lead to pseudo-obstruction.
- There is an association with thyroid disease, PBC, and rare neurological involvement (neuropathy).
- The vascular disturbance may lead to ischaemia of the ends of digits that, if not treated rapidly, will lead to dry gangrene and progressive reabsorption of the terminal phalanges.
- Systemic forms are often accompanied by a prodrome of malaise and fatigue.
- Rarely, there may be renal and lung involvement without cutaneous involvement.

SSc: diagnosis and treatment

Diagnosis

- Screening for ANAs may reveal the presence of nucleolar staining patterns, or speckled patterns due to the presence of anti-centromere antibodies (specific for CREST). HEp-2 cells give the best differentiation of the staining patterns and these should be followed up by specific tests for Scl-70 (specific for SSc).
- Assays for individual nucleolar antigens are not routinely available, apart from RNA Pol III.
- In the CREST syndrome there may also be antibodies to the M2 antigen (25%). 30% will be positive for rheumatoid factor.
- ESR/CRP will be low.
- All patients should be screened for thyroid disease.
- All patients with Raynaud's should also be checked for cryoglobulins.
- Thermography is useful to confirm abnormal responses to cold challenge.
- Nailfold capillaroscopy is valuable for diagnosis and objective monitoring of progression.
- Baseline lung function, including gas transfer, chest radiograph ± CT scanning should be carried out for all systemic forms.
- Echocardiography should be carried out to monitor for the development of pulmonary hypertension.
- Renal function needs to be assessed at presentation and then monitored regularly.
- No immunological tests are valuable for monitoring.

Treatment

- Many drugs have been tried in scleroderma but few have stood the test of proper double-blind, placebo-controlled trials.
- NSAIDs and steroids should be avoided if possible as they may worsen or trigger the development of renal crises.

- Penicillamine and colchicine have been used, with some evidence that they slow progression.
- Steroids only help with active inflammatory problems such as myositis or arthritis (but watch for renal deterioration) and use for short periods only.
- Cytotoxics such as azathioprine and cyclophosphamide may have some benefit; low-dose methotrexate may be better.
- Anti-TNF agents may be helpful in selected patients.
- Ciclosporin may be of benefit (but watch renal function!).
- High-dose immunosuppression with autologous stem cell support has been tried; however, survival was poor!
- Anti-TNFs, rituximab, and anti-TGFs have been tried without much evidence of benefit.
- Tyrosine kinase inhibitors (imatinib and analogues) may show some promise.
- Raynaud's may be difficult to control. Avoidance of cold and wearing warm clothing and heated gloves may help. Low-dose aspirin may improve circulation. Other treatments to be tried include:
  - high-dose fish oil or evening primrose oil;
  - slow-release or long-acting calcium channel blockers (nicardipine, felodipine, amlodipine, nimodipine);
  - ACE inhibitors; angiotensin-II receptor blockers;
  - topical GTN (glyceryl trinitrate) ointment;
  - oxypentifylline;
  - 5-HT antagonist (ketanserin, not a licensed drug);
  - SSRIs such as fluoxetine;
  - phosphodiesterase inhibitors (sildenafil and analogues) are valuable for severe cases.
- Acute ischaemia should be treated with prostacyclins analogue infusions (epoprostenol, iloprost): although the half-life is only seconds, the clinical effect may last for months (reasons unknown). Bosentan may also be helpful.
- Infection in sclerodermatous skin needs aggressive treatment, often with intravenous antibiotics.
- Malabsorption should be sought and treated.
  - Continuous oxytetracycline may reduce bacterial overgrowth.
- Omeprazole, low-dose erythromycin, or octreotide may help with reflux and improve motility.
- Pulmonary artery hypertension can be treated with phosphodiesterase inhibitors (sildenafil and analogues) and endothelin-1 receptor antagonists (bosentan).
- Avoid calcium channel blockers if possible where there is oesophageal involvement as they make the reflux worse.

Testing
- See Table 12.11.

Table 12.11 Testing for SSc

Tests for diagnosis	Tests for monitoring
FBC	FBC
Cr & E	Cr & E
Creatinine clearance/isotopic clearance	Creatinine clearance/isotopic clearance
Tests for malabsorption	Tests for malabsorption
TFTs	TFTs
LFTs	LFTs
Lung function, diffusing capacity	Lung function, diffusing capacity
Echocardiogram	Echocardiogram
Pulmonary imaging (HR-CT)	Pulmonary imaging (HR-CT)
ANA (HEp-2 screen)	
Anti-Scl-70	
Anti-mitochondrial antibodies	
Cryoglobulins	
CRP, ESR	

Scleroderma mimics

A number of conditions mimic scleroderma.

Nephrogenic systemic fibrosis (nephrogenic fibrosing dermatopathy)
- Occurs in patients with renal failure.
- Similar to eosinophilic fasciitis.
- May be triggered by gadolinium or erythropoetin.

Scleromyxedema (papular mucinosis)
- Occurs is patients with malignancy, or alone.
- Waxy skin thickening.
- Paraprotein often present.

Scleredema
- Occurs in patients with diabetes.
- May be associated with presence of a paraproteins.

Eosinophilia-myalgia syndrome
- Pathology is similar to eosinophilic fasciitis (see ➲ 'Eosinophilic fasciitis', p. 318).
- Has been associated with consumption of L-tryptophan as a food supplement.

Toxic oil syndrome
- Caused by aniline-contaminated cooking oil.
- Prominent eosinophilia.
- Limb oedema with scleroderma-like changes.
- Arthritis with joint contractures.
- Myalgia with elevated CK.
- Pulmonary involvement with infiltrates.

Eosinophilic fasciitis (Shulman's syndrome)

Rare disease with limb and trunk erythema and oedema with induration due to increased collagen deposition and eosinophilic infiltration.

Aetiology and immunopathology
- Cause is uncertain.
- Infiltration of fascia with lymphocytes, plasma cells, and eosinophils.
- Increased IFN-γ, IL-5 and IL-10.
- Increased circulating histamine.
- Increased collagen gene expression.

Clinical features
- Non-pitting oedema, often with peau d'orange.
- Woody induration of deep tissues.
- Muscle pain and weakness—perimyositis may be present.
- No sclerodactyly.
- Arthritis in 40%.
- May be associated with thyroiditis.
- Association with myeloma, lymphoma, and leukaemia.
- Distinguish from Churg–Strauss syndrome and other hyper-eosinophilic syndromes.

Diagnosis
- Peripheral blood eosinophilia (60–90%).
- Raised ESR.
- Paraproteins and cryoglobulins may be present.
- MRI imaging of soft tissues will be abnormal.
- Biopsy essential for confirmation of diagnosis.

Management
- Corticosteroids are first-line treatment.
- Hydroxychloroquine may be an alternative.
- Methotrexate, PUVA, ciclosporin, and hdIVIg have been used in resistant cases.

Anti-phospholipid syndrome (APS)

This set of syndromes (now sometimes referred to as Hughes's syndrome) is associated with antibodies against a range of biologically relevant phospholipids.

Aetiology and immunopathology

- Both sexes may be affected, although it appears to be more common in females.
- One-third of patients with SLE may have APL antibodies.
- MHC association has been reported (DR4, DR7, among others). Why the antibodies arise is not known, although non-pathogenic antibodies may be induced by infection.
- Appearance of APL antibodies can be triggered by viral infection (EBV, HIV, hepatitis viruses), bacterial infections, malaria, leishmaniasis, syphilis, and *Pneumocystis*.
- APL antibodies may also be seen in association with malignancy (lymphoma, solid tumours), Klinefelter's syndrome, and other autoimmune diseases (pernicious anaemia, diabetes, inflammatory bowel disease, ITP).
- Antibodies appear to recognize a variety of different phospholipids, but pathogenic antibodies seem to require the presence of a cofactor, β_2-glycoprotein-I (apolipoprotein H). Antiphospholipid antibodies that arise secondary to infection (such as syphilis, EBV infection) do not require the presence of β_2-glycoprotein-I, and do not seem to cause a clotting disorder.
- Spectrum of antibodies includes both anti-cardiolipin antibodies and lupus anticoagulants. Either may be found in the absence of the other, but the clinical significance is identical.
- Activity of the antibodies *in vivo* is complex, but includes activation of platelets, interference with endothelial cell function (reduced prostacyclin production, reduced thrombomodulin function), complement activation, and reduced levels of proteins C and S, leading to a pro-coagulant effect.
- A 'second hit' may be required to trigger thrombosis (OCP, pregnancy, malignancy, etc.).
- Other APL antibodies which may be found include:
  - anti-prothrombin;
  - anti-annexin V;
  - antibodies to phosphatidylserine, phosphatidylinositol, phosphatidylethanolamine.

Clinical features

- Anti-phospholipid antibodies can occur either as an isolated finding or in association with other connective tissue disease, usually SLE.
- Major clinical features are arterial and venous thromboses, with pulmonary emboli, recurrent miscarriage, and thrombocytopenia. As the arterial system can be affected, strokes in young people should always be investigated.

- Recurrent minor cerebrovascular occlusions may lead to a multi-infarct dementia.
- Recurrent fetal loss is common.
- APS is associated with ITP and haemolytic anaemia.
- Other clinical syndromes associated include the Budd–Chiari syndrome, chorea, transverse myelitis, pulmonary hypertension (recurrent asymptomatic PEs), and cardiac valve lesions.
- Livedo reticularis is a useful cutaneous marker, and may be associated with Sneddon's syndrome (hypertension, cerebrovascular disease, and livedo).
- Catastrophic APS (CAPS): multi-organ failure due to DIC-like picture, associated with adult respiratory distress syndrome (ARDS).

Diagnosis

- Clinical suspicion should lead to testing for IgG and IgM anti-cardiolipin antibodies (ACAs) and clotting studies for lupus anticoagulants (LACs), which should include APTT (prolonged) and a dilute Russell's viper venom test (dRVVT; prolonged).
- 85% of patients will have both ACAs and LACs, but either can be present alone.
- FBC should be checked for thrombocytopenia.
- The significance of IgM anti-cardiolipin antibodies alone is uncertain, but, if associated with clinical features of recurrent thrombosis, this should be treated seriously.
- IgA ACAs have been described: they may be associated with thrombosis.
- IgG ACAs are most strongly associated with thrombosis.
- False-positive VDRL test may be noted, but this is not diagnostically helpful.
- Assays for β_2-glycoprotein-I are available and may help to distinguish between antibodies of no significance triggered by infection and those of pathogenic significance. At present it is not clear that they are necessary for routine management.
- There is no correlation between the numerical value of ACAs detected by ELISA and the severity of symptoms, although there has been a suggestion that levels may correlate with neurological disease in SLE.
- To determine whether there is a primary or secondary APS, a full search should be done for other markers of connective tissue diseases.
- Assays for antibodies to individual phospholipids are available in research centres for investigations of atypical cases.
- There is no indication that routine monitoring of levels of anti-phospholipid antibodies is helpful in determining treatment.

Management

- Asymptomatic patients require no treatment; there is no evidence of benefit from either low-dose aspirin or warfarin in preventing thrombosis.
- Once thrombosis has occurred there is no role for aspirin alone.

- Symptomatic patients should be warfarinized for life. The optimum INR is not known but should be at least 2.5. If thrombotic events continue then a higher INR can be used (> 3), or low-dose anti-platelet agent can be added (beware of haemorrhagic complications—aim for INR of 2–3).
- Direct acting oral anticoagulants have a predictable anticoagulant effect and require no monitoring. Rivaroxaban, dabigatran, and apixaban have all been used but not in direct head-to-head comparisons with vitamin K antagonists.
- Role of steroids ± cytotoxics is controversial, but may be tried where there are continuing catastrophic thrombotic events: do not expect there to be much change in antibody levels.
- Hydroxychloroquine may be helpful (prevents platelet activation and arachidonic acid release).
- Statins, which have anti-inflammatory and anti-thrombotic effects, can be usefully used as an adjunct but are not recommended as primary therapy.
- Sirolimus has been used in APS nephropathy.
- Plasmapheresis may be tried, but beware of rebound rises in antibody.
- Thrombocytopenia is rarely severe but, if it is, hdIVIg and steroids may help. Splenectomy may increase the thrombotic tendency if the platelet count rebound is very high, and so needs to be considered carefully. Danazol may also be of benefit.
- Catastrophic APS (50% mortality) is treated with pulse IV methylprednisolone 1 g/day × 3, with full heparinization. Plasmapheresis and hdIVIg have also been used. Rituximab 375 mg/m^2 can be used as an alternative. Eculizumab has also shown benefit. ITU support is required.

Management in pregnancy

- For management of pregnancy, no treatment or low-dose aspirin is recommended for those with either no history or a history only of first-trimester loss.
- Where there is a history of second/third-trimester loss the treatment is low-dose aspirin ± subcutaneous heparin.
- Low molecular weight heparins (LMWHs) are preferred due to lower risk of heparin-induced thrombocytopenia (HIT) and osteopenia, compared to unfractionated heparin.
- If there is a previous history of thrombosis, then low-dose aspirin and heparin/LMWH are suggested, even for first pregnancies.
- Consideration should be given to post-partum prophylaxis.
- Hydroxychloroquine may be beneficial and is associated with a higher rate of live births, and reduced placental insufficiency.
- IVIg may also be valuable.

Testing

- See Table 12.12.

Table 12.12 Testing for APS

Tests for diagnosis	Tests for monitoring
FBC	FBC
IgG and IgM anti-cardiolipin antibodies	INR (warfarin)
APTT	
dRVVT	
Anti-β_2-glycoprotein I	
ANA	
dsDNA	
ENA	
C3, C4	
Thrombophilia screen (exclude other thrombophilic disorders)	
Exclude homocystinuria	

Raynaud's phenomenon

Raynaud's phenomenon refers to an exaggerated vascular response to cold (and sometimes emotion). Common in women without evidence of underlying disease (primary) but may be associated with connective tissue diseases (SLE, RhA, dermatomyositis, scleroderma, limited scleroderma), arterial occlusive diseases (cervical ribs), pulmonary hypertension, neurological diseases, paraproteinaemias (including cryoglobulinaemia, HCV infection, Waldenström's macroglobulinaemia), trauma, electrical shocks, drugs (ergot derivatives, β-blockers, bleomycin, vinblastine, and cisplatin). Primary Raynaud's tends to be less severe.

Clinical features

- Cold-induced colour change (blue→white→red on rewarming).
- May affect ears and nose if severe.
- May be associated with migraine.
- Severe cases may lead to ischaemic ulceration and gangrene if left untreated.
- Cutaneous ulceration may occur.
- Distinguish from acrocyanosis and erythromelalgia.
  - Acrocyanosis affects predominantly young women and causes persistent cyanotic discoloration; it does not cause long-term damage and treatment is not required.
  - Erythromelalgia affects predominantly men and causes burning red discoloration of the feet and hands. It may be primary or associated with polycythaemia rubra vera, essential thrombocytosis, connective tissue diseases, and drug therapy (bromocriptine and analogues). It may respond to aspirin.

Diagnosis

- Exclude secondary causes, e.g. autoimmune disease and paraproteinaemia.
- Check for cryoglobulins and evidence of HCV infection.
- Thermography with cold challenge is useful.
- Capillaroscopy will identify early vascular features of scleroderma.
- Check for cervical ribs and consider MR angiography.

Testing

- See Table 12.13.

Treatment

- See also p. 313 under ➲ 'Systemic sclerosis'.
- Avoid cold exposure, particularly rapid temperature change.
- Thermal gloves and socks (battery operated gloves are useful but usually patients complain they are too bulky).
- No smoking!
- Low-dose aspirin and omega-3 fish oils may be helpful for mild cases.
- Topical glyceryl trinitrate ointment is very helpful pre-exposure.
- Calcium channel blockers (nifedipine, nicardipine, nimodipine, amlodipine, diltiazem) are the first line. Preferable to use slow-release formulations or long-acting drugs.
- ACE inhibitors and angiotensin-II inhibitors can be used.
  - ❶Most patients with Raynaud's have low BP and tolerate anti-hypertensives poorly.
  - High-dose vitamin E is a useful alternative.
- Hydroxychloroquine may be useful because of its anti-platelet effect.
- Alprostadil (PGE1) and epoprostenol (PGI2) infusions can give prolonged relief. Essential if there is critical digital ischaemia.
- Heparin (unfractionated or LMW) may also be helpful (probably due to its rheological and anti-inflammatory properties) in severe cases.

Table 12.13 Testing for Raynaud's phenomenon

Tests for diagnosis	Tests for monitoring
FBC & ESR	As for underlying disease
Immunoglobulins & serum electrophoresis	Serial capillaroscopy
Autoantibody screen	
ENA	
Cryoglobulins (cold agglutinins)	
Viscosity (if available!)	
HCV status	
Capillaroscopy	
Thermography	

- Sildenafil and analogues are effective.
- Bosentan may be helpful where the prostanoids are ineffective.
- Surgery may be required for compressive lesions or to perform sympathectomy. Amputation of ischaemic digits may be required.

Livedo reticularis

A mottled net-like discoloration of the skin, which is worse on cold exposure. The primary benign form is commoner in women. Secondary forms may be associated with connective tissue diseases and may be associated with ulceration. It is particularly seen with the APS and with SLE and with Sneddon's syndrome (see ➲ 'Anti-phospholipid syndrome (APS)', p. 319, ➲ 'Systemic lupus erythematosus (SLE) and variants', p. 293, and ➲ 'Vasculitis secondary to connective tissue and other autoimmune diseases', Chapter 13, p. 358). It may be seen in cryoglobulinaemia and hyperviscosity syndromes. Treatment is for underlying disease.

Rheumatic fever

After a period of decline, rheumatic fever is now on the increase again, paralleling the rise in infection with group A streptococci.

Aetiology and immunopathogenesis
- Disease is due to molecular mimicry between streptococcal M proteins and N-acetyl-β-D-glucosamine found in particular strains of group A streptococci (GAS) and myocardial proteins (cross-reactive autoimmune response).
- Pharyngitis is an essential precursor.
- Expression of CD44 in the pharynx may be important—binds GAS.
- There is weak association in some racial groups with MHC class II antigens.

Clinical features
- Major criteria: carditis, migratory polyarthritis, chorea, subcutaneous nodules, erythema marginatum.
- Minor criteria: pyrexia, arthralgia, elevated acute-phase proteins, prolonged PR interval.
- Plus evidence of recent group A streptococcal infection (increased ASOT, anti-DNAse B, positive culture, or antigen detection).

Diagnosis
- No specific immunological tests.
- Diagnosis is clinical, supported by serology/bacteriology.

Treatment

- Treat acutely with high-dose aspirin, together with anti-streptococcal antibiotics.
- Steroids may be used in carditis (prednisolone 2 mg/kg for 1–2 weeks, then tapering off).
- Long-term prophylactic phenoxymethylpenicillin 500 mg bd for at least 10 years.
- Streptococcal vaccines may be useful but difficult to develop because of the cross-reactivity.

Fibromyalgia

Condition characterized by widespread muscular and joint pain, with typical point tenderness. Strongly associated with chronic fatigue syndrome (see ➲ Chapter 14). May accompany other autoimmune connective tissue diseases (beware of over-treating these because of fibromyalgia symptoms). No specific diagnostic tests. Current research points to 'miswiring' of pain perception centrally. Defects associated with serotonin transport, metabolism, and receptors have been associated, as well as polymorphisms in β-adrenrenoreceptor and dopamine receptor have been implicated.

Websites

American College of Rheumatologists: ✍ www.rheumatology.org
Arthritis Research Council: ✍ www.arc.org.uk
Raynauds & Scleroderma Association: ✍ www.raynauds.org.uk
Lupus UK: ✍ www.lupusuk.com

Vasculitis

Causes of vasculitis

The term vasculitis implies inflammation affecting predominantly the blood vessels. The effects of the process depend on the location of the inflammatory change and the size and type of the vessel involved. It is unclear why there is selectivity for vessels of a certain type, size, or location. Although at present vasculitis is divided into primary and secondary, it is likely that, with the passage of time, we shall identify environmental triggers for most of the so-called primary vasculitides.

Primary

Many classifications have been proposed for primary vasculitis, but the most satisfactory is that based on the size of the vessel involved and on the presence or absence of granulomata (see Table 13.1). However, there is considerable overlap in the size of vessels involved.

Since the previous edition, Wegener's granulomatosis has been renamed as 'granulomatosis with polyangiitis' and Churg–Strauss syndrome as 'eosinophilic granulomatosis with polyangiitis'. Both names will be used for clarity.

Table 13.1 Classification of primary vasculitis

Small artery	Medium artery	Large artery	Veins
No granulomata			
Buerger's disease	Buerger's disease	Takayasu's disease	Buerger's disease
Henoch–Schönlein purpura	Kawasaki syndrome		Behçet's disease
Microscopic polyarteritis	Polyarteritis nodosa		
Primary angiitis of the CNS	Cogan's syndrome		
Behçet's disease			
Hypergammaglobulinaemic purpura of Waldenström			
With granulomata			
	Wegener's granulomatosis	Takayasu's disease	
	Churg–Strauss syndrome	Giant-cell arteritis	
	Lymphomatoid granulomatosis		

Secondary

There are many causes of secondary vasculitis and the following is not an exhaustive list.

- Infections: bacterial (streptococci; bacterial endocarditis), spirochetes (syphilis, *Borrelia*), fungal (histoplasma), mycobacterial, rickettsial, viral (EBV, HIV, VZV, CMV, hepatitis A, B, and C, influenza), with and without cryoglobulins.
- Malignancy: hairy-cell leukaemia, lymphoma, acute myeloid leukaemia, with and without cryofibrinogens.
- Drugs: biologicals (serum sickness), oral contraceptive, sulfonamides, penicillins, minocycline, propylthiouracil, hydralazine, thiazides, aspirin, illicit drugs (cocaine, amphetamines, LSD).
  - Cocaine vasculitis is thought to be due to adulteration of the street drug with levamisole.
- Secondary to other autoimmune diseases: primary biliary cirrhosis, Goodpasture's syndrome, SLE, RhA, systemic sclerosis, Sjögren's syndrome, polymyositis/dermatomyositis, hypocomplementaemic urticaria, relapsing polychondritis.
- Secondary to inflammatory bowel disease: ulcerative colitis, Crohn's disease; also intestinal bypass surgery.
- Complement component deficiency; α_1-antitrypsin deficiency.
- Silica exposure (e.g. after Kobe earthquake in 1995).
- Mimics of vasculitis: cholesterol embolus, myxoma embolus, ergotism.

The lines between primary and secondary are blurred, as a number of environmental factors have been potentially associated with the development of ANCA-associated vasculitis (AAV). These include smoking, infectious disease (staphylococcal infection), heavy metal exposure, and ultraviolet light.

Diagnostic tests

Biopsy

- The most important diagnostic test is often biopsy of the affected organ, which is particularly convenient if the skin is involved. Some vasculitides may mimic neoplasia, e.g. Wegener's and lymphomatoid granulomatosis, and may therefore be difficult to distinguish on imaging.
- Small biopsies are frequently non-diagnostic if vessels are not included.
- Temporal artery biopsy is essential in giant-cell arteritis.

Imaging

- Imaging is an essential source of diagnostic information in cranial vasculitis (MRI is better than CT), unless invasive biopsy is considered justified. PET-CT may be helpful.
- Angiography is particularly helpful in identifying large- and medium-vessel disease. MR angiography is less invasive than conventional angiography.
- Temporal artery ultrasound is valuable in the diagnosis of giant-cell arteritis, and can be used to target biopsies to affected areas.
- Where there is suspected involvement of the coronary arteries, ECG, echocardiography, and coronary angiography will be required.

Immunological tests

- Immunoglobulin measurements contribute very little to diagnosis, being on the whole non-specifically elevated.
- Electrophoresis is necessary to identify paraproteins.
- Consider the possibility of cryoglobulinaemia and cryofibrinogenaemia (samples taken at 37°C required).
- Complement measurements (including complement breakdown products or other tests of complement turnover) are essential, particularly in secondary vasculitis.
- Autoantibody testing should include ANA, ENA, dsDNA, and ANCA (including MPO and PR3). The routine role of other ANCA-specificities is unclear
- Role of anti-endothelial cell antibodies (AECA) is not determined as these antibodies do not seem to be disease-specific.

Acute-phase response

- Acute-phase response (CRP) is mostly high (except in the case of SLE (although the ESR is high) and scleroderma).
- In some vasculitides, the caeruloplasmin is significantly elevated: this accounts for the greenish colour of the serum from patients with active vasculitis.
- Ferritin is high (> 1000) in adult Still's disease.
- Complement levels will be elevated: both C3 and C4 are acute-phase proteins.
- Serum electrophoresis will show reduced albumin (negative acute-phase protein) and elevated α_2 band (α_2-macroglobulin).
- Fibrinogen levels will also be elevated.
- Regular monitoring of the acute-phase response provides useful information on the response of the disease to treatment.

Blood count

- Full blood count will often show the anaemia of chronic disease, together with a thrombocytosis.
- There is often a lymphopenia.

Henoch–Schönlein purpura (HSP)

Aetiology and immunopathogenesis

- HSP is a disease of the small blood vessels, characterized by palpable purpura, triggered by infections, drugs, foods, insect bites, and, occasionally, malignancy (see Table 13.2).
- IgA-containing immune complexes can be detected in affected tissues, including glomeruli. These involve both IgA_1 and IgA_2 but contain mostly polymeric IgA.
- IgA rheumatoid factors are also detectable and the levels are highest in the acute phase of the disease; IgA ANCA may occur in some patients (but not frequently enough to be diagnostically valuable).
- Polyclonal increase in IgA.

Table 13.2 Causes of HSP

Infections	Drugs
Streptococci	Cefuroxime
Hepatitis B	Vancomycin
Herpesviruses	Enalapril
Parviovirus B19	Captopril
Coxsackieviruses	Diclofenac
Adenoviruses	Ranitidine
Helicobacter pylori	
Measles	
Mumps	
Rubella	

- Complement C3 and C4 are normal but C3d is increased, indicating an increase in complement turnover. Properdin levels are decreased while C1q levels are normal, suggesting alternate pathway activation. Properdin and C3 deposits can be detected in affected kidneys. There is an increased incidence of HSP in patients with C2 and C4 deficiency.

Clinical presentation
- Mainly disease of small children, with a peak age of onset at around 3 years, although it can occur at any age and does occur in adults, in whom it is possibly more chronic.
- Male predominance.
- Often a history of a preceding upper respiratory tract infection.
- Typical clinical feature is palpable purpura especially at sites of pressure (socks). These occur in crops, often with an urticarial component, and may become confluent. There is GI involvement, often with GI haemorrhage and associated with colic, vomiting, and intussusception (3%).
- Renal disease with nephritis occurs in 50%, although in most cases this recovers spontaneously and does not lead to long-term renal damage. It may recur in transplanted kidneys in the small proportion who do have progressive renal damage (4–14%). Renal disease may be more common in adult forms.
- Testicular involvement, pulmonary haemorrhage, pancreatitis, and CNS involvement are all very rare complications.
- Myocardial involvement occurs in adults but rarely in children.
- Fever in 45–75% and often a migratory arthralgia.
- Attacks may recur every few weeks to months and are thought to be triggered by β-haemolytic streptococci.

Diagnosis
- Diagnosis is based on the signs and symptoms; if there is doubt biopsy will assist.
- In practice, only complement C3, C4, and total immunoglobulins will be measured.

- Raised IgA in only 50%.
- Assays for IgA immune complexes and IgA rheumatoid factors are not routinely available.
- Acutely, the CRP/ESR will be elevated.
- HSP nephritis is similar to that of IgA nephropathy but with additional fibrin deposition.

Treatment

- Treatment is most often not required as HSP is a self-limiting disease.
- Aspirin should be avoided as it will exacerbate the bowel bleeding.
- Steroids reduce symptoms but do not shorten the illness; they may reduce the risk of developing nephritis.
- Factor XIII, which is required for healing of the bowel wall, has been used experimentally by infusion to reduce GI haemorrhage.
- Steroids, mycophenolate, azathioprine, ciclosporin, cyclophosphamide, and rituximab have all been used for the treatment of progressive nephritis.

Testing

- See Table 13.3.

Table 13.3 Testing for HSP

Tests for diagnosis	Tests for monitoring
Urinalysis	Urinalysis
FBC	FBC
Cr & E	Cr & E
CRP, ESR	CRP, ESR
C3, C4	C3, C4
ASOT	
Biopsy (skin, kidney)	

IgA nephropathy (Berger's disease)

- IgA nephropathy (Berger's disease) is probably closely related to HSP, and may be HSP with renal disease but no rash, as the glomerular lesion is identical (IgA deposition, with C3).
- Male preponderance.
- Often a history of a preceding upper respiratory tract infection.
- Unlike HSP, it may be familial but no unique genes identified.
- GWAS has identified abnormalities in complement, MHC, regulation of IgA secretion, and innate immunity genes.
- It is commoner in Asia than Europe.
- Family members often have urinary abnormalities and higher levels of galactose-deficient IgA.

- Bowel involvement and arthralgia may occur.
- Associated with IgA immune complexes and IgA RhF.
- Galactose-deficient IgA_1 is present, which may generate an autoimmune response to glycan (N-acetylgalactosamine).
- *Haemophilus parainfluenzae* membrane antigens have been detected in the kidney and it is thought that this may be the candidate triggering antigen.
- Persistent polyclonal elevation of IgA present.
- Relapses and remissions are common, but long-term prognosis is good.
- Can recur in transplanted kidney.

Buerger's disease (thromboangiitis obliterans)

- Affects predominantly small- and medium-sized arteries and veins.
- Occurs mainly in male smokers above 30 years of age (less than 5% of patients are non-smokers).
- Presents as a migratory thrombophlebitis with claudication in the lower limbs, and less commonly in the upper limbs.
  - Raynaud's phenomenon is common.
  - Ischaemic features will arise with peripheral gangrene.
  - Systemic features are usually absent.
- No acute-phase response.
- Histology shows infiltration of blood vessels by neutrophils early; then mononuclear cells later. Eventually fibrosis of the vessel supervenes.
- Active inflammatory lesions improve when smoking ceases, suggesting a direct toxic effect, although fibrotic lesions will not improve.
- Diagnosis is on the history backed up by angiography.
- The most important therapeutic intervention is cessation of smoking.
- There is no role for corticosteroids or immunosuppressives.
- Iloprost, sildenafil and analogues, endothelin receptor blockers (bosentan), immunoadsorption, and IL-18 inhibitors have all been used with variable benefit (few good-quality trials).
- Stem cell infusions/injections (intramuscular and intra-arterial) in affected limbs have been reportedly of benefit.
- Amputations may be required.

Hypersensitivity ('allergic') vasculitis

- This is a generic term, which is less used now, for small-vessel cutaneous vasculitis (leukocytoclastic vasculitis).
- It is not a discrete disease and may be caused by:
  - drugs;
  - infections;
  - SLE/SS;
  - cryoglobulins;
  - inflammatory bowel disease;
  - HSP.

- Typical features include:
  - purpura;
  - urticaria;
  - ulceration;
  - bullae;
  - systemic features (fever, arthralgia, myalgia).
- Drugs causing small-vessel vasculitis include:
  - hydralazine, propylthiouracil, allopurinol, thiazides, sulfonamides, phenytoin, gold, penicillin;
  - some drugs also trigger the appearance of anti-MPO ANCA (hydralazine, propylthiouracil).

Microscopic polyarteritis (MPA)

Aetiology and immunopathogenesis

- MPA is an aggressive small-vessel vasculitis, which is distinct from polyarteritis nodosa. It is thought that ANCA play a pathogenic role in the development of the renal disease.
- May occur in families, suggesting either a transmissible agent or a genetic background.

Clinical features

- Illness is often of relatively sudden onset with a short prodrome of fever, malaise, and myalgia/arthralgia, followed by onset of glomerulonephritis with hypertension and renal insufficiency.
- There may be pulmonary haemorrhage mimicking Goodpasture's syndrome: this has a high (75%) mortality.
- Extra-renal complications include:
  - weight loss;
  - mononeuritis multiplex;
  - cutaneous vasculitis;
  - episcleritis;
  - rarely, coronary artery involvement;
  - lung and upper airway involvement does not occur.

Diagnosis

- Renal biopsies show a necrotizing glomerulonephritis without evidence of granulomata.
  - Renal lesions are similar to those found in Wegener's granulomatosis.
  - There is a paucity of immunoglobulin and complement in the biopsy (pauci-immune GN).
- Granulomata are not found in biopsies.
- Angiography of the mesenteric vessels does not show microaneurysms, thus distinguishing MPA from polyarteritis nodosa (PAN).
- P-ANCA, with anti-myeloperoxidase specificity on ELISA, can be detected in the serum of 75% of patients; a few patients have C-ANCA with proteinase 3 specificity; some patients may also have anti-GBM antibodies.

- C3, C4 will be normal or high.
- ESR/CRP will be elevated.
- Normochromic normocytic anaemia is to be expected.
- Creatinine will be elevated.
- Microscopic haematuria is constant and there will be proteinuria (> 3 g/24 hours).
- Other reported abnormalities include eosinophilia (14%).

Treatment

- Treatment is with high-dose (usually pulsed IV) steroids and cyclophosphamide (pulse IV or continuous oral).
- There may be an acute role for plasmapheresis in preserving renal function.
- Rituximab may be an effective alternative to cyclophosphamide.
- Azathioprine, mycophenolate, or methotrexate may be used as maintenance therapy once remission has been obtained.
- Pneumocystis prophylaxis is required.

Testing

- See Table 13.4.

Table 13.4 Testing for MPA

Tests for diagnosis	Tests for monitoring
Urinalysis (casts, protein)	Urinalysis (casts, protein)
FBC	FBC & differential WBC
Cr & E	Cr & E, LFTs (MTX, Azathioprine)
ANCA (MPO, PR3) and titre	ANCA titre
Anti-GBM	
ESR, CRP	ESR, CRP
Renal biopsy	

Primary angiitis of the CNS (PACNS)

Aetiology and clinical features

- Primary cerebral vasculitis is very difficult to diagnose ante-mortem without recourse to biopsy, which has significant hazards.
- It is a diagnosis of exclusion in patients with an acquired neurological deficit.
- Infections such as HIV and VZV must be excluded.
- Similar features have been found following the use of cocaine, amphetamines, and phenylpropanolamine; in ergotism; and with phaeochromocytomas, suggesting a vasospastic origin.

- An association with viral (herpesviruses) and mycoplasma infections has also been postulated: turkeys infected with *Mycoplasma gallisepticum* develop a very similar illness.
- Disease is a rare one, primarily of small arteries of the cortex and meninges.
- Presents in older patients with headache, disturbance of higher mental function, and strokes. Males are more commonly affected.
- A more benign variant has also been described (benign angiitis of the CNS, BACNS), found more commonly in females.
- Systemic symptoms are absent (if they are present then it is likely that there is a systemic vasculitis with cerebral involvement).

Diagnosis

- Histology shows that most cases have a granulomatous infiltrate around the blood vessels (granulomatous angiitis of the CNS, GACNS).
- CSF may be normal or show elevated protein and cell count.
- MRI scanning and angiography may be required to establish the extent of the disease.
- No specific immunological tests are helpful: test for systemic vasculitis (ANA, ANCA) as part of exclusion criteria.

Treatment

- Treatment is with steroids, rituximab, and cyclophosphamide, as for Wegener's granulomatosis. Azathioprine, methotrexate, and mycophenolate may be used to maintain remission.
- The use of cerebral vasodilators (nimodipine, nicardipine) has also been advocated to relieve vasospasm.

Testing

- See Table 13.5.

Table 13.5 Testing for PACNS

Tests for diagnosis	Tests for monitoring
Infection screen (HIV, syphilis, herpesviruses, mycobacteria, *Borrelia*, *Bartonella*)	FBC & differential WBC
FBC	Cr & E, LFTs
Cr & E	(MTX, Azathioprine)
ANCA (MPO, PR3) and titre	ESR, CRP
ANA, ENA, dsDNA	
Immunoglobulins & electrophoresis	
C3, C4	
ESR, CRP	
Brain biopsy	

Behçet's disease

This is a multisystem vasculitis that, unusually, also involves veins as well as arteries. Agreed international criteria for diagnosis are:
- recurrent oral ulceration with at least two of the following:
  - recurrent genital ulceration;
  - eye lesions;
  - skin lesions;
  - pathergy (sterile pustule formation at sites of skin trauma, e.g. needle puncture sites).

Aetiology and immunopathogenesis

- Histology shows transmural vascular inflammation with arterial and venous involvement.
- Disease is common in eastern Mediterranean countries where there is a strong association with HLA-B5 (B51) and also an increase in DR2, DR7, and DR52.
- Sporadic cases occur and these do not have the same MHC associations.
- Polymorphisms have been identified in IL-10, IL-23R, CCR1, STAT4, and KLCR4.
- GWAS screening has shown upregulation of multiple genes for pro-inflammatory molecules.
- Cause of the disease is unknown.
- An abnormal response to antigens from *Streptococcus mutans* and possibly *Helicobacter pylori* antigens has been postulated.
- Immunological features:
  - Excessive response of polymorphs to fMLP.
  - IgA antibodies to the 65 kDa heat-shock protein of bacteria.
  - Detectable anti-endothelial cell antibodies (these are non-specific).
  - Reduced mannose-binding lectin levels are associated with more severe disease.
  - There are alterations in both Th1 (increased) and Th2 subsets and cytokine production.
  - Raised TNFα, IL-8, IL-21, and IL-17; increased Th17.
  - Autoantibodies have been identified to a range of antigens, including anti-*Saccharomyces cerevisiae* (ASCA), as in inflammatory bowel disease, Retinal-S antigen, other retinal antigens, and anti-kinectin. None are specifically diagnostic.

Clinical features and presentation

- Disease is characterized by recurrent orogenital ulceration, similar to aphthous ulceration but deeper, which may heal with scarring.
- Erythema nodosum may occur.
- Eye disease is often present, including:
  - anterior and posterior uveitis;
  - hypopyon;
  - retinal vasculitis;
  - optic atrophy.

- Vascular features include:
  - thrombophlebitis;
  - deep vein thrombosis (DVT);
  - arteritis (large vessel).
- Arthralgia/arthritis which is often asymmetric and typically affects large joints, especially the knees.
- CNS disease is due to vasculitis and typically causes pontine lesions.
- Other CNS complications include:
  - pseudotumour cerebri;
  - myelitis;
  - meningitis;
  - dural sinus thrombosis;
  - organic brain syndromes.
- CNS disease is rare but a poor prognostic marker.
- Pulmonary haemorrhage (with diffuse infiltrates).
- Nephritis (rare).
- Gastrointestinal disease: inflammatory bowel disease clinically and histologically similar to Crohn's disease.
- Venous thrombosis may lead to a Budd–Chiari syndrome and vena caval obstruction.
- Epididymitis.
- Amyloidosis is a long-term complication (see ⊙ Chapter 14).

Diagnosis
- There are no routine diagnostic markers: diagnosis is clinical.
- There is a significant acute-phase response.
- Complement C9 is often increased.
- There are high circulating levels of von Willebrand factor (vWF).
- Anti-cardiolipin antibodies may be raised in some cases.
- 25% of patients may have cryoglobulins.
- Immunoglobulins are polyclonally increased.
- The MHC-associated cases, but less often sporadic cases, show the phenomenon of pathergy: deliberate testing for pathergy can be used as a diagnostic test.

Treatment
- Treatment is difficult and is mainly aimed at symptom control.
- In the UK, specialist Behçet's Treatment Centres have been established with funding for biological agents.
- Ulceration of the mouth may be treated with topical steroids (hydrocortisone pellets, triamcinolone paste, steroid sprays for asthma sprayed directly at ulcers).
- Genital ulceration can be treated with topical steroid creams.
- Arthritis is usually treated with NSAIDs.
- Ulceration may be helped with colchicine or thalidomide.
  - Colchicine causes diarrhoea in large doses.
  - Thalidomide should not be used in women of child-bearing age without discussion of the teratogenic risks.
    —It causes a neuropathy.
    —Detailed consent is required.

- —Supplier in the UK requires participation in a formal monitoring programme.
- —Baseline nerve conduction studies are mandatory.
- —Risks are significant and the benefits often slight.
- —May be used for gastrointestinal ulceration.
- —Oxypentifylline is an alternative (weak!) oral anti-TNF agent.
- Corticosteroids have a beneficial short-term effect, but there is little evidence for long-term benefit and chronic use should be avoided.
- Systemic vasculitis warrants the use of ciclosporin, tacrolimus, azathioprine, mycophenolate mofetil, or low-dose weekly oral methotrexate.
- Eye and CNS involvement carry a poor prognosis and azathioprine, mycophenolate, ciclosporin, or tacrolimus have been shown to be of significant benefit, although the disease usually relapses when the drugs are withdrawn.
- Anti-TNF drugs (etanercept, infliximab, adalimumab) are valuable in severe disease.
- Interferon alfa is beneficial for intractable ulceration and in ocular or neurological disease.
- Other drugs that have been used include dapsone and clofazimine.
- ❶Anticoagulants need to be used with care and are probably contraindicated if there is retinal disease—seek specialist ophthalmological advice.

Testing

- See Table 13.6.

Table 13.6 Testing for Behçet's disease

Tests for diagnosis	Tests for monitoring
FBC	FBC
Cr & E	Cr & E
ESR/CRP	ESR/CRP
Anti-cardiolipin antibodies	Drug monitoring (ciclosporin, tacrolimus levels, LFTs)
Lupus anticoagulant (dRVVT)	
Exclusion tests (ANCA, ANA, ENA, dsDNA)	

Polyarteritis nodosa (PAN)

Aetiology and immunopathogenesis

- Very strong association with hepatitis B infection.
- Very high incidence in areas where HBV is endemic.

- 10–30% of cases are associated with HBV, although this figure is higher in endemic areas.
- Incidence is declining with the increasing use of HBV vaccines.
- Immunofluorescence demonstrates HBV antigens, IgM, and complement in vessel walls.
- Also associated with tuberculosis and HIV infections.
- There is a very strong link with hairy-cell leukaemia, and a PAN-like vasculitis may be the first feature of the leukaemic process.
- It is not an uncommon disease, with a prevalence of 63 per million.
- Necrotizing inflammation of medium-sized arteries, causing aneurysmal dilatation.

Clinical features and presentation
- Main clinical features of PAN include:
  - fever;
  - weight loss;
  - painful nodular skin lesions (which need to be distinguished from those of erythema nodosum);
  - hypertension (often with a tachycardia);
  - abdominal pain (cholecystitis may be a feature);
  - myalgia;
  - arthralgia;
  - mononeuritis multiplex, peripheral neuropathy;
  - orchitis; epididymitis.

Diagnosis
- The major diagnostic features are the presence of micro-aneurysms on mesenteric and renal angiography and the absence of ANCA.
  - The latter is a relatively new definition as older studies claimed that ANCA was present in a proportion of cases of PAN.
- Biopsies show that inflammatory change is limited to small- to medium-sized arteries and there is no evidence of small-artery involvement, which if present would indicate a diagnosis of MPA.
- Testicular and/or muscle biopsy may be required.
- There is a profound acute-phase response and usually a leucocytosis.
- Poor prognosis is indicated by proteinuria, > 3 g/24 hours, renal insufficiency, pancreatitis, and cardiomyopathy.

Treatment
- Treatment is with corticosteroids and cyclophosphamide. Rituximab can be used. Azathioprine and mycophenolate can be used for maintenance once remission has been established (as for Wegener's granulomatosis).
- It has been suggested that vidarabine ± interferon alfa (antiviral agents) be used for HBV-associated disease in conjunction with plasmapheresis to reduce the antigenic load: this is still experimental.
- < 10% relapse after successful treatment.

Testing
- See Table 13.7.

Table 13.7 Testing for PAN

Tests for diagnosis	Tests for monitoring
FBC	FBC
Cr & E	Cr & E
LFTs	LFTs
Urinalysis	Urinalysis
Creatinine clearance (or isotopic equivalent)	Creatinine clearance (or isotopic equivalent)
ESR/CRP	ESR/CRP
Hepatitis serology	
ANCA (PR3/MPO)	
Exclusion antibodies (ANA, ENA, dsDNA)	
Biopsies (skin, muscle, nerve, testicle)	
Imaging (MRA, MRI)	

Churg–Strauss syndrome (CSS)/ eosinophilic granulomatosis with polyangiitis (EGPA)

Aetiology and immunopathogenesis
- CSS/EGPA is thought to be a subset of PAN in atopic individuals.
- Usually an allergic prodrome that lasts several years, typically causing asthma, before the onset of vasculitis.
- May occur in asthmatics treated with leukotriene-antagonists although this may be due to steroid withdrawal in undiagnosed CSS/EGPA patients.
- Coincidence of upper and lower airway disease suggests that an inhaled antigen is the trigger, although none has been identified so far.
- Histology shows necrotizing vasculitis of small–medium arteries and there is intimal inflammation with eosinophilic infiltrate. Eosinophilic granulomata will be seen.
- Levels of eosinophil cationic protein (ECP) are raised in active disease. This protein is known to be neurotoxic and therefore may account for some of the neurological sequelae.

Clinical features and presentation

- Onset of the vasculitis is heralded by fever, malaise, and weight loss.
- Mononeuritis multiplex is common (up to 80%).
- Other systemic features include:
  - GI involvement with bleeding, inflammatory bowel-like symptoms;
  - cholecystitis;
  - cardiac involvement with an eosinophilic myocardial fibrosis, endocarditis, or pericarditis;
  - cutaneous vasculitic lesions;
  - sinuses and upper airways are often involved.

Diagnosis

- Diagnosis is mainly one of clinical suspicion, backed up by biopsies.
- Chest radiograph may show infiltrates.
- Echocardiography may show pericardial effusions, altered left ventricular function, and endocarditis.
- Lung function testing is required.
- Imaging of sinuses is useful (CT).
- Normochronic, normocytic anaemia is present.
- Marked peripheral blood eosinophilia (> 1.5×10^9/l).
  - Measurement of ECP (if available) may be helpful in monitoring the disease, although it is not a specific marker for CSS.
- Total IgE is also often raised, although this is less helpful as a diagnostic or monitoring tool.
- ESR and CRP are markedly elevated.
- Autoantibodies to eosinophil peroxidase may be present, which may give an atypical fluorescent staining pattern on neutrophil cytospins. The diagnostic value of this remains uncertain.
- 60% have anti-myeloperoxidase antibodies (P-ANCA) and 10% anti-proteinase 3 antibodies (C-ANCA).

Treatment

- Treatment is with steroids and cytotoxics, usually cyclophosphamide or azathioprine, as for other types of vasculitis.
- Rituximab has been used for remission induction in refractory cases.
- Hydroxycarbamide may be considered, as this has potent anti-eosinophil activity.
- Mepolizumab (anti-IL-5) and more recently benralizumab (anti-IL-5Rα) have shown significant benefit.
- Therapy with steroids may need to be continued long term to control asthma. Relapses are common.

Testing

- See Table 13.8.

Table 13.8 Testing for CSS

Tests for diagnosis	Tests for monitoring
FBC including eosinophil count	FBC including eosinophil count
Cr & E	Cr & E
LFTs	LFTs
Urinalysis	Urinalysis
Echocardiography & ECG	Echocardiography & ECG
ESR/CRP	ESR/CRP
Lung function	Lung function
ANCA (PR3/MPO), titre	ANCA
Exclusion antibodies (ANA, ENA, dsDNA)	CXR
Biopsies (nerve)	
Imaging (CXR, CT sinuses, lungs)	

Cogan's syndrome

- This is a rare syndrome of deafness due to cochlear damage leading to audiovestibular dysfunction, keratitis, and vasculitis.
- Other ocular features include conjunctivitis, episcleritis, uveitis, and glaucoma.
- Systemic features include fever, headache, polyarthralgia, myalgia, anorexia, and gastrointestinal symptoms.
- 72% of cases have a systemic necrotizing vasculitis indistinguishable from PAN.
  - Affects particularly large blood vessels, especially the aorta and coronary vessels (similar to Takayasu's arteritis).
  - Vasculitis may be florid.
- Although the trigger is not known, the syndrome has been linked to infections, including *Chlamydia* and *Borrelia*.
- No specific diagnostic tests.
  - Antibodies may be detected to inner ear antigens including Hsp-70 and DEP-1/CD148 (density-enhanced protein tyrosine phosphatase 1, which has homology to laminin and connexin 26).
  - These antigens share homology with Ro antigen and also with Reovirus III major core protein λ1.
- Monitoring of hearing and vision is essential.
- Paraproteins may be detected in the serum.
- Treatment is high-dose steroids, with steroid-sparing agents (methotrexate, cyclophosphamide, azathioprine, and ciclosporin).
- Infliximab is being used as first-line therapy in some cases. Adalimumab appears ineffective. Tocilizumab has been used in resistant cases. Rituximab does not appear beneficial.
- Cochlear implants may be required to restore hearing.
- Mesenchymal stem cell transplants are being tested in experimental models.

Kawasaki syndrome (mucocutaneous lymph node syndrome)

Aetiology and immunopathogenesis
- Kawasaki syndrome was first described in Japan, although it is now known to occur throughout the world.
  - Endemic form is associated with HLA-B51.
- Sometimes also referred to as infantile PAN.
- Histological features of the vascular lesions are identical to those of PAN.
- Aetiology is obscure but the clustering of cases strongly suggests an infectious agent. Rates increased in siblings of cases. Commoner in winter and early spring.
- Reported possible association with parvovirus B19.
- Has also been suggested, on the basis of T-cell receptor gene usage, that the disease may be due to superantigenic stimulation, possibly due to staphylococcal or streptococcal superantigenic toxins.
- It may be associated with polymorphisms in the *ITPKC* gene, a negative regulator of T cell activations.
- GWAS has identified associations with *FCGR2A*, *CASP3*, MHC class II, *BLK*, and *CD40*.

Clinical features and presentation
- Characterized by a high spiking fever for more than 5 days, accompanied by:
  - bilateral conjunctivitis;
  - mucosal damage (lips, tongue);
  - rash on the hands and feet with desquamation;
  - diffuse macular exanthem;
  - cervical lymphadenopathy.
- Other infectious causes must have been excluded.
- Most feared complication is the development of coronary artery aneurysms, which have a mortality of 1–2% (higher if not recognized).
- Myocardial infarction may occur.
- Aneurysms may also occur elsewhere.

Diagnosis
- There is currently no specific diagnostic test.
- Both ANCA and AECA are detectable but these may also be found in other febrile childhood illnesses.
- High levels of circulating soluble TNF receptor have been noted, but this is not a routinely available test.
- There is often a thrombocytosis, but it may not be present until the second week of illness.
- ESR/CRP significantly elevated.
- Echocardiography and occasional angiography are required to evaluate the coronary arteries for evidence of aneurysms.

Treatment

- Treatment of choice is hdIVIg (1 g/kg/day for 2 days or 2 g/kg as a single dose) together with aspirin (80–100 mg/kg/day for 14 days with monitoring of blood levels), which should be begun immediately the diagnosis is suspected.
  - hdIVIg will elevate the ESR, so it cannot be used as a monitoring tool!
- This regimen prevents the development of coronary artery aneurysms if begun early, but has no effect once they are established.
- 10% of patients are resistant to IVIg.
- Corticosteroids are not usually used, but may be valuable in resistant cases.
- If aneurysms are documented, then low-dose aspirin ± anticoagulants should be continued.
- Infliximab, anakinra, ciclosporin, cyclophosphamide, and plasma exchange have been used for resistant cases.
- Coronary artery bypass grafting and cardiac transplantation have been required.
- Although, mostly, the disease does not recur, it has been suggested (although not proven) that treatment with IVIg increases the risk of recurrence (about 3% get recurrent disease).

Wegener's granulomatosis (granulomatosis with polyangiitis, GPA)

Wegener's granulomatosis is a multisystem granulomatous vasculitis.

Aetiology and immunopathogenesis

- Cause is unknown.
- Reports that co-trimoxazole may influence the course of the disease have raised the possibility that it is triggered by an infection.
- Associated with development of specific autoantibodies against proteinase-3 (Pr3, neutrophil granule enzyme).
- Autoantibodies are known to penetrate intact cells and to inhibit the function of the enzyme by binding near its catalytic site, as well as by interfering with its inactivation by α_1-antitrypsin.
- Autoantibody also potentiates neutrophil functions:
  - chemotaxis in response to fMLP;
  - adhesion to endothelium;
  - nitric oxide production.
- PR3 may also be expressed by endothelial cells.
- C-ANCA may increase adhesive and activation molecules (E-selectin, VCAM-1, ICAM-1) as well as IL-8 production.
- All of these effects will enhance the inflammatory interaction between neutrophils and endothelium.

Clinical features and presentation

- Wegener's granulomatosis occurs in two forms:
  - systemic disease, which always includes a necrotizing glomerulonephritis;
  - limited form in which the disease tends to be localized (upper and lower respiratory tract) without renal involvement.
- In both forms there is often a prolonged prodrome of malaise, arthralgia, and myalgia.
- The limited form presents typically with involvement of the upper and lower respiratory tracts.
  - Sinusitis and otitis are common.
  - Nasal crusting, ulceration, and bleeding occur.
  - Nasal cartilage is often eroded, leading to gradual collapse of the bridge of the nose.
  - Subglottic stenosis is very typical and leads to acute presentation with stridor.
  - There may be haemoptysis and the chest radiograph may show multiple 'cannon ball' lesions, often with cavitation.
  - Endobronchial disease may also occur, causing lower respiratory obstruction.
  - More central involvement of the head may lead to proptosis and obstruction to the draining veins.
  - Erosion into main head and neck arteries may also occur.
  - Skin involvement may include a leucocytoclastic vasculitis.
  - Other complications include parotid enlargement, endocarditis (similar to Libman–Sacks endocarditis), transverse myelitis, peripheral neuropathy, and granulomatous bowel disease. Episcleritis and uveitis may occur.
  - The limited form rarely develops into the systemic form.
  - The limited form may be locally invasive with considerable morbidity and mortality.
- The systemic form tends to present as fulminant renal failure, often with pulmonary involvement, high fever, arthralgia, and malaise.
  - Features seen in limited disease will also be found.
- Lung lesions may be mistaken for tumours.

Diagnosis

- Diagnostic test is presence of ANCA.
- Major target antigen is proteinase 3.
- 95% of patients with Wegener's granulomatosis will have detectable ANCA, of whom 85% will have C-ANCA (anti-proteinase 3) and 10% P-ANCA (anti-myeloperoxidase).
- Anti-neutrophil elastase antibodies have also been detected (P-ANCA pattern on immunofluorescence).
- Approximately 5% of cases are seronegative.
- Peristent ANCA positivity after induction therapy is a risk factor for relapse.
- Biopsy is also important and will show the granulomatous vasculitis, often with fibrinoid necrosis.

- Renal biopsy will usually show a necrotizing glomerulonephritis.
- Other features include:
  - normochromic, normocytic anaemia;
  - thrombocytosis;
  - leucocytosis (occasional leukaemoid reactions);
  - slight eosinophilia (distinguish from CSS).
- Acute-phase responses (ESR/CRP) are marked.
- Rheumatoid factors are detectable in about 50%.
- Immunoglobulins are usually normal.
- Monitor disease with acute-phase markers (CRP/ESR) and serial ANCA measurements.
  - Antibody titre does not correlate with the degree of disease activity.
  - Rising titre may herald relapse, but not always.
  - This is not affected by secondary infection, which will elevate the CRP.
  - ANCA remain positive for many years after clinical remission has been obtained and treatment withdrawn.
- Disease activity is also marked by an increase in soluble CD25 (IL-2 receptor), vWF, soluble ICAM-1, and thrombomodulin, but none of these additional markers have been critically evaluated.
- Renal function must be monitored regularly, and the urine sediment inspected for evidence of glomerular damage.
- Indium-labelled leucocyte or gallium-67 scanning may be useful for defining sites of disease activity.

Testing

- See Table 13.9.

Table 13.9 Testing for Wegener's granulomatosis

Tests for diagnosis	Tests for monitoring
FBC	FBC
Cr & E	Cr & E
LFTs	LFTs
Urinalysis (casts)	Urinalysis (casts)
Renal function (creatinine or isotope clearance)	Renal function (creatinine or isotope clearance)
ESR/CRP	ESR/CRP
Lung function (laryngeal/tracheal obstruction)	Lung function (laryngeal/tracheal obstruction)
ANCA (Pr3/MPO)	ANCA
Exclusion antibodies (ANA, ENA, dsDNA)	CXR
Biopsies (lung, sinuses, kidney)	Serial CT/MRI (monitor locally invasive disease)
Imaging (CXR, CT sinuses, lungs; MRI)	
Indium-labelled leucocyte/gallium-67 scanning	Indium-labelled leucocyte/gallium-67 scanning

Treatment

- The gold standard of treatment is steroids, given either orally or as intravenous pulses, with cyclophosphamide, which is given either as continuous oral therapy or as pulsed intravenous/oral therapy.
- Continuous oral cyclophosphamide therapy may be more effective but may increase risk of long-term side-effects (bladder neoplasia, myeloid leukaemia).
- IV cyclophosphamide must be accompanied by mesna to prevent haemorrhagic cystitis.
- Rituximab is an alternative induction agent and repeated courses may be used for maintenance (watch for hypogammaglobulinaemia).
- Azathioprine and mycophenolate mofetil are not used for induction of remission but may be used for maintenance therapy.
- Low-dose weekly methotrexate (20–30 mg/week) has also been effective as maintenance therapy (avoid where there is liver disease or renal impairment).
- Co-trimoxazole may have a disease-modifying effect, but should only be used as sole agent where there is upper airway disease only.
    - All patients should receive low-dose treatment with this agent as prophylaxis against *Pneumocystis jirovecii* pneumonia secondary to immunosuppression. Do not use with methotrexate. Azithromycin or atovaquone are alternatives.
    - Co-trimoxazole may have a negative impact on renal function.
- Ciclosporin (up to 5 mg/kg/day, with monitoring of blood levels) may be effective in combination with steroids.
- High-dose IVIg (0.4 g/kg/day for 5 days, repeated monthly) has been suggested as an alternative in small uncontrolled trials, and one small controlled trial.
- Belimumab (anti-BLyS), abatacept, and tocilizumab are being studied. Anti-TNF agents appear ineffective.
- Avacopan, an oral anti-C5a receptor antagonist, has shown benefit in trials, including induction trials where it enabled the dose of prednisolone to be reduced.
- Tracheostomy may be required for laryngeal disease.

Lymphomatoid granulomatosis

Aetiology and immunopathogenesis

- An unusual condition in which there is a lymphocytic proliferation and infiltration affecting mainly small arteries and veins.
- May mimic Wegener's granulomatosis, but it is not a true vasculitis.
- EBV+ B-cell lymphoproliferation, accompanied by T-cell reaction.
- Occurs in patients with autoimmune diseases and in association with HIV.
- May be difficult to distinguish from angiocentric lymphoma; may be an unusual lymphoma variant.

Clinical features

Key clinical features include the following:

- Lung involvement with breathlessness and cough.
- Radiographic evidence of multiple nodules.
- Upper airways involvement, including sinuses, is common and may mimic lethal midline granuloma.
- Skin lesions, including nodules and ulcers, are present in > 50% of patients.
- Renal involvement with proteinuria and haematuria.
- CNS involvement is either due to mass lesions or as a more diffuse process due to vascular infiltration.
- Lymph node and splenic enlargement are very rare and the lack of these helps distinguish the condition from true lymphoma.
- Myalgia and arthralgia occur.

Diagnosis

- No specific diagnostic test other than biopsy.

Treatment

- Treatment comprises steroids plus cyclophosphamide, although the difficulty in distinguishing the disease from lymphoma has meant that aggressive lymphoma protocols have also been used.
- Irradiation may be useful for localized disease.

Giant-cell arteritis (GCA) and polymyalgia rheumatica (PMR)

Aetiology and immunopathogenesis

- These two diseases are closely associated and predominantly affect the elderly, with a peak incidence in the over 70s.
- May occur in younger patients where the diagnosis may not be considered.
- Almost exclusively Caucasian diseases.
- Female predominance of 3:1.
- Rare in black people.
- Incidence is > 170 per million, making them common diseases.
- Known association with HLA-DR4.
- Cause is unknown, although they may occur in association with acute myeloid leukaemia and with HTLV-1 infection.
- Limited clonality of T cells suggests localized antigenic stimulus.
- Macrophages produce high levels of IL-1 and IL-6.

Clinical features and presentation

- Typical presentation of GCA is with headache, fever, and an anaemia of chronic disease.
- Temporal arteries are often swollen, red, and tender.

- Other features of GCA include:
  - jaw/tongue claudication;
  - sudden blindness (occurs in 10% through retinal artery occlusion or cortical blindness);
  - extraocular muscle palsies;
  - ischaemic symptoms in arms and legs;
  - stroke;
  - myocardial infarction;
  - inflammatory aneurysms of the aorta and large branches;
  - pyrexia of unknown origin (PUO) in the elderly.
- GCA is a systemic vasculitis, not just a localized (temporal artery) vasculitis.
- Features of PMR include:
  - limb girdle pain;
  - marked morning stiffness;
  - mild synovitis without erosive disease.

Diagnosis
- No specific immunological tests at present.
- Diagnosis is clinical backed up by temporal artery biopsy.
  - A reasonable length of artery should be removed as the disease process is often patchy.
  - Pan-arteritis is present.
  - There is an infiltrate of T cells, predominantly CD4+ T cells, and macrophages, with giant cells.
  - Infiltrating T cells are of limited clonality.
  - Pre-treatment for up to a week with steroids will not abolish the typical appearances.
- Scanning (MRI) and angiography (MRA) may be required to delineate the extent of disease in major vessels (aorta and branches). CT-PET scanning is also useful.
- Ultrasound of shoulder/hip joints may be valuable in PMR.
- Acute-phase response (CRP/ESR) is marked.
  - Occasional patients lack an acute-phase response, despite evidence of disease on biopsy.
- Normochromic, normocytic anaemia is usual.
- Immunoglobulins and complement are normal.

Treatment
- For GCA, use high-dose steroids (60–100 mg/day initially), which are reduced rapidly to maintenance levels (7.5–10 mg/day) and continued for 18–24 months.
- The minimum required to keep the disease suppressed is used, as determined by suppression of the acute-phase response and clinical symptoms.
- CRP is more useful for monitoring than the ESR.
- Failure to control the disease with high-dose steroids may require the use of cytotoxic agents such as methotrexate, azathioprine, or cyclophosphamide.
- Infliximab and adalimumab are ineffective.

- Tocilizumab is beneficial.
- Treatment of PMR in the absence of GCA requires lower-dose steroids, usually not more than 20 mg/day.
- Methotrexate (12.5–25 mg/weekly) may be used as a steroid-sparing agent.
- The diseases usually burn out over several years and treatment can be withdrawn, although some cases grumble on for even longer periods.

Takayasu's disease (aortic arch syndrome)

Aetiology and immunopathogenesis

- Predominantly a disease of Asian patients.
- Strong association with HLA-B52, also B39.
- 85% of cases are women.
- Age of onset is usually below 40 years, often in teenage girls and young women.
- Histology shows a granulomatous infiltrate of multinucleate giant cells with a patchy distribution.
- Disease begins in media and there is intimal proliferation.
- Circulating immune complexes have been demonstrated.
- In the late phase (pulseless), there is transmural sclerosis.

Clinical features and presentation

- There is a pre-pulseless phase with exertional dyspnoea, cough, and tachycardia.
- After a variable interval, there is a subacute presentation with fever, malaise, night sweats, nausea, and upper/lower limb claudication.
- Examination will reveal widespread arterial bruits.
- Erythema nodosum may occur.
- There is often an arthralgia with a synovitis.
- Disease may be associated with adult or juvenile rheumatoid arthritis or spondylitis.
- May involve the coronary arteries.
- Aorta and/or pulmonary arteries are involved in 50% of patients.
- Other complications include headache, stroke, visual loss, aneurysms, interstitial lung disease, pulmonary hypertension, renovascular hypertension, and glomerulonephritis.
- Takayasu's retinopathy is due to ischaemia.
- Five types are recognized, dependent on arterial involvement:
  - type IA: ascending aorta, aortic arch, and arch vessels without aneurysms;
  - type IB: as for IA but with aneurysms;
  - type II: thoraco-abdominal aorta;
  - type III: aortic arch and thoraco-abdominal aorta;
  - type IV: pulmonary arteries.
- In pregnancy, disease may be accelerated, with marked hypertension.
- Disease may burn out after 5 years, leaving vascular scarring with multiple bruits.

Diagnosis

- No diagnostic test, apart from angiography (MRA), CT-PET scanning, and biopsy.
- The acute-phase response, ESR/CRP, is high in the early acute inflammatory phase of the disease.
- Immunoglobulins are elevated in some cases.
- Anaemia and leucocytosis are present on full blood count.
- Anti-aorta antibodies and AECA have been demonstrated.
- Proteinuria (mild) and haematuria may occur.

Treatment

- In the inflammatory stage, the disease responds to high-dose steroids.
- Cytotoxic agents (cyclophosphamide, mycophenolate, methotrexate) may be used when there is a poor response to steroids.
- Anti-TNFs appear effective, but rituximab and tocilizumab have been disappointing.
- Surgery or percutaneous angioplasty with stenting may be required to bypass sclerotic narrowed arteries in the end-stage of the disease.

Urticarial vasculitis (hypocomplementaemic urticarial vasculitis, HUV)

Aetiology and immunopathogenesis

- Three types are recognized:
  - normocomplementaemic variant: idiopathic and benign;
  - hypocomplementaemic variant in association with other CTD;
  - hypocomplementaemic variant in association with autoantibody to C1q.
- Marked female predominance.
- An autoantibody to the collagenous region of C1q may be found and activates the classical pathway of complement. A similar syndrome may also occur with C3-nephritic factor (see Part 2).
- May occur with SLE.

Clinical features and presentation

- Recurrent bouts of prolonged atypical urticaria, persisting for > 24 hours (may be up to 72 hours) and fading to leave brown pigmentation due to extravasated red cells.
- Skin lesions tend to be painful and burn rather than itch.
- Often accompanied by arthritis (non-erosive); glomerulonephritis in 40%.
- Frequently occurs in association with other connective diseases, SLE, Sjögren's syndrome, and cryoglobulinaemia.
- Obstructive lung disease (worse in smokers) and cardiac valve disease may occur.
- Ocular inflammation.

Diagnosis

- Typical skin lesions—biopsy will confirm evidence of vasculitis (leukocytoclastic).
- Increased acute-phase response.
- Renal biopsies show granular IgG along the glomerular basement membrane.
- CH_{100} is low/absent, and C1q, C2, and C4 are reduced.
- Detection of antibody to C1q.

Treatment

- Steroids, antimalarials, colchicine, or dapsone (impairs chemotaxis and lysosomal activity of neutrophils and neutrophil adherence—check G6PD levels first!).
- Immunosuppressive therapy: corticosteroids, azathioprine, cyclophosphamide, methotrexate, and mycophenolate have all been used in severe cases.
- Plasmapheresis may be used (beware rebound if not combined with B-cell immunosuppression).
- Severe cases may respond well to rituximab.
- Omalizumab has been demonstrated to be effective.

Erythema elevatum diutinum

- An exceptionally rare disease, mainly in the elderly (although it may occur in girls in childhood).
- Characterized by:
  - cutaneous purpuric lesions accompanied by persistent red/orange plaques (like xanthomata);
  - violaceous nodules over extensor surfaces.
- Histology of fresh lesions shows a leucocytoclastic vasculitis.
- Older lesions show evidence of lipid deposition, with histiocytes.
- Immunoglobulins are increased.
- May occur in HIV infection (mimics Kaposi's sarcoma), and in association with myeloma (especially IgA), hairy-cell leukaemia, cryoglobulinaemia, and coeliac disease.
- Thought to be due to an aberrant immune response to a pathogen (undefined).
- First-line treatment is dapsone.
- Sulfapyridine and corticosteroids also used.
- Cyclophosphamide and chlorambucil used where IgA is elevated.

Degos's syndrome

- Rare syndrome of occlusive vasculitis with multiple cutaneous, mesenteric, and CNS infarcts.
- Skin lesions typically crops of painless papules evolving into 'porcelain drop' lesions.
- Mainly occurs in older Caucasians.

- Histology shows multiple infarcts with infiltrates of scant lymphocytes and monocytes.
- Cause is uncertain; activated T cells may play a role.
- A viral aetiology has been proposed.
- Treatment is unsatisfactory: steroids and cytotoxics are unhelpful; aspirin and anticoagulation may help.

Erythema nodosum

Aetiology and immunopathogenesis
- This is a form of small-vessel vasculitis particularly affecting the fat of the subcutaneous tissue.
- It is invariably secondary to an infective or toxic insult.
- The causes are multitudinous, but worldwide the commonest cause is mycobacterial infection (TB and leprosy).
- In the UK the most common causes are:
  - streptococcal infection;
  - sarcoidosis.
- It may also be caused by other infections:
  - viral (EBV);
  - fungal (histoplasma, blastomycosis);
  - bacterial (Yersinia, tularaemia, cat scratch disease, lymphogranuloma venereum).
- It is also associated with:
  - inflammatory bowel disease;
  - Behçet's disease;
  - leukaemia and lymphoma;
  - pregnancy;
  - oral contraceptive pill;
  - sulfonamides.

Clinical features and presentation
- Characteristic features are of red, hot, painful swellings on the shins, and less commonly on the arms.
- These resolve slowly, often with desquamation of the skin, leaving a brown pigmented area.
- May recur if the underlying disease is not identified.
- There is often fever, malaise, and arthralgia.

Diagnosis
- The most important investigation is the patient's history, including drugs and travel, followed by a chest radiograph.
- Other investigations will be determined by the type of precipitant suspected.
- Acute-phase response will be markedly elevated.

Treatment
- Treatment is primarily for the underlying disease.
- NSAIDs relieve the discomfort.
- Corticosteroids also relieve the pain but do not speed resolution.

Weber–Christian disease (relapsing febrile panniculitis)

Aetiology and immunpathogenesis
- Rare infiltrative inflammatory disease of fat.
- Typically occurs in young white females.

Clinical features
- Tender skin nodules.
- Fever.
- Arthralgia.
- Myalgia.

Diagnosis
- Skin biopsy.
- Small-vessel vasculitis may be present.

Treatment
- No gold standard treatment.
- NSAIDs, corticosteroids, tetracycline, antimalarials, thalidomide, and immunosuppressive drugs have been tried

Relapsing polychondritis

Aetiology and immunpathogenesis
- Rare autoimmune disease affecting cartilage.
- Disease of middle age and older, but has been described in children.
- Sex incidence is equal.
- 20% of patient have antibodies to type II, IX, and XI collagen, but these have little diagnostic or predictive value.
- Matrilin-1 may also be a target antigen.
- May be associated with other autoimmune diseases.
- HLA-DR4 is present in 56% of patients compared to 25% of controls, but there is no association with particular HLA-DRB1 alleles and no association with HLA-B27, despite the similarities to ankylosing spondylitis.
- There is a mononuclear cell infiltrate of cartilage.
- There is a necrotizing vasculitis of small-/medium-sized blood vessels, accompanied by a cutaneous vasculitis.
- Immunoglobulin and complement deposits are found at sites of inflammation.

Clinical features and presentation
- Typically affects the cartilage of the nose and the pinna of the ear, which become red and exceedingly painful.
- More rarely, it is associated with damage to the cartilage of the trachea (causing respiratory failure), larynx (causing hoarseness), cardiac valve rings (causing aortic incompetence), and costochondral junctions.

- There is often a non-deforming arthritis, hearing loss, fever, and malaise.
- It is a rare cause of PUO.
- Eye involvement includes episcleritis, iritis, and conjunctivitis.
- Course may be fluctuating.
- It is important to distinguish it from Wegener's granulomatosis, Cogan's syndrome, infectious causes, and chondrodermatitis nodularis chronica helicis, which is limited to ear.
- A focal chondritis may be seen in SLE.

Diagnosis
- The acute-phase response is marked (ESR and CRP and complement).
- Full blood count shows the anaemia of chronic disease and leucocytosis.
- Low-titre RhF, C-ANCA, P-ANCA, and ANA may be seen.
- Regular lung function with flow–volume loop is required to demonstrate tracheomalacia.
- MRI of the upper airways is valuable.
- CT-PET may identify active inflammation.

Treatment
- NSAIDs where the disease is mild.
- Steroids ± cyclophosphamide or ciclosporin where the disease is more widespread.
- Dapsone has also been used.
- Infliximab, abatacept, and tocilizumab all appear to be beneficial, but anakinra and rituximab were not.
- Aortic valve replacement and tracheal stents and laryngeal reconstruction may be required. Plastic surgery may be needed to restore external cosmetic appearance.

Cystic fibrosis
- Patients with CF may develop a vasculitis.
- This has been associated with the presence of atypical ANCA.
- Specificity of these ANCAs has been shown to be against the bactericidal/permeability increasing (BPI) protein of neutrophil granules.
- Disorder is likely to be triggered by the chronic infection present in CF patients, although the precise relationship remains to be determined.
- Vasculitis is a poor prognostic marker.

Infection as a trigger of vasculitis
- Many of the vasculitides discussed in this chapter are suspected, or known to be triggered by infection.
- Causes include the following.
    - Direct microbial invasion of the vascular tree: cryptococcal aortitis, *Aspergillus, Salmonella, Pseudomonas*.
    - Septic emboli.

- Replication of the pathogen in the endothelial cells: rickettsial vasculitis (rickettsia are found in endothelial cells of gangrenous limbs).
- VZV in immunosuppressed patients with lymphoma (cutaneous vasculitis with VZV in endothelial cells).
- HIV is recognized to cause a wide range of vasculitis responses, including PAN and HSP-like small-vessel vasculitis (leucocytoclastic and neutrophilic), and may include cerebral vasculitis.
- Tuberculosis may cause a PAN-like disease.
- CMV vasculitis accounts for gastrointestinal ulceration, pneumonitis, and skin lesions (ulcers).
- Syphilis (now rare in the UK) causes an endarteritis.
- *Borrelia* is associated with a vasculitis, particularly accounting for the CNS features (Lyme disease).
- *Bartonella* is also associated with a vasculitis.
- Mechanisms may include:
  - immune complex deposition and complement activation, with secondary recruitment of inflammatory cells;
  - type IV hypersensitivity with granuloma formation and activation of T cells, with either direct tissue damage or cytokine release;
  - cross-reactive antibodies against pathogens may directly damage host components: this may involve the generation of cryoglobulins (e.g. in HBV).

Malignancy-associated vasculitis

- Vasculitis may occur as a paraneoplastic phenomenon.
- Examples include:
  - association of PAN with hairy-cell leukaemia (strong association; vasculitis resolves with HCL treatment, which includes α-IFN);
  - leucocytoclastic vasculitis has been associated with myelomonocytic leukaemia, T-cell lymphoma, Wilm's tumour, and renal cell carcinoma;
  - vasculitis is strongly associated with chronic NK-cell lymphocytosis (urticarial vasculitis, PAN, and acute glomerulonephritis).
- Neoplasms may also present as 'vasculitis':
  - myxoma (diagnose by demonstration of myxomatous material on biopsy);
  - angiocentric T-cell lymphoma (cutaneous lesions, mainly in the elderly) mimics PAN, Wegener's granulomatosis, and LG.
- Vasculitis may present as a neoplasm:
  - Wegener's and lymphomatoid granulomatosis.
  - PAN: a testicular presentation of PAN is often confused with testicular tumours. Biopsy will distinguish between the two and prevent unnecessary orchidectomy.

Drug-related vasculitis

- Drug-related vasculitis accounts for 10–20% of all dermatological vasculitis.
- Presentation may be at any time after the drug has been started, including after many years of therapy.
- Often accompanied by fever, arthralgia, hepatitis, and lymphadenopathy.
- Systemic vascular involvement is variable and may include lung, heart, CNS, and kidney.
- There may be typical features of serum sickness.
- Any drug is potentially capable of triggering a vasculitic reaction.
- More common causes include:
  - aspirin;
  - penicillin;
  - thiazides;
  - sulfonamides;
  - AZT;
  - cytokines: interferon alfa (which may actually be used to treat vasculitis associated with HBV and HCV); colony-stimulating factors such as G-CSF (the vasculitis is related to the increasing neutrophil count).
- Rare cases have been reported with illicit drugs (amphetamines, cocaine (contaminated with levamisole), heroin, LSD) but in many of the reports the role of hepatitis viruses has not been excluded.

Vasculitis secondary to connective tissue and other autoimmune diseases

- Vasculitis is a well-recognized feature of all of the connective tissue diseases.
- Rheumatoid vasculitis is a small-vessel vasculitis and characterized by:
  - very high levels of rheumatoid factor;
  - atypical ANCA against elastase and lactoferrin (P-ANCA): not specific for rheumatoid vasculitis.
- Sjögren's syndrome is associated with vasculitis in 5–10% of cases. This is characterized by:
  - purpura;
  - recurrent urticaria;
  - skin ulceration;
  - mononeuritis multiplex;
  - Raynaud's is common;
  - bowel infarction from systemic vasculitis (rare);
  - glomerulonephritis (rare);
  - hypergammaglobulinaemia;
  - high-titre RhF;
  - anti-Ro antibodies (especially with purpuric lesions);
  - cryoglobulins are usual (mixed, type II with IgMκ paraprotein);
  - treatment is with steroids ± cyclophosphamide.

- SLE, systemic sclerosis, dermatomyositis/polymyositis, inflammatory bowel disease, PBC, and Goodpasture's syndrome are all associated with a medium- to small-vessel vasculitis.
- Sneddon's syndrome is a complex of livedo reticularis and endarteritis obliterans, especially of medium-sized cerebral arteries, leading to strokes. It is often associated with anti-phospholipid antibodies (LAC or ACA).

Cryoglobulinaemia and cryofibrinogenaemia

Cryoglobulinaemia

- Mixed essential mixed cryoglobulinaemia (type II, see Part 2) is associated with:
  - purpura (leucocytoclastic vasculitis);
  - Raynaud's phenomenon;
  - arthralgia;
  - severe peripheral neuropathy;
  - Sjögren's syndrome;
  - glomerulonephritis;
  - liver disease.
- There is usually an IgMκ paraprotein with RhF activity and evidence for a low-grade lymphoproliferative disease.
- Disease is very common in northern Italy, where there is a major association with chronic HCV infection.
- Less commonly found in HBV and EBV infections.
- Other chronic bacteraemic infections, such as shunt nephritis and low-grade endocarditis, may also lead to cryoglobulin formation.
- Complement studies show low C1, C2, and C4.
- Plasma viscosity is increased.
- Some patients with glomerulonephritis have an antibody to a 50 kDa renal antigen, although the nature of the antigen is unknown.
- Plasmapheresis may be required and peginterferon alfa, with ribavirin, sofosbuvir, or daclatasvir, may be tried in order to eliminate HCV.
- Low-dose rituximab has been used for relapses.

Cryofibrinogenaemia

- This behaves in a very similar manner to cryoglobulinaemia, with cold-related purpura, haemorrhagic ulcers, and thrombosis of superficial blood vessels in exposed extremities.
- It may be idiopathic or associated with malignancy (see Part 2).

Hypergammaglobulinaemic purpura of Waldenström and cholesterol emboli

Hypergammaglobulinaemic purpura of Waldenström

- Benign disease characterized by purpuric lesions and a polyclonal increase in immunoglobulins, high-titre rheumatoid factor, and anti-Ro antibodies.
- Recurrent bouts of purpura, often triggered by prolonged standing/ walking. Associated fever, arthralgia, malaise, weight loss, and rarely renal involvement.
- Mainly seen in females.
- High levels of immune complexes can be detected.
- There is neutrophilic infiltration around small blood vessels with C3 and IgG deposition.
- Cause is unknown, but other conditions (hypersensitivity vasculitis, HSP, cryoglobulinaemia, HUVS, and secondary vasculitis) need to be excluded.
- May be seen in cystic fibrosis.
- Optimum treatment is unclear: hydroxychloroquine, indometacin, and colchicine have been used. Short courses of prednisolone may be required.

Cholesterol emboli

- These may mimic vasculitis, with a PAN-like pattern of skin lesions.
- Fever, myalgia, high ESR, hypertension, and eosinophilia also occur.
- Skin biopsy demonstrates the presence of cholesterol clefts.
- May arise following invasive vascular investigations as well as spontaneously.
- Symptoms may be chronic.
- Statins and aspirin may be tried. Severe cases may respond to iloprost infusions.

Atrial myxoma and serum sickness

Atrial myxoma

- Atrial myxomas mimic vasculitis when emboli are shed.
- Emboli appear in distal small blood vessels and give the typical appearances of small cutaneous vasculitic lesions, with multiple splinter haemorrhages.
- More major embolic lesions are the major complication (strokes).
- Appearances are very similar to those of SBE.
- Tumour 'plop' associated with prolapse of the tumour through the mitral valve may be identified on cardiac auscultation.
- Tumours may secrete high levels of IL-6 and are therefore accompanied by malaise, fever, an elevated CRP/ESR, and a polyclonal increase in immunoglobulins.
- The diagnostic test is echocardiography.
- Treatment is surgical removal.
- As the tumours are benign, removal is curative and recurrence unlikely.

Serum sickness
- Characterized by fever, polyarthritis, lymphadenopathy, and urticaria 7–14 days after primary exposure and 1–3 days after secondary exposure to foreign proteins, or drug-modified self-proteins (e.g. with penicillin).
- Acute venulitis and occasionally systemic vasculitis may occur.
- CRP will be high and ESR will rise during the illness.
- Complement levels may fall acutely and there will be an increase in C3 breakdown products.
- Renal function may deteriorate temporarily.
- Treatment is symptomatic; corticosteroids may help.
- The illness is usually self-limiting as the immune complexes are cleared.

Websites

American College of Rheumatology: ℘ www.rheumatology.org
Arthritis Research Campaign: ℘ www.arc.org.uk
Behçet's Society: ℘ www.behcets.org.uk
Wegener's Association: ℘ www.wgassociation.org

Miscellaneous conditions, including autoinflammatory syndromes

Sarcoidosis

Sarcoidosis is a multisystem disease characterized by non-caseating granulomata.

Presentation

- Common presentations include:
  - asymptomatic bihilar lymphadenopathy;
  - erythema nodosum, arthritis, uveitis, and bihilar lymphadenopathy (Löfgren's syndrome);
  - uveo-parotid fever (von Heerfordt's syndrome);
  - primary cerebral involvement;
  - multisystem presentation, which can affect all organs in the body.
- Other clinical features include erythema nodosum, arthralgias, skin involvement (lupus pernio), and symptoms and signs of hypercalcaemia.

Cause and immunopathogenesis

- Formation of non-caseating granulomata is typical, but not by itself diagnostic.
- Differential diagnosis of non-caseating granulomata is extensive and includes:
  - infections (*Toxoplasma, Bartonella*);
  - lymphoma;
  - carcinoma;
  - berylliosis, due to beryllium exposure;
  - vasculitis and connective tissue diseases;
  - Crohn's disease;
  - chronic granulomatous disease.
- Granuloma comprises a central area of macrophages, epithelioid cells, and Langerhans giant cells surrounded by lymphocytes (mainly CD4$^+$ cells and plasma cells), monocytes, and fibroblasts.
- Macrophages are activated and release enzymes and 1,25-dihydroxycholecalciferol—hence the tendency to hypercalcaemia.
- IL-12 is released; IL-18 associated with granuloma formation.
- Peripheral blood lymphopenia (T and B cells), cutaneous anergy, and poor *in vitro* tests of lymphocyte proliferation.
- T cells have an 'activated' phenotype and T-cell receptor studies show skewing of the V_β chain usage, and this might be compatible with a response to a single, as yet unidentified, pathogen.
- Disease manifestations are of a Th1 phenotype.
- Serum immunoglobulins are elevated and, as a result, low-level autoantibodies may be present. IgM anti-T-cell antibodies may be detected.
- Tregs reduced; increased Th17 activity.
- Bronchoalveolar lavage specimens show a lymphocytosis (predominantly CD4$^+$ T cells with high levels of activation and adhesion markers) and monocytes/macrophages (also activated with elevated MHC class II).
- Soluble activation markers, such as sIL-2R, are raised.

- Multiple susceptibility and protective MHC genes depending on racial background.
- Disease associated:
  - DR3, DRB1*11:01 (African Americans, Caucasians), DRB1*15:01 (Caucasians).
  - DR14, DR15 associated with severe disease.
- Protective:
  - DR1, DR4.
  - DRb1*03:01 and DQB1*02:01 associated with favourable outcomes.
- Other genes also identified that contribute to disease: *TNF* gene polymorphisms, chemokine receptors, *RAGE*, *NOD2* (early-onset sarcoid in children only), butyrophilin-like 2 (*BTNL2*).

Investigations

- No specific diagnostic tests are available for sarcoidosis.
- Raised ACE levels in about 40–90% of patients (released by epithelioid cells in the granulomata).
- Hypercalcaemia (and hypercalciuria).
- Serum immunoglobulins show a polyclonal elevation of all classes, but predominantly IgG.
- Low-titre rheumatoid factors and ANAs may be present.
- Peripheral blood lymphocyte analysis will show a generalized lymphopenia, with a proportional reduction in all cell types.
- DTH testing will show anergy. There is no clinical need to assess lymphocyte proliferation *in vitro*, although it will be reduced.
- Biopsy with appropriate immunohistochemical staining is helpful.
- Kveim test, in which an extract of sarcoid spleen is injected under the skin and biopsied 4–6 weeks later, has been used in the past: a granuloma forms at the site of injection. This test, which uses human material, is no longer considered appropriate.
- BAL studies are helpful where there is interstitial lung disease, although the changes are not specific.
- Gallium-67 scanning or FDG-PET are helpful in identifying granulomata. Contrast MRI is helpful for neurological disease.
- CSF oligoclonal bands may be present (again not specific) in cerebral sarcoidosis.
- Lung function testing and appropriate radiological studies are essential.

Treatment

- Asymptomatic disease picked up by chance on chest radiography requires no specific treatment.
- Treat erythema nodosum with NSAIDs initially.
- Symptomatic disease requires low- to moderate-dose steroids.
- Neurosarcoid requires high-dose steroids.
- Occasionally patients require other immunosuppressive drugs as steroid-sparing agents (cyclophosphamide, methotrexate, and azathioprine).
- Hydroxychloroquine may be helpful through its effects on T-lymphocyte activation and may reduce hypercalcaemia.

- Infliximab has a small effect on lung function, and was more effective for extra-pulmonary disease. Adalimumab may be more effective in some patients. Etanercept, golimumab, and ustekinumab were not effective in pulmonary disease.
- Patients with uveitis may require aggressive treatment to preserve vision.
- Progressive lung disease may be an indication for lung transplantation, but disease recurs in 30–80% of cases.

Prognosis
- Asymptomatic disease usually resolves spontaneously over several years.
- Symptomatic disease is frequently chronic.

Treatment
- See Table 14.1.

Table **14.1** Testing for sarcoidosis

Tests for diagnosis	Tests for monitoring
Serum ACE	Serum ACE
Vitamin D levels	CRP/ESR
CRP/ESR	Calcium
Serum immunoglobulins	FBC
Calcium and urinary calcium excretion	Cr & E
FBC	Imaging (CXR, CT, gallium-67, PET, MRI)
Cr & E	
Imaging (CXR, CT, gallium-67; PET, MRI)	
Biopsy	
BAL	

Amyloidosis

This group of conditions that cause multisystem disease is often overlooked clinically. The diseases are characterized by the deposition of polymerized proteins in an insoluble β-pleated sheet form, either generally or in a single organ, depending on the type of polymerizing protein. Once established, it is virtually impossible to eliminate the deposits. Multiple proteins have been associated with amyloid formation (see Table 14.2). Hereditary forms occur.

Table 14.2 Types of amyloid*

Amyloid protein	Protein precursor	Clinical syndrome
AL, AH	Light or heavy chain of immunoglobulin	Idiopathic, multiple myeloma, gamma-heavy chain disease
AA	Serum amyloid A	Secondary, reactive: inflammatory arthritis, familial Mediterranean fever, hyper-IgD syndrome, TRAPS (periodic fever), Behçet's, Crohn's disease
Aβ2M	β_2-microglobulin	Dialysis amyloid (cuprophane membranes)
Acys	Cystatin C	Hereditary cerebral angiopathy with bleeding (Iceland)
Alys, AFibA	Lysozyme, fibrinogen Aα	Non-neuropathic hereditary amyloid with renal disease
AIAPP	Islet amyloid polypeptide	Diabetes mellitus type II; insulinoma
AANF	Atrial natriuretic peptide	Senile cardiac amyloid
Acal	Procalcitonin	Medullary carcinoma of the thyroid
Ains	Porcine insulin	Iatrogenic
ATTR	Transthyretin	Familial amyloid polyneuropathy, senile cardiac amyloid
Aβ	Aβ-protein precursor	Alzheimer's disease
AprP	Prion protein	Spongiform encephalopathies

* Abbreviated list—27 amyloidogenic protein fibrils identified in humans so far.

AL amyloid

Presentation
- Typical clinical features include:
  - hepatosplenomegaly;
  - cardiac failure due to infiltration;
  - malabsorption;
  - nephrotic syndrome;
  - peripheral neuropathy (especially carpal tunnel syndrome); mixed motor/sensory neuropathy; autonomic neuropathy;
  - macroglossia may be present;
  - deposits may occur in the skin;
  - bleeding tendency due to selective absorption of clotting factors;
  - periorbital purpura triggered by Valsalva manoeuvre.
- It is a disease predominantly of older people.

Cause and immunopathogenesis

- In this type of amyloid the deposited protein is derived from immunoglobulin light chains (λ:κ = 2:1—the opposite of that found in myeloma).
- Often associated with evidence of lymphoproliferative disease.
- 20% of AL amyloid patients only have myeloma; the rest have other paraproteinaemias.
- Rarely, AL amyloid has been associated with heavy chain deposition.

Investigations

- Serum and urine should be checked for the presence of monoclonal immunoglobulins and free light chains: sensitive techniques may be required to demonstrate the paraproteins, which are present in up to 80% of cases.
- Paraprotein levels are often low.
- Serum free light chain analysis is very valuable.
- Some paraproteins may not be detected as the light chain is highly abnormal or polymerized in circulation, such that it does not react with the usual antisera, or the band overlaps on electrophoresis with other protein bands.
- Biopsy of an affected organ and Congo red staining, which gives apple-green birefringence, is helpful. More specific immunostaining with anti-light chain antisera may give reactions, although the distorted protein structure may prevent reactivity.
- Bone marrow examination is essential.

Testing

- See Table 14.3.

Treatment

- No curative treatment, but steroids, melphalan, and colchicine may slow down the rate of progression; symptomatic organ-specific treatment will be required.
- HSCT may be necessary.
- Iododoxorubicin binds to AL amyloid and promotes resorption.
- Bortezomib (Velcade®), a proteasome inhibitor, may be helpful.

Table 14.3 Testing for AL amyloid

Tests for diagnosis	Tests for monitoring
Serum immunoglobulins and electrophoresis, immunofixation (isoelectric focusing)	Paraprotein quantitation
	Serum free light chains
Urinary electrophoresis	
Paraprotein quantitation	
Serum free light chains	
Bone marrow examination	
Biopsy (Congo red stain)	

AA amyloid

Presentation
- Presents predominantly with hepatosplenomegaly, nephrotic syndrome, and malabsorption.
- Cardiac and nerve involvement is rare.

Cause and immunopathogenesis
- Caused by the polymerization of serum amyloid A protein (SAA), an acute-phase protein, whose levels rise in response to IL-1 and IL-6.
- Is a complication of chronic infection or inflammation (TB, bronchiectasis, rheumatoid arthritis, ankylosing spondylitis, etc.).
- There is some evidence that it may be transmissible, due to a seeding mechanism.
- Is a complication of periodic fever syndromes (see respective sections later in this chapter):
  - familial Mediterranean fever;
  - hyper-IgD syndrome;
  - TRAPS;
  - Muckle–Wells syndrome;
  - familial cold urticaria.

Investigations
- Biopsies will confirm the presence of the amyloid deposits, and the serum will contain high levels of acute-phase proteins (e.g. CRP).
- SAA can be measured routinely, especially in amyloidogeneic conditions such as the autoinflammatory diseases on treatment.
- SAP scans may help localize deposits.

Treatment
- Treatment is aimed at the underlying disease to eliminate the drive to high levels of SAA, using anti-cytokine agents (anti-IL-6).
- Agents that interfere with heparin sufate, which binds to SAA, may be effective. A sulfonate, eprodisate (Kiacta®), has entered clinical trials.
- Colchicine is a valuable prophylactic agent in some periodic fever syndromes.

Other acquired amyloidoses

Dialysis amyloid
- Caused by the polymerization of β_2-microglobulin ($A\beta_2MG$).
- Related to failure of certain older (cuprophane) haemodialysis membranes to clear β_2MG. Current membranes do not have this problem to the same extent.
- Widespread deposition of β_2MG occurs but these deposits may resolve slowly with a successful transplant or on switching to dialysis with more permeable membranes.
- Serum β_2MG levels will rise to very high levels (> 20 mg/l).
- Doxycycline is being trialled as an agent that disrupts beta-pleated sheets.

Prion disease

- Amyloid deposition has been associated with prions in Creutzfeldt–Jakob disease, where the prion protein, PrP, is mutated and becomes amyloidogenic.

Alzheimer's disease

- β-amyloid protein has also been identified in certain cases of Alzheimer's disease and is associated with the typical neurofibrillary tangles.
- Protein is derived from a larger precursor amyloid β-precursor protein (AβPP), and in Alzheimer's it appears that the processing is defective, leading to an abnormal β-amyloid.

Diabetes

- Amyloid deposits are found in patients with type II maturity-onset diabetes.
- Amyloidogenic protein is thought to be islet amyloid polypeptide (AIPP), which is normally co-secreted with insulin.
- This type of amyloid may occur in association with insulinomas.

Senile cardiac amyloid

- Senile cardiac amyloid is very common in the elderly and is due to deposition of polymerized atrial natriuretic factor.

Medullary thyroid carcinoma

- Medullary thyroid carcinoma may be associated with a form of amyloid derived from pro-calcitonin and calcitonin.

Inherited amyloidosis

- There are a number of rare inherited amyloid deposition diseases related to rare mutations in proteins. These include:
  - transthyretin;
  - apolipoprotein A-I;
  - gelsolin;
  - fibrinogen;
  - cystatin C;
  - lysozyme.
- Clinical features are variable but renal and neurological involvement, both central and peripheral, are common.
- Diagnosis is by identification of the mutated genes.
- Hereditary transthyretin-associated amyloid (hATTR) causes familial amyloid polyneuropathy. Mutations cause instability of the tetramer of TTR.
  - This can now be treated with patisiran, a small interfering RNA which reduces wild-type and mutated transthyretin, which stabilizes and even reverses the condition.
  - A drug which stabilizes TTR, tafamidis (Vyndaqel®), is being trialled.
  - Tetracyclines such as doxycycline disrupt beta-pleated sheets and may be useful.

Introduction
to autoinflammatory diseases

- Broad spectrum of diseases, often monogenic, with predominant features of autoinflammation, with some overlap with autoimmunity.
- Most are rare, and may affect specific racial groups (e.g. familial Mediterranean fever, FMF).
- Can be broken down into inflamasome-related conditions and type I interferonopathies.
- Genetic studies are assisting in identifying the causes of autoinflammatory diseases of unknown origin.

Familial Mediterranean fever (FMF)

Presentation

- Inherited disease, most common in Jewish and Arab people, Italians, Turks, and Armenians, especially those living around the Mediterranean basin.
- Clinical features include attacks of abdominal pain with high fever, mimicking acute peritonitis but settling over 24–48 hours. Pleuritic chest pain, arthritis (which may be destructive and mimic RhA), and erythematous skin rashes also occur. Pericarditis may occur rarely.
- Attacks usually begin before the age of 20 (90% of cases).
- Typical attacks last 24–72 hours and can be triggered by physical exertion, stress, and menstruation.
- Periodicity is variable and unpredictable.
- AA amyloid may be a long-term complication of repeated attacks, especially in Jewish people (up to 75%).

Cause and immunopathogenesis

- Inherited as an autosomal recessive.
- Associated with mutations in the *MEFV* gene (16p13.3), encoding pyrin (also known as marenostrin), a protein that regulates caspase 1 and IL-1 secretion.
- Inheritance of the M694V/M694V genotype is associated with more severe disease (earlier onset, more arthritis, and long-term complications).
- A specific mutation in exon 2 (p.S242R) of the *MEFV* gene is associated with a separate illness: pyrin-associated autoinflammation with neutrophlic dermatosis (PAAND).

Investigations

- There is a peripheral blood leucocytosis, mild anaemia, and the ESR and CRP rise during attacks. Fibrinogen levels are high (> 5 g/l).
- Serum immunoglobulins are non-specifically polyclonally elevated.

- Involved serosal surfaces have an inflammatory infiltrate, mainly neutrophils. Joint fluid also shows a high neutrophil count during an acute attack.
- Autoantibodies are not found.
- Biopsies need to be considered if AA amyloid is suspected.
- Genetic diagnosis is confirmatory.

Treatment

- Colchicine in a daily dose of 1–1.5 mg will reduce the frequency and severity of attacks markedly and reduce the risk of developing amyloidosis.
- Colchicine taken inadvertently by pregnant women may increase the risk of Down's syndrome.
- 5–10% of cases are resistant to colchicine.
- Anakinra (anti-IL-1) is beneficial. Canakinumab (anti-IL-1β) and rilonacept (dimeric IL-1-receptor-IgG Fc fusion protein) are also used.

TNF receptor-associated periodic syndrome (TRAPS, familial Hibernian fever)

Presentation

- Recurrent attacks of pleurisy, peritonitis, pericarditis, erythematous rash, arthritis, and myalgia, beginning in childhood.
- Monocytic fasciitis.
- Conjunctivitis, rarely uveitis.
- Pericarditis, lymphadenopathy.
- 25% develop amyloidosis.
- Attacks usually prolonged > 7 days.

Cause and immunopathogenesis

- Dominant mutations in the *TNFRSF1A* gene (12p13), encoding the TNF receptor.
- Mutations occur in external domains and prevent the normal shedding of the receptor.

Diagnosis

- Demonstration of TNF receptor mutations.

Treatment

- Colchicine is not effective in TRAPS.
- Corticosteroids can be used in short courses for flares.
- Anti-TNF agents appear to be less effective than anti-IL-1 treatments (anakinra, canakinumab, rilonacept).
- Anti-IL-6 (tocilizumab) may be effective in anakinra-resistant disease.

Hyper-IgD syndrome (mevalonate kinase deficiency)

Clinical features

- Rare autosomal recessive syndrome comprising bouts of fever, lymphadenitis, and occasionally oligoarthritis. Diffuse rash.
- Peritonitis and pleurisy are common.
- Oral and vaginal ulcers may occur.
- Attacks last 3–7 days.
- Severe immunization reactions are a particular feature.
- Severe form (mevalonic aciduria) presents at birth with psychomotor retardation, ataxia, failure to thrive, cataracts, dysmorphism, with episodic fever and inflammation. Frequently fatal.

Cause and immunopathogenesis

- Mutations in the *MVK* gene (12q24) encoding mevalonate kinase.
- Predominantly occurs in Dutch and other northern European peoples.
- 24% of cases do not have mutations in the coding part of the gene.
- Defects in the gene cause defective prenylation of proteins. Mitochondria are abnormal and accumulate in the cytoplasm and may activate NLRP3.
- Mutations in *MVK* in other conditions (ulcerative colitis, retinitis pigmentosa) without evidence of decreased mevalonate kinase activity—significance is uncertain.

Investigations

- Humoral immune responses may be poor, with reduced IgM, raised IgG_3, and very high IgD levels. IgA may also be elevated.
- IgD can be measured with commercial RID assays.

Treatment

- NSAIDs for fever.
- Anakinra and anti-IL-1 treatments—preferred option.
- Anti-TNFs may be tried, but may not give complete response.
- Tocilizumab may be effective.
- Statins have now been abandoned as ineffective (mevalonate kinase is part of the HMG-CoA reductase pathway).
- HSCT has been used in a few cases.

Muckle–Wells and related syndromes

Three hereditary febrile syndromes have been described in association with dominant mutations in the gene *NLRP3* (*NALP3*, *PYPAF1*, *C1AS1*), coding for cryopyrin. These are gain-of-function mutations causing increased NLRP3 activity.

- Muckle–Wells syndrome.
  - Episodic symptoms lasting up to 48 hours. Urticaria (not cold associated), arthralgia, myalgia, headache, conjunctivitis, episcleritis; may lead to amyloidosis (25%).

- Neonatal-onset multisystem inflammatory disease (NOMID, also known as CINCA = chronic infantile neurologic cutaneous and articular syndrome).
  - Chronic disease, diffuse urticaria, epiphyseal overgrowth, conjunctivitis, uveitis (blindness), sensorineural deafness. Amyloidosis may occur as late feature.
- Familial cold autoinflammatory syndrome (FCAS).
  - Fever, rigors, headache, arthralgia, conjunctivitis, and urticaria in response to cold exposure.
  - Has also been associated with mutations in *NLRP12*, as well as *NLRP3*.
- Familial cold urticaria.
  - This is a milder variant of FCAS and also maps to the *NLRP3* gene.

Treatment
- NSAIDs are usually used.
- Anakinra (IL-1-RA), canakinumab (anti-IL-1β), and rilonacept are very effective.
- Experimental caspase-1 inhibitor VX-765 (belnacasan) has been shown to reduce IL-1 and is undergoing trials.

Periodic fever with aphthous ulcers, pharyngitis, and cervical adenopathy (PFAPA)

- A rare syndrome characterized by periodic fever, aphthous ulceration, pharyngitis, and adenitis.
- So far does not appear to be a monogenic syndrome.
- Starts early in childhood but improves as child grows up.
- Cause uncertain—no gene identified yet.
- During flares IFN/IL-1 genes upregulated; can be abolished by a pan-caspase inhibitor.
- Treat with corticosteroids, colchicine, or IL-1 inhibition.
- Cimetidine has been shown to resolve fever in some cases.
- Adenotonsillectomy has resolved some cases.

Schnitzler's syndrome

- A rare syndrome characterized by urticaria, skin papules, intermittent fever, bone pain, arthritis/arthralgia, and monoclonal IgM monoclonal gammopathy.
- Severe anaemia of chronic disease is common.
- IL-6 levels are elevated. ESR is raised.
- Mosaicism in myeloid cells for somatic mutations in *NLRP3* has been reported.
- Evolves into lymphoma or Waldenström's macroglobulinaemia in 15–20%.

- Treatment may involve corticosteroids, colchicine, thalidomide, or anakinra. Preferred treatment is anakinra.
- Tocilizumab may be effective in anakinra-resistant disease.
- Pefloxacin, a quinolone antibiotic, may reduce complete remission in some patients (mechanism unknown).
- Anti-TNF therapy may make it worse.
- Antihistamines, rituximab, and hdIVIg are ineffective.

Mullins' syndrome

- A variant of Schnitzler's syndrome.
- Monoclonal gammopathy (not necessarily IgM).
- Fever, rash, hypotension.
- Complement consumption, with reduced C3/C4 (normal in Schnitzler's syndrome).
- Leucopenia and thrombocytopenia.
- Resistant to anakinra, but acute attacks respond to steroids.
- No gene identified.

Blau syndrome

- Familial early-onset granulomatous arthritis, anterior and posterior uveitis, cutaneous granulomata.
- Autosomal dominant gain-of-function mutations in *NOD2/CARD15*.
- Overlaps with sarcoidosis and Crohn's disease.
- Treated with TNF and IL-1 antagonists.

Deficiency of the interleukin-1 receptor antagonist (DIRA)

- A rare autosomal recessive autoinflammatory syndrome.
- Severe anaemia of chronic disease is common.
- Sterile multifocal osteomyelitis, periosteitis, cutaneous pustulosis, from birth.
- Mutations in IL-1 receptor antagonist gene, *IL1RN*.

Pyogenic sterile arthritis, pyoderma gangrenosum, acne (PAPA)

- Autosomal dominant condition.
- Presents with early arthritis (destructive), pyoderma gangrenosum (variable), and nodulocystic acne and hidradenitis suppurativa.
- Mutations identified in CD2 binding protein 1 gene (*PSTPIP1, CD2BP1*) gene, located on chromosome 15.
- Treat with anti-TNF or anti-IL-1 agents.

Chronic recurrent multifocal osteomyelitis (CRMO) and Majeed syndrome

- Multiple syndromes associated with CRMO in childhood. Recurrent sterile osteomyelitis.
- Majeed syndrome is autosomal recessive CRMO with dyserythropoetic anaemia and neutrophilic dermatosis (Sweet's syndrome), associated with mutations in *LPIN2* (lipin-2).
- Other associations of CRMO include psoriasis, palmar-plantar pustulosis, Crohn's disease, and arthritis.
- Multiple other gene mutations identified in CRMO (*Pstpip2, IL1RN, FBLIM1*).
- IL-1 inhibition is beneficial (anakinra, cankinumab).

Other autoinflammatory conditions

- All of the following are very rare with small numbers of cases recorded worldwide. However, they give insights into hitherto unknown inflammatory pathways.
- PLAID (PLCg2-associated antibody deficiency and immune dysregulation).
  - Gene is *PLC2G*—autosomal dominant gain-of-function mutation.
  - Presents with cold urticaria, autoimmunity, blistering skin disease, lung and bowel disease, hypogammaglobulinaemia, and auto-inflammatory changes.
- A20 haploinsufficiency.
  - Autosomal dominant loss-of-function mutations in *TNFAIP3*.
  - Defective inhibition of NF-κB pathway.
  - Presents with early-onset inflammation, arthritis, orogenital ulceration, and eye inflammation (similar to Behcet's syndrome).
  - Mutations have also been linked to SLE.
- COPA defect.
  - Autosomal dominant.
  - Autoimmune inflammatory arthritis, interstitial lung disease. Th17 dysregulation.
- Otulin-related autoinflammatory syndrome.
  - Autosomal recessive loss-of-function mutations in Met 1 deubiquitinase *OTULIN* (*gumby*) which impairs NF-κB activation.
  - Neonatal-onset severe inflammatory disease with prolonged fevers, arthritis, diarrhoea, and failure to thrive. Pustular or nodular skin rash (neutrophilic dermatosis).
  - Anti-TNF therapy is effective.
- NLCR4 macrophage activation syndrome.
  - Autosomal dominant gain-of-function mutations in *NLCR4*, leading to increased IL-1β and IL-18, with macrophage activation.
  - Severe enterocolitis and macrophage activation, triggered by cold exposure.

- ADA2 deficiency syndrome.
  - Autosomal recessive mutations in *CECR1*.
  - Presents with polyarteritis nodosa (vasculopathy); childhood/early-onset ischaemic stroke and fever. Livedo reticularis, hypertension, leg ulcers, Raynaud's.
  - Anti-TNFs, recombinant ADA2, and HSCT have been used.
- ADAM17 deficiency syndrome.
  - Autosomal recessive mutations in ADAM17.
  - Defective TNFα production.
  - Early-onset diarrhoea with skin lesions, including pustular psoriasis and cardiomyopathy.
- NLRP1 deficiency syndrome.
  - Autosomal recessive mutations in *NLRP1*.
  - Elevated IL-18 and caspase 1.
  - Dyskeratosis, autoimmunity, and arthritis.
- NLRP12 deficiency syndrome.
  - Autosomal dominant mutations in *NLRP12*.
  - Increased caspase 1 activation.
  - Periodic fever syndrome.
- TNSFRSF11A (RANK) deficiency syndrome.
  - Autosomal recessive mutations in *TNFRSF11A*.
  - Similar to TRAPS.
- SLC29A3 deficiency syndrome.
  - Autosomal recessive mutations in *SLC29A3*.
  - Presents with hyperpigmentation, hypertrichosis, hepatosplenomegaly, cardiac abnormalities, hypogonadism, and recurrent fever.
  - Homozygous mutations present as autoinflammatory disease.
- Cherubism.
  - Autosomal dominant mutations in *SH3BP2*.
  - Symmetrical cysts in maxillae and mandible, filled with osteoclasts. TNFα is involved, but inhibition does not appear helpful.

Type I interferonopathies

- All are rare.
- Aicardi–Goutieres syndrome.
  - Multiple genetic abnormalities described (*TREX1* (autosomal dominant or recessive), *RNASEH2B, RNASEH2C, RNASEH2A, SAMHD1, ADAR1* (all autosomal recessive), *IFIH1* (gain-of-function).
  - All lead to increased production of type I interferons.
  - Leukodystrophy with brain calcification and intellectual impairment. Evidence of CSF inflammation; painful chilblains; lupus-like disease with vasculitis.
  - Raised CFS IFN-α at the time of flares is diagnostic.
  - No effective treatment at present.
- Spondyloenchondrodysplasia with immune dysregulation syndrome (SPENCD).
  - Mutations in *ACP5*, leading to upregulation of IFN production.

- Short stature, multiple haematological autoimmune cytopenias.
- Recurrent viral and bacterial infections.
- SAVI syndrome.
  - STING-associated vasculopathy with onset in infancy.
  - Mutations in STING (stimulator of interferon gene)/*TMEM173*.
  - Onset in infancy with cutaneous vasculopathy, with necrosis and progressive interstitial fibrosis.
  - May respond to azathioprine or JAK 1/2 inhibitors.
- X-linked reticulate pigmentary disorder.
  - Mutations in *POLA1*, leading to upregulation of IFN production.
  - Characteristic appearance, hyperpigmentation. Lung and gut involvement.
- CANDLE syndrome.
  - Autosomal dominant and recessive forms.
  - Multiple genes: *PSMBR8* is most important.
  - *PSMB8* encodes β5i subunit of immunoproteasome.
  - Contractures, panniculitis, pernio, lipodystrophy, fevers, and intracranial calcification.
  - Disorder of proteasome.
  - Similarities to C1q-deficient SLE.
  - Treated with corticosteroids for acute attacks; JAK 1/2 inhibitors may help.

Xanthogranulomatosis, juvenile xanthogranulomatosis, Erdheim–Chester disease, Rosai–Dorfman disease

Adult xanthogranulomatosis

- Syndrome is characterized by subcutaneous xanthogranulomatous plaques, typically around the eyes, and associated with hard subcutaneous nodules.
- There is an association with the development of paraproteins and eventually with lymphomas.
- Paraproteins seem to associate with apo-B lipoproteins, which are then taken up by macrophages in the lesions.
- Diagnosis is made by appearance and biopsy features.
- The disease responds well to corticosteroids.
- Regular monitoring of serum immunoglobulins and electrophoresis is required.

Juvenile xanthogranulomatosis (JXG)

- Benign paediatric histiocytosis which usually resolves spontaneously.
- Multiple mutations identified.
- Lesions usually limited to skin but disseminated severe form may occur (4%).
- Ocular involvement may occur.

- Lesions arise from dermal dendrocytes.
- Treat by surgical excision of localized lesions.
- Systemic disease treated with steroids plus vinblatine or cladribine.

Erdheim–Chester disease (ECD)

- Rare multisystem lipoid granulomatosis.
- May involve long bones.
- Cardiac involvement, including aorta.
- Orbital infiltration.
- Diabetes insipidus due to pituitary involvement.
- Can be distinguished from JXG by the surface marker expression on biopsies.
- Mainly affects adults.
- About half of the cases have *BRAF-V600E* mutations (also seen in melanoma).
- Peginterferon alfa is preferred treatment.
- Cladribine and sirolimus with steroids have been used.
- BRAF inhibitor vemurafenib has been used successfully in refractory ECD.

Rosai–Dorfman disease

- Histiocytic syndrome characterized by benign proliferation of S100$^+$ histiocytes in sinuses of lymph nodes and lymphatics, leading to massive lymphadenopathy, fevers, night sweats, and weight loss.
- Similar histology may be seen in ALPS (Fas deficiency), SLE, and JIA.
- Mainly affects children and young adults.
- Probably not a single entity.
- No specific genetic abnormality (some cases have mutations in MAPK/ERK pathway) and no confirmation of infective trigger.
- May occur with some malignancies (leukaemias and lymphomas).
- Similar histology in congenital Faisalabad syndrome. Rare autosomal recessive presenting with joint deformities, deafness, and lymphadenopathy. Associated with mutations in *SLC29A3* gene, coding for equilabrative nucleoside transporter ENT3.
- Treatment is steroids, with chemotherapy. Interferon alfa, imatinib, and cladribine have been used.

Kikuchi's syndrome

- A rare syndrome of lymphadenopathy seen in children and young adults, usually self-limiting.
- Clinical features include fever, lymphadenopathy, skin rashes, and headache.
- May be triggered by viral infections (CMV, EBV, HSV, VZV, parvovirus).
- Possible association with autoimmune diseases, including SLE.
- May also be a cause of haemophagocytosis.
- Responds to NSAIDs; corticosteroids for severe disease.

Satoyoshi syndrome (Komura–Guerri syndrome)

- A very rare syndrome of progressive muscle spasms, alopecia, diarrhoea, endocrinopathy with amenorrhoea, and skeletal abnormalities, first described in Japan.
- Possibly linked to mutations in *ZNF808* gene.
- Spasms are painful and can affect breathing; myoclonus may occur. There are similarities to stiff-person syndrome.
- Thought to be autoimmune; may be associated with antibodies to GAD.
- Treated with steroids and immunosuppressants (azathioprine).

Castleman's syndrome

- Syndrome of diffuse lymphadenopathy, fever, malaise, and weight loss.
- May be unicentric or multicentric.
- Many cases appear to be due to HHV-8 infection. Also seen with POEMS syndrome (see ➔ Chapter 4) and SLE.
- TAFRO syndrome.
  - Thrombocytopenia, anasarca, fevers, reticulin myelofibrosis, organomegaly.
  - Part of idiopathic multicentric Castleman's syndrome spectrum.
  - VGEF may be more important than IL-6.
  - Hypergammaglobulinaemia is not marked.
- IL-6 levels may be elevated (?direct effect of virus).
- Characteristic 'onion-skin' appearance in lymph nodes. Angiofollicular lymph node hyperplasia.
- Usually treated with corticosteroids; role of antivirals uncertain.
- TAFRO syndrome treated with steroids, rituximab, tocilizumab (anti-IL-6), cyclophosphamide, and etoposide. Outcome may be poor.

Cheilitis granulomatosa (Miescher–Melkersson–Rosenthal syndrome; orofacial granulomatosis)

- Rare syndrome presenting with non-tender swelling of the lips (upper lip more common than lower lip).
- Melkersson–Rosenthal syndrome presents with the triad of orofacial oedema, relapsing facial paralysis, and a fissured tongue.
- Initially attacks are intermittent, but eventually the swelling becomes permanent and progressive.
- Must be distinguished from angioedema (more persistent).
- Attacks of swelling may be accompanied by low-grade fever.
- Swellings may also appear on other parts of the face.
- Lymph nodes may be enlarged.

- Biopsies may show granulomata in established cases.
- May have a genetic basis but no specific gene identified. Cause is unknown; may be a localized form of Crohn's disease.
  - ❶Consider a labelled white cell scan to look for other evidence of Crohn's disease.
- Patch testing may show positive reactions to cinnamon and benzoates and occasionally metals; trial of dietary avoidance may help a few patients.
- Granulomatous reactions to dental amalgam have been noted.
- Treatments suggested include clofazimine, metronidazole, intra-lesional steroid, azathioprine, sulfasalazine, and other antibiotics.

Chronic fatigue syndromes (CFS) 1

Chronic fatigue is a major presentation to doctors; causes are multiple and establishing a diagnosis time-consuming. CFS is a diagnosis of exclusion. ME (myalgic encephalomyelitis) is an inappropriate term as there is no evidence for an encephalomyelitis. It is not a new syndrome and has been well described from Victorian times onwards (neurasthenia).

Presentation

- Significant debilitating fatigue (not tiredness!) is that lasting beyond 6 months.
- About half have a sudden onset often after an acute infectious event; remainder have gradual onset (unclear if these types differ).
- Excess of 'major life events' in year preceding presentation.
- Other symptoms include:
  - unrefreshing sleep; sleep disturbance;
  - poor short-term memory and poor concentration; word-finding difficulty;
  - non-specific arthralgia, without arthritis;
  - myalgia; fibromyalgia;
  - headaches;
  - disturbed temperature perception;
  - sensory intolerance (noise, light, touch, smell, taste);
  - sore throats and swollen glands;
  - debilitating fatigue;
  - secondary depression;
  - alcohol intolerance;
  - activity makes all symptoms worse ('post-exertional malaise').
- Weight loss is *not* a feature and should always prompt a detailed search for an underlying medical or surgical cause.
- Patients often self-diagnose CFS/ME: this is dangerous.
- Patients may acquire bizarre beliefs about the cause and treatment of their symptoms, obtained from alternative practitioners, lay publications, and the internet. These include:
  - multiple allergies, including multiple chemical sensitivity;
  - reactions to mercury amalgam fillings;
  - chronic *Candida* overgrowth.

- There is no evidence to support these aetiologies.
- The CFS is a hotch-potch of miscellaneous syndromes, dependent on the speciality of the 'expert'! Included within the spectrum are:
  - irritable bowel syndrome;
  - food allergy;
  - fibromyalgia;
  - somatization disorder;
  - effort syndrome;
  - overtraining syndrome (see ⟶ 'Sports immunology 2', p. 389);
  - patients with medically unexplained symptoms;
  - patients with significant medical/psychiatric disorders (up to 47% of referrals to hospital).

Differential diagnosis

In hospital practice, up to 47% of patients may turn out to have other medical or surgical problems: the differential diagnosis is long but includes:

- chronic infections: EBV, HIV, coxsackievirus, *Toxoplasma, Brucella, Yersinia, Borrelia*;
- connective tissue diseases: SLE, Sjögren's syndrome, rheumatoid arthritis, polymyositis, polymyalgia rheumatica often have a long prodrome of fatigue;
- other autoimmune diseases: especially thyroid disease, Addison's disease, diabetes mellitus, pituitary disease;
- gastrointestinal disease: PBC, autoimmune hepatitis, coeliac disease;
- neurological disease: MS, degenerative disease (including CJD), Parkinson's disease (early stages), primary muscle disease;
- sleep apnoea, other primary sleep disorders, incl. restless legs, idiopathic hypersomnolence, circadian rhythm disorder, REM sleep disorder;
- cardiac disease: cardiomyopathy (alcohol, thiamine deficiency);
- poisonings: carbon monoxide, heavy metals, prescription drugs (e.g. β-blockers, opiate analgesics);
- malignancy;
- primary psychiatric disorders: depression (but a secondary depression is common), bipolar disorder, autistic spectrum disorders, somatization disorder, stress;
- malingering (rare but usually perpetuated by obvious financial benefit from maintenance of sick role).

UK and US case definitions for CFS

The UK criteria have evolved out of the need to identify homogeneous groups of patients for research trials. Not all patients will fit the criteria.
- Severe disabling fatigue affecting physical and mental functioning.
- Minimum duration of symptoms = 6 months.
- Functional impairment = disabling.
- Mental fatigue required.
- No other symptoms required.
- No evidence for other medical illness.
- Normal screening blood tests.

The North Americans have a similar case definition, with minor differences.
- Physical causes of fatigue excluded.
- Psychiatric disorders excluded, including:
  - psychosis;
  - bipolar disorder;
  - eating disorder;
  - organic brain disease.

Epidemiology
- Institutional epidemic outbreaks (Royal Free disease): these differ substantially from sporadic disease.
- 'Chronic fatigue', loosely defined, is very common in the community: prevalence of 20–30%.
- 10–20% of attenders in primary care complain of chronic fatigue (loosely defined).
- For 5–10% this will be the primary reason for consultation.
- Only a minority fulfil the case definition for CFS (as previously described).
- Female to male ratio = 2:1.
- The prevalence of CFS/ME is much lower, but similar figures have been obtained from the USA and UK (using the different criteria):
  - point prevalence, 0.08–1% range using restrictive criteria;
  - point prevalence of up to 2.6% using UK (Oxford) criteria;
  - there are no reliable data on incidence.
- It has been estimated that there may be as many as 150 000 cases in the UK.

CFS 2: cause and immunopathogenesis, assessment, and investigations

Cause and immunopathogenesis

Virology
- Antecedent history of acute infection can be documented in about 50% of CFS/ME patients.
- Definable fatigue syndromes are well documented after:
  - EBV: persistent EBV IgM positive (chronic EBV); only occurs in 10% of EBV-infected individuals;
  - *Toxoplasma*;
  - cytomegalovirus;
  - other infectious agents (non-specific response): severe bacterial infections.
- Association with enteroviral infections is unproven (VP1 test is not reliable).
- Association with XMRV (murine retrovirus) has been discounted.

Immunology
- Autoantibodies have been described against adrenergic receptors; plasmapheresis and rituximab have been claimed to be beneficial.
- Immunological abnormalities described are:

- minor abnormalities of IgG subclasses;
- increased CD5+ CD19+ B cells;
- poor B-cell function;
- low levels of autoantibodies (RhF);
- reduced CD4+ T cells; increased CD8+ T cells;
- increased markers of T-cell activation;
- abnormalities of NK cells and monocytes;
- no clear changes in cytokine production;
- antibodies against nuclear pore antigens were found in 60–70% of CFS patients in one study.

🅘 Significant immunological abnormalities should raise doubts about a diagnosis of CFS.

Genetic abnormalities
- Likely to be a genetic predisposition to develop the disease.
  - Other family members may be affected.
  - Multiple genes involved (brain, immune system).

Muscle abnormalities
- No characteristic abnormalities.
  - CK may be mildly elevated.
  - NMR studies demonstrate abnormal metabolism, with failure to clear lactate.
  - Cardiomyopathy may occur in a small subset.
  - Clinical studies have shown benefit from co-enzyme Q10 and NADH, suggesting possible mitochochondrial defect.

Neurological abnormalities
- No diagnostic abnormalities. However, a range of abnormalities has been documented, the significance of which are uncertain at present.
- MRI scanning may show white matter abnormalities.
- Single-photon emission tomography (SPET) reflects abnormalities of regional cerebral perfusion.
- SPET abnormalities identified in brainstem; lesser abnormalities are reported in patients with depression.
- Autonomic abnormalities are frequent and may occur in other disorders with fatigue (PBC); postural orthostatic tachycardia syndrome (POTS) is a variant of CFS with marked autonomic abnormalities. Severity of autonomic disorder correlates with fatigue.

Endocrine abnormalities
- Dynamic tests of the hypothalamic–pituitary–adrenal axis demonstrate abnormal responses.
- Subgroup of CFS patients may have low cortisols (usually high in depression): exclude Addison's disease.
- Testosterone and oestrogen levels may be reduced: supplementation does not improve symptoms, so changes are likely to be secondary.

Psychiatric changes
- No convincing evidence to show that CFS is purely a psychiatric disorder.
- Depression is usually secondary.

- There is an increased risk of developing psychiatric disorder in CFS patients (2- to 7.5-fold compared to chronic disease controls).
- There is overlap with somatization disorders.

Assessment

- Assess the patient objectively (and try to ignore the long-standing patient's interpretation of events).
- Are criteria for CFS met?
- What is the degree of disability?
- What are the patient's beliefs about his/her illness?
- Are there any symptoms/signs of other medical problems?
- Low-grade fever, muscle wasting, orthostatic hypotension, pallor, breathlessness, tremor allowable (deconditioning due to prolonged rest).
- Marked weight loss, lymphadenopathy, and fever > 38°C require further investigation and should *not* be accepted as part of CFS.

Investigations

- There are *no* specific diagnostic tests despite attempts to find a biomarker or combination of biomarkers.
- Basic screen must include:
  - FBC, differential white count;
  - acute-phase response (evidence for inflammatory disease—ESR/ CRP);
  - LFTs, Cr & E, TFTs, blood sugar, CK;
  - endomysial/tissue transglutaminase (tTG) antibody;
  - urine (protein/sugar).
- Other tests should only be carried out if there are suspicious findings on history or examination.
- These may include:
  - viral serology (EBV, HIV);
  - cortisol, short tetracosactide (Synacthen®) test;
  - ferritin, vitamin D, folate, vitamin B_{12};
  - screening for connective tissue disease.

❶ There is *no* role for *routine* viral serology, lymphocyte subsets, or auto-antibody screens: test only against clinical indications.

CFS 3: management, outcome, and children with CFS

Management

An holistic approach is required ('Mindfulness'—see ➔ *Wherever You Go, There You Are* by Jon Kabat-Zinn).
- Evaluate the contribution of life events and psychological background.
- Identify significant secondary depression and deal with this.
- Deal with bizarre beliefs (⌨ http://www.quackwatch.com is a useful website with robust rebuttals of bizarre beliefs); ⌨ http://www. neurosymptoms.org/ is another useful site for patients with non-organic neurological symptoms.

- Reassurance early that no serious medical condition has been identified.
- Detailed explanation of current theories of CFS.
- Expected prognosis.
- Limit investigation (and control multiple referrals!).
- Management by the smallest possible team who are familiar with the illness.
- Physical reconditioning.
- Graded activity and pacing.
- Sleep hygiene.
- Drug therapy is symptomatic (not curative).
  - Management of pain is problematic: avoid long-term use of opiates (ineffective and contribute to central sleep apnoea).
  - Gabapentenoids may be used, but current evidence suggests that they too become ineffective over time and increase weight.
  - Amitryptiline in very small doses may help sleep and fibromyalgia pain.
  - Duloxetine is recommended for fibromyalgia, but is often not tolerated.
  - Melatonin is useful for teenagers with CFS and sleep disturbance (need to have a break every 4–6 weeks as effect wears off).
  - Antidepressants for reactive depression: use smallest possible dose as these drugs are usually poorly tolerated. No drug appears better than any other in practice.
- Psychological support.
- Cognitive behaviour therapy (often resisted by patients).
- Lightning therapy, an accelerated form of psychotherapy based on neurolinguistic programming (NLP), helps some patients significantly.
- General support from a *sympathetic* medical team.
- *Fighting Fatigue* by Sue Pemberton and Catherine Berry is an excellent self-help guide for patients.
- A recent study from Norway has suggested a response to rituximab—blinded trials showed no benefit.
- Plasmapheresis has been used with benefit in a German trial, linked to detection of adrenergic autoantibodies.
- ❶ There is currently *no* place in management for:
  - immunoglobulin (intravenous or intramuscular);
  - antihistamines;
  - interferons (usually make the symptoms worse);
  - antivirals (except where there is a proven persistent EBV infection);
  - antifungals;
  - magnesium;
  - colonic irrigation;
  - anti-*Candida* diets;
  - low-allergen diets;
  - enzyme-potentiated desensitization.
- Homeopathy, aromatherapy, reflexology, acupuncture may provide symptomatic relief.
- Multiple medical referrals perpetuate illness.
- Deal with need for support for benefits, occupational advice.

Outcome

- The prognosis is variable.
  - Most patients show significant improvement over 2 years if identified early and entered into a management programme.
  - 'Cure' rate is probably 6–13% (several different series).
  - If there is no improvement by 2 years then recovery is unlikely (assuming that no perpetuating features are identified).
- It is important to discuss adaptation of the patient's lifestyle to his or her illness early on.
- There are no laboratory markers that predict outcome.
- Progression of symptoms may mean that the original diagnosis is wrong—be prepared to re-evaluate.
- ❶ Treat all new symptoms on their merits—just because a patient has a diagnosis of CFS/ME doesn't mean that they will not develop other unrelated illnesses.
- A poor outcome is associated with:
  - late presentation;
  - unaddressed psychosocial factors;
  - poor management ('there is nothing wrong with you—it's all in your mind');
  - inadequate rehabilitation (failure to encourage exercise perpetuates deconditioning);
  - secondary gain;
  - perpetuation of bizarre beliefs (*Candida* syndrome, total allergy syndrome).

Children with CFS

- Syndrome is not as rare in children as previously thought!
- Early assessment of a tired child is appropriate.
- Beware of 'Munchausen syndrome by proxy'.
- Management is more complicated and must address family issues.
- Depression is common (60–80% of childhood CFS cases).
- The same principles as those identified earlier in this section apply to investigation and management.
- Psychosocial factors (bullying) and psychiatric problems must be dealt with.
- Deal with peer-relationship problems and school avoidance.
- Avoid home tuition as this encourages social isolation.
- Aim for a recovery programme including graded physical and intellectual exercise, with identification of recovery goals.

Idiopathic oedema

- A syndrome of non-menstrually related swelling of face, hands, abdomen, and feet, with no identifiable causes.
- Associated with affective, somatic, and functional symptoms including debilitating fatigue.
- Overlaps with CFS/ME, fibromyalgia, and irritable bowel syndrome.
- May respond to spironolactone or bromocriptine (dopaminergic mechanism?).

Shoenfeld's syndrome and macrophagic myofasciitis

Shoenfeld's syndrome

- Also known as autoimmune/inflammatory syndrome induced by adjuvants (ASIA).
  - The condition has been associated with adjuvants, particularly aluminium-based, in vaccines.
  - Also associated with leakage of silicone breast implants; symptoms may remit when implants are removed.
  - Features may mimic connective tissue diseases, including Still's disease, SLE, and scleroderma.
  - Autoantibodies may be detected, including nuclear and related antibodies.
- The relation with vaccine adjuvants and silicone is not unequivocally accepted and mechanism is uncertain.

Macrophagic myositis

- Rare muscle disease, said to be triggered by aluminium salts in vaccines.
- Focal infiltration of vaccinated muscles with PAS⁺ macrophages.
- Associated with systemic features:
  - Fatigue
  - Malaise
  - Generalized arthralgia and myalgia
  - Muscle weakness
  - Fever.
- Muscle biopsy & MRI may show abnormalities.
- No specific treatment—manage as for CFS/ME.

Burning mouth syndrome

- Characterized by intraoral burning sensation without evidence of medical or dental disease.
  - Need to exclude xerostomia, aphthous ulceration, vitamin deficiencies, intraoral infections including HSV.
  - Patch testing particularly to nickel, amalgam components, and dental products (cinnamon, benzoates) may identify delayed hypersensitivity in a small number of patients.
- Is one of a family of medically unexplained facial pain syndromes, which may have psychological elements.
- May present as 'oral allergy'—testing to prove to the patient that allergy is NOT the cause may be required.
- ❗Allergy does not cause continuous burning pain.
- Treat with tricyclic antidepressants, gabapentin, clonazepam, or possibly pramipexole (non-ergot dopamine D_2 receptor agonist; unlicensed indication).

Postural orthostatic tachycardia syndrome (POTS)

- Condition seen predominantly in young women, often but not exclusively with CFS/ME; may be associated with vasovagal syncope.
- Clinical features include postural dizziness, excessive thirst, and palpitations, as well as other CFS/ME symptoms.
- Key clinical finding is inappropriate tachycardia on asking the patient to stand after resting horizontally. Pulse should rise to > 120 bpm.
- Diagnosis requires formal tilt-table testing.
- ❶It is important to recognize this syndrome as it is amenable to treatment (and in the context of CFS this reduces overall fatigue). Treatments (often off-licence) include:
  - increase fluid and salt intake;
  - avoid alcohol;
  - fludrocortisone;
  - midodrine;
  - β-blockers (not well tolerated in CFS/ME);
  - ivabradine (experimental).

Sports immunology 1

- The immunology of sport is interesting because of the increased susceptibility to infection that high-level sporting activity generates.
- Changes may be due to acute effects of training/competition and longer term adaptive changes.
- Changes may be secondary to neurohumoral changes.
- Chronic change is usually related to hard training (see ➋ 'Sports immunology 2: overtraining syndrome', p. 391).
- Illicit drug use should be considered, as this may affect immune function.

Acute-phase response

- Exercise increases acute-phase proteins (CRP, fibrinogen, haptoglobin), although considerable amounts of exercise (> 2 hours) are required.
- Levels of IL-1 (although this is contentious), IL-6, α- and γ-interferon, and TNFα in serum are increased (with caveats about serum measurements of cytokines).
- LPS-stimulated release of cytokines by monocytes is also increased by adrenaline, present in high levels during exercise.
- IL-2 levels are reduced.

Innate immune response

- C3a increases significantly following exercise, and the greater the duration of exercise the greater the rise.
- Damage to muscle fibres may be the trigger for alternate pathway activation.
- A leucocytosis is present after quite short bursts of exercise, due to increased mobilization.

- After marathons, a persistent marked neutrophil and monocyte leucocytosis is apparent.
- Adrenaline may play a role in the mobilization, although it may still occur in the presence of β-blockade.
- Neutrophils are also activated, and granule components may be detected in the circulation.
- NK-cell numbers are increased in absolute and percentage terms and NK activity is increased, except in high-intensity exercise (such as a marathon), when it is reduced.

Specific immunity
- Many effects on the specific immune system have been described, although the relationship to clinical status is often obscure.
- The following changes have been documented in B cells during and immediately after acute exercise:
  - no significant change in B-cell numbers;
  - reduced salivary IgA after long-duration exercise;
  - reduction of circulating antibody-producing cells;
  - monocyte-induced suppression (indometacin inhibitable), suggesting role for prostaglandins.
- The following changes have been documented in T cells during and immediately after acute exercise:
  - increase in T cells (CD8+ > CD4+);
  - altered CD4:CD8 ratio;
  - increased CD4+ CD45RO+ T cells (?activation or altered trafficking);
  - reduced proliferative response to PHA and ConA;
  - increased proliferative responses to IL-2, LPS, PWM;
  - increased soluble activation markers after long-duration exercise (sIL-2R, sCD8, sICAM-1, sCD23, sTNF-R, neopterin).
- Many of the effects on the immune system are mediated by the combination of changes in circulating and local hormones:
  - catecholamines;
  - growth hormone;
  - endorphins;
  - cortisol (which may be responsible for late effects).
- Hypoxia and hyperthermia may also contribute.
- Glutamine reduction due to increased muscle demand for glutamine as an energy source starves the immune system of an essential metabolic precursor, leading to impaired function.

Adaptive changes during training
- Resting immunology of athletes during training does not normally show very dramatic changes.
- During low-intensity training there is a reduction of total lymphocyte count, with a reduction of CD4:CD8 ratio.
- More intense training tends to have less effect.
- NK-cell numbers increase slightly.
- Most trained athletes show slightly higher neutrophil counts, although some long-distance runners may have a neutropenia.

- Neutrophil (and monocyte) function is normal.
- Acute changes in immunological parameters seen in trained athletes are less than in sedentary individuals undertaking a similar workload.

Exercise and infection
- Acute changes as noted previously may give a window of opportunity to pathogens accounting for increased susceptibility to infection post-exercise.
- Window may last up to 2 weeks.
- Risks seem to be mainly in extreme athletes (marathon and ultra-runners, iron-man triathletes etc.).

Sports immunology 2: overtraining syndrome

- There is a J-shaped curve relating overall immune function to exercise. Low and moderate levels of exercise improve immunological function; high levels lead to immunological impairment.
- It is difficult to ascertain for any given individual what level of exercise will be compromising immune function.
- Overtraining syndrome has many features in common with the chronic fatigue syndrome (CFS; see relevant sections, this chapter).
- Short-term fatigue is a normal consequence of exercise.
- Prolonged fatigue is usually a marker for overtraining.
- This can usually be attributed to inappropriate training and/or competitive programmes that do not allow adequate recovery periods.
- Nature of the overtraining syndrome is uncertain, but might relate to chronic overproduction of acute-phase cytokines (e.g. TNF), hormones (cortisol and thyroid hormones are increased while testosterone is decreased).
- Interference with the neurohumoral axis may occur, and patients may have features of anxiety and depression.
- Chronic glutamine deficiency may be a minor contributing factor.
- Illicit drugs and inappropriate supplements may contribute (seek information by direct questioning).

> ❶High-intensity exercise may be a surrogate form of anorexia in young females particularly: such athletes are at high risk of serious complications of exercise due to inadequate nutrition and over-exercising: stress fractures; premature osteoporosis; iron-deficiency anaemia.

Immunology
- Immunological changes of optimum training are difficult to analyse, but include:
  - increased NK-cell numbers and activity;
  - minor changes in T- and B-cell numbers;

- little change in serum immunoglobulins;
- levels of soluble markers such as IL-2R, sCD8, sICAM-1, sCD23, and sTNF-R are all increased.
- Very heavy training and/or competition tend to lead to a reduction in cell numbers and function and reductions in antibody levels.
- Exercise itself tends to mobilize cells from storage pools (spleen, marginated cells) but this effect is transient.
- In the overtraining syndrome:
  - lymphocyte and NK-cell numbers are reduced;
  - there is evidence of *in vivo* activation on the basis of expression of activation markers CD25, CD69, and HLA-DR (on T cells);
  - *in vitro* mitogen responses are reduced (a common finding where there is evidence of increased *in vivo* activation);
  - phagocytic cell function is impaired.

Investigation
- Similar to that for chronic fatigue (see ➜ 'CFS 2', p. 383).
- Investigation should be geared towards excluding other contributors to fatigue:
  - full blood count including differential white count;
  - acute phase (ESR/CRP);
  - glucose and thyroid and liver function tests;
  - serological tests for chronic infection (EBV, *Toxoplasma*);
  - vitamin and mineral status (vitamin D, iron, especially in women, folate, vitamin B_{12});
  - serum immunoglobulins and lymphocyte surface markers if there is a history of significant infections.
- Routine diagnostic use of lymphocyte subset analysis and *in vitro* tests of NK- and T-cell function are not normally required for management.

Treatment
- Explain the cause of the problem.
- Advise a period of reduction of training to basal levels for a period of several months, followed by a gradual increase.
- Emphasizing the need to have peaks and recovery troughs in the training programme is essential ('periodization').
- Attention to diet and vitamin and mineral supplementation may be required.
- There is no good scientific evidence that high-dose vitamin C helps, but many sportspeople have empirically found that it reduces the susceptibility to infection. It may, however, cause renal stones as it is metabolized to oxalate. This may be a particular problem in athletes who are prone to dehydration during competition so it is important to emphasize the need for adequate hydration.
- Refer high level athletes to sports medicine specialist (English Institute of Sport can advise: ✎ http://www.eis2win.co.uk/pages/Sport_Medicine.aspx).

Depression and immune function

- There is a close link between mental state and immune function.
- Lymphocytes have receptors for certain neurotransmitters (catecholamines) as well as neurohormones (endorphins).
- Cytokines such as IL-1 affect cerebral function (fever, hormone release).
- Chronic or severe acute stress may both be immunosuppressive and lead to an increased risk of infection, through multiple neurohumoral pathways.
- Similar changes are seen in prolonged depressive illness.
- Findings may include:
  - minor lymphopenia and reduced NK cells;
  - poor NK function;
  - reduced immunization responses.
- Routine investigation of the immune system is not warranted unless there is evidence of a major susceptibility to bacterial or viral infection.
- Recognition and treatment of underlying cause is essential.

Immunology of infection

Dealing with infection is the primary function of the immune system and the reader is referred to the standard immunology textbooks for details of this. There are, however, certain clinically important points that need to be borne in mind when interpreting immunological tests taken in patients with active infection.

Neutrophils

- A neutrophilia, often with a left shift (i.e. immature cells newly emigrating from the marrow) and toxic granulation is a major early feature of bacterial infection.
- Severe neutropenia may also result from overwhelming sepsis due to consumption exceeding the marrow capacity for production.
- This must be distinguished from a primary neutropenia causing the infection. Bone marrow examination may help.
- If severe, G-CSF may speed recovery.

Monocytes

- Monocytosis is often seen in viral infections.
- Compensatory monocytosis is also seen during infective episodes in neutropenic patients.

Eosinophils

- Marked eosinophilia is a feature of parasitic infections.
- In the UK, marked eosinophilia with fever is more likely to be due to a hypereosinophilic syndrome with or without vasculitis, rather than an infection.
- Eosinophilia $> 10 \times 10^9$/l will be due to hypereosinophilic syndromes not parasites.
- Hodgkin's lymphoma may cause eosinophilia (and fever).

- Levels of eosinophil cationic protein (ECP) may be significantly raised and are important in diseases like Churg–Strauss vasculitis (eosinophilic granulomatosis with polyangiitis), as high levels of ECP are neurotoxic.

Lymphocytes
- Acute viral and bacterial infections often lead to a generalized proportional lymphopenia.
- In viral infections this will be followed by a rise in the CD8$^+$ cytotoxic T cells and a fall in CD4$^+$ T cells, leading to a marked reversal of the CD4:CD8 ratio.
- There is usually an increase in activation markers (CD25, HLA-DR).
- Lymphocyte subset analysis is not suitable as surrogate testing for HIV for this reason.
- EBV infection often leads to a marked lymphocytosis, with B cells followed by CD8$^+$ T cells.
- Very high B-cell counts may occur following EBV infection in bone marrow transplant patients where there are insufficient T cells to control the EBV-driven B-cell proliferation (B-lymphoproliferative disease).

Serum immunoglobulins
- Acute bacterial infection may lead to severe panhypogammaglobulinaemia; this may lead to erroneous diagnosis of a primary antibody deficiency.
- Repeat testing after infection has been treated.
- ❶Do *not* start IVIg until confirmatory tests have been carried out.
- More commonly, there will be an initial rise in IgM followed by a polyclonal rise in IgG which then returns to normal.
- Chronic infection will lead to significant polyclonal increases in immunoglobulins and may be accompanied by the appearance of monoclonal bands in the serum (from anti-pathogen clones).
- Bands are often multiple on a polyclonally increased background.
- Excess free light chains may also be found in the urine.
- Bands will disappear within a few months of satisfactory treatment.
- Persistently raised IgM or IgA may be found in tuberculosis.

Complement
- Viral infection tends to have little effect on complement.
- Acute bacterial infection will often lead to reductions of C3 and C4 (as well as factor B if measured).
- As complement components are acute-phase proteins, there may be normal levels despite significant consumption.
- Complement breakdown products will be increased.
- Haemolytic complement assays may show reduced activity related to critical reductions in one or more component(s) (usually in the terminal lytic sequence).
- Patients with bacterial endocarditis often show marked reductions of C3 and C4.
- In patients with suspected post-streptococcal nephritis, persistence of a low C3 beyond 6 weeks should prompt a check for a C3-nephritic

factor, an autoantibody that stabilizes the alternative pathway C3-convertase and leads to unregulated C3 cleavage.
- In patients with meningococcal disease, assay of haemolytic complement to look for complement deficiency should be deferred for at least 4 weeks: doing the tests early often leads to confusing results.

CRP
- Highest levels of CRP (> 300 mg/l) are seen in bacterial infection.
- Very highest levels (> 400 mg/l) are seen in *Legionella* infection.
- Beware of elevated CRP in infection with herpesviruses, especially EBV (levels up to 100 mg/l).
- High levels may also be seen in certain malignancies, including lymphoma and hypernephroma (may present as PUO).

Immunological diseases of pregnancy 1

Pregnancy is a form of allograft and non-rejection is a complex multifactorial process: readers are referred to major texts for detailed discussion.
- Immunological changes can be documented during pregnancy.
  - Reduction in T cells (mainly CD4⁺) which reaches a nadir around the seventh month.
  - Reduced NK-cell numbers.
  - B-cell numbers and function remain static.
  - Antibody synthesis and serum immunoglobulin levels are essentially unchanged.
- Despite the change from Th1 to Th2, there is no evidence for increased susceptibility to infection, with the exception of *Listeria*, which has a tropism for the placenta and requires macrophages and T cells for clearance (these are locally suppressed).
- There are no changes in solid organ allograft tolerance during pregnancy.
- Autoimmune diseases may behave unpredictably.
- Lupus may get worse or better during pregnancy, but may relapse immediately after delivery due to the sudden hormonal changes.
- Vaccine responses are normal.

Pre-eclampsia
- See 'Pre-eclampsia', p. 398.

Recurrent miscarriages
There are many immunological theories for recurrent miscarriages, but many have little in the way of supportive evidence.
- Antibody-mediated theory:
  - Anti-phospholipid antibodies—well substantiated.
  - Anti-sperm antibodies—not substantiated.
  - Anti-trophoblast antibodies—not substantiated.
  - Blocking antibody deficiency (anti-paternal antibodies): these antibodies are well documented but appear to be irrelevant to pregnancy outcome (agammaglobulinaemic women and mice have normal pregnancies).

- Absence of complement regulatory proteins CD55 and CD59 on trophoblast as a cause of recurrent miscarriage—no evidence so far.
- Cell-mediated theory:
  - Excessive Th1 response: some evidence of increased Th1 cytokines (γ-IFN and TNFα, both of which are abortifacient in mice) and Th1 responses to trophoblast antigens in recurrent aborters—this is a strong possibility.
  - Deficiency of Th2 cells/cytokines: no human evidence yet.
  - Deficiency of decidual 'suppressor' cells: uncertain whether this is cause or effect.
  - Inappropriate MHC class I and II expression: evidence in mice only; none from humans.
  - HLA homozygosity: no convincing evidence as inbred mouse strains reproduce normally.
  - Mutations in C3 have been associated with recurrent spontaneous pregnancy loss.

Laboratory investigation
- Screen for anti-phospholipid antibodies (cause microthrombi in placenta with placental failure):
  - Anti-cardiolipin IgG and IgM antibodies: IgM anti-cardiolipin antibodies are significant if persistent.
  - Anti-β_2 glycoprotein-1 antibodies.
  - Lupus anticoagulant: prolonged APTT—check dRVVT.
- Platelet count (APS patients have moderate thrombocytopenia, 80–120 $\times$ 10^9/l).
- Anti-thyroid peroxidase (microsomal) antibodies, anti-nuclear antibodies, antibodies to ENA (especially Ro and La) and dsDNA.
- C3 and C4.
- These tests should identify otherwise 'silent' cases of SLE.

Management
- Joint obstetric and medical management is required for such patients.
- Low-dose aspirin or heparin may be required.
- Treat APS patients with no previous history of thrombosis or pregnancy loss with low-dose aspirin alone.
- Those with a prior history of thrombosis should go on to heparin.
- Those with recurrent miscarriages and a previous history of thrombosis should go on to aspirin plus heparin.
- Heparin is associated with occasional severe osteoporosis in pregnancy. It is not yet clear whether this effect is also seen with low molecular weight heparins.
- Discuss the risks of these therapies fully with the patient.
- If these treatments are unsuccessful, then consider high-dose IVIg as an immunoregulatory agent. Counsel concerning potential infective risks (hepatitis, spongiform encephalopathies) and record information given in the notes.
- For recurrent miscarriages not associated with anti-phospholipid antibodies, the optimal treatment is unknown.

- Many manipulations have been tried but there are few good clinical trials. In 58% of untreated patients successful pregnancy may ensue, and this figure rises to 85% with good supportive psychotherapy.
- No convincing evidence that leucocyte transfusions, steroids, ciclosporin, progesterone (immunosuppressive in high doses), or other drugs make a significant difference.

Blood group incompatibility
- See ➲ Chapter 9 (haemolytic anaemia).

Alloimmune thrombocytopenia
- See ➲ Chapter 9.

Immunological diseases of pregnancy 2: autoimmune diseases and immunodeficiency

Autoimmune diseases
- Autoimmune diseases in the pregnant mother that are accompanied by IgG autoantibodies may occur in the fetus/neonate due to placental transmission of the antibody.
  - Myasthenia gravis.
  - Thyroid disease.
- This also confirms the pathogenicity of some antibodies.
- Mothers with SLE who are anti-Ro or anti-La antibody positive are at increased risk of having babies affected with:
  - neonatal lupus: photosensitive rash (made worse if the baby is given phototherapy for jaundice): self-limiting and disappears over first 6 months as maternal IgG is catabolized;
  - development of in utero complete heart block (Ro^+ = 2%; Ro^+/ La^+ = 5%).
- Congenital complete heart block is caused by anti-Ro antibodies crossing the placenta between 8 and 12 weeks' gestation and causing inflammation and subsequent fibrosis of fetal cardiac conduction system.
  - Death may occur in utero.
  - Survivors require immediate pacemaker insertion at birth (and require lifelong pacemakers).
  - Dexamethasone given during pregnancy crosses placenta and may reduce inflammation: it must be given early to be effective. Prednisolone is metabolized by the placenta and is ineffective.
  - 1 in 20 Ro^+ mothers will be affected; if there has been an affected pregnancy then risk rises to 1 in 4.
  - Anti-La may also be associated with congenital complete heart block.
- Children with neonatal lupus or congenital complete heart block are at increased risk of developing lupus in their own right.

Immunodeficiency

- Primary antibody deficiency may be diagnosed during pregnancy when routine testing fails to identify isohaemagglutinins in the pregnant mother.
- Replacement therapy should be started at once to ensure approximately normal levels of placental transfer.
- Failure to treat means that the neonate will be at significant infective risk during the first 6–9 months of life.
- If no maternal replacement has been undertaken, then the infant should be given at least 6 months of IVIg in normal replacement doses, while continuing to receive the normal childhood immunizations.
- Maternal infection (including rubella and the herpesviruses; see ➔ Chapter 2) during pregnancy, particularly peripartum, may also lead to neonatal immunodeficiency due to *in utero* or neonatal infection.
- HIV infection poses particular risks of vertical transmission.
- Schedules of prophylactic treatment with antiretroviral drugs are now used to reduce the risk of transmission.
- Congenital HIV infection may cause hypogammaglobulinaemia and unsuspected cases may present with recurrent bacterial infections rather than the opportunist infections seen in adults.

Pre-eclampsia and HELLP (haemolysis, elevated liver enzymes, low platelets) syndrome

- A syndrome of late pregnancy (5–7%) with severe hypertension, peripheral oedema, which if untreated causes fits and multi-organ failure.
- Cause is unknown, but excessive IL-6 release and a placental tyrosine kinase may contribute to maternal endothelial activation.
- Risk factors include:
  - anti-phospholipid antibody syndrome;
  - nulliparous women;
  - presence of anti-thyroid antibodies;
  - extremes of maternal age;
  - diabetes;
  - pre-existing hypertension and/or renal disease.
- Complement C4 is reduced.
- HELLP syndrome is a form of severe pre-eclampsia with haemolysis, elevated liver enzymes, low platelets.
- Urgent control of hypertension and rapid delivery are required for control of the syndrome.

Transplantation

Haematopoietic stem cell transplantation (HSCT) 1: clinical indications and types of HSCT

Clinical indications

- Severe combined immunodeficiency (SCID): all types (see
  ➲ Chapter 1).
- Combined immunodeficiency where there is reason to suspect progression, including:
  - Wiskott–Aldrich syndrome;
  - hyper-IgM syndrome;
  - activation defects (ZAP70 kinase deficiency, etc.);
  - MHC antigen deficiency (class I, class II);
  - X-linked lymphoproliferative disease;
  - purine nucleoside phosphorylase deficiency;
  - cartilage–hair hypoplasia;
  - DiGeorge syndrome (severe; thymic transplants also used);
  - chronic mucocutaneous candidiasis;
  - CD40 ligand deficiency.
- Neutrophil disorders, including:
  - chronic granulomatous disease;
  - leucocyte adhesion molecule deficiency (LFA-1 deficiency);
  - Chediak–Higashi syndrome (in accelerated phase);
  - Griscelli syndrome;
  - Shwachman–Diamond syndrome.
- Inherited metabolic diseases, including:
  - osteopetrosis;
  - Gaucher's disease;
  - adrenoleucodystrophy;
  - metachromatic leucodystrophy;
  - mucopolysaccharidoses (Hurler's syndrome, Maroteaux–Lamy syndrome, Hunter syndrome);
  - Lesch–Nyhan syndrome.
- Marrow failure due to:
  - Fanconi anaemia;
  - aplastic anaemia;
  - thalassaemia major;
  - congenital anaemia (Diamond–Blackfan syndrome).
- Lymphoma, leukaemias, myeloma, usually when in remission.
- Solid tumours (Ewing sarcoma, neuroblastoma, germ cell tumours, breast and ovarian cancer).
- Juvenile chronic arthritis.
- The use of stem cell transplantation is now being extended to a range of degenerative conditions.
- HSCT is now approved in the UK for adults with PID, subject to national MDT approval and restricted to a small number of centres with experience.

Types of HSCT

HSCT involves the reconstitution of the full haematopoietic system by transfer of pluripotent stem cells. This may be as unpurified bone marrow or manipulated to enrich stem cells.

- It may be classified according to donor source and site of harvest of stem cells.
  - Allogeneic—another genotypically matched individual acts as donor of stem cells. May be a sibling or matched unrelated donor (MUD).
  - Autologous—patient acts as own source for stem cells.
  - Bone marrow stem cells procured from direct puncture and aspiration of bone marrow before intravenous re-infusion.
  - Peripheral stem cells—stem cells liberated into peripheral circulation and then collected by apheresis.
  - Cord blood stem cells—stem cells collected from umbilical cord blood after delivery; these may come from cord blood stem cell banks.

All sources of bone marrow/stem cells may undergo *in vitro* manipulation to remove mature T cells (T-cell depletion) or accomplish stem cell (CD34$^+$) enrichment.

- T-cell depletion may be achieved by:
  - soya bean lectin and sheep erythrocyte agglutination;
  - alemtuzumab (Campath$^®$) antibody plus complement;
  - sheep erythrocyte agglutination;
  - depletion with antibodies to Tcr$\alpha\beta$ and CD19 (B cells).
- T-cell depletion and CD34$^+$ stem cell enrichment may also be achieved by magnetic bead separation.
- Type of manipulation may depend on underlying condition.
- Stem cells sourced from peripheral blood have 10-fold more mature T cells than stem cells isolated from bone marrow.

HSCT 2: conditioning and matching

Conditioning

- Conditioning is required to eliminate residual immune system and allow incoming stem cells to engraft.
- Recipient is treated with cytoreductive therapy including busulphan and cyclophosphamide.
- This leads to a severe aplastic phase during which isolation to laminar flow isolation and supportive transfusion are required.
- Complications of this phase include:
  - veno-occlusive disease;
  - alopecia;
  - severe mucositis;
  - immune suppression predisposing to wide variety of potentially fatal infections.
- Prophylactic IVIg, antibiotics, antifungals, and antivirals are used routinely.
- Regular surveillance and prompt treatment of infection is mandatory.

- Long-term complications include:
  - infertility;
  - hypothyroidism;
  - secondary malignancy;
  - late sepsis due to hyposplenism;
  - psychological disturbance.
- Reduced intensity or non-myeloablative conditioning regimens may be used in patients unable to tolerate the more toxic myeloablative chemotherapy.
- For many patients with SCID, donor stem cells may engraft without conditioning due to lack of recipient T-cell numbers and function normally required to reject a stem cell graft.

Matching

For all allogeneic transplants, MHC matching is required.
- Success of the transplant is dependent on the match. Preferred sources are ranked in the following order:
  1 Identical sibling matches.
  2 Matched unrelated donors.
  3 If neither are available, then haplo-identical parental bone marrow can be used or less well-matched unrelated donors.
- Where a SCID baby requires a haplo-identical marrow, paternal marrow is preferred, to eliminate any residual maternofetal engraftment.
- Fully matched whole marrow can be used from an identical sibling.
- Where there are mismatches, *in vitro* or *in vivo* T-cell depletion is used to remove mature T cells that are capable of producing GvHD.

Matching procedures
- (See ➜ Chapter 21.)
- Confirmation of the suitability of the chosen donor is checked pre-transplant by molecular typing.
- Mixed lymphocyte reactions (MLR) and CTLP or HTLP frequency (see ➜ Chapter 21) have been used in the past but are not commonly used now.
  - High levels of reactivity in these tests are good predictors of the development of GvHD.
- Immunosuppressants, including ciclosporin, methotrexate, mycophenolate mofetil, and steroids, are administered to reduce the risks of development of GvHD.

Marrow donation
- Donors are assessed medically and screened for transmissible infections, including EBV, HIV, CMV, and parvovirus.
- If there is a mismatch of viral status between donor and recipient, then prophylactic antivirals may be used.
- Whole marrow donors have to undergo a general anaesthetic for harvest, so cardiorespiratory fitness is essential.
- Marrow is now tested routinely for stem cell numbers, to assess the quality of the graft.

Stem cell harvesting
- Peripheral stem cell harvesting is also being used for patients with marrow that would be unsuitable for harvesting (i.e. infiltrated with tumour).
- In the autologous setting the advantages are:
  - better stem cell yield;
  - less contamination with tumour cells.
- In the allogeneic setting the advantages are:
  - easier to collect from the donor's perspective;
  - faster engraftment.
- This may be augmented by administration of CSFs to donor prior to apheresis.
- Donors of the bone marrow may also be used as apheresis donors for neutrophils to provide cover due to the aplastic phase post-transplant.

Procedural considerations
- Use of growth factors (G-CSF, GM-CSF) post-BMT in the recipient may speed up the reconstitution process and shorten the aplastic phase in the recipient.
  - There are concerns about long-term leukaemic risk from use of CSFs.
- All recipients must receive irradiated cellular blood products, to prevent accidental engraftment of viable donor lymphocytes until there is evidence of satisfactory immunological recovery.
- All blood products should be CMV negative unless the recipient is known to be CMV positive.
- *In utero* HSCT (injection of CD34$^+$ stem cells into the peritoneum of the fetus) is associated with lower risk of graft rejection but there is a risk of fetal loss and GvHD.

HSCT 3: post-transplant monitoring

Post-transplant immunological monitoring has an important role in optimizing management and, in particular, for assessing the return of adaptive immunity. Frequency of monitoring is dependent on clinical status. Monitoring should include the following.

Full blood count
- Indicates need for red cell and platelet support.
- Rise of the neutrophil count gives a good indication of when adequate protective innate immunity has returned.
- Neutropenia post BMT may last between 9 and 21 days.
- Neutropenia beyond 21 days suggests stem cells have failed to engraft.

Lymphocyte subsets
- Demonstrate when safe levels of CD4$^+$ T and B cells have returned.
- Rising NK-cell counts often precede infection and GvHD.
- Very rapid rises in B cells in the absence of T cells usually indicate B-lymphoproliferative disease secondary to EBV.

- These should be done at least monthly, or more often if there are problems.
- A basic panel will include CD4, CD8, CD3, CD16/56, CD25, HLA-DR, CD19, or CD20.
  - Other markers in combination (CD45RA, CD45RO, CD27) may be helpful in monitoring immune reconstitution in greater depth.

Acute-phase proteins (CRP)
- Provides early warning of infection.
- Regular monitoring is required.

Immunoglobulins
- Trough immunoglobulins—to assess adequacy of IVIg replacement (patients may be hypercatabolic and require increased doses) where IVIg is being used.

Lymphocyte proliferation assays
- Optimum panel of mitogens should include PHA, anti-CD3 (OKT3), and ConA.
  - PHA responses are the last to return.
  - ConA responses return earlier, followed by anti-CD3 responses.
- Flow cytometric assays involving CD69 expression do not correlate well with formal proliferation assays.
- Assays should only be requested when T cells can be detected in the peripheral blood.

Chimerism studies
- Genetic techniques (RFLP, FISH, karyotype) now allow analysis of the origin of separated cell lineages (using monoclonal antibody coupled to magnetic beads).
- In suitable patient–donor pairs, use of fluorescent anti-MHC antibodies may provide rapid information on origin of cells (host or donor).
- B-cell recovery is often host even when T cells are donor.
- Despite this, there is usually full immunological recovery of B-cell function, even if there is an MHC mismatch between T and B cells.

Other functional tests
- The use of specific tests may determine the return of function known to be defective pre-transplant and confirm the success of the transplant, e.g.:
  - flow cytometric analysis of oxidative metabolism of neutrophils in CGD transplants, where autologous reconstitution may be a concern;
  - CD40 ligand expression in transplants for hyper-IgM syndrome. *Note:* this assay is inhibited by prophylactic ciclosporin!
- Once prophylactic IVIg has been stopped, the development of IgG subclasses and specific antibodies can be followed.
- Formal humoral responses to immunization can be evaluated.
- Clues to satisfactory B-cell function include the return of IgM isohaemagglutinins, and rising IgA and IgM levels, as well as satisfactory B-cell numbers in peripheral blood.

HSCT 4: immunological reconstitution

- Rate of immunological development is dependent on:
  - the age at transplant: transplants at less than 3.5 months have superior thymic output;
  - conditioning regimen;
  - stem-cell dose;
  - donor source;
  - use of and type of T-cell depletion;
  - matching of MHC;
  - development of GvHD;
  - use of immunomodulation post-transplant;
  - infection: both pre-existing, which may lead to a furious response from the incoming graft, and infection acquired post-BMT.
- Under optimum conditions, evidence of lymphocyte engraftment is usually present within 28 days, but may be delayed up to 90 days.
- Long-term monitoring of humoral immune function and cellular reconstitution is required, as the very long-term outlook is as yet unknown.

T cells

- CD3$^+$ T cells are absent in the first month post-transplant and then gradually rise to normal by 3 months in an uncomplicated transplant.
- Early post-transplant period is characterized by rapid expansion of post-thymic derived T cells leading to uneven clonal expansion and skewed Tcr V gene expression.
- Reduced CD4$^+$ T-cell numbers may persist for a year or more.
- CD8$^+$ T cells reconstitute rapidly resulting in a reversed CD4/CD8 ratio.
- Thymic-derived 'naïve' CD4$^+$CD45RA$^+$RO$^-$ T cells are required for restoration of T-cell repertoire and start to appear after 6 months.
- Presence of T-cell receptor excision circles (TRECs) identify recent thymic emigrants.
- Complete regeneration takes up to 2 years and in some cases never fully recovers, with immune competence partly derived from the post-thymic T-cell compartment.
- T-cell function returns sequentially, with anti-CD3/IL-2 responses returning early and PHA responses occurring late (90–120 days).
- T-cell proliferation may be suboptimal for up to 1 year post-transplant.
- Drugs used for GvHD prophylaxis may affect T-cell proliferation assays.

B cells

- CD19$^+$ (CD20$^+$) B cells increase only slowly over the first 3 months post-transplant.
- Thereafter numbers increase to a plateau at 6–9 months.
- Early appearance of large numbers of B cells indicates either:
  - autologous reconstitution;
  - EBV-driven lymphoproliferative disease.
- During the first year post-engraftment, the majority of circulating B cells express an undifferentiated phenotype.

- Return of class-switch memory B cells (IgM–IgD–CD27$^+$) is slow.
- Recovery of normal B-cell numbers and function will take at least 2 years.
- Post-transplant Ig gene rearrangements are polyclonal and normalize at around 3 months.
- Gene rearrangements exhibit many fewer somatic mutations compared to normal.
- There is differential recovery of Ig isotypes:
  - IgM normalizes by 6 months;
  - IgG normalizes by 12 months;
  - IgA normalizes by 2 years.
- IgG$_2$ subclass levels rise only very slowly after transplantation, mirroring normal ontogeny.
- Return of isohaemagglutinins and a rising IgA and IgM are early signs that can be readily detected despite IVIg.
- IVIg is usually continued for at least a year (longer if there have been complications such as GvHD) and then stopped if there is evidence of Ig production.
- Occasionally B cells fail to engraft and autologous B-cell reconstitution does not take place: such patients need to remain on IVIg.

NK cells
- Massive expansion occurs within a few weeks with NK activity reaching normal within 1 month.

Poor outcome
- Some patients may have long-term evidence of immunodeficiency with recurrent bacterial infections, low serum immunoglobulins, poor specific antibacterial responses, and lymphopenia.
- These patients require long-term monitoring and prophylaxis, including IVIg.

HSCT 5: immunization post-transplant and results

Immunization post-transplant
- Current recommendations for post-HSCT vaccination schedules are based on good theoretical but limited study data.
- Donor antibody status is associated with response to vaccines, suggesting at least short-term adoption of donor memory cells.
- Killed vaccines are usually administered after IVIg has cleared from the circulation.
- A full course of 'childhood' immunizations is required.
- Live viral vaccines should not be given until there is evidence of good responses to killed or subunit vaccines and good *in vitro* T-cell function.
- Live vaccines should not be given in the 24 months after HSCT, and only in patients without ongoing chronic GvHD or immunosuppression.

- HSCT recipients are at particular risk of life-threatening encapsulated bacterial infections due to functional hyposplenism.
- BCG is contraindicated post-HSCT.

Results
- HSCT for acute leukaemia and lymphomas gives a 50–60% disease-free survival in first complete remission, falling to 30% in second remission and 15% in refractory disease.
- For SCID, the figures for long-term survival are dependent on the closeness of the match, age at transplant, and the presence or absence of infection at the time of transplant.
- In the best centres, over 90% survival is now regularly achieved for early matched sibling transplants, falling to 30% survival for late transplants in infected recipients with poor matches.
- Results are less good in adults.
- Potential developments:
  - Use of anti-CD117 (C-kit) mAb to displace autologous stem cells and enahance engraftment.
  - Improving thymic stromal function with keratinoctyte growth factor (KGF).
  - Acceleration of engraftment with IL-7 (currently in mouse models).
  - Reduction of post-transplant mortality using virus-specific cytotoxic T cells (CTLs).
- IgG_2 subclass levels rise only very slowly.

Gene therapy

- This is the holy grail of transplantation: engineering of the patient's own cells (preferably stem cells) to correct the genetic defect and cure the disease.
- Complications such as GvHD are avoided and prolonged immunosuppressive therapy is not required.
- The normal gene is delivered to the target cell using viral vectors (range of viruses tried).
- Problems have been identified with controlling the sites of integration of the inserted gene.
  - The retroviral vector used to correct XL-SCID inserted close to the *LMO2* gene (transcription factor involved in haematopoetic cells development) and the retroviral long terminal repeat activated the gene causing a T-cell leukaemia.
- For immunodeficiency, gene therapy has been successful in XL-SCID, ADA-SCID, CGD. Wiskott–Aldrich syndrome is also a potential target.
- Some transfers fail due to inadequate engraftment of transfected stem cells.
- Where there is a matched sibling donor, standard stem cell transplantation is still the preferred option.

Graft-versus-host disease (GvHD)

- GvHD occurs when transplanted immunocompetent donor T cells recognize HLA-mismatch and initiate an immune response.
- Major risk factor for development of GvHD is MHC disparity between donor and recipient.
- GvHD may occur, despite good matching by molecular techniques due to:
  - differences in the minor histocompatibility antigens;
  - non-MHC-encoded gene polymorphisms;
  - cytokine polymorphisms.
- A disease resembling GvHD may be seen in autologous transplants, possibly due to the development of autoreactive T cells.

Acute GvHD (aGvHD)

- Severe aGvHD is now rare due to improved matching and better T-cell depletion, in combination with stem cell enrichment.
- aGvHD is defined as occurring before an arbitrary 100-day period.
  - Manifestations of aGvHD may occur after day 100 post-transplant.
  - Classic chronic GvHD (cGvHD) may be present before day 100 and is better defined by clinical manifestations than timing.
- Development of aGvHD is a cause of significant morbidity and mortality.
  - Most deaths occur due to infection.
  - Infection occurs in aGvHD due to immunosuppression used to treat it.
  - aGvHD is itself immunosuppressive.
- aGvHD causes damage mainly to rapidly dividing tissues, particularly affecting:
  - skin;
  - liver;
  - gut.
- It is graded from I (mild) to IV (severe).
- Skin is the most commonly affected site with typical distribution of rash affecting palms and soles initially, progressing to face, head, and body.
- Main sign of GI involvement is diarrhoea (may be profuse).
- Hyperbilirubinaemia and raised ALP are seen with hepatic involvement.
- Diagnosis is usually obvious clinically.
- May be confirmed on biopsy, showing infiltrates of mature T cells with increased tissue MHC class II expression.
- Donor T cells in graft are causative.
  - aGVHD may be reduced by T-cell depletion.
- Tissue damage occurs due to direct cellular toxicity and high cytokine production (IL-1, TNFα, γ-IFN).
- Reduced intensity conditioning and cord donors are associated with a decreased incidence of aGvHD.

Prevention of aGvHD

- aGvHD prevention is attempted using immunosuppression and T-cell depletion.
- Prophylactic T-cell suppression is achieved with combinations of methotrexate, ciclosporin, tacrolimus, and mycophenolate mofetil.
- T-cell depletion is associated with higher engraftment failure and decreased graft-versus-tumour effect.

Treatment of aGvHD

Treatment of established aGvHD is difficult.
- First-line therapy is high-dose steroids ± ciclosporin or tacrolimus.
- Second-line therapy is anti-thymocyte globulin (ATG), alemtuzumab (Campath®-1H), anti-CD25, and/or anti-TNF monoclonal antibodies.
- Aggressive therapy early is important to prevent cGvHD.

Chronic GvHD (cGvHD)

- cGvHD is the most common non-relapse problem post-allogeneic transplantation and may occur in up to 10–15%.
- Risk factors for cGvHD include:
  - aGvHD (most important);
  - increasing age;
  - donor–recipient gender mismatch;
  - MHC mismatch;
  - lack of T-cell depletion.
- Disease may evolve:
  - directly from aGvHD ('progressive');
  - following a period of resolution ('interrupted');
  - de novo in patients with no history of aGvHD.
- De novo form has a good prognosis.
- Progressive form has a grim prognosis.
- Interrupted form has an intermediate prognosis.
- cGvHD has many features in common with systemic sclerosis and collagen vascular disorders.
- Features occurring most commonly are:
  - skin (lichen planus, pigmentation, scleroderma);
  - liver (raised bilirubin, transaminases, and ALP);
  - mouth (lichen planus, xerostomia, ulcers);
  - eyes (keratoconjunctivitis sicca, corneal ulcerations).
- Any organ may be affected.
- Complications:
  - gastrointestinal involvement results in fibrosis, abnormal motility, and malabsorption;
  - lung involvement may cause bronchiolitis obliterans and bronchiectasis;
  - infection is the major cause of mortality.
- Dysregulation of the immune system and cGvHD therapy lead to severe immunosuppression.

- Dysregulation leads to:
  - autoantibody formation;
  - hypo- or hypergammaglobulinaemia;
  - CD8$^+$ T-cell numbers are usually markedly increased.
- Steroids, mycophenolate mofetil, tacrolimus, and ciclosporin are used for first-line treatment.
- Second-line therapies include thalidomide, azathioprine, and monoclonal antibody therapy.
- Response rates to treatment are generally poor.
- Untreated, all patients will die.

Graft-versus-tumour (GvT) effect

- Antitumour activity is seen after stem cell transplantation in many patients, including those with CML, CLL, acute leukaemia, multiple myeloma, lymphoma, and renal cell carcinoma.
- GvT effect is dependent upon minor and major histocompatibility mismatch between donor and recipient.
- GvT is mediated by T cells and NK cells through receptors including killer cell Ig-like receptors (KIR).
- Patients with mismatch have an increased risk of GvHD.
- Current GvHD prophylactic therapies also reduce GvT.
- Strategies to exploit genetic differences to improve GvT whilst minimizing GvHD are being explored.

Graft failure

- Graft failure is associated with high mortality.
- Risk of failure is low with matched sibling but rises with degree of MHC mismatch.
  - < 5%, matched sibling;
  - 15–25%, 2–3 antigen mismatch.
- Failure can be defined as early (< 1 month) and late (> 1 month).
- Key factors are:
  - MHC mismatch;
  - conditioning (risk of graft failure reduced by increased conditioning);
  - T-cell depletion;
  - post-transplant immunosuppression;
  - pre-transplant alloantigen sensitization (non-PID) by blood transfusion, platelet transfusion.
- Graft rejection is mediated by T cells and NK cells.

Solid organ transplantation 1

Routine solid organ transplantation now includes kidney, liver, heart, lung, and pancreas. The shortage of donor organs is the major barrier to transplantation. Frequently, organs are less than ideal in terms of matching and infection status of the donor.

- For cardiac transplantation and liver transplantation, MHC matching is rarely carried out, due to the need to proceed quickly with the transplant procedure.
- Pancreatic transplants are matched for MHC and ABO status.
- For renal transplants more extensive matching is performed, including testing for pre-formed antibodies.
- Eventual outcome is dependent on the following:
  - Minimizing transplant immunogenicity by optimizing care of donor.
  - Reducing ischaemic time.
  - Limiting reperfusion injury.
  - Delay in retrieval of organs may increase the risk of contamination of the organ with candida.
- Screening and matching for CMV status should be performed if possible.
- High-dose IVIg, in combination with immunosuppressive therapy and plasmapheresis, has been used in highly sensitized patients, to reduce anti-donor antibodies, especially antibodies against MHC class II antigens.
- Anti-rejection therapy is usually commenced with three drugs (prednisolone, azathioprine, ciclosporin, tacrolimus, sirolimus (rapamycin), or mycophenolate mofetil).
- Treatment is reduced to two drugs after an initial period of up to 6 months (depending on progress).
- It has been observed for many years that both random and donor-specific pre-transplant blood transfusions improve the outcome (precise mechanism unclear).

Solid organ transplantation 2: immunology of rejection

Solid organ rejection is divided into four phases, and these are applicable to all types of organ.

Hyperacute rejection (< 24 hours)

- Mediated by pre-formed complement-fixing antibodies (usually anti-MHC class I or anti-ABO).
- These cause neutrophil recruitment and vessel thrombosis through platelet activation.
- There is fever and rapid loss of organ function.
- Often the organ is affected immediately, as soon as the clamps are removed and the organ is revascularized.
- Eculizumab (anti-C5 mAb, which prevent C5 activation) is being used experimentally to treat hyperacute rejection but if this fails the organ must be removed.
- C1-esterase inhibitor may also be beneficial.

Accelerated rejection (3–5 days)

- Mediated by non-complement-fixing antibodies, and recruitment of FcR-bearing cells.
- There is fever, swelling of the graft, and loss of function.
- Immunosuppression is only partially effective.

- Repeated attacks occur.
- Graft removal is usually required.

Acute rejection (6–90 days)
- Mediated by T cells ($CD4^+$ and $CD8^+$ T cells involved).
- Phagocytes are recruited.
- Antibody may play a role.
- Endothelium of the graft is a major target, along with interstitial elements such as tubules.
- There is loss of function, graft swelling, and tenderness, but less fever.
- Early recognition and aggressive immunosuppression with pulsed steroids, and anti-T-cell monoclonal antibody therapy is often effective.
- It may recur and progress to chronic rejection.

Chronic rejection (> 60 days)
- Precise mechanism is unknown.
- There is usually evidence of progressive fibrosis, with vascular damage, glomerular obliteration, 'vanishing bile ducts', bronchiolitis obliterans, or accelerated coronary artery occlusion, depending on the organ grafted.
- Treatment is relatively ineffective and graft function is progressively lost.

Prophylaxis of rejection
- In addition to the orally administered drugs, treatment with biologicals may be valuable (see ⮑ Chapter 16).
  - Anti-CD3 mAb: OKT3 has now been withdrawn, but other antibodies are being developed.
  - Anti-IL-2 (CD25): basiliximab and daclizumab are both used for prophylaxis of acute rejection.
  - Alemtuzumab (Campath®, (anti-CD52)) depletes T cells and has been used as induction therapy to reduce the requirement for other immunosupressive agents.
  - Belatacept, which blocks the B7 co-stimulatory pathway, is also being used as induction therapy.

Solid organ transplantation 3: immunosuppression and infection after transplantation

- To maintain transplant tolerance, solid organ grafts are supported with high levels of continuing immunosuppression over many years.
- This significantly increases the long-term risk of:
  - infections (including opportunistic);
  - EBV-associated post-transplant lymphoproliferative disease (PTLD);
  - malignancy (particularly skin).
- Grafting organs from CMV-positive donors into CMV-negative recipients may cause acute CMV infection in the post-transplant period.
  - Latent CMV may reactivate even in recipients who are CMV status matched.

- Valganciclovir or ganciclovir prophylaxis may reduce the incidence and severity of such episodes.
- Severe infection may be difficult to treat in patients who remain on high-dose immunosuppression.
  - A decision may be required to reduce immunosuppression and risk losing the graft.
- Improved chemotherapy regimens: PTLD treatment has been improved with the primary use of anti-CD20 mAb (rituximab) combined with antivirals, which has decreased immunosuppression.
- Preliminary data suggest that the use of autologous or allogeneic EBV-specific CTLs may have a significant role in treatment.

Immune function post-transplant

- Immune function post-transplant should be considered.
- Azathioprine may produce a persistent humoral immunodeficiency when used in high doses over long periods.
  - Patients may then start to develop recurrent bacterial infections and should be treated with replacement IVIg.
- Transplantation in early childhood (e.g. heart transplants) followed by immunosuppression may cause problems by interfering with normal immunological maturation, particularly with regard to the development of anti-polysaccharide antibody responses.
  - This is a problem mainly in those transplanted under the age of 2, when these responses will not have developed.
  - Surgery damaging the thymus in the under twos will also severely impact on subsequent immunity.

Solid organ transplantation 4: laboratory tests

- In the immediate post-transplant period the major clinical question is the presence or absence of rejection or infection.
- Biopsy with immunostaining is the mainstay of diagnosis.
- Markers such as β_2-microglobulin, sICAM-1, and sCD25 (IL-2R) may have a certain predictive value, but also tend to rise in infection as well.
- Procalcitonin appears to be sensitive for bacterial sepsis and is not elevated in rejection.
- Clinical assessment, knowledge of the temporal association of complications, and tissue histology remain the key indicators to distinguish infection from rejection.
- Patients on high-dose immunosuppression require monitoring of peripheral lymphocyte subsets to ensure that drugs such as anti-CD3 and anti-CD20 are effective.
  - ATG, in particular, suffers from batch-to-batch variation.
  - Enumeration of T cells and B cells identifies effective therapy with B- and T-cell depleting agents.
  - CH_{100} or assays of C5a–C9 will identify effective blockade of C5 by eculizumab.

- Failure of therapy with xeno-antibodies may be due to development of anti-mouse or anti-rabbit antibodies, which can be monitored.
- Patients on long-term chronic immunosuppression require monitoring of T- and B-cell numbers.
  - Full investigation of T- and B-cell function may be necessary when there are problems of recurrent infection in those on chronic immunosuppression (see ➲ Chapter 2).
  - This is particularly important in children receiving transplants followed by immunosuppression early in life (under 2 years of age).

Immunotherapy

Introduction

The aim of this chapter is to give an overview of the very complex but exciting area of immunotherapy. Despite great advances in the basic science, the results of clinical immunotherapy have not been as good as had been hoped. Nonetheless, the advances in basic immunology continue to provide new avenues to explore.

Major mechanisms of immunomodulation

- Immunization:
  - active;
  - passive.
- Replacement therapy:
  - immunoglobulin (IM, SC, IV);
  - C1-esterase inhibitor;
  - α_1-antitrypsin;
  - plasma.
- Immune stimulants:
  - drugs;
  - cytokines.
- Immune suppressants:
  - drugs;
  - monoclonal antibodies;
  - cytokines and antagonists;
  - IVIg;
  - antibody removal (plasmapheresis).
- Desensitization:
  - bees and wasps;
  - other allergens.
- Anti-inflammatory agents:
  - NSAIDs;
  - anti-cytokines (anti-TNF); IL-1ra;
  - anti-complement mAbs;
  - anti-endotoxin mAb;
  - anti-T cell/anti-B cell mAbs.
- Adoptive immunotherapy:
  - bone marrow transplantation;
  - stem-cell transplantation;
  - ?thymic transplants.

Passive immunization

Protection is provided by transfer of specific, high-titre antibody from donor to recipient. The effect is transient (maximum protection 6 months). Protection is immediate (unlike active immunization).

Problems

- Risk of transmission of viruses.
- Serum sickness (including demyelination); acute reactions.

- Development of antibodies against infused antibodies reduces effectiveness.
- Identification of suitable donors (Lassa fever; rabies).

Types
- Pooled specific human immunoglobulin, selected for high-titre antibodies.
- Animal sera (antitoxins, antivenins).
- ?Monoclonal antibodies (anti-endotoxin).

Uses
- Hepatitis A prophylaxis (but new vaccine provides active immunization and longer prophylaxis).
- Hepatitis B (for needlestick injuries), tetanus (Tetagam®), rabies, Lassa fever.
- Botulism, VZV (especially during pregnancy and in the immunocompromised), diphtheria, snake bites (post-exposure).
- CMV (transplant setting).
- Rhesus incompatibility (post-delivery anti-D).

Active immunization

The purposes of active immunization are to:
- stimulate the production of protective antibody (opsonization, complement fixation, enhanced phagocytosis, blocking uptake (virus neutralization));
- stimulate antigen-specific T cells: whether these are Th1 or Th2 cells depends on the type of pathogen and the optimal protective response;
- produce long-lasting immunological memory (T and B cells):
  - mediated by the retention of antigen on follicular dendritic cells in lymph nodes, leading to a long-term depot;
  - hence antibody levels often persist years after the primary course of immunizations have been completed, rather than decaying to zero;
- produce 'herd immunity': the generation of a sufficiently large pool of immune individuals reduces the opportunity for wild-type disease to spread, increasing the effectiveness of the immunization programme;
  - over 75% immunization rates are required to achieve this.

Active immunization can use:
- purified component, e.g. toxin (inactivated = toxoid);
- subcomponent;
- live attenuated pathogen (e.g. BCG, polio).

Active immunization can be combined with passive immunization (although this may reduce the development of long-term immunological memory).
- This approach is used for tetanus and rabies as a strategy for treatment, post-exposure.

Toxoid/subcomponent vaccines
- Immune response frequently requires augmentation with adjuvants.
- May be side-effects from adjuvants.
- No risk that disease will be produced.
- Inactivation may damage key epitopes and reduce protection.
- Safe to use in the immunocompromised but responses (and protection) unpredictable.

Attenuated vaccines
- Usually more immunogenic and do not require adjuvants.
- Risk of reversion to wild type (e.g. polio).
- Side-effects from culture contaminants (demyelination from duck embryo rabies).
- May produce mild form of disease (measles, mumps).
- Contraindicated in immunosuppressed (paralytic polio in antibody deficiency).
- Unexpected viral contaminants (SV40 and polio; hepatitis B and yellow fever).

General problems of active immunization

Active immunization has a number of problems, including the following:
- Allergy to any component (e.g. residual egg protein, often in viral vaccines from the growth media).
- Reduced/absent responses in immunocompromised (including splenectomy).
- Delay in achieving protection (primary and secondary immune responses require multiple injection schedules).
- Preferred route of administration (site of IM; SC, ID):
  - route of administration may determine the type of immune response;
  - route to be relevant for the route of infection of the pathogen (e.g. need for mucosal immunity to enteric organisms).
- Storage: most live vaccines require refrigerated storage to maintain potency; this may be a problem, especially in tropical countries.
- Age at which a vaccine is administered may alter the response, e.g. responses to polysaccharide antigens are poor in:
  - children under the age of 24 months;
  - the elderly.
- Maternal antibody, passive immunization, concomitant medical illness, and associated drug therapy may reduce the response.
- Ideally, responses should be checked serologically in patients where there may be a poor response.
- Serological unresponsiveness does not preclude good T-cell immunity (hepatitis B).
- Anti-self immune response to immunization (e.g. autoimmunity after meningococcus group B polysaccharide administration).
- Multiple immunogenic strains of target organism (e.g. *Meningococcus*, *Pneumococcus*).

Additional stimulation of the immune system

Poorly immunogenic antigens may be used if combined with agents that non-specifically increase immune responses ('adjuvants'). Adjuvants mimic PAMPs (pathogen-associated molecular patterns) and increase the innate immune response via TLR and augment the activity of dendritic cells macrophages and lymphocytes.

- Adjuvants:
  - 'depot' of antigen (alum-precipitated; oil); squalene;
  - non-specific stimulation (Freund's; MDP); Freund's adjuvant is too potent to be used in humans! It has however been safely used in microlitre quantities;
  - polymerization (liposomes; ISCOMS—Quil A);
  - ds DNA and ss DNA (which encourage endocytosis);
  - unmethylated CpG dinucleotides;
  - expression in vectors (e.g. use of vaccinia; chimeric viruses; BCG, *Salmonella*);
  - virosomes (membrane-bound haemagglutinin and neuraminidase from influenza virus)—facilitates uptake into antigen-presenting cells.
- Use of immunogenic carrier proteins conjugated to primary antigen:
  - tetanus toxoid;
  - diphtheria toxoid.

Modern approaches to vaccine development

Development of more potent but safer vaccines is always the goal.

- Molecular techniques have been used to modify pathogens through site-specific mutation, reducing pathogenicity, or by inserting the gene into a carrier (vaccinia, *Salmonella*).
  - Development of the host response to the carrier organisms means that it can only be used once.
- Molecular techniques allow the safe synthesis of bulk quantities of antigen (e.g. hepatitis B surface antigen).
  - Recombinant technique needs to be selected carefully to ensure appropriate post-translational glycosylation of the antigen.
- Recombinant organisms may also be used to target antigens to particular cells, for example:
  - *Salmonella* are rapidly taken up by macrophages;
  - inserted gene products will also be directed straight to antigen-presenting cells.
- Conjugation of poorly immunogenic antigens (such as polysaccharides) to immunogenic proteins (tetanus, diphtheria toxoids).
  - Humoral immune response to the polysaccharide switches from IgG_2 to IgG_1 and IgG_3.

- Specific peptides are being used experimentally to try to stimulate specific T-cell responses.
  - Epitope mapping of antigens to determine the T- and B-cell epitopes is required.
- Direct injection into muscle of nucleic acid (RNA, DNA) coding for specific genes, coupled to gold microsphere carriers or in plasmids, generates an immune response.
  - Nucleic acid is not degraded but is taken up into myocytes and specific protein production can be detected for several months thereafter, leading to an excellent depot preparation.
  - Concern over risk of bystander attack by the immune system on myocytes containing the injected DNA.

Generation of effective response

To generate an effective immune response, both host and pathogen factors need to be taken into account. Factors encouraging the development of an effective vaccine involve both infectious agent factors and host factors.

- Infectious agent factors:
  - one or a small number of serotypes; little or no antigenic drift;
  - pathogen is only moderately or poorly infectious;
  - antigens for B- and T-cell epitopes are readily available;
  - the immune response can be induced readily at the site of natural infection;
  - wild-type infection is known to produce protective immunity;
  - availability of animal models to test vaccine strategies.
- Host factors:
  - humoral and cellular immunity is readily induced;
  - MHC background of population is favourable to a high response;
  - proposed antigens induce appropriate Th1 or Th2 response.

Factors in the infectious agent that mitigate against an appropriate immunization response and therefore prevent the development of good vaccines include the following.

- Marked antigenic variation/drift; many serotypes causing disease: this limits the ability to generate an effective vaccine (e.g. pneumococcal disease).
- Potential for change in host range of the pathogen (e.g. change in cell tropism of viruses such as HIV).
- Infection may be transmitted by infected cells that are not recognized by the immune system even after immunization.
- Integration of viral DNA into the host genome (latency).
- Natural infection does not induce protective immunity.
- Pathogen uses 'escape' mechanisms:
  1 resistant external coats, e.g. mycobacteria;
  2 poorly immunogenic capsular polysaccharides;
  3 antigenic variation in response to host immune recognition, e.g. influenza virus, malaria;

4 camouflage with host proteins, e.g. CMV and β_2-microglobulin;
5 production of proteins similar to host proteins, e.g. enterobacteria; may give rise to autoimmunity;
6 extracellular enzyme production to interfere with host defence (staphylococcal protein A);
7 production of molecules that disrupt immune responses, e.g. superantigens.
- Pathogen-induced immunosuppression (HIV).
- Failure to form appropriate response (e.g. complement-fixing antibodies).
- No suitable animal model.

Host factors that mitigate against an appropriate immunization response and therefore prevent the development of good vaccines include the following.
- Immune response is inappropriate, e.g. antibody when cellular response is required (e.g. leishmaniasis).
- Immune response enhances infection, e.g. antibody formation may enhance infection through increased uptake into macrophages (yellow fever; ?HIV).
- Cells of immune system are target of infection.
- 'Wrong' MHC background predisposes to a low response or autoimmunity.

The ultimate goal of any immunization programme is the eradication of the disease. This requires that:
- the infection is limited only to humans;
- there is no animal or environmental reservoir;
- absence of any subclinical or carrier state in humans;
- a high level of herd immunity can be established to prevent person-to-person spread:
  - this requires considerable infrastructural support to ensure that all at-risk populations are targeted for immunization and that this is maintained (decline in herd immunity leads to resurgence of disease, e.g. diphtheria in Russia);
  - this has only been achieved for smallpox;
  - immunity for smallpox has waned as the immunization programme have stopped; bioterrorism with smallpox is a significant threat.

'Replacement' therapy

This is used for treatment of primary and some secondary immune deficiencies. See Table 16.1.

Table 16.1 Replacement therapies for some primary and secondary immune deficiencies

Type of deficiency	Replacement therapy
Antibody deficiency	Immunoglobulin (IV, SC)
α_1-AT deficiency	α_1-AT
Mannan-binding lectin deficiency	MBL (experimental—value uncertain)
Complement deficiency	C1-esterase inhibitor
	Fresh-frozen plasma (virally inactivated)?
Cellular immune deficiency	Bone marrow transplantation (stem cell transplant)
	Cord blood transplant
	Thymic transplant
Combined immune deficiency (SCID)	Bone marrow transplantation (stem cell transplant)
	Cord blood transplant
	Thymic transplant
	Gene therapy (ADA)
	Red cells (ADA)
	PEGylated-ADA
	Immunoglobulin (IV, SC)
	Cytokines (IL-2, γ-IFN)
Phagocytic defects	Bone marrow transplantation (stem cell transplant)
	Cord blood transplant
	Granulocyte transfusions
	Cytokines (G-CSF, GM-CSF, IL-3)

Intravenous immunoglobulin (IVIg) for replacement therapy 1

Manufacture and specification

- IVIg is a blood product, prepared by cold ethanol precipitation of pooled plasma.
- Donors are screened for transmissible infections (HIV, HCV, HBV).
- UK plasma is not used currently (risk of prion disease); no test currently available to identify prion disease in donors.
- Donated plasma is usually quarantined until donor next donates (avoids undetected infection at time of first donation).
- Donor pool usually > 1000 donors, to ensure broad spectrum of antibody specificities.
- Subsequent purification steps vary between different manufacturers but all are based on the original Cohn fractionation process.

- The IgA content is variable.
  - Significant levels of IgA may be important when treating IgA-deficient patients, who may recognize the infused IgA as foreign and respond to it, leading to anaphylactoid responses on subsequent exposure.
  - Uncertain how much of a problem this, and there is no standardized method for detecting clinically significant anti-IgA antibodies.
  - All current UK products have low/undetectable IgA.
  - Product must have low levels of pre-kallikrein activator, Ig fragments, and aggregates as these three can cause adverse events on infusion.
- Variations of IgG subclasses do not seem to make significant differences to the effectiveness as replacement therapy.
- Comparing the presence of functional antibodies in individual products is difficult as there are no internationally standardized assays, but IVIg must have intact opsonic and complement-fixing function.
- All licensed products must have at least two validated antiviral steps:
  - cold ethanol precipitation;
  - pH4/pepsin;
  - solvent/detergent treatment;
  - pasteurization;
  - nanofiltration.
- Model viruses are used to demonstrate that the process is effective.
- No product should be viewed as virally 'safe'.
  - Full counselling about risks and benefits must be given to patient, with written information, and this must be recorded in the medical notes.
  - Written consent must be obtained prior to therapy and retained in the medical notes.
  - A pre-treatment serum sample should be stored, to facilitate 'look-back' exercises if required.
- Liquid preparations are now preferred for ease of administration.
- Most manufacturers are moving to 10% solutions, with more rapid infusion times. For SCIg, 20% solutions are now available; standard SCIg is 16%.
- IVIg/SCIg is stabilized with sugars (maltose) or proline.
- IVIg and SCIg are in short supply due to the proliferation of uses (mainly high doses).

Supply issues

- Manufacturers are struggling to keep up with demand, both obtaining suitable plasma from safe/reliable sources and the manufacture. Viability of plasma fractionation for immunoglobulin is also dependent on sale of other plasma derived factors. However, the increasing use of recombinant clotting factors has reduced saleable yield from plasma and has impacted on the cost of immunoglobulin.
- Some countries have introduced strict guidance on approved uses of immunoglobulin (UK, Australia). In the UK, use has to be approved by a local/regional immunoglobulin committee according to a prioritization regime (Red = highest priority, Blue = intermediate, Grey = low, Black = not to be used). Data on use including batch numbers is collected on a central database.

- Problems for the NHS have arisen due to the initiation of central tendering for products to control cost: this has led to the suppliers of the cheapest products being overwhelmed by demand that they have been unable to meet and suppliers of more costly products that have not been endorsed by NHS-E withdrawing altogether from the UK market. All of this was entirely predictable and has resulted in severe supply disruption in the UK.
- Notwithstanding NHS-E guidance, products should NOT be changed except for clinical reasons. Anaphylaxis has been reported on product change. Changes cause unnecessary anxiety to patients and make look-back exercises in the event of infectious incidents much harder.
- Where change is required due to supply disruption, patients must be counselled and pre-change checks HIV/HCV status carried out. Samples should be stored against look-back exercises.
- Hospitals should ensure that they use a range of products, rather than relying on a single product, to reduce risk in the event of supply difficulty.

Uses

- IVIg (or SCIg—see ⊃ 'IVIg for replacement therapy 3: monitoring and home therapy', p. 428) is mandatory for:
  - replacement in the major antibody deficiencies (XLA, CVID);
  - in combined immunodeficiencies (pre- and immediately post-BMT).
- IVIg is also recommended in patients with secondary hypogammaglobulinaemia, such as CLL and myeloma, post-chemotherapy, etc. (see ⊃ Chapter 2).
- The role of IVIg in IgG subclass and specific antibody deficiency is less secure, and regular prophylactic antibiotics might be tried first, with IVIg reserved for continuing infection despite therapy (assess risk–benefit).
- Where there is doubt, a 1-year trial is reasonable, with monitoring of clinical effectiveness through the use of symptom diaries.
- To ensure a realistic trial, adequate dosing and frequency of infusions must be undertaken to ensure that benefit will be obvious.

Dose regimen

- Treatment should provide 0.2–0.6 g/kg/month given every 2–3 weeks for primary antibody deficiency, or as an adjunct in combined immunodeficiency.
- Older patients with CLL may manage on monthly infusions.
- Most patients on monthly schedules become non-specifically unwell or develop breakthrough infections after 2–3 weeks.
  - Under these circumstances the interval should be shortened.
- Rare hypercatabolic patients, or those with urinary or gastrointestinal loss, may require weekly infusions of large doses to maintain levels.
- Adjust dose according to the trough IgG level, aiming to achieve a trough IgG level within the normal range (6–16 g/l).
- Aim for higher trough in patients with established bronchiectasis or chronic sinusitis (target trough 9 g/l), as this will reduce lung damage.
- Breakthrough infections are an indication to re-assess interval and target trough level.

IVIg for replacement therapy 2: adverse reactions and risks of infection

Adverse reactions

- Most adverse reactions are determined by the speed of infusion and the presence of underlying infection.
- Untreated patients receiving their first infusions are most at risk.
- Reactions are typical immune complex reactions such as:
  - headache;
  - myalgia;
  - arthralgia;
  - fever;
  - bronchospasm;
  - hypotension;
  - collapse;
  - chest pain.
- Pre-treatment of the patient with antibiotics for 1 week prior to the first infusion reduces antigenic load and reaction risk.
- Hydrocortisone (100–200 mg IV) and an oral antihistamine (cetirizine, fexofenadine) given before the infusion are also of benefit.
- The first infusion should be given at no more than two-thirds of the manufacturer's recommended rate.
- Start slowly and increase rate in steps every 15 minutes.
- Similar precautions may be required before the second infusion.
- Reactions may occur in established recipients if:
  - there is intercurrent infection;
  - there is a batch or product change.
- Other adverse events include:
  - urticaria;
  - eczematous reactions;
  - delayed headache and fatigue (responds to antihistamines!);
  - medical problems from transferred antibodies (e.g. ANCA—uveitis);
  - aseptic meningitis—usually seen with hdIVIg, but occasionally with replacement doses.
- Products should only be changed for clinical not financial reasons.
  - Severe anaphylactoid reactions have been reported after switching products.
  - IVIg products are NOT interchangeable.

Risks of infection

- Infection remains a major concern.
  - Hepatitis B is no longer an issue.
  - There have been a significant number of outbreaks of hepatitis C.
  - Other hepatitis viruses (HGV) may cause problems.
  - No risk of HIV transmission, as the process rapidly destroys the virus.
  - Safety in respect of prion disease is not known but risk will be cumulative with continuing exposure.
  - Antiviral steps reduce but do not eliminate risk.
- Batch exposure needs to be kept to a minimum.
- Batch records must be kept to facilitate tracing recipients. In the UK batch data must be entered onto the national database.

IVIg for replacement therapy 3: monitoring and home therapy

Monitoring

- Check HCV PCR and baseline LFTs pre-treatment.
- Store pre-treatment serum long-term.
- Monitor trough IgG levels on all patients regularly (alternate infusions).
- Monitor liver function (alternate infusions, minimum every 3–4 months)—transmissible hepatitis.
  - Repeat HCV PCR if any unexplained change in LFTs.
- Monitor CRP—evidence of infection control.
- ▶Record batch numbers of all IVIg administered. This should be done through the MDSAS National Database in the UK.
- Use symptom diaries in appropriate patients to monitor infective symptoms, antibiotic use, and time off work/school.
- In the event of a significant adverse reaction:
  - immediate blood sampling for evidence of elevated mast-cell tryptase, complement activation (C3, C4);
  - consider sending sample for anti-IgA antibodies (if IgA deficient): value is uncertain;
  - screen for infection (CRP, cultures);
  - rare antibody-deficient patients seem to react persistently to IVIgs: changing to a different product or using SCIg may sometimes assist. Occasionally continued prophylactic antihistamines, paracetamol, or even steroids may be required before each infusion to ensure compliance with therapy.

Home therapy

- For patients with primary immunodeficiencies, home treatment is a well-established alternative to hospital therapy.
- This can be either with IVIg or more commonly SCIg, due to ease of administration of the latter.
- Most products can now be stored at room temperature, avoiding the need for refrigerators, and come as liquids ready to use.
- Criteria for entry to home therapy programmes are laid down in approved guidelines (see Table 16.2).
- Specific centres in the UK are recognized as being able to provide appropriate training.
- Patients should not be sent home on IVIg without formal training and certification by an approved centre.
- The centres will also arrange for long-term support, with trained home therapy nurses and support from community pharmacy suppliers.
- The patient support organizations (PID-UK: ℘ http://www.piduk.org/ and UKPIPS: ℘ http://ukpips.org.uk/) or UK Primary Immunodeficiency Network (℘ http://www.ukpin.org.uk) can provide details of approved centres in the UK. IPOPI (℘ https://ipopi.org/) can provide details of overseas contacts.
- Home therapy is not available in all countries for legal and/or financial reasons.

Table 16.2 Criteria for home therapy

Criteria for home therapy	Comments
4–6 months hospital therapy	Must be reaction-free
Must have good venous access (IVIg)	Consider SCIg if venous access poor
Patient must be motivated	
Patient must have a trainable long-term partner	Infusions must *never* be given alone
Patient must have access to telephone at site where infusions will be given	To call for assistance if problems
GP must be supportive	Rare for GP to be called
Patient must accept regular follow-up at training centre	Regular supervised infusions are advisable
Patient must agree to keep infusion logs with batch records	Essential for dealing with batch recalls, look-back exercises
Patient and partner must complete training programme, with written assessment	Training manual must be provided

Intramuscular and subcutaneous immunoglobulins for replacement therapy

Intramuscular immunoglobulin (IMIg)

There is no role for IMIg in replacement therapy. IMIg is still used for passive immunization (e.g. tetanus, VZV, rabies).

Subcutaneous immunoglobulin (SCIg)

For those with poor venous access, high-dose SCIg replacement is at least equivalent to IVIg in terms of maintaining adequate trough IgG levels and preventing infection.

- 16–20% solution of immunoglobulin is used.
- An SCIg with hyaluronidase to facilitate much higher dosing is available (Hyqvia®).
- Specific licensed SCIg preparations are now available from several manufacturers.
- It is administered in a weekly dose of 100 mg/kg via a syringe driver, in multiple sites. Daily push can be used as an alternative.
- One or two infusion pumps may be used, depending on type and availability.
- Rate is usually set to the maximum; some pumps use restrictors on the giving sets.
- 10 ml per site is the usual maximum tolerated dose per site.
- Tolerability is reasonable, with local irritation being the only significant side-effect.

- Home therapy can be undertaken (see ➲ 'IVIg for replacement therapy 3', p. 428, for guidance).
- Regular trips to hospital or GP will be required for trough IgG and LFT & CRP monitoring.
- Trough levels tend to run approximately 1 g/l higher than the same dose given as IVIg on a 2–3-weekly cycle.
- Electronic syringe drivers must be checked at least annually by a qualified medical electronics technician. Clockwork drivers require no servicing, but the springs may break.

C1-esterase inhibitor for replacement therapy

Deficiency of C1-esterase inhibitor causes episodic angioedema, which may be fatal if involving the upper airway (see ➲ Chapter 1).
- Purified C1 inhibitor is available in the UK as Berinert®, Cinryze®, Rhucin®/Ruconest®.
- Berinert® and Cinryze® are blood-derived products and carry the same risks as IVIg in respect of transmissible infections.
- Products undergo viral inactivation steps (steam treatment).
- Patients should have samples checked for LFTs and HCV status prior to each course of treatment.
- Appropriate consent should be obtained if possible.
- Batch numbers must be recorded.
- Indications for treatment include:
  - attacks above the shoulders;
  - surgical prophylaxis (including major dental work).
- Weekly administration has been used in pregnancy where there are frequent severe attacks.
- It is less effective against bowel oedema, but if pain is severe one dose should be given.
- Attacks involving the bowel should be treated with fluids, analgesics, and NSAIDs.
  - Surgery should be avoided unless there is good evidence for pathology unrelated to HAE.
- Dose is 10–20 u/kg administered as a slow bolus IV.
  - Manufacturer's information and guidelines suggest the higher dose is required, but this is not always true.
  - Levels of C1-esterase inhibitor level in the serum should rise to above 50% for several days.
  - Same dose is used for prophylaxis.
- ❶When used as treatment, it will prevent attacks progressing, but does *not* lead to a dramatic resolution of symptoms; accordingly, laryngeal oedema may require other measures, such as tracheostomy, as urgent procedures.

- Recombinant C1-esterase inhibitor, produced in rabbit milk (Rhucin®/Ruconest®) is now available; known allergy to rabbits precludes treatment because of a risk of anaphylaxis. Recipients must be screened annually for the development of anti-rabbit IgE antibodies. It has a shortened half-life compared to Berinert®, and is therefore suitable only for acute treatment.
- Purified blood-derived, nanofiltered C1-esterase inhibitor, Cinryze®, is also now licensed. As it is blood derived, unlike Rhucin®/Ruconest®, normal precautions relating to the use of blood products should be observed, as for Berinert®.
- Home therapy is possible and subcutaneous versions are available in some countries.
- Plasma can be used if the purified concentrate is unavailable, but is less effective and may even increase the oedema by providing fresh substrate for the complement and kinin cascades.
  - Pooled virally inactivated FFP is now available, and may carry a reduced risk of infection, although this is debated.
  - On the whole, plasma should be avoided unless there is no alternative in the emergency situation.

Other uses for C1-esterase inhibitor

C1-inh is being trialled in other indications including:
- adjunct to acute ischaemic stroke treatment (animal studies);
- treatment of acute antibody-mediated graft rejection.

Other immunotherapies for hereditary angioedema (HAE)

Other therapies are now available for the acute treatment of HAE, which avoid the use of blood-derived and recombinant C1-esterase inhibitor.
- Icatibant (Firazyr®) is a bradykinin B2 receptor blocking drug, which is effective at reducing the symptoms of acute attacks of HAE.
  - It is administered as a subcutaneous injection of 30 mg (repeated once, if necessary, after 6 hours).
  - It is now licensed for self-administration at home in the UK, and there is a home support programme in place.
  - It has a short half-life and is therefore not suitable for prophylaxis for surgery.
  - Injections can be painful and may limit uptake.
- Lanadelumab is a monoclonal antibody targeting kallikrein, now licensed for prophylactic use in HAE.
- Ecallantide (Dy88) is an inhibitor of plasma kallikrein and is licenced in the USA but not Europe for treatment of acute attacks.
  - The main concern is the risk of anaphylaxis from the drug (not good in patients with angioedema!).

α_1-Antitrypsin (α_1-AT) for replacement therapy

α_1-AT deficiency leads to progressive emphysema and to liver disease. Purified α_1-AT is now licensed for treatment, although its efficacy is still debated. No good prophylactic trials have been undertaken in asymptomatic patients, so it is not yet known how effective the drug is in preventing complications. Supplementation may also be useful during acute infections when high local levels of trypsin are released by activated neutrophils. Infusions need to be given at least weekly to maintain enzyme activity.

Mannan-binding lectin (MBL) for replacement therapy

Trials of MBL replacement therapy in deficient patients have not shown any significant clinical benefit.

Immune stimulation

- Specific immunostimulation.
- Specific immune stimulation = immunization (see ➜ 'Passive immunization' and 'Active immunization', pp. 418–19).

Non-specific immunostimulation

- A number of agents are now available that act as non-specific immune stimulators and have significant clinical benefit.
- Specialist literature should be consulted for current dose regimens.

BCG

- Direct stimulant of immune system; activates macrophages.
- Only found to be of value in bladder cancer.
- As it is a live agent, it should *not* be administered to those with concomitant immunosuppression (lymphoid malignancy, drug induced).
- Derivative of cell wall muramyl dipeptide (MDP) licensed in Japan to enhance bone marrow recovery after chemotherapy.
- Other bacterial products are under investigation (extracts of *Corynebacterium*) as immunostimulants.

Cimetidine

- Known to have immunoregulatory properties, not related to anti-H2 activity, as actions do not appear to be shared with other anti-H2 drugs such as ranitidine.
- Thought to reduce T-suppressor activity.
- Has been used with success in the hyper-IgE syndrome to reduce IgE and in CVID to increase IgG production.

Glatiramer

- An immunostimulatory drug, comprising synthetic peptides, administered by injection.
- Used in the treatment of relapsing and remitting multiple sclerosis.
- Side-effects include chest pain, allergic reactions, and lymphadenopathy.

G-CSF/GM-CSF

- Act on bone marrow precursors to increase production of mature neutrophils.
- Used as adjuncts to chemotherapy to prevent or reduce neutropenic sepsis.
- Used to mobilize stem cells for apheresis.
- Used to treat congenital neutrophil disorders: Kostman's syndrome, cyclic neutropenia, idiopathic neutropenia.
- PEGylated form of G-CSF available to increase duration of action.
- May increase the risk of myeloid malignancy.
  - Do not use in Kostman's syndrome where there are cytogenetic abnormalities, as risk of malignant transformation is increased.
- Bone pain may be a side-effect.

Interleukin-2 (aldesleukin)

- Licensed for use in metastatic renal cell carcinoma.
- Can produce tumour shrinkage, but no increase in survival.
- Intravenous administration is associated with a severe capillary leak syndrome.
- Rarely used.

Interferon alfa

- Main use now is in treatment of hepatitis C, in combination with ribavirin.
- PEGylated interferon is available, to increase duration of action.
- Also valuable in carcinoid tumours, hairy-cell leukaemia and lymphomas, myeloma, melanoma, and hepatitis B.
- Side-effects can be severe and include severe flu-like symptoms and a severe depressive state (suicide may be provoked): patients with a history of depression should *not* receive interferon alfa.
- Dose is determined by the condition treated.

Interferon beta

- Used in the treatment of relapsing and remitting multiple sclerosis (although support from NICE has been equivocal at best).
- Side-effects similar to those of interferon alfa but may also cause humoral immune abnormalities, and monitoring of serum immunoglobulins pre- and post-treatment is recommended.

Interferon gamma-1b (Immukin®)

- Interferon gamma-1b is used as adjunctive therapy in patients with chronic granulomatous disease for prevention and treatment of infections.
- It can also be used to increase response rate to HBV vaccination in poor responders.
- Side-effects include severe flu-like symptoms.
- Dose is usually 50–100 $\mu g/m^2$ three times a week.

Levamisole
- Originally introduced as an anti-parasitic drug.
- Found to increase circulating T cells, activate macrophages, and enhance DTH reactions.
- Used in RhA and as adjuvant in colonic cancer (FDA approved).
- May cause agranulocytosis (in HLA-B27⁺ patients).

Imiquimod
- This drug possesses antiviral and antitumour activity.
- Acts via TLR-7 receptor.
- Stimulates α-IFN production and NK-cell activity (switch to Th1 pattern).
- Used topically to treat genital HPV infection, actinic keratosis, basal cell carcinoma, and molluscum contagiosum.

Immunosuppressive/immunomodulatory drugs: corticosteroids

These drugs are based on endogenous products of the adrenal cortex and form the mainstay of immunosuppressive therapy; synthetic compounds are more potent. Natural steroids are highly plasma bound (corticosteroid-binding globulin; albumin). Actions of corticosteroids are manifold.

Actions
- Transiently increased neutrophils (decreased margination and release of mature neutrophils from marrow).
- Decreased phagocytosis and release of enzymes (lysosomal stabilization).
- Marked monocytopenia and reduced monokine (IL-1) production.
- Alteration of cellular gene expression (high-affinity cytoplasmic receptor translocated to nucleus) via NF-κB inhibition through increased cytoplasmic concentrations of IκBa.
- Release of lipomodulin (inhibits phospholipase A2 with reduction of arachidonic acid metabolites).
- Lymphopenia due to sequestration in lymphoid tissue and interference with recirculation (CD4⁺ T cells > CD8⁺ T cells > B cells) and lymphocytotoxic effects (high doses).
- Decreased T-cell proliferative responses (inhibit entry into G1 phase).
- Reduced serum IgG and IgA.
- No effect on NK or antibody-dependent cell-mediated cytotoxicity (ADCC) activity.

Side-effects
- Carbohydrate metabolism: poor cellular glucose uptake; increased hepatic gluconeogenesis; and glycogen deposition.
- Increased lipolysis and free fatty acid (FFA); increased selective fat deposition.
- Inhibit protein synthesis and enhance protein catabolism.

- Increase glomerular filtration rate (GFR) and sodium retention; decrease calcium absorption, inhibit osteoblasts.
- Clinical side-effects are multitudinous:
  - diabetes;
  - hyperlipidaemia;
  - obesity;
  - poor wound healing;
  - growth arrest (children);
  - myopathy;
  - hypertension;
  - purpura and skin thinning;
  - cataracts;
  - glaucoma;
  - peptic ulcer;
  - allergy (synthetic steroids);
  - avascular necrosis;
  - psychiatric complications;
  - thrush.
- Patients on medium- to long-term treatment require regular checks of blood pressure, blood sugar, and bone mineral density.
- Prophylactic therapy against bone loss is highly desirable, especially in females and all older patients.
  - Optimal therapy is yet to be determined but includes hormone replacement therapy (HRT; if not contraindicated by underlying disease), vitamin D and calcium, or oral bisphosphonate.
- Doses of over 20 mg/day for long periods may also increase the risk of opportunist infection with *Pneumocystis jirovecii*; consideration should therefore be given to the use of low-dose co-trimoxazole or alternative as prophylaxis.

Uses

- Autoimmune diseases, e.g. SLE, vasculitis, rheumatoid arthritis.
- Polymyalgia rheumatica, giant-cell arthritis.
- Allergic diseases (asthma, hay fever).
- Inflammatory diseases (Crohn's disease).
- Malignant disease (lymphoma).
- Allograft rejection.
- Other immunological diseases (ITP, glomerulonephritis).

Dosage regimens

- Variable according to the disease being treated, and up-to-date literature should always be consulted.
- Prednisolone is the stock drug. Other steroids have little advantage but the BNF has equivalency tables.
- Enteric-coated tablets are kinder to patients, but may lead to erratic absorption and are more expensive.
- If plain steroids are used, gastroprotection with either an H2-antagonist or proton-pump inhibitor is most effective in preventing ulceration.
- Low-dose steroids for RhA (prednisolone 7.5 mg/day) have been used: most patients are now on methotrexate or anti-TNF agents.

- For SLE higher doses (up to 30 mg/day) are required (larger doses for cerebral lupus).
- Life-threatening immunological disease requires much higher doses, 1–2 mg/kg, orally or IV.
- Various pulsed regimens using IV methylprednisolone have been advocated, especially in acute vasculitis. The evidence is split over their effectiveness: 10 mg/kg is advocated, pulsed at varying intervals, often in combination with IV cytotoxics.
- Topical steroids with limited absorption are invaluable in controlling local allergic symptoms (asthma, hay fever).
- Where patients who have been on long-term steroids are being tailed off, adrenal suppression may persist for up to 6 months after cessation of therapy: patients should therefore have steroid cover for illnesses, operations, etc. Short tetracosactide (Synacthen®) testing should be carried out. Patients should carry warning cards.

Immunosuppressive/immunomodulatory cytotoxic drugs: azathioprine

Azathioprine is converted *in vivo* to 6-mercaptopurine and acts to inhibit the synthesis of inosinic acid (precursor of purines) thus inhibiting DNA synthesis and reducing cell replication.

Actions

- Preferentially inhibits T-cell activation rather than B-cell activation.
- Reduces the circulation of large 'activated' lymphocytes, but has little effect on small resting lymphocytes.
- Long-term use causes significant lymphopenia (T and B cells).
- Hypogammaglobulinaemia, due to inhibition of B-cell proliferation (less or no effect on T-cell proliferation).
- Suppression of monokine production.

Side-effects

- Causes profound bone marrow suppression: this is related to deficiency alleles of the enzyme thiopurine methyltransferase (TPMT) involved in its metabolism.
  - Screening for enzyme levels is widely available.
- Toxic hepatitis (?related to TPMT deficiency).
- Opportunist infections (including HSV, papillomaviruses).
- Gastric upset (probably unrelated to TPMT deficiency).
- Teratogenicity.
- ?Malignancy (lymphoma).
- PUO syndrome (hypersensitivity).

Uses

- Autoimmune diseases (SLE, rheumatoid arthritis, vasculitis, liver disease, myasthenia, inflammatory bowel disease).
- As a 'steroid-sparing' agent.

Dosage

- In view of the potential for severe/fatal side-effects, azathioprine must be introduced carefully.
- Initial dose should not exceed 1 mg/kg and the patient should receive weekly full blood counts with a differential white count for the first month of therapy.
- If there is any decrease in platelets or white cells, it is unsafe to continue with therapy.
- Deficiency alleles for TPMT are present in 1 in 300 of the population: pre-treatment screening is helpful.
- If it is tolerated, then the dose can be increased to 2.5 mg/kg (or in special circumstances to 4 mg/kg).
- The need for continuing therapy needs to be reviewed regularly.
- Hypogammaglobulinaemia may be severe and require replacement therapy, although recovery may eventually occur over several years.
- Liver function tests must also be monitored.

❶Allopurinol is contraindicated with azathioprine as it interferes with elimination and raises blood levels.

Immunosuppressive/immunomodulatory cytotoxic drugs: cyclophosphamide and chlorambucil (alkylating agents)

These drugs bind to and cross-link DNA and possibly also RNA, thus interfering with DNA replication and transcription. Effects are dependent on the phase of the cell cycle during exposure and the competence of the DNA repair mechanisms.

Actions

- Dose-dependent lymphopenia (T (CD8 > CD4) and B cells).
- Reduced B-cell proliferation and antibody synthesis (reduced IgG and IgM).
- Lesser effect on T cells (CD8 >> CD4, which may actually enhance T-cell responsiveness under certain circumstances).

Side-effects

- Bone marrow depression.
- Alopecia.
- Haemorrhagic cystitis (caused by acrolein)—ensure good hydration and use mesna for doses above 200 mg/kg. May be less risk with pulsed IV therapy.
- Sterility (males and females—offer males sperm banking; warn all patients of reproductive age and record in notes).
- Secondary lymphoid neoplasms (especially NHL (11-fold increase), bladder tumours (10% long-term), skin tumours (fivefold increase), and acute myeloblastic leukaemia).

- Opportunist infections (use co-trimoxazole, or alternative, and antifungal prophylaxis).
- Nausea and vomiting (high dose).

Major uses
- Vasculitis, especially Wegener's granulomatosis, PAN, MPA, CSS.
- SLE and RhA.
- Glomerulonephritis (including Goodpasture's).

Dosage
- There is considerable debate over the optimal regimens for use of cyclophosphamide.
  - Continuous low-dose oral cyclophosphamide (2–4 mg/kg/day).
  - Intravenous pulse therapy (10 mg/kg/pulse or 0.75–1 g/m² body surface area; intervals determined by protocol and blood counts).
- Long-term side-effects may be higher with continuous oral therapy, but this may reflect the higher total dose, and lower doses may be effective.
- Cumulative total dose of cyclophosphamide should be monitored, as long term risks of malignancy relate to high cumulative dose.
- In life-threatening conditions, high-dose IV pulses, with IV steroids, will have a faster effect (remember mesna cover and IV fluids).
- Chlorambucil is used orally in doses of 0.03–0.06 mg/kg/day and is less toxic to the bladder than cyclophosphamide, but probably equally toxic to the marrow in therapeutic doses.
- Dosages of both drugs will require adjustment in renal impairment. Regular blood counts are required, according to current local protocols.
- New haematuria in a patient treated with cyclophosphamide should trigger investigation for bladder cancer.

Immunosuppressive/immunomodulatory cytotoxic drugs: methotrexate (MTX)

Methotrexate is a competitive inhibitor of the enzyme dihydrofolate reductase and impairs synthesis of tetrahydrofolate from folic acid (required as cofactor for thymidine synthesis). It therefore interferes with DNA synthesis. It is also thought to interfere with other intracellular enzymes. As an immunosuppressive agent it is used in low weekly doses (much lower than the doses used as an antineoplastic agent). Low-dose MTX probably inhibits the enzyme 5-amino-imidazole-4-carboxamide ribonucleotide (AICAR) transformylase, leading to the accumulation of AICAR and increased adenosine.

Actions
- Variable effects on lymphocyte numbers in peripheral blood.
- Possible inhibition of monokine production.
- Inhibition of lipoxygenase pathway.
- Reduction in antibody synthesis.
- Converted to methotrexate polyglutamates, which persist long term intracellularly and are potent inhibitors of AICAR transformylase and dihydrofolate reductase.

Side-effects

- Mucositis, nausea, and vomiting.
- Bone marrow suppression (megaloblastic—may be reversed by folinic acid rescue): may be worse if other anti-folate drugs are co-administered, e.g. sulfasalazine, co-trimoxazole.
- Hepatic fibrosis (dose related).
- Pneumonitis (5% of patients), a hypersensitivity reaction.
- Sterility.

Uses

- RhA; psoriatic arthropathy.
- Polymyositis/dermatomyositis.
- GvHD in BMT.
- Adjunctive therapy with infliximab (see ➋ 'Immunosuppressive/immunomodulatory biologicals: anti-TNF agents', p. 451).

Dosage

- The drug is given *weekly* either orally or IM.
- Initial dose is 7.5 mg (adult), increased stepwise depending upon side-effects and clinical benefit to a maximum of 20–30 mg/week.
- Dose may need reducing in renal impairment.
- Care needs to be taken with co-administration of other drugs.
- Folinic acid may reduce risk of bone marrow toxicity and mucositis (given 24–36 hours later). Folic acid will not be effective as MTX inhibits its conversion to the active form.

⊙: The most frequent cause of side-effects, including death, is the inadvertent daily administration of the drug—always check prescriptions carefully. Do not rely on pharmacy systems to spot errors.
- Baseline tests should include FBC, LFTs, chest radiograph, and lung function.
- Monitor weekly (initially) pre-dose full blood counts and regular liver function tests.
  - If abnormal LFTs are noted, the drug dose should be reduced or the drug stopped.
  - It is thought that the risks of monitoring for liver disease by biopsy outweigh any benefit.
- Development of pneumonitis is an absolute indication for withdrawing the drug: high-dose steroids may be required.

Immunosuppressive/immunomodulatory cytotoxic drugs: cladribine (2-chlorodeoxyadenosine, 2CDA) and fludarabine

- Mode of action is by inhibition of adenosine deaminase, i.e. effectively producing ADA-deficient severe combined immunodeficiency.
- Primary use is in the treatment of haematological malignancy (B-cell tumours), but they have the potential, with careful use, to be potent immunosuppressive agents.

- Both produce a profound and long-lasting B-cell and CD4+ T-cell lymphopenia.
- Prophylactic antibiotics (co-trimoxazole) and antifungals are advisable.
- Long-term monitoring of lymphocyte surface markers and serum immunoglobulins is advisable after treatment.

Immunosuppressive/immunomodulatory drugs: ciclosporin (CyA)/tacrolimus (FK506)/sirolimus (rapamycin)

These three agents are macrolide antibiotics derived from fungi. They act specifically on T-helper cells, but leave other cell types unaffected. Target cells are inhibited but not killed (therefore effects are fully reversible on cessation of treatment).

Modes of action

- Ciclosporin (CyA) interacts with cyclophilin, a 17 kDa protein (peptidyl-prolyl *cis–trans* isomerase) and tacrolimus interacts with FK-BP12, a 12 kDa protein, similar to cyclophilin.
- Complex prevents calcineurin, a calcium- and calmodulin-dependent protein, from dephosphorylating the nuclear factor of activated T cells (NF-AT), reducing transcription of the *IL2* gene.
- Immunosuppressive activity is not directly related to this activity.
- CyA and tacrolimus inhibit *IL2* and *IL2RA* gene expression and prevent T-cell activation (cells arrested at G0/G1).
- Sirolimus has no effect on IL-2 production; it binds FK-BP12, but the complex does not inhibit calcineurin; it appears to block calcium-independent signalling (via CD28) and inhibits mTOR.
- May interfere with macrophage function (lymphokine release and receptor synthesis).
- CyA interferes with B-cell proliferation and antibody production.
- Pimecrolimus is an analogue of tacrolimus which is available for topical use.

Side-effects

- Hypertension.
- Hirsutism.
- Nephrotoxicity.
- Hepatotoxicity.
- Lymphomas (NHL—85% EBV+).
- Opportunist infections (CMV, papillomaviruses, HHV-8).
- Neurotoxicity.
- Multiple drug interactions (CyA and tacrolimus induce cytochrome P450(IIIEI)).
- Diabetes (inhibition of insulin release).
- Headache.

Uses

- Combination therapy for allografts.
- RhA, SLE.
- Autoimmune diseases (uveitis, Behçet's, inflammatory bowel disease).
- Topical tacrolimus and pimecrolimus are used to treat atopic dermatitis and other immunological skin conditions, as they are small molecules that penetrate the skin.

Dosage

- CyA and tacrolimus are available orally and intravenously.
- Dosage for CyA depends on the circumstances, but 10–15 mg/kg/day may be required for allograft rejection, while 5 mg/kg may suffice for autoimmune disease.
- Tacrolimus dosage is 0.1–0.3 mg/kg/day for allograft rejection; experience of this drug is less in autoimmune disease, but doses up to 0.1 mg/kg/day in divided doses appear to be effective.
- Monitoring of drug levels is desirable for both drugs: this can prevent toxicity and monitor compliance.
- Sirolimus dosage is 6 mg as a stat dose followed by 2 mg daily, with drug monitoring and appropriate dosage changes, in allografts. Dosages for use in autoimmune disease are not defined—check for local protocols.
  - Because it operates on different activation pathways it may make a useful combination treatment.
- Creatinine and electrolytes, liver function, and blood pressure should be monitored regularly.
- ❶Now that generic versions are available it is essential that the brand is specified, especially in the transplant setting, as the bioavailability of the different products is NOT the same; transplanted organs have been lost because of inadvertent product switches.

Immunosuppressive/immunomodulatory drugs: mycophenolate mofetil (MMF)

This drug is a prodrug of mycophenolic acid. In its actions it is similar to azathioprine and can be used as a replacement. It is usually well tolerated. Mycophenolic acid (Myfortic®) can be used as an alternative and may be tolerated where MMF is not.

Mode of action

- Blocks inosine monophosphate dehydrogenase and blocks synthesis of guanine, but has no effect on salvage pathway.
- It acts predominantly on lymphocytes, to prevent proliferation, but has little effect on non-lymphoid cells.

Side-effects

- Lymphopenia.
- Opportunist infections (CMV, HSV); PML.

- Lymphoma.
- Hepatotoxicity; pancreatitis.
- Electrolyte disturbance (hyperkalaemia, hypomagnesemia, hypocalcaemia).
- Breathing problems and pleural effusions; pulmonary fibrosis.
- Recognized to be teratogenic to males and females. Advise appropriate contraception and check local drug regulatory authority advice (MHRA in UK).

Uses
- Prophylaxis of allograft rejection.
- Autoimmune disease: SLE nephritis; uveitis.

Dosage
- Dosage is 0.5–1 g twice a day, increased to maximum of 1.5 g twice daily.
- It is also available for intravenous infusion.
- Mycophenolic acid (Myfortic®) is given in a dose of 720 mg twice daily (equivalent to MMF 1 g twice daily).
- FBC and LFTs should be monitored regularly.

Immunosuppressive/immunomodulatory drugs: leflunomide

- After oral administration is converted to an active metabolite that inhibits dihydro-orotate dehydrogenase (involved in pyrimidine synthesis and required by T cells).
  - T-cell proliferation is blocked.
- Used in RhA: as effective as methotrexate.
- Teriflunomide, an activate metabolite, is now marketed for the treatment of MS.
- Onset of action is slow (4–6 weeks).
- Side-effects include severe hepatotoxicity and Stevens–Johnson syndrome.
  - Drug can be 'washed-out' with colestyramine or activated charcoal (binds it in the gut).
- It is teratogenic: effective contraception is required.
- Dose is 100 mg daily for 3 days; then 10–20 mg daily.
- Monitoring with regular FBC and LFTs mandatory.

Immunosuppressive/immunomodulatory drugs: penicillamine and gold

Penicillamine
This enigmatic drug comes and goes in terms of its utility as an immunomodulator.

- Precise immunological actions are not known.
  - It decreases antibody production.
  - It inhibits T-cell proliferation, possibly through enhanced hydrogen peroxide production or through sulphydrylation of the surface receptors of the lymphocytes.
  - Neutrophil chemotaxis and oxidative function are impaired.
  - Macrophage antigen-presenting function and monokine production are reduced.
- Also believed to inhibit collagen synthesis; hence its use in scleroderma.
- Very slow in its onset of action.
- Main side-effects include a range of autoimmune diseases, including myasthenia gravis, renal disease (nephrotic), SLE, polymyositis, and Goodpasture's syndrome.
- Mainly used in RhA and scleroderma, but has fallen out of favour due to side-effects.
- Dosage is 250 mg daily increased to 1 g daily.
- Regular monitoring (every 1–2 weeks initially) of renal function, urinalysis, and FBC required.
- Penicillin-allergic patients may be at increased risk of reacting to penicillamine.

Gold

- Gold may be given either as IM injections or orally: evidence suggests that parenteral therapy is more effective.
- Concentrated selectively in macrophages, and reduces monokine production (IL-1); hence also reducing T- and B-cell responses.
- Impairs endothelial expression of adhesion molecules and hence reduces cellular traffic to sites of inflammation.
- Profile of side-effects is similar to that of penicillamine, and the onset of action is also slow.
- It is used only in RhA: now mainly replaced by anti-TNF agents and methotrexate.
- Dosage is dependent on the route and expert advice on current regimens should be sought from a clinician experienced in its use.
- ❶Both gold and penicillamine are strongly associated with the development of late secondary hypogammaglobulinaemia.

Immunosuppressive/immunomodulatory drugs: hydroxychloroquine/mepacrine

- Antimalarials have a particular role to play in the management of joint and skin complaints in connective tissue diseases.
- Effective in relieving the fatigue experienced in association with connective tissue diseases such as SLE and Sjögren's syndrome.
- Mode of clinical action is uncertain.
  - Interfere with the production of cytokines and reduction of production of granulocyte lysosomal enzymes; drug accumulates in lysosomes

- Decrease chemotaxis, phagocytosis and superoxide production in neutrophils
- Inhibit TLR9 and reduce antigen presentation by dendritic cells to T cells.
- Anti-platelet action demonstrated: may be valuable in anti-phospholipid syndrome.
- Onset of action is slow.
- Well tolerated with few side-effects.
- Haemolysis may occur in G6PD-deficient patients.
- Retinal toxicity is possibly a problem with hydroxychloroquine, and definitely a problem with chloroquine (not used in rheumatic disease now).
  - Evidence that there is a significant risk of ocular toxicity from hydroxychloroquine is minimal in normal doses. Cumulative dose > 1000 g is associated with risk.
  - Annual follow-up by optometrist recommended.
  - Near vision should be recorded with test type before starting treatment; then at 6–12-month intervals thereafter.
  - Loss of colour discrimination may be an early sign.
- Hydroxychloroquine may cause nausea and vomiting which can be severe and usually occurs during the initiation phase.
- Haemolysis may occur in G6PD-deficient individuals—this affects children more than adults.
- Mepacrine stains the skin yellow.
- Preferred antimalarial is hydroxychloroquine.
  - Starting dose for hydroxychloroquine is 400 mg/day (adult), reducing to maintenance of 200 mg/day. Alternatively the maximum daily dose is calculated as 6.5 mg/kg lean body mass.
- Mepacrine is an unlicensed drug in the context of autoimmune disease, and the dose is 50–100 mg per day.

Immunosuppressive/immunomodulatory drugs: thalidomide and analogues/ oxypentifylline

- Thalidomide is an interesting drug that reduces the severity of conversion reactions due to treatment of lepromatous leprosy.
- Mechanisms of action:
  - Potent inhibition of TNFα production by monocytes, due to interference with gene transcription.
  - Decrease in the expression of adhesion molecules.
  - Reduction of circulating CD4$^+$ T cells.
  - Inhibition of γ-interferon production by T cells, due to preferential stimulation of Th2 cells.
  - Inhibition of angiogenesis.
  - Inhibition of IL-6 production.
  - Activation of apoptotic pathways via caspase 8.

- Side-effects include its well-documented teratogenicity, neuropathy, and drowsiness (which may limit dose).
- It is used in the management of ulceration in Behçet's syndrome and in reducing the severity of GvHD.
- It is used with benefit in multiple myeloma, with dexamethasone.
- Dosage is 100 mg/day, reducing to 50 mg on alternate days.
- It is an unlicensed drug in the UK and is only available from the manufacturer if the patient is enrolled in a monitoring programme.
- Nerve conduction studies should be carried out as a baseline pre-treatment, and at intervals on treatment.
- Women of child-bearing age must be formally counselled over the risks and agree to take appropriate contraceptive measures. This must be recorded in the notes.
- Lenalidomide is a derivative of thalidomide, introduced for treatment of multiple myeloma and myelodysplastic syndromes. It has direct anti-tumour effects (apoptosis), inhibition of the microenvironment via anti-angiogenic and anti-osteoclastic activity.
- Pomalidomide is another derivative of thalidomide undergoing clinical trials.
- Oxypentifylline is a drug originally introduced for peripheral vascular disease. It has similar but weaker actions to thalidomide in inhibiting TNFα production. Clinical benefit may be difficult to discern, but it is non-toxic.

Immunosuppressive/immunomodulatory drugs: sulfasalazine and colchicine

Sulfasalazine
- Sulfasalazine was originally introduced as an antibiotic.
- It comprises sulfapyridine coupled to 5-aminosalicylic acid via a diazo bond that can be split by enteric bacteria.
- The precise mode of action as an immunomodulatory agent is uncertain.
- It has minor immunosuppressive activities, mainly localized to the gut, but little effect on peripheral blood lymphocyte numbers or function.
- It is used predominantly in inflammatory bowel disease, rheumatoid arthritis, and seronegative arthritides, in doses of 500–2000 mg/day in divided doses.
- It has a significant array of side-effects including male infertility (azoospermia), macrocytic anaemia, rash, Stevens–Johnson syndrome, and secondary hypogammaglobulinaemia.
- Regular monitoring of FBC is required.

Colchicine
- Colchicine is a useful anti-inflammatory.
- Precise immunological role is uncertain, but it inhibits microtubule assembly and therefore inhibits mitosis.
- Concentrated in neutrophils and inhibits chemotactic activity, thus reducing the accumulation of non-specific inflammatory cells.

- Valuable in Behçet's syndrome and familial Mediterranean fever; may be helpful in other autoinflammatory diseases.
- Value is limited by side-effects at therapeutic doses (diarrhoea and gastrointestinal discomfort).
- Usual dose is up to 0.5 mg four times daily, if tolerated.
- Grapefruit juice may increase toxicity.

Immunosuppressive/immunomodulatory drugs: dapsone

- Used to treat dermatitis herpetiformis, urticarial vasculitis, and IgA dermatoses.
- Inhibits β-integrin-mediated neutrophil adherence to endothelium by binding to intracellular G-protein.
- Inhibits myeloperoxidase.
- Main side-effect is haemolysis, which is marked in G6PD-deficient patients.
  - Always check G6PD status prior to use and monitor FBC for signs of haemolysis (reduced haptoglobins are a sensitive indicator of haemolysis; reticulocyte count).
- Dose is usually 1–2 mg/kg/day.

Immunosuppressive/immunomodulatory drugs: fingolimod

- Analogue of sphingosine and phosphorylated by sphingosine kinases.
- Inteferes with lymphocyte trafficking via sphingosine 1 phosphate receptor (S1PR1) and also acts on endogenous cannabinoid receptors (cPLA2).
- Approved for use in MS, but appears active in other autoimmune diseases.

Immunosuppressive/immunomodulatory drugs: dimethyl fumarate (DMF, Tecfidera®)

- Mechanism of action is uncertain. Rapidly metabolized to monomethyl fumarate, so is actually a prodrug.
- Both DMF and MMF activate a transcription factor erythroid-2-like 2 (Nrf2) pathways, which may be neuroprotective and act as a nicotinic acid receptor agonist.
- It depletes reduced glutathione and increases DNA fragmentation and lymphocyte apoptosis. It is anti-proliferative, causing cell cycle arrest.
- IL-6 and IL-12 production are reduced.

- Can cause significant CD4 and CD8 lymphopenia: regular monitoring of lymphocyte subsets is advisable. Th1 and Th17 subsets are reduced.
- The compound is a potent allergic sensitizer and was associated with severe allergic reactions to leather sofas, where it was used as a mould inhibitor. Now banned in the EU in consumer products.
- Used in MS (Tecfidera®) and psoriasis.

Immunosuppressive/immunomodulatory drugs: Janus kinase inhibitors/tyrosine kinase inhibitors

- Cytokine type I and type II receptors signal via Janus kinase enzymes, which phosphorylate the activated receptor and activate STAT transcription factors,
- As JAK2 knock-out is embryonically lethal in mice, caution has been observed in developing JAK2 inhibitors. Primary polycythaemia and myelofibrosis are associated with gain-of-function mutations in JAK2, indicating that inhibitors may be clinically useful.
- Inhibitors interfere with cytokine signalling.
- Used to treat cancers and leukaemias, but also valuable for other conditions such as hypereosinophilia.
- Imatinib is the prototype and is active against the active form of the oncogene Abl, a tyrosine kinase.
- Tofacitinib is a specific JAK3 inhibitor which is useful in rheumatoid arthritis and psoriasis.
- Ruxolitinib is active against JAK1/JAK2 and is active in psoriasis, rheumatoid arthritis, and myelofibrosis.
- Oclatinib is active against JAK1 and controls the pruritus associated with allergic dermatitis.
- Baricitinib is active against JAK1/JAK2 and has been approved for use in rheumatoid arthritis.
- A huge range of other kinase inhibitors are in clinical trials for autoimmune disease (rheumatoid arthritis, Crohn's disease) and haematological diseases (myelofibrosis, polycythaemia rubra vera, essential thrombocytosis), including among others filgotinib, gandotinib, lestaurtinib, momelotinib, pacritinib, upadacitinib, peficitinib, fedratinib.

Immunosuppressive/immunomodulatory drugs: Syk inhibitors/PKC inhibitors

Fostamatinib
- Inhibitor of Syk.
- Undergoing trials as treatment for immune thrombocytopenia and IgA nephropathy.

Sotrastaurin
- Inhibitor of multiple isoforms of PKC.
- Inhibits T-cell proliferation, IL-2, and γ-IFN production.
- Undergoing trials as a treatment for B-cell lymphoma and psoriasis.

Immunosuppressive/immunomodulatory drugs: bortezomib

- Bortezomib is used to treat myeloma.
- It inhibits the catalytic site of the 26S proteasome, which may allow apoptosis of the malignant myeloma cells.
- It increases the risk of shingles and prophylactic acyclovir is advisable.
- It also causes neuropathy and myelosuppression.

Immunosuppressive/immunomodulatory drugs: apremilast

- Apremilast is an oral phosphodiesterase 4 inhibitor.
- It regulates inflammation by raising intracellular cAMP in immune cells, which decreases expression of pro-inflammatory cytokines such as IL-10.
- Effective in psoriatic arthritis and Behçet's syndrome.

Immunosuppressive/immunomodulatory drugs: avacopan

- Avacopan is a small molecule oral C5a receptor antagonist.
- It blocks the effects of C5a.
- It has been shown to prevent the development of glomerulonephritis in ANCA-associated vasculitis.
- It is likely to be effective in other conditions where activation of the terminal lytic sequence of complement occurs (atypical HUS).

Immunosuppressive/immunomodulatory biologicals: overview

Since the last edition there has been an explosion of biological agents to treat a whole range of conditions especially autoimmune disorders and cancer. This has included the introduction of 'generic' biologicals, replicating the function of branded ones: these are known as biosimilars. Caution should be exercised, as there may be small differences which alter the side-effect profiles and they should not be assumed to be automatically interchangeable without consideration. The following sections should not be viewed as exhaustive and I have not included details of the biosimilars.

Immunosuppressive/immunomodulatory biologicals: high-dose IVIg

High-dose IVIg is widely used as an immunomodulatory agent in auto-immune diseases. Unfortunately, many of the uses have not been well supported by proper double-blind placebo controlled trials and, in view of the potential risks of infection (increased in response to volume exposure in these groups; see ➔ 'IVIg for replacement therapy', pp. 424–28) and supply issues, this cannot be condoned. The precise mechanisms of action clinically are uncertain, although many mechanisms have been postulated.

Actions
- Fc-receptor blockade on phagocytic cells.
- Inhibition of cytokine production.
- Inactivation of pathogenic autoantibodies (anti-idiotypes).
- Inhibition of autoantibody production by B cells.
- Decreased T-cell proliferation.
- Actions of soluble cytokines, cytokine receptors, and antagonists present in IVIg.
- Inhibitory actions of stabilizing sugars.

Side-effects
- Aseptic meningitis (elevated lymphocytes and protein in CSF) ?secondary to sugars.
- Renal failure (secondary to osmotic load from sugars).
- Massive intravascular haemolysis (secondary to IgG isoagglutinins).
- Hyperviscosity (CVAs, MI).
- Immune complex reactions in patients with high-titre rheumatoid factors, cryoglobulins (types II and III), or other immune complex disease, e.g. SLE.
- Anaphylactoid reactions (IgA deficiency; infected).

Main uses
- Replacement therapy for primary and secondary immunodeficiencies (see ➔ 'IVIg for replacement therapy 1', p. 424).
- Autoimmune cytopenias (ITP, AIHA).
- Vasculitis: Kawasaki syndrome; Wegener's granulomatosis.
- Neurological diseases (acute Guillain–Barré, CIDP, pure motor neuropathy, myasthenia gravis, LEMS, MS).
- Factor VIII and factor IX inhibitors.
- Anti-phospholipid antibodies in pregnancy.
- Autoimmune skin disease (pemphigus, pemphigoid, epidermolysis bullosa acquisita).
- Eczema.
- Polymyositis, dermatomyositis.

Dosage
- Dosage regimens range from 0.4 g/kg/day for 5 days, through 1 g/kg/day for 2 days to 2 g/kg/day as a single dose.
- Minimal evidence is available to distinguish between the schedules.

- Fewer doses may be required for ITP (1g/kg effective).
- My own practice is to start all high-dose regimens on the 5-day schedule to assess tolerability and then increase to 1 g/kg/day for 2 days subsequently.
- In adults and children, risks of renal impairment and aseptic meningitis are highest with the ultrarapid infusion schedule of 2 g/kg/day, and I avoid this if possible.
- Rapid infusions should be avoided in all elderly patients because of the risks of hyperviscosity.
- Pre-treatment IgA deficiency and high-titre rheumatoid factors should be excluded, and renal function assessed.
- Pre-treatment FBC, LFTs, and hepatitis serology (HBV, HCV) should also be measured.
- IgA-deficient patients require special care, and should be on products low in IgA.
- If there is renal impairment to start with, a daily creatinine should be measured and, if there is a rise of 10% or more, then therapy should be discontinued.
- FBC should be repeated during the course to ensure that haemolysis does not take place (haptoglobin is a sensitive indicator of intravascular haemolysis).
- Infusion rates should follow manufacturers' guidelines.
- There should be no switching of products, unless unavoidable.

▶Batch numbers *must* be recorded (in the UK on the MDSAS Database).

Immunosuppressive/immunomodulatory biologicals: polyclonal antibodies, high-dose anti-D immunoglobulin, and blood transfusion effect

Polyclonal antibodies

- Xenogeneic antisera raised by the immunization of animals with purified human T cells or thymocytes (rabbit anti-thymocyte globulin (ATG) and rabbit anti-lymphocyte globulin (ALG)) are potent immunosuppressive agents.
- They cause a profound lymphopenia.
- They are difficult to standardize and have significant batch-to-batch variation.
- They also contain cross-reactive antibodies that react with other cells types, including platelets.
- Utility is limited by the development of a host anti-rabbit response, which both neutralizes the xeno-antiserum and also gives rise to a serum sickness reaction.

Actions

- Complement-mediated lymphocyte destruction.
- Cause marked but variable lymphopenia.
- Reduced T-cell function.

Uses
- Acute graft rejection or GvHD.
- Diamond–Blackfan syndrome.

Dosage
- Dosage depends on batch but is usually within the range of 5–30 mg/kg/day.
- Effect can be monitored by absolute lymphocyte counts or flow cytometric analysis of peripheral blood lymphocytes.

High-dose anti-D immunoglobulin
- High dose anti-D immunoglobulin can be used to control autoimmune haemolytic anaemia in rhesus D$^+$ patients.
- Mechanism of action is unclear.

Blood transfusion effect
- In renal allografts it has been well documented that both donor and random blood transfusions reduce the risks of graft rejection.
- Immunological mechanism is uncertain.

Immunosuppressive/immunomodulatory biologicals: anti-TNF agents

Since the second edition of this book there has been an explosion of monoclonal antibodies, now mainly chimeric or humanized molecules, and these are replacing murine monoclonal antibodies, which have a high rate of induction of anti-mouse antibodies, which abolish the effectiveness.

Infliximab (Remicade®)
- Chimeric monoclonal antibody to TNFα.
- Licensed for use in Crohn's disease, rheumatoid arthritis, ankylosing spondylitis, psoriasis, juvenile arthritis.
- Major hazard of use is significant increase in TB.
  - Screening for TB prior to administration is advised.
  - Use of Quantiferon Gold may be valuable in establishing previous TB infection.
  - Development of PUO, cough, weight loss should trigger search for TB.
- Induces development of anti-nuclear antibodies.
- Must be used in combination with MTX to prevent the development of anti-chimera antibodies.
- Dose 3 mg/kg as IV infusion, repeated at 2-, 6-, and then 8-week intervals.
- Cessation of therapy in Crohn's disease may lead to loss of effect when re-introduced.

Adalimumab (Humira®)
- Another monoclonal antibody to TNFα.
- Side-effects, dosing, and indications are similar to those for infliximab.
- Co-therapy with MTX is recommended.
- Dose is 40 mg on alternate weeks subcutaneously.

Golimumab (Simponi®)
- Another monoclonal antibody to TNFα, recently licensed for use in rheumatoid arthritis.

Certolizumab (Cimzia®)
- Another monoclonal antibody to TNFα.
- Pegylated Fab' fragment of humanized anti-TNF mAb.
- Marketed for use in Crohn's disease.

Etanercept (Enbrel®)
- Etanercept is a soluble fusion protein of the ligand binding portion of the type 2 TNF receptor (p75) coupled to the Fc portion of human IgG_1.
- It binds both TNFα and TNFβ.
- It is synergistic with MTX.
- It is licensed for use in RhA, psoriatic arthritis, and juvenile arthritis.
- It may be of value in Behçet's disease and uveitis.
- Demyelination has been reported; risk of immunosuppression is significant.
- Dose is 25–50 mg twice a week by subcutaneous injection for 12 weeks, reducing to 25 mg twice a week with a maximum duration of therapy of 24 weeks.
- If there is no response by 12 weeks, then it should be discontinued.

Immunosuppressive/immunomodulatory biologicals: other cytokines

Ustekinumab (Stelara®)
- Human monoclonal antibody directed against IL-12 and IL-23.
- Approved for treatment of psoriasis and possibly psoriatic arthropathy. Also used in inflammatory bowel disease.
- Associated with possible increased infection risk (TB) and increased cancer risk.
- Allergic reactions reported.

Secukinumab (Cosentyx®)
- A neutralizing humanized monoclonal antibody against IL-17A.
- Currently undergoing trials for treatment of psoriasis, psoriatic arthritis, rheumatoid arthritis, and uveitis.
- Not effective against inflammatory bowel disease.
- Probable increase in infections.

Ixekizumab (Taltz®)
- A humanized IgG_4 monoclonal antibody against IL-17A.
- Currently undergoing trials in psoriasis, rheumatoid arthritis, and uveitis.

Anakinra (Kineret®)

- A recombinant version of the naturally occurring IL-1 receptor antagonist.
- Blocks the action of IL-1.
- Has been used in RhA, but evidence of benefit is not compelling and NICE no longer recommends it.
- Effective in autoinflammaory syndromes, including cryopyrin-associated periodic syndromes (familial cold autoinflammatory disease, Muckle–Wells syndrome, and NOMID—see ➲ Chapter 14).
- Causes neutropenia and headache.
- Dose is 100 mg daily subcutaneously.

Canakinumab (Ilaris®)

- Human monoclonal antibody against IL-1β.
- Approved for use in cryopyrin-associated periodic syndromes (familial cold autoinflammatory disease, Muckle–Wells syndrome, and NOMID—see ➲ Chapter 14).

Rilonacept (IL-1-Trap, Arcalyst®)

- Dimeric fusion protein comprising extracellular domain of IL-1R and Fc of human IgG_1, binds and neutralizes IL-1.
- Approved for use in cryopyrin-associated periodic syndromes (familial cold autoinflammatory disease, Muckle–Wells syndrome, and NOMID—see ➲ Chapter 14).

Tocilizumab (Actemra®)

- Humanized monoclonal antibody against IL-6 receptor.
- Mainly developed and now approved for use in rheumatoid arthritis, but likely to be effective in a range of antibody-mediated diseases, including myeloma, Castleman's syndrome.
- Administered monthly in a dose of 8 mg/kg by IV infusion.
- Other anti-IL6 and Il6-R mAbs are being trialled.

Anifrolumab

- A humanized monoclonal antibody against the interferon alpha receptor 1 (IFNAR1), which blocks the binding of the interferon.
- Currently undergoing trials in moderate to severe SLE.

Immunosuppressive/immunomodulatory biologicals: anti-T-cell agents

Since the first edition of this book there has been an explosion of monoclonal antibodies.

OKT®3 (muromonab-CD3)

- Murine antibody against T-cell CD3 ε-chain.
- Used to treat allograft rejection.

- Associated with high incidence of the development of HAMA (human anti-mouse antibodies) that reduce its effect and cause a serum sickness reaction.
- Now withdrawn, a humanized variant is in development; other anti-CD3 antibodies are available.

Otelixizumab (TRX4)
- Chimeric humanized antibody against T-cell CD3 ε-chain.
- In trials for type I diabetes.

Ruplizumab (Antova®)
- Anti-CD154 (gp39, CD40 ligand) blocks the binding of CD154 on activated but not resting T cells with CD40 on B cells and APCs.
- Of possible benefit in SLE and nephritis.
- Complications have included thrombosis and thrombocytopenia.

Zanolimumab (HuMax-CD4®)
- Anti-CD4 humanized monoclonal antibody.
- Of possible benefit in rheumatoid arthritis, psoriasis, and T-cell lymphomas.

Immunosuppressive/immunomodulatory biologicals: anti-CD25 agents

These are now being introduced to prevent graft rejection in solid organ transplantation.

Basiliximab (Simulect®)
- A humanized monoclonal IgG$_1$antibody that binds to the α-chain of the high-affinity IL-2 receptor (CD25) and prevents T-cell proliferation.
- Used in the prophylaxis of acute organ rejection in renal allografts, in combinations with ciclosporin and corticosteroids.
- Main side-effect is severe hypersensitivity.
- Dose is 20 mg 2 hours before transplant and 20 mg 4 days after surgery.

Daclizumab (Zenapax®)
- A humanized monoclonal antibody that binds to the γ-chain of the IL-2 receptor and prevents T-cell proliferation.
- Used in the prophylaxis of acute organ rejection in renal allografts, in combinations with ciclosporin and corticosteroids.
- Has been shown to benefit birdshot chorioretinopathy and MS.
- Main side-effect is severe hypersensitivity.
- Dose is 1 mg/kg by IV infusion in the 24 hours pre-transplant, then continued daily for 14 days.
- Daclizumab beta (Zenbryta®) has been associated with an increased risk of potentially fatal encephalitis when used in MS as well as hepatotoxicity. Its marketing authorization has been suspended.

Immunosuppressive/immunomodulatory biologicals: anti-co-stimulatory agents

Abatacept (Orencia®)

- A fusion protein of CTLA-4 and immunoglobulin that binds to B7; inhibits co-stimulation of T cells.
- Approved for use in rheumatoid arthritis and is being tested in inflammatory bowel disease, lupus nephritis, and type I diabetes.

Belatacept (Nulojix®)

- A fusion protein of CTLA-4 and immunoglobulin that binds to B7; inhibits co-stimulation of T cells.
- It differs from abatacept by only two amino acids.
- It is being studied in renal transplantation.
- It appears to increase the risk of post-transplant lymphoproliferative disease.

Ipilimumab (Yervoy®)

- A human monoclonal antibody against CTLA-4.
- Being trialled for melanoma (approved by FDA), small cell lung cancer, and prostate cancer.

TGN1412

- Humanized antibody against CD28.
- Caused a severe cytokine release syndrome in first human trial in normal volunteers (approved by MRHA); not predicted by prior studies.
- Predicted that administration may have caused long-term immune damage.
- Company became insolvent as a result of the adverse publicity.

Check-point inhibitors (pembrolizumab (Keytruda®) and nivolumab (Opdivo®))

- These antibodies inhibit the programmed cell death receptors normally expressed by antigen-stimulated T cells (PD1).
- Tumours express the ligand for PD1 (PD-L1) and switch off T cells.
- Pembrolizumab and nivolumab reactivate T cells and have been shown to be effective in augmenting the immune response to some tumours, including melanoma.
- Atezolizumab, an antibody to PD-L1, is effective against a range of tumours.

Immunosuppressive/immunomodulatory biologicals: anti-B-cell agents

Alemtuzumab (MabCampath®)

- Humanized anti-CD52 monoclonal (Campath®).

- Lytic antibody: targets predominantly B cells, but also T cells, macrophages, NK cells, and some neutrophils.
- Used in B-cell lymphomas, B-CLL, and B-lymphoproliferative disease (EBV[+]) in the immunosuppressed.
- Causes tumour lysis and cytokine release syndrome (capillary leak), as for rituximab.
- Secondary autoimmunity common (thyroid).

Rituximab (MabThera®)

- A humanized anti-CD20 monoclonal antibody: CD20 is strongly expressed on normal and malignant B cells.
- Licensed for use in non-Hodgkin's B-cell lymphomas.
- Can cause massive tumour lysis syndrome, with cytokine release (antibody-complement mediated lysis) and capillary leak syndrome 1–2 hours after infusion.
  - Fever and chills, nausea and vomiting, and hypersensitivity reactions are common.
  - Analgesic and antihistamine should be administered before treatment.
  - Full resuscitation facilities should be available.
- Synergistic with chemotherapy.
- Likely to be valuable in the treatment of autoimmune diseases where autoantibody plays a significant role (autoimmune haemolytic anaemia, ITP).
- Also showing promise as adjunctive therapy in SLE and other antibody-mediated autoimmune diseases.
- Side-effects include severe and prolonged hypogammaglobulinaemia due to destruction of normal B cells. Reduced IgM is an early sign.

Ofatumumab (Humax-CD20, Arzerra®)

- A humanized anti-CD20 monoclonal antibody.
- Recognizes different epitopes to rituximab.
- Licensed for the treatment of resistant CLL but has also shown promise in lymphoma, rheumatoid arthritis, and MS.
- Administration can be complicated by a cytokine release syndrome and pre-medication with analgesics, antihistamines, and corticosteroids is recommended.

Belimumab (LymphoStat-B, Benlysta®)

- A human monoclonal antibody against B-lymphocyte stimulator (BLyS, also known as BAFF—B cell activation factor of TNF family).
- Approved for use in SLE in N. America and Europe, although not trialled in severe SLE. Cost likely to be about £35 000 per annum per patient.
- Side-effects include nausea, diarrhoea, and allergic reactions. Increased risk of infections noted in clinical trials (avoid live vaccines during treatment).

Inebilizumab

- A humanized monoclonal antibody against CD19.
- Depletes plasma cells, which are not targeted by anti-CD20 mAbs.
- Undergoing trials in systemic sclerosis, MS, neuromyelitis optica, and B cell malignancies.

Brentuximab vedotoxin (Adcentris®)

- A humanized monoclonal antibody against CD30, covalently coupled to the anti-tubulin agent monomethyl auristatin E.
- CD30 is expressed on subpopulations of T cells and B cells and, importantly, Reed–Sternberg cells found in Hodgkin's disease.
- Approved for use in Hodgkin's disease and non-Hodgkin's lymphoma where CD30 is expressed.
- Because increased CD30 is seen on activated T cells in SLE, the drug is currently being trialled in this condition.

Atacicept

- A recombinant human fusion protein containing the ligand-binding domain of TACI and a modified human IgG Fc.
- Binds to BLys (BAFF) and APRIL, preventing activation via these molecules.
- Also interferes with Ig class switching and may cause long-term hypogammaglobulinaemia.
- Currently being trialled in SLE.

Daratumumab

- A monoclonal antibody targeting CD38, a plasma cell marker over-expressed on plasma cells, which causes the cells to apoptose.
- Used to treat myeloma and certain types of lymphoma.
- Interferes with cross-matching, as it is expressed on red cells, and with flow cytometric evaluate of plasma cells.

Immunosuppressive/immunomodulatory biologicals: anti-allergic agents

More biologicals are now available to treat allergic diseases.

Mepolizumab (Bosatria®)

- A humanized monoclonal antibody against IL-5.
- Shown to be useful in treatment of eosinophilic conditions, including asthma and possibly F1P1L1/PDGFRA-negative hypereosinophilic syndromes.
- Herpes zoster may be increased in treated patients.

Reslizumab (Cinqair®)

- A humanized monoclonal antibody against the IL-5R binding region on IL-5.
- Approved by the FDA for treatment-resistant asthma with eosinophilia.

Benralizumab (Fasenra®)

- A humanized monoclonal antibody against IL-5R (CD125).
- Also depletes IL-5R+ eosinophils and basophils via ADCC.
- Shown to be useful in treatment of asthma with a similar effectiveness to mepolizumab.

Dupilumab (Dupixent®)

- A humanized monoclonal antibody against the shared alpha-chain of IL-4 and IL-13 receptors.
- Shown to be useful in treatment of atopic eczema and in asthma, especially where the eosinophil count is elevated.

Omalizumab (Xolair®)

- A humanized monoclonal antibody against IgE Fc region that prevents binding to the high-affinity IgE receptor (FcεR1).
- FcεR1are downregulated on basophils and this provides a useful flow cytometric test for efficacy.
- Now validated as a treatment for moderate to severe asthma.
- In the UK, severity is marked by repeated attendances at hospital, penalizing those who have severe disease but self-manage at home.
- Local primary care commissioner approval for treatment is variable, giving rise to postcode prescribing.
- Approved for use in severe urticaria (fixed dose).
- It is being investigated as adjunctive therapy to desensitizing immunotherapy.
- Dose is determined by serum total IgE, meaning that those with very high IgE levels cannot be treated.
- It is administered subcutaneously every 2–4 weeks.
- Anaphylaxis to treatment has been reported.

Immunosuppressive/immunomodulatory biologicals: anti-integrin agents

A number of agents have been produced against integrins. Those against CD11/CD18 have all been disappointing and have been associated with severe side-effects. Efalizumab (anti-CD11a) was introduced for psoriasis, but its licence has been withdrawn in the USA because of concerns over the risk of progressive multifocal leukoencephalopathy (PML).

Natalizumab (Tysabri®)

- A humanized monoclonal antibody against α4-integrin.
- Thought to work by preventing inflammatory cell migration, particularly through the blood–brain barrier.
- Used for treatment of MS and Crohn's disease.
- Associated with PML and was temporarily withdrawn from the market; cases of PML may be linked to combined therapy with other agents.

Vedolizumab (Entyvio®)

- A humanized monoclonal antibody against the integrin α4β7.
- Inhibits lymphocyte trafficking to the gut.
- Effective in both Crohn's disease and ulcerative colitis for both induction and maintenance of remission.
- Concern about long-term risk of GI malignancy due to reduced immune surveillance.
- No evidence for PML risk.

Immunosuppressive/immunomodulatory biologicals: miscellaneous agents

Gemtuzumab (Mylotarg®)
- A monoclonal antibody against the CD33 antigen expressed on myeloid leukaemic blasts and normal myeloid cells.
- Used to treat AML in first relapse.

Trastuzumab
- A humanized antibody against the epidermal growth factor receptor Her-2.
- Blocks and downregulates the receptor.
- Valuable in the treatment of metastatic breast cancer where the tumour overexpresses Her-2.
- Her-2 is also expressed on other tumours.

Abciximab (ReoPro®)
- Monoclonal antibody binding to platelet glycoprotein IIb/IIIa receptors.
- Used once only as an adjunct to heparin and aspirin in high-risk patients undergoing percutaneous transluminal coronary artery interventions to prevent thrombotic complications.

Digoxin-specific antibody (Digibind®)
- Fab′ fragments of antibody against digoxin.
- Used to treat digoxin poisoning by binding to the drug.

Bevacizumab (Avastin®)
- Humanized monoclonal antibody that inhibits vascular endothelial growth factor A (VGEF-A).
- Approved to treat a variety of cancers especially with metastases, although effects may be small.
- Also used to treat macular degeneration.

Emapalumab
- A human monoclonal antibody against γ-IFN.
- Currently being trialled in haemophagocytic lymphohistiocytosis.

Eculizumab (Soliris®)
- Monoclonal humanized antibody binding to complement C5 and preventing its activation by C5 convertase, thus preventing the generation of the terminal lytic sequence.
- Licensed for the treatment of paroxysmal nocturnal haemoglobinuria and haemolytic–uraemic syndrome (in the UK cases must be referred to supraregional specialist service).
- Undergoing investigation as a drug for treatment of acute complement-mediated graft rejection.
- Increases risk of meningococcal disease (as expected from primary complement deficiency): patients should be immunized with quadrivalent conjugated meningococcal vaccine at least 2 weeks prior to receiving drug. This will not provide protection against group B meningococci.

Total lymphoid irradiation (TLI)

- TLI is experimental as an immunosuppressive therapy, having been used previously for the treatment of lymphoid malignancies.
- Produces profound impairment of T-cell numbers and function, although there is a small population of radioresistant small lymphocytes.
- A more modern variant is to use UV sensitizing agents (psoralens) and then irradiate leucocytes in an extracorporeal circulation (photopheresis).
- TLI may be of benefit in intractable rheumatoid arthritis, multiple sclerosis, and severe SLE.

Side-effects
- Severe leucopenia
- Thrombocytopenia
- Opportunist infections
- Lymphoma (NHL).

Photopheresis

- Extracorporeal phototherapy, using sensitizing agents, is used for the treatment of GvHD, inflammatory bowel syndrome.
- 8-Methoxypsoralen is used as the sensitizer, which when activated binds to lymphocyte DNA.

Thoracic duct drainage

- Has been used in the past for treatment of severe RhA.
- Causes a severe and long-lasting immunosuppression.
- Similar effects are seen from accidental thoracic duct damage in oesophageal and cardiac surgery, where a chylous effusion is allowed to drain unchecked.
  - A profound and persistent lymphopenia of both T and B cells is caused.
  - Recovery of immune function may occur over a long period.
  - Prophylaxis against *Pneumocystis jirovecii* pneumonia and fungal infections will be required if the drainage is accidental.
  - Immunoglobulin replacement therapy may be required.

Plasmapheresis

- Plasmapheresis is the removal of plasma constituents using automated cell separators; the plasma components are removed by either centrifugation or membrane filtration.
- Erythrocytes and other cellular components are re-infused and the removed plasma replaced with either FFP or FFP + IVIg to maintain circulating volume.

- About 50% of the plasma is removed each time.
- A therapeutic course is usually 3–5 daily treatments.
- The amount of antibody removed depends on volume of distribution.
  - 90% of IgM but only 20% of IgG is removed each time as only 40% of the IgG is within the vascular space.
- Plasmapheresis also has the advantage of the removal of immune complexes and small mediators (toxins, anaphylotoxins, cytokines, etc.), in addition to the antibodies.
- Plasmapheresis is only suitable for urgent therapy, as antibody levels return rapidly and frequently overshoot to higher levels after plasmapheresis is discontinued.
  - It is important to commence conventional immunosuppression at the same time.

Side-effects

- Leakage/air embolism.
- Anticoagulation (citrate toxicity)/thrombocytopenia.
- Reactions to replacement fluids.

Uses

- Hyperviscosity (Waldenström's macroglobulinaemia, IgA myeloma).
- Goodpasture's syndrome/Wegener's granulomatosis.
- Cryoglobulinaemia.
- Myasthenia gravis.
- Guillain–Barré syndrome (but IVIg is as good).
- It has been tried in other autoimmune diseases (RhA, FVIII antibodies, MS, lupus nephritis) with variable anecdotal success.
- A limiting factor in its use is access to appropriate equipment, particularly in the urgent setting.

Immunoadsorption

- Selective removal of autoantibodies has been attempted using an extracorporeal circuit including a column of inert beads coated with protein A or protein G for specific adsorption of IgG.
- This treatment is experimental and it is not widely used in clinical practice.

Allergy interventions: drugs

Treatment for allergic disease is divided into three major target areas: mast cells, released mediators, and the specific immune response. Treatment can be topical or systemic: topical is preferred if this is effective. The underlying chronic inflammatory component, especially of asthma, needs always to be addressed rather than just using symptomatic agents. Corticosteroids and antihistamines are more effective as prophylactic agents, taken before allergen exposure.

Mast-cell active drugs
- Corticosteroids (interfere with synthesis of leukotrienes).
- Mast-cell stabilization: cromoglicate/nedocromil/ketotifen (prevent allergen-triggered calcium flux and hence prevent degranulation).

Released mediators
- β-Agonists (smooth muscle relaxation, ?some anti-inflammatory effect (salmeterol)).
- Antihistamines: use long-acting high-potency non-sedating drugs without cardiotoxicity (loratadine, desloratadine, levocetirizine, cetirizine, fexofenadine).
- Corticosteroids.
- Anti-PAF drugs (clinical results disappointing).
- Leukotriene (LTD_4) antagonists, montelukast, zafirlukast (useful adjunctive treatment in asthma).
- 5-Lipoxygenase inhibitor, zileuton (asthma).
- Kinin antagonists: icatibant (anti-bradykinin B2 receptor antagonist), WIN64338, FR173657 (orally active B2 antagonist).

Specific IgE
- Desensitization.
- Peptide therapy (experimental but not successful clinically).
- Anti-FcRε therapy (experimental).
- Omalizumab, anti-IgE, see ➜ 'Immunosuppressive/immunomodulatory biologicals: anti-allergic agents', p. 458.

Allergy interventions: desensitization (immunotherapy)

Mechanism of benefit
- Mechanism of desensitization is uncertain: specific IgE may rise in early stages of treatment, then fall.
- The role of 'blocking antibodies' (IgG_4) is unknown.
- One hypothesis suggests that sequential exposure gradually switches the $CD4^+$ T-cell response from Th2 to Th1, reducing IgE production and the levels of the pro-allergic cytokines IL-4 and IL-5.

Indications
- Desensitization should be considered for patients with:
  - anaphylaxis to insect venoms;
  - rhinoconjunctivitis not controlled with maximal medical therapy, used correctly, and including repeated courses of oral steroids;
  - asthma may be amenable to treatment but carries high risks.
- In the UK, most vaccines are available only on a named patient basis.

Exclusions
- Current UK guidelines suggest that desensitization is *inappropriate* for those with:
  - multiple allergies;

- severe asthma (FEV_1 < 75% predicted): seasonal wheeze only induced by pollen is not a contraindication to desensitization out of the pollen season;
- heart disease;
- hypertension requiring β-blockade (difficult to resuscitate in emergencies!);
- use of ACE inhibitors (increased risk of angioedema, local and systemic);
- during pregnancy;
- excess alcohol consumption (increased risk of side-effects).
- Age > 50 years is associated with poorer responses (exception is venom immunotherapy).

Subcutaneous immunotherapy (SCIT)

- Traditional desensitization is done with weekly subcutaneous injections of increasing doses of aqueous allergen until maintenance doses are reached at 14–18 weeks.
- Once on maintenance doses, intervals between injections are spaced out to 4–6 weeks for 3 years.
- Short course (4 or 6 injections over the winter) of adsorbed allergens (Pollinex® and Pollinex Quattro®) are as effective for pollen allergies: course is repeated annually for 3 years.
- Some authorities recommend up to 5 years of treatment. However, the additional benefit from the extra 2 years may be minimal.
- Retreatment is possible.
- Allergens available in the UK include:
  - venoms: bee, wasp, bumblebee (for market gardeners who use bumblebees for pollination!);
  - pollens: grass, birch pollen, ragweed (USA mainly);
  - animals: cat (potent allergen associated with high incidence of side-effects), horse, dog (but this is not as effective as the others);
  - house dust mite;
  - some moulds.
- Highly purified allergens should always be used: whole insect extracts or multiple allergens combinations are not recommended in the UK.
- All except Pollinex® are unlicensed at present and are therefore administered on a named-patient basis.
  - Formal written consent is required.
- Precise protocol and total duration of therapy varies depending on the allergen.
- All require long-term commitment from patients.
  - Schedules are onerous and the leeway for changes to accommodate holidays are minimal.
  - Patients must not undertake vigorous exercise after injections (increased risk of side-effects).
  - Injections cannot be given if patient is unwell.
- Pre-treatment with antihistamines reduces risk of local reactions.
- Peak flow should be monitored pre- and 30 minutes post-injection.
- All patients must stay for at least 1 hour post-injection (no exceptions).
- Rush and ultra-rush schedules have been devised for venom allergy, but are rarely required in practice and significantly increase the risks of reactions.

🛑Desensitization must be carried out in hospital and staff must be conversant with emergency management of anaphylaxis and cardiac arrest procedures.

Side-effects
- Main side-effects are pain and swelling at site of injections (pre-treat with antihistamine and supply oral steroid).
- Systemic reactions may occur (cough is often the first sign): treat as for any acute allergic reaction.
- Risk of reactions is increased:
  - during the up-dosing period (aqueous allergens);
  - in patients treated with cat allergen;
  - if patient has intercurrent infection (defer injection);
  - if patient is extremely anxious (use sedation if necessary);
  - if patient is exposed to allergen naturally during the up-dosing period;
  - if patient is drinking excess alcohol;
  - if patient is started on ACE inhibitor.

Venom immunotherapy
- Immunotherapy is only indicated for those with systemic reactions. Large local reactions are not an indication and do not predict risk of future anaphylaxis.
- Decisions about immunotherapy will be influenced by factors that influence risk of further stings such as occupation (forestry workers, gardeners, pest controllers), hobbies (bee-keepers).
- Difficulties in decision making occur if there have been multiple simultaneous stings, as this may give rise to systemic venom toxicity rather than allergy.
- Risks of anaphylaxis decline steadily over time without further stings. Whether this reaches the population baseline of 3% by 10–20 years is debated.
- Mast cell tryptase should be checked: patients with mastocytosis are at high risk of severe anaphylaxis.
- Prior to desensitization, clear documentation of the primary triggering venom is required.
- This requires skin prick testing, if necessary backed up by specific IgE.
- Recombinant allergens are available for key bee and wasp venom allergens and cross-reacting carbohydrate determinants (not important for immunotherapy).
- Immunotherapy is available to bees, bumblebees, and wasps. For allergy to hornets, wasp venom is recommended.
- The role of sting challenges before and after immunotherapy is debated.
- Duration in the UK is usually 3 years, but up to 5 years may be used. The latter may be helpful in those who struggle to reach normal maintenance dosage because of repeated reactions.
- Adrenaline autoinjectors should be provided, but the need for them should be reviewed after completion of immunotherapy.

Sublingual therapy (SLIT)
- Sublingual desensitization is widely practised in Europe.
- Allergen drops or tablets are placed under the tongue on a daily basis.
- Local tingling and minor swelling may occur.
- Experience from Europe suggests that this is safe and effective and can be administered at home.
- Grazax®, a sublingual tablet for grass pollen allergy, is licensed in the UK, but treatment should be initiated and supervised by a trained allergist/immunologist. Shellfish allergy is a contraindication due to the nature of the coating on the tablet.
- Acarizax®, a house dust mite tablet, is shortly to be licensed in the UK.
- 3 years of treatment is still required.
- First dose of sublingual treatment should be administered in hospital; thereafter, self-treatment at home is appropriate.
- Eosinophilic oesophagitis has been reported after sublingual grass pollen immunotherapy.

Adoptive immunotherapy

Stem cell transplantation
- See ➲ Chapter 15.

Adoptive cell therapy
- LAK therapy (lymphokine-activated killer cells) has been proposed as a treatment for malignant disease.
- Peripheral blood lymphocytes are harvested and then stimulated *in vitro* with high-dose IL-2 and re-infused into the patient with additional cytokine cocktails.
- Side-effects can be severe and tumoricidal activity limited.
- A better approach may be to expand tumour-invading lymphocytes (TIL), derived from lymph nodes or from tumours. These are expanded *in vitro* and then infused back after conditioning.
- The therapy is moderately toxic in therapeutic doses (fluid retention; capillary leak syndrome).
- There is evidence of benefit in melanoma, with long-lasting tumour regression and renal cell carcinoma (salvage therapy).

Part 2

Immunochemistry

Techniques

Electrophoresis, immunoelectrophoresis, immunofixation, isoelectric focusing, and immunoblotting

Serum electrophoresis

The most basic technique for the detection of serum proteins.

- Serum is applied to an electrolyte containing agarose gel and a current applied across the gel. Proteins are separated largely on the basis of their surface charge.
- Separated proteins are then visualized by incubating the gel with a protein-binding dye. As the amount of dye bound is proportional to the protein present, the amount of protein present in each band can be calculated from the absorbance of the dye if the total protein concentration is known. This is the method used for paraprotein quantitation.
- Faster semi-automated systems use capillary zone electrophoresis (CZE)

Immunoelectrophoresis/immunofixation

Techniques for identifying the nature of the proteins separated in an electrophoretic strip.

- Individual proteins may be identified by immunoelectrophoresis, in which troughs cut parallel to the electrophoretic strip are filled with antisera, which is allowed to diffuse towards the separated proteins.
- Reaction at the point of equivalence gives an arc of precipitation.
- A faster technique is immunofixation, in which the antisera are laid over the electrophoretic separation and unreacted proteins washed out before staining with a protein-binding dye.
- Both these techniques are used principally to identify monoclonal immunoglobulins. Serum is preferred as the mobility of fibrinogen is such that it runs in the same region as some immunoglobulins.
- CZE can also be adapted to immunofixation.

Isoelectric focusing and immunoblotting

More sensitive techniques are required for CSF, as the concentrations of immunoglobulins are lower.

- Electrophoretic separation is carried out by isoelectric focusing. The gel contains ampholytes, which move under the current to set up a pH gradient across the gel.
- Proteins applied subsequently then move to the part of the gel where the pH ensures that they become electrically neutral. They then cease to move in the current.
- The gel is then blotted on to nitrocellulose filters, which are reacted with antisera against immunoglobulins (immunoblotting).

Radial immunodiffusion (RID)

A simple, although slow, method for the measurement of any protein for which an antiserum exists.

- Antiserum is incorporated into an agar gel, which is poured on to a plate and allowed to set. Regular holes are then cut into the gel and the serum containing the protein of interest placed in the holes. The serum diffuses into the gel and forms an immunoprecipitate that can be seen as a white halo around the well.

- The log[concentration] is proportional to the diameter of the ring. The ring diameter can be measured using an eyepiece graticule.
- If this method is used to measure concentrations of immunoglobulins, caution is required as variations in molecular weight (e.g. if serum contains monomeric rather than polymeric IgM, as may happen in Waldenström's macroglobulinaemia) or the presence of immune complexes may cause falsely low or falsely high values.
- IgA-deficient individuals often have antibodies to ruminant proteins, including immunoglobulins, and, as the antisera that are incorporated in the gel are often raised in ruminants, this may cause reverse precipitation in the gel and lead to entirely spurious results.

Ouchterlony double diffusion

A technique used for non-quantitative identification of proteins.

- Wells are cut in agar and test serum and antisera placed in the wells and allowed to diffuse towards each other.
- Lines of precipitation will form, which can be seen using a light box. Where multiple samples are tested, lines of identity and partial identity may be recorded between sample wells.
- Technique is sensitive and can be used for low-level IgA detection.
- A variant in which the antigen and antibody are forced together by application of a current speeds the process up, but is dependent on the electrophoretic mobility of the antibodies and antigens—it is used for detection of antibodies to ENA (see ➲ Chapter 18)—this is called countercurrent immunoelectrophoresis.

Nephelometry and turbidimetry

These techniques are the mainstay of automated specific protein measurement.

- As with other techniques, they rely upon immune complex formation when antibodies and antigens react. This alters the optical properties of the solution and the light absorbance or scatter can be measured.
- The reactions can be enhanced by using reaction diluents containing polyethylene glycol (PEG), which stabilizes the immune complex.
- Accuracy may be enhanced by using kinetic assays (rate nephelometry).
- This technique is suitable for automation, but is dependent on high-grade monospecific antisera of high potency. Monoclonal antibodies are rarely suitable for this type of system.
- Anything that causes the serum to be turbid before the reaction begins, or interferes with the optical properties of the solution, will cause difficulties. This includes lipaemic sera or haemolysed samples with excess free haemoglobin (with haemoglobin–haptoglobin complexes).

α₁-**Acid glycoprotein**

- Units: g/l.
- Normal range:
  - male, 0.6–1.2 g/l;
  - female, 0.4–1.0 g/l.

Principles of test
- Measured by nephelometry/turbidimetry.

Indications for testing
- Also known as orosomucoid, an acute-phase protein, induced by IL-1, IL-6, and TNFα.
- It used to be used extensively in the diagnosis and monitoring of inflammatory bowel disease, and it was felt that it was more specific for this category of disease. There is no strong evidence to support this assertion and CRP probably provides all the information required.
- Dynamic range is only twofold, compared to > 100-fold for CRP.
- There is a sex difference, with levels in females being lower. Levels are also reduced in pregnancy and in patients receiving oestrogens.
- It is known to bind certain drugs such as propranolol.
- There are no routine indications for its regular measurement at present.

α_1-Antichymotrypsin

- Units: g/l.
- Normal adult range: 0.3–0.6 g/l.

Principles of test
- Measured by nephelometry/turbidimetry.

Indications for testing
- This protein is one of the SERPIN family (serine protease inhibitors) whose major role is the protection of tissues from proteolysis by neutrophil and macrophage enzymes. It is particularly active against cathepsin G.
- It rises rapidly during an acute-phase response (within 8 hours) and has a dynamic range of fivefold (much less than CRP). It remains elevated for longer.
- It has been suggested as a useful marker for inflammatory bowel disease, but there is little evidence to support this and it is not widely used.

α_1-Antitrypsin (α_1-AT)

- Units: g/l.
- Normal adult range: 1.0–1.9 g/l.

Principles of test
- α_1-AT is measured by nephelometry/turbidimetry.

Indications for testing
- α_1-AT is a proteolytic inhibitor with a wide range of inhibitory activities. It is a member of the SERPIN family.

- Low levels are associated with cirrhosis, emphysema, and neonatal jaundice, and also adult liver disease. Deficiency may also be associated with vasculitis (particularly of the skin) and with membranoproliferative glomerulonephritis.
- There are a number of deficiency alleles and, when a low value is detected, the phenotype should be determined. Other members of the family should be screened and phenotyped. This represents the only clinical utility of α_1-AT measurements.

Interpretation

- α_1-AT comprises the major part of the $\alpha1$ fraction on serum electrophoresis and major deficiency may be detected readily on an electrophoretic strip.
- Occasionally split α_1 bands may be noted due to allelic variants of α_1-AT with different mobilities.
- In conditions where there are high levels of circulating proteases, protease α_1-AT complexes may form, with loss of the $\alpha1$ band; the complex moves in the α_2–β region of the electrophoretic strip.
- High levels are seen as part of the acute-phase response, and particularly in chronic infections (bronchiectasis).
- Levels are also increased in pregnancy, in patients on oestrogens, and in certain malignant diseases, including some germ-cell tumours. However, it is not useful clinically in any of these situations.
- It has been suggested that measurement of α_1-AT in faeces may give information on gut protein loss, as it is resistant to degradation, although there appears to be a high false-negative rate. It may be a useful alternative to radioisotopic methods for proving the presence of a protein-losing enteropathy. Normal levels are < 5 mg/g dry weight of faeces.

α_1-Antitrypsin (α_1-AT) genotype (*PI* typing)

- Gene for α_1-AT is located on chromosome 14, close to the immunoglobulin heavy chain locus (*PI* gene system, for protease inhibitor). A large number of variant alleles have been described.
- The identification is usually undertaken by isoelectric focusing, but for some rare alleles functional studies may also be required.
- In the UK, deficiency alleles occur with an incidence of about 1 in 2000. Many variants are seen in other racial groups and, as a consequence, are found only exceedingly rarely in the UK.
- The important deficiency alleles include *S, P, W, Z, Mmalton*, and *null* (no expressed α_1-AT). Homozygosity for one or heterozygosity for any two of these alleles leads to severe deficiency. Heterozygosity with any non-deficiency alleles leads to a reduction but not absence of α_1-AT.
- The allele *Mduarte* gives rise to a functional deficiency with normal antigenic concentrations.

- Studies should always be undertaken on family members and referring clinicians should always be asked for a family tree.
- Antenatal diagnosis is also possible, by *PI* typing a fetal blood sample.
- In the UK, *PI* typing is undertaken by the Protein Reference Units (PRUs) in Birmingham and Sheffield, and their excellent handbook gives more detail on the genetic system (see ➋ 'Introduction', p. xix, for details).

α_2-Macroglobulin

- Units: g/l.
- Normal ranges (quoted by PRU):
  - < 15 years. 2.8–6.7 g/l;
  - > 15 years, 1.3–2.0–3.5–5.0 g/l depending on age and sex.

Indications for testing

- No value in routine measurement at present.

Interpretation

- α_2-macroglobulin has anti-protease activity. It is an acute-phase protein and also acts as the carrier for IL-6.
- In adults, levels are slightly lower in females and fall with age.
- It is a major component of the $\alpha2$ band on electrophoresis and contributes significantly to the elevation of $\alpha2$ seen in chronic inflammatory conditions.
- As it is a very high molecular weight protein (725 kDa), it is preferentially retained in the nephrotic syndrome, giving a relative increase in relation to other areas of the electrophoretic strip.
- Levels are also reported to be elevated in ataxia telangiectasia, diabetes mellitus, oestrogen therapy, and pregnancy.
- Reduced levels have been found in pre-eclampsia and acute pancreatitis. Deficiency has been reported but is exceptionally rare.

Acute-phase proteins (CRP, ESR, SAA)

- Units:
  - CRP, mg/l;
  - ESR, mm/h;
  - SAA, mg/l.
- Normal ranges:
  - CRP, 0–6 mg/l;
  - ESR, 0–25 mm/h;
  - SAA, 0–10 mg/l.

Principles of test

- As serum proteins, C-reactive protein (CRP) and serum amyloid A (SAA) are amenable to measurement by nephelometry or turbidimetry.
- Measurement of the ESR is by timing the rate of fall of erythrocytes in a graduated tube.

Indications for testing

- Acute and chronic infections, vasculitis, connective tissue disease, arthritis, autoinflammatory diseases.

Interpretation

- CRP is member of the pentraxin family of proteins.
- CRP is a bacterial opsonin and binds free DNA.
- Clinicians are usually confused by ESR and CRP—they do not give the same information and should be used together.
- ESR is largely dependent on elevation of fibrinogen, a long-lived serum acute-phase protein, and of serum macroglobulins (α_2-macroglobulin, IgM). It is also affected by red cell morphology.
- CRP is like blood glucose while ESR is like glycated Hb in relation to measurement of the inflammatory response.
- CRP rises within hours of onset of inflammation/infection and falls quickly once treatment is instituted. Half-life is 6–8 hours. It is therefore useful for rapid diagnosis and for monitoring response.
- Common associations for levels of CRP are given in Table 17.1.
- The ESR rises slowly, being dependent in part on fibrinogen, a long-lived protein, and falls equally slowly. Half-life of fibrinogen is approximately 1 week.
- In active SLE, the ESR is high, but the CRP is not elevated.

Table 17.1 Levels of CRP and their common associations

Level of CRP	Common associations
Little or no change (< 4–100 mg/l)	Most viral infections
	Active SLE
	Systemic sclerosis and CREST
	Inactive RhA
	Myeloma
	Most tumours
Moderate elevation (100–200 mg/l)	EBV/CMV infection
	Bacterial infection
	Active rheumatoid arthritis
	Polymyalgia rheumatic
	Temporal arteritis
	Lymphoma
	Hypernephroma
Large elevation (> 200 mg/l)	Severe bacterial sepsis
	Legionella
	Active vasculitis (Wegener's, rheumatoid)
Huge elevation (> 400 mg/l)	Overwhelming sepsis (deep tissue abscess)
	Fulminant legionella
	At this level, death is the usual outcome

- CRP is driven by IL-6, as well as IL-1 and TNFα, and may be elevated in myeloma: measurements of CRP reflect serum IL-6 levels: there is no additional value to measuring IL-6 directly.
- Levels in very young children may be much lower for a given stimulus.
- A very small number of patients do not make inflammatory responses that exceed the normal range, but seem to run on a lower 'normal' range (10-fold less): ultrasensitive assays for low-level CRP are available.
- Some patients with giant cell arteritis never show an 'elevated' CRP.
- SAA, which is the circulating precursor of the secondary (AA) type of amyloid and whose physiological function is currently unknown, is an acute-phase protein with a very wide dynamic range (1000-fold).
- Monitoring of SAA is said to be valuable in disease known to predispose to the development of AA amyloid, such as chronic infections and inflammation, particularly autoinflammatory syndromes. CRP test is more widely available and probably gives the same information.
- In allograft rejection, CRP and SAA may move independently.
- Serum amyloid P (SAP) is related to CRP structurally and is a member of the pentraxin family. Despite this similarity, its function is not fully understood and it does not function as a major acute-phase protein. Routine measurement is not justified at present, although labelled SAP has been used as a tracer for amyloid deposits.

Amyloid proteins

- Amyloid refers to the deposition of altered proteins in tissues in an insoluble form (see also Table 17.2).
- The precursor protein varies according to the cause, and can often be measured specifically.
- Amyloid is usually confirmed by special stains on histological examination of biopsies.
- Measurement of serum immunoglobulins and electrophoresis, serum free light chains, β_2-microglobulin, and CRP is essential if amyloid is suspected.

Table 17.2 Clinical syndromes and associated amyloid proteins and protein precursors

Amyloid protein	Protein precursor	Clinical syndrome
AL, AH	Light or heavy chain of immunoglobulin	Idiopathic, multiple myeloma, gamma-heavy chain disease
AA	Serum amyloid A	Secondary, reactive: inflammatory arthritis, familial Mediterranean fever, hyper-IgD syndrome, TRAPS (periodic fever), Behçet's, Crohn's disease
Aβ_2M	β_2-microglobulin	Dialysis amyloid

Table 17.2 (Contd.)

Amyloid protein	Protein precursor	Clinical syndrome
ACys	Cystatin C	Hereditary cerebral angiopathy with bleeding (Iceland)
ALys, AFibA	Lysozyme, fibrinogen Aα	Non-neuropathic hereditary amyloid with renal disease
AIAPP	Islet amyloid polypeptide	Diabetes mellitus type II; insulinoma
AANF	Atrial natriuretic peptide	Senile cardiac amyloid
ACal	Procalcitonin	Medullary carcinoma of the thyroid
AIns	Porcine insulin	Iatrogenic
ATTR	Transthyretin	Familial amyloid polyneuropathy, senile cardiac amyloid
Aβ	Aβ-protein precursor	Alzheimer's disease
AprP	Prion protein	Spongiform encephalopathies

Avian precipitins

- Units: reported semi-quantitatively.
- Normal range: healthy adults exposed regularly to birds may demonstrate precipitins.

Principles of test

- Usually carried out by double diffusion. Fluorescence assays and ELISA are also used and Thermo-Fisher has an ImmunoCAP® available.

Indications for testing

- Used in the investigation of bird fancier's lung (extrinsic allergic alveolitis).

Interpretation

- IgG-precipitating antibodies to avian antigens are found in cases of bird-fancier's lung. These react particularly with avian serum and faecal proteins.
- Presence of precipitins is a marker of exposure and does *not* automatically mean that disease will be present.
- Presence of multiple precipitin lines tends to be a feature of disease.
- Any bird species is capable of inducing precipitins, but the most common causes of problems are pigeons (in pigeon-breeders), psittacine cage birds, and domestic poultry (as an occupational disease).

Bacterial and viral antibodies (specific antibodies; functional antibodies)

- Units are variable: u/l, IU/ml, µg/ml.
- Ranges are variable: check with reporting laboratory.
  - Pneumococcal antibodies, > 20 u/l (asplenics > 35).
  - Serotype specific pneumococcal antibodies, ≥0.35 mg/l.
  - Tetanus antibodies, > 0.1 IU/ml (minimum protective level).
  - *Haemophilus influenzae* type B, > 1.0 µg/ml (full protection; asplenics > 1.5).
  - Diphtheria antibodies, minimum protective level > 0.01 IU/ml; optimum protective level 0.1 IU/ml.
  - Viral antibodies, usually qualitatative, semi-quantitative, or titre.

Principles of test

- Measurement of antibody production against defined pathogens or antigens purified from pathogens plays an important role in the investigation of suspected immunodeficiency.
- Most assays carried out by enzyme-linked immunoassay, but some viral antibodies are still measured by haemagglutination or complement fixation.
- Pre- and post-immunization samples should be run on the same run for direct comparison as the coefficients of variation for the assays tend to be high: 15–25%!
- An EQA scheme exists for tetanus, pneumococcal, and Hib antibodies, and internationally agreed standards are available for tetanus and Hib; a UK standard exists for pneumococcal antibodies.
- Post-immunization samples should be taken at 3–4 weeks to see optimum response.
- Assays have tended to focus on agents for which there are safe and effective vaccines.
- ⚕: Live vaccines should *never* be given to any patient in whom immunodeficiency is suspected.
- Antibodies normally run in immunology laboratories include: pneumococcal polysaccharides, which may be further differentiated as IgG_1 and IgG_2; *Haemophilus influenzae* type B (Hib); and tetanus.
- Assays to individual serotypes of *Pneumococcus* are available in reference laboratories: this is a time-consuming and expensive test, but can be automated using multiplex systems, and should only be used by experienced immunologists investigating suspected immune failure.
  - Serotypes are of different immunogenicity.
  - Cut off for response is debated (between 0.15 and 0.35). Most immunologists accept 0.35 mg/l.
  - Criteria for a response when comparing pre- and post-vaccination samples is also debated: an absolute increase of 0.3 mg/l to eight or more serotypes tested (and present in the vaccine!) or ≥ 2-fold rise (provided that it exceeds threshold).

- Diphtheria antibodies are not run by many laboratories as the assay's EQA performance has been so poor. However, they are available if required.
- Antibodies to *Pseudomonas* and *Burkholderia* are used in cystic fibrosis.
- Antibodies to *Salmonella* Vi antigens are being studied as a potential for evaluating immune response to polysaccharide antigens (alternative to pneumococcal antibodies).
- Meningococcal C polysaccharide antibodies are run by a few specialized laboratories, but correspondence with known clinical status has been poor and there is no EQA.
- ASOT may be helpful; antibodies to staphylolysin are not useful and in most centres no longer available.
- Viral antibodies may be valuable—to natural exposure and immunization antigens such as polio, measles, mumps, rubella, chickenpox, EBV, and hepatitis B (if immunized).
- Isohaemagglutinins are naturally occurring IgM antibodies (in patients of suitable blood group) and can be measured as part of a functional antibody screen. Doubt has been cast on their value as a routine test. However, I am aware of several cases of antibody deficiency identified in pregnancy by a lack of appropriate isohaemagglutinins.

Indications for testing

- These assays should be used in the work-up of patients with suspected immunodeficiency, or in monitoring change in such patients.
- Anti-*Pseudomonas*/*Burkholderia* antibodies are used in some centres for monitoring CF patients.
- Responsiveness to immunization is a helpful marker of immunological recovery post-bone marrow transplant.
- Annual monitoring of levels may be valuable in asplenic patients, as such patients lose immunity more rapidly than a eusplenic population.

Interpretation

- Interpretation is entirely dependent on the context!
- Assays for pneumococcal polysaccharides measure a composite of responses to the 23 strains in the Pneumovax® 23 vaccine. This can be misleading as not all strains represented in the vaccine are equipotent as immunostimulators. This means that a 'normal' response may actually mean a good response to the immunogenic strains masking failure of response to the less immunogenic strains.
- Evaluation of the response to conjugated pneumococcal vaccines and the measurement of serotype-specific responses may be helpful.
- For this reason, evaluation of such patients should be carried out by an immunologist with an interest in immunodeficiency. More weight should be placed on changes in response to immunization than to actual values—hence the need to run pre- and post-immunization samples together.
- A 'normal' response to immunization has never been standardized; publications frequently use different criteria, rendering comparison impossible. The following is a useful working definition:
  - ▶A fourfold rise in titre that rises to well within the normal range.

- All antibody responses must be interpreted in the light of the clinical history and previous infections/immunizations.
- Some patients lose specific antibody rapidly, within 3–6 months of immunizations (i.e. poor long-term immunological memory): if this is suspected then repeat testing after 6 months.
- Measured responses if conjugated pneumococcal vaccines (Prevenar 13®), which contain fewer serotypes, are used may be lower if the laboratory uses assays based on Pneumovax® 23 as the test antigen mix.

Bence Jones proteins

See ➔ 'Urine electrophoresis and immunofixation' and 'Urine free light chains', pp. 506–7.

β_2-Microglobulin (β_2MG)

- Units: mg/l.
- Normal range: 1–3 mg/l.

Principles of test

- Test measures free β_2-microglobulin, which normally forms the light chain of HLA class I molecules but is shed when there is increased lymphocyte turnover and is therefore present in the serum in soluble form. It is usually rapidly cleared by the kidneys.
- It has a molecular weight of 11–12 kDa.
- Measurement is usually by automated analyser, nephelometry, or turbidimetry.
- RID is still used but it is slow.

Indications for testing

- The main indication is as part of the routine monitoring of patients with myeloma, lymphoma, and HIV. However, its non-specific nature and the influence of renal function on results mean that it is less widely used.
- Serum-free light chains are replacing β_2MG in the monitoring of myeloma.
- Elevated levels can be seen in dialysis patients and are a risk factor for β_2MG amyloid.

Interpretation

Levels are elevated in the following:
- HIV infection (surrogate marker of progression).
  - In HIV disease, β_2MG is said to be a useful surrogate predictor of disease progression, and gives similar information to the absolute CD4+ T-cell count. However, the dynamic range in HIV is small compared to that in lymphoproliferative diseases. The CD4+ T-cell count and viral load are preferred in the UK.
- Other viral infections.

- Myeloma (marker of tumour mass).
  - In myeloma, serial measurement of β_2MG is a useful adjunct in terms of monitoring tumour burden and cell turnover. Interpretation of levels is complicated by the need to consider renal function, particularly as free light chains are nephrotoxic and may damage tubules, thus inhibiting reabsorption, and there may also be glomerular damage preventing filtration: the effects on β_2MG serum levels in myeloma are therefore complex.
  - Levels below 4 mg/l are associated with a good prognosis, while levels above 20 mg/l are associated with a poor prognosis, although this may well represent the effects of renal damage.
  - Treatment with α-interferon elevates serum levels, which needs to be considered in monitoring levels.
- Lymphoma.
- Common variable immunodeficiency (correlation with severity): it appears most highly correlated with granulomatous disease.
- Renal dialysis (depending on type of membrane): very high levels may be associated with amyloid.
- High levels may also be seen in renal tubular dysfunction, such as damage from aminoglycoside drugs.
- Allograft rejection (beware of intercurrent viral infections); levels will fall with treatment.
- Elevated levels of β_2MG are seen in connective tissue diseases such as Sjögren's syndrome and rheumatoid arthritis, and in granulomatous diseases such as sarcoidosis. Levels fall when patients are treated with corticosteroids or other lymphocytotoxic chemotherapy.
- Measurement of urinary β_2MG is of no value as it is rapidly degraded in urine.

Biologicals: drug levels and anti-drug antibodies

Routine monitoring of drugs levels for adalimumab and infliximab and anti-drug antibodies are available through a number of centres including the PRU in Sheffield. Caution may need to be exercised with both types of assays where biosimilars are used, as the assays may only be calibrated for one molecule. Assays for both drugs and anti-drug antibodies are carried out by ELISA, interferon beta-2 is used in the treatment of MS and during treatment clinically significant antibodies to the drug may develop. Not all patients develop the antibodies, but in those that do the antibodies are persistent.

- Infliximab drug level units: mg/l.
  - Subtherapeutic: < 3 mg/l;
  - Therapeutic: 3–7 mg/l;
  - Supratherapeutic: > 7 mg/l.
- Anti-infliximab antibodies: normal = negative.
- Adalimumab drug level units: mg/l.
  - Subtherapeutic: < 3 mg/l;
  - Therapeutic: 3–7 mg/l;
  - Supratherapeutic: > 7 mg/l.

- Anti-adalimumab antibodies: normal = negative.
- Neutralizing antibodies to β_2-interferon: normal = negative.
- Low levels may be due to under-dosing, poor compliance, or anti-drug antibodies. Low levels should trigger checking for antibodies. Antibodies should also be checked if there are adverse reactions to the drugs.

Caeruloplasmin

- Units: g/l.
- Normal adult range: 0.19–0.71 g/l.

Principles of test

- Caeruloplasmin is measured by nephelometry.

Indications for testing

- Clinically, the most important indication for measurement is in suspected Wilson's disease.
- It has been proposed as a useful marker in the monitoring of vasculitis, although it is doubtful whether it gives any additional information over measurement of CRP (it is the cause of green serum in vasculitis!).

Interpretation

- Caeruloplasmin is a copper-binding protein, of molecular weight 150 kDa, with an $\alpha 2$ mobility on electrophoresis.
- Levels are reduced in most cases of Wilson's disease (hepatolenticular degeneration), although a few patients will have normal values, usually when there is an intercurrent stimulus to the acute-phase response.
- As it is synthesized in the liver, levels will be reduced in severe liver disease (hepatitis and primary biliary cirrhosis).
- Levels are reduced in severe malabsorptive syndromes where there is copper deficiency.
- Levels will be elevated in acute-phase responses, in particular in rheumatoid arthritis and vasculitis, and in pregnancy, oral contraceptive use, and thyrotoxicosis.

Complement C3, C4, and factor B

- Units: g/l or mg/l.
- Normal ranges:
  - complement C3, 0.68–1.80 g/l;
  - complement C4, 0.18–0.60 g/l;
  - complement factor B, 295–400 mg/l.

Principles of test

- C3, C4, and factor B are usually measured by rate nephelometry or turbidimetry.
- Care needs to be taken with samples as venepuncture and transportation may lead to *in vitro* activation, which may reduce levels of C3 and especially C4 and lead to spurious increases in breakdown

products. This may be prevented by taking samples into EDTA, as breakdown is calcium dependent.

Indications for testing

- Valuable in:
  - suspected SLE (C3, C4, C3d);
  - suspected complement deficiency (C3, C4, haemolytic complement);
  - suspected anaphylaxis (anaphylotoxins C4a, C5a);
  - suspected hereditary angioedema (C3, C4, C1q, C1 esterase inhibitor, immunochemical *and* functional);
  - monitoring SLE and immune complex disease (SBE, serum sickness);
  - atypical HUS.
- Measurement of all three components allows analysis of both classical and alternate pathway activation; factor B is not usually measured routinely.
- See Table 17.3.

Interpretation

- Complement deficiency is common (especially C4 and C2 deficiency); predisposes to recurrent neisserial disease, bacterial infections (C3 deficiency), and immune complex disease (lupus-like).
- Measurement of C3 is valuable in monitoring SLE. C4 null alleles are common and affect the baseline level of C4: it is not possible to use C4 levels as a marker of activity in SLE without knowing how many null alleles there are.
- It is useful in the diagnosis of SBE (reduced C3), post-streptococcal glomerulonephritis (low C3), and other conditions of complement activation.
- A persistently low C3 may indicate the presence of a C3-nephritic factor (see ➲ Chapter 18).
- In patients with angioedema, a low C4 may indicate C1-esterase inhibitor deficiency, but a normal C4 does not exclude the diagnosis.
- Both C3 and C4 are acute-phase proteins, and may therefore be normal even at times of rapid consumption: assessment of C3 breakdown products is advised.
- C4 is often reduced in pre-eclampsia.

Table 17.3 Levels of C3 and C4—indications for testing

Low C4, normal C3	Normal C4, low C3	Low C4, low C3
Genetic deficiency	Post-streptococcal GN	Sepsis
SLE (active)—check C3 breakdown products	C3-nephritic factor (persistent low C3)	SLE (active)
Hereditary angioedema	Gram-negative sepsis (alternate pathway activation)	RhA (rare)
Type II cryoglobulins		SBE
Eclampsia		

Complement allotypes

The locations for the complement genes are known. C2, factor B, C4A, and C4B form part of the MHC genes (class III) encoded on chromosome 6, linked to HLA-DR. C3 is encoded by an autosomal co-dominant system on chromosome 19. Null alleles are common, particularly for C2 and C4. Determination of the complement allotypes is sometimes undertaken as part of extended MHC phenotyping/genotyping when looking at disease association and specifically at complement deficiency states. It may also be used as an additional test during tissue typing. C4 null alleles confer an increased risk of developing SLE and also drug-induced lupus. C4 null alleles have also been associated with systemic sclerosis, rheumatoid arthritis, common variable immunodeficiency, and selective IgA deficiency. Complement allotypes are available through the PRUs—see their website for further details of sample requirements and indications.

$CH_{100}/APCH_{100}$ (haemolytic complement; lytic complement function tests)

- Units: can be reported in arbitrary units, or percentage of normal plasma but better reported as 'normal', 'reduced', or 'absent', when used for the diagnosis of primary complement deficiencies.
- Normal range: present (80–120% of reference plasma).
- Quantitative assays are available for CH_{50}.

Principles of test

- Haemolytic complement assays screen for the integrity of the classical, alternate pathways and the terminal lytic sequence, and use either antibody-coated sheep cells (CH_{100}, classical pathway) or guinea-pig red cells ($APCH_{100}$, alternate pathway). Either a gel or liquid assay can be used. If a liquid-based assay is performed the results are reported at the point of 50% lysis (CH_{50}, $APCH_{50}$). These can now be automated.
- Liposomal lysis in the presence of complement to produce a colour change.
- Kinetic CH_{50} plate assays are available and are more appropriate for use when monitoring the response of aHUS to eculizumab, where rapid turnaround of tests is required.
- For the investigation of complement deficiency both CH_{100} and $APCH_{100}$ must be performed in parallel.
- In both types of assay the classical pathway activity is detected by using antibody-coated sheep red cells, while, for the alternate pathway, guinea-pig red cells are used, as these are susceptible to direct lysis via the alternate pathway.
- Both assays are dependent on the terminal lytic sequence.
- Activity can be reported in terms of units/ml or compared to a standard serum and reported as a percentage. However, it is probably adequate to report as 'normal', 'low', or 'absent'.

Indications for testing
- Any patient in whom deficiency of a complement component is suspected.
- Any patient with recurrent neisserial disease or infection with an unusual strain of *Neisseria*.

Interpretation
- Reduced levels of haemolytic activity will be seen during infections and during immune complex diseases such as serum sickness and SLE. It will also be seen after treatment with eculizumab.
- Testing for absence of a component needs to be undertaken at a minimum of 4–6 weeks after recovery from infection.
- Absence in both CH_{100} and $APCH_{100}$ indicates a deficiency in the terminal lytic sequence C5–C9 (C9 deficiency will give slow lysis).
- Absence in CH_{100} indicates a missing component in the classical pathway C1–C4.
- Absence in $APCH_{100}$ indicates deficiency in alternate pathway (factor D, factor B, C3).
- Follow-up testing to identify missing component must be undertaken if there is absence of activity in one or both of the assays.
- Serial monitoring of haemolytic complement activity has been used to monitor disease activity in SLE, but is not a reliable or accurate measure. C3 breakdown products of C5b–C9 assays are better, if available.

❶Critical action: anyone who has a single episode of neisserial meningitis with an unusual strain or a second episode *must* be assumed to have a complement deficiency until proven otherwise. Investigation of haemolytic complement after recovery is mandatory.

C1-esterase inhibitor (immunochemical and functional)
- Units:
  - immunochemical, g/l;
  - functional, reported as percentage activity compared to normal fresh plasma.
- Normal range:
  - immunochemical, 0.18–0.54 g/l (paediatric ranges not well defined, but lower than adult ranges);
  - functional, 80–120% normal plasma.

Principles of tests
- Immunochemical measurement carried out by RID or nephelometry; functional assay is usually a colorimetric assay.
- If C4 is low in a patient with angioedema and immunochemical C1-esterase inhibitor is normal or high, suspect type II HAE and measure C1-esterase inhibitor function.
- If immunochemical C1-esterase inhibitor is low/absent, there is no additional value to measuring functional C1-esterase inhibitor.

- There are a number of specific assays for functional C1-esterase inhibitor, including commercial colorimetric assays. Some require citrated plasma while others require serum, and it is important to check which samples are required by the local laboratory.
- The inhibitor is labile and samples should be separated as soon as possible to avoid artefactually reduced levels.
- EQA scheme for both immunochemical and functional inhibitor levels is available in UK.

Indications for testing

- Key indication is angioedema occurring *without* urticaria at any age. If urticaria is present, diagnosis is *never* C1-esterase inhibitor deficiency.
- C4 is a useful screen: normal C4 during an attack makes C1-inhibitor deficiency less likely; however, normal C4 does not exclude the diagnosis.

Interpretation

- C1-esterase inhibitor is a control protein of the classical pathway. C1-esterase inhibitor deficiency causes hereditary angioedema.
- Two main types of HAE are recognized, related to C1-inhibitor deficiency (other types exist—see ➲ Chapter 1):
  - type I (common, 80%); absence of immunochemical C1-esterase inhibitor;
  - type II (rare 20%); presence of non-functional C1-esterase inhibitor; due to point mutations affecting enzyme active site; immunochemical levels normal or high.
- Both are inherited as autosomal dominants.
- HAE presents with angioedema, usually with *no* urticaria; may involve larynx and gut, usual onset at puberty.
- C4 usually absent during acute attacks. See ➲ Chapter 1 for treatment.
- Rare acquired form due to autoantibody to C1-esterase inhibitor (SLE, myeloma, splenic villous lymphoma); C1q levels are reduced and a paraprotein may be present.
- The development of new angioedema in an older patient should lead to a search for such a paraprotein (immunoglobulins, electrophoresis, paraprotein, and β_2-microglobulin) and for its source (look for spleen, lymph nodes, and consider CT scan), as well for evidence of complement consumption.
- Some centres are able to identify autoantibodies to C1-inhibitor.

Complement breakdown products

Measurements of specific complement breakdown products such as factor Bb, C3bi, and C3d are more valuable as markers of complement turnover. Several tests are available.
- Units:
  - C3d, mg/l;
  - SC5b–9, μg/l.

- Normal range:
  - C3d, < 5 mg/l;
  - SC5b–9, < 60 μg/l.

Principles of tests
- C3d is measured by NanoRID (Binding Site) sC5b–9 by sandwich ELISA.
- There is no gold standard. There is no EQA.
- Because some activation of C3 occurs with blood clotting, it is essential that samples are taken into EDTA, which chelates the calcium required for C3 degradation. EDTA plasma must be separated within 60 minutes of venepuncture and stored/transported frozen.

Indications for testing
- Testing for C3 breakdown products is essential in any condition in which complement consumption is suspected or when anti-complement therapy is in use (eculizumab).
- As C3 (and other complement proteins) is an acute-phase protein, levels may be normal even with consumption: measurement of breakdown is therefore the only reliable way of detecting the complement-consuming process.

Interpretation
- C3d levels correlate with disease activity in SLE, and are also elevated in patients with severe diffuse cutaneous disease associated with systemic sclerosis.
  - They are valuable because, as noted previously, C3 is an acute-phase protein and levels may remain within the normal range despite significant consumption if there is an acute phase.
- Other assays have been studied: the best seems to be a multistage sandwich ELISA to detect the terminal lytic complex C5b–C9. This also correlates well with disease activity, but is a more expensive and complicated assay.

C1q
- Units, mg/l.
- Normal range, adults 50–250 mg/l (PRU).

Principles of test
- Measurement is usually by RID.

Indications
- Abnormal CH_{100}, with normal $APCH_{100}$.
- Suspected acquired angioedema.

Interpretation
- Low C1q is supposedly associated specifically with acquired but not hereditary angioedema.
- Familial deficiency may occur, causing recurrent bacterial infections, SLE, and glomerulonephritis.

Other individual complement components

- Units: mg/l.
- Normal ranges (taken from the PRU, Sheffield):
  - C2, 10–30 mg/l;
  - C5, 80–150 mg/l;
  - C6, 40–80 mg/l;
  - C7, 50–80 mg/l;
  - C8, 40–280 mg/l
  - C9, 50–250 mg/l.

Principles of tests

- Measurement of individual complement components requires the availability of specific antisera.
- They are usually detected by either double diffusion or RID.
- It may be necessary to carry out functional assays, with complementation by other sera with known complement deficiencies.
- Measurement of individual components should follow, not precede, a functional evaluation by $CH_{100}/APCH_{100}$, to determine the location of the missing component.

Indications for testing

- Testing is of value in the investigation of recurrent meningococcal disease, glomerulonephritis (C1q, C2, C3), pyogenic infections (C3, factors D, P, I), and atypical lupus (C1q, C2, C4, C5–8), where deficiency of a complement component is suspected.

Interpretation

- C2 levels will be reduced in activation of the classical pathway. However, C2 deficiency is the most common deficiency of the complement pathway, with C2 null alleles occurring at a frequency of between 1 in 100 to 1 in 500.
- C2 deficiency often leads to an atypical form of lupus in which skin manifestations are common.
- As active lupus will lower C2 levels through consumption, it is often difficult to be sure whether complete C2 deficiency is present.
- However, in complete deficiency the CH_{100} will be absent.
- Genetic studies may be necessary to confirm the diagnosis.
- Other complement components may be absent in atypical lupus, glomerulonephritis, and pyogenic infections.

C3a, C4a, and C5a (anaphylotoxins)

- Units: µg/l.
- Normal ranges:
  - C3a, 10–570 µg/l (EDTA plasma);
  - C4a, 102–212 µg/l;
  - C5a, < 10 µg/l.

Principles of test

- Assays are not readily available (radioimmunoassay), but the PRUs offer testing.
- Samples need special handling as the anaphylotoxins are labile: special collection tubes are required containing a protease inhibitor, nafamostat, as well as EDTA. The commercial source of these tubes has now ceased production. Immediate separation and freezing of the plasma is required for accurate measurement.

Indications for testing

- Anaphylotoxins are released as part of the activation process of the complement cascade, being cleaved off their parent molecules. All share a terminal arginine, which is essential for biological activity and which is removed by carboxypeptidase-N, the enzyme responsible for their inactivation.
- All are potent triggers for histamine release and smooth muscle constrictors, and they increase vascular permeability. They also act as chemotactic factors and aggregate neutrophils.
- Clinical utility of measurements of the anaphylotoxins is limited, although they may be valuable in monitoring shocked patients, patients with respiratory distress syndrome, and in patients undergoing extracorporeal circulation.
- Although they change in other conditions with complement activation, such as SLE, there are other, more convenient assays that will give the same information.

Complement factors H and I

- Units: g/l and mg/l.
- Normal range:
  - factor H, 0.35–0.59 g/l;
  - factor I, 21–40 mg/l.

Principles of test

- RID is used to measure factors H and I.

Indications for testing

- Haemolytic–uraemic syndrome (HUS).

Interpretation

- Deficiency of either of these factors may lead to HUS. Measurement is possible in specialized centres, with follow-up genetic testing.

C4-binding protein (C4BP)

- Units: µg/l.
- Normal range, adults: 140–220 µg/l.
- C4BP is an acute-phase regulatory protein of the complement system, as a cofactor for factor I.

- It binds to protein S and serum amyloid P (SAP).
- Familial deficiency has been associated with atypical Behçet's syndrome.
- Raised levels are seen in young patients with strokes (reduced free protein S), in pregnancy, nephrotic syndrome, DIC, SLE, and recurrent thromboses.

Cryoglobulins

- Units: usually reported qualitatively but a 'cryocrit' can be measured in a similar way to a manual haematocrit using capillary tubes. The cryocrit will be reported as a percentage of the serum volume.
- Normal range: tiny amounts of cryoglobulins may be found in normal individuals.

Principles of test

- Cryoglobulins are immunoglobulins that precipitate when serum is cooled. The temperature at which this occurs determines whether disease will result. If the blood circulates through a part of the body where the temperature is below the critical temperature, then the protein will precipitate in the capillaries causing obstruction, vascular damage, and eventually necrosis.
- The reason for cold insolubility is unknown but may be due to abnormal amino acid structure (paraproteins) and abnormal glycosylation (connective tissue disease).
- All immunoglobulins will precipitate to a small extent in the cold.
- The temperature of the hand is approximately 28°C at ambient room temperature: immunoglobulins that precipitate at or above 28°C will cause clinical problems (obviously lower if ambient temperature is reduced).
- To detect cryoglobulins, take blood using a warmed syringe into a warmed bottle and transport to laboratory at 37°C, using a thermos flask with either pre-warmed sand or water at 37°C. The laboratory will allow the blood to clot at 37°C and then cool the serum to 4°C.
- Cryoglobulins will form a precipitate as the temperature drops. This usually occurs within 24 hours, but occasionally longer is needed.
- The precipitate is then washed and redissolved for analysis by electrophoresis and immunofixation.
- The redissolved cryoprecipitate should be tested for rheumatoid factor activity.
- Measurement of immunoglobulin in sera with cryoglobulins will give misleading results on nephelometers and turbidimeters: RID carried out at 37°C is required.
- Cryoglobulins are *not* the same as cold agglutinins (a feature of *Mycoplasma pneumoniae* infection).

Indications for testing

- All patients with Raynaud's phenomenon of new onset, or with winter onset of purpuric or vasculitic lesions on the extremities.
- Chronic hepatitis C infection is often accompanied by type II cryoglobulinaemia and a characteristic syndrome: 'mixed essential cryoglobulinaemia' = autoimmune phenomena, arthritis, ulceration, glomerulonephritis, neuropathy. C3 normal; C4 reduced.
- Patients with myeloma, SLE, Sjögren's syndrome, and rheumatoid arthritis.

Interpretation

- See Table 17.4.
- Most cryoglobulins are IgG or IgM; IgA and free light chain cryoglobulins are rare.
- HCV-associated cryoglobulins are very common in northern Italy.
- In infection-triggered cryoglobulinaemia, the immunoglobulins may have specificity against the infecting agent.

Table 17.4 Interpretation of cryoglobulin tests

Type of cryoglobulin	Nature of cryoprecipitate
Type I	All monoclonal immunoglobulin: myeloma, lymphoma
Type II	Monoclonal immunoglobulin with rheumatoid factor activity: myeloma, lymphoma, connective tissue diseases, infections (especially HCV, SBE)
Type III	Polyclonal rheumatoid factor: connective tissue diseases, infections

Cryofibrinogen

- This is found less commonly than cryoglobulins, and presents with typical cold-induced vasculitic lesions on exposed areas.
- To detect a cryofibrinogen, paired EDTA and clotted samples (*not* heparin) must be taken at 37°C and transported at that temperature to the laboratory, where the serum and plasma will be separated warm and then cooled to 4°C. The cryoprecipitate will form only in the EDTA plasma. This will be washed, redissolved, and its identity confirmed either by direct measurement or by immunofixation on electrophoresis.
- The main association is with occult malignancy and thrombophelebitis migrans. Commonest tumours include myeloma, leukaemia, and carcinoma of the prostate.
- Also associated with IgA nephropathy, connective tissue disease, pregnancy, OCP use, diabetes mellitus, and cold urticaria.
- A separate form may also be seen in heparin-treated patients, when the heparin acts as a cofactor for the precipitation.

C-reactive protein (CRP)

See ➔ 'Acute-phase proteins', p. 474.

CSF proteins

- Units: g/l.
- Normal adult range:
  - IgG, 0.01–0.05 g/l;
  - albumin, 0.06–0.26 g/l;
  - IgG:albumin ratio, < 22%.

Principles of test

- IgG and albumin measured by nephelometry.
- Oligoclonal bands detected by isoelectric focusing (IEF) and immunoblotting of paired serum and CSF.

Indications for testing

- Measurement of CSF IgG, albumin, and detection of oligoclonal bands are useful as adjunctive tests in the diagnosis of multiple sclerosis.
- Other CSF proteins can be measured at PRUs (myelin basic protein and tau proteins); these may provide other confirmatory evidence in suspected demyelination.

Interpretation

- When the blood–brain barrier is intact, mainly low molecular weight proteins are found in the CSF.
- Any inflammatory disease increases the passage of proteins into the CSF, including those of higher molecular weight.
- Certain conditions are associated with the presence of plasma cells within the brain, leading to local immunoglobulin production, which is oligoclonal.
- Contamination of the CSF with blood through poor lumbar puncture (LP) technique renders the test uninterpretable.
- Elevation of the CSF IgG or a ratio of CSF IgG/CSF albumin > 22% is strongly suggestive of intrathecal synthesis.
- Intrathecal synthesis of IgG is present if IEF bands are detected in CSF but not serum.
- Oligoclonal IgG bands in the CSF are found in MS but may also occur in encephalitis, neurosarcoid, neurosyphilis, meningitis, polyneuritis, subacute sclerosing panencephalitis, SLE, and tumours.
- If a paraprotein is present in serum, then this may also be found in the CSF.
- By international consensus, five types of CSF analysis are accepted:
  - Type 1: normal.
  - Type 2: oligoclonal IgG restricted to CSF.
  - Type 3: oligoclonal IgG in CSF with additional bands in serum and CSF.
  - Type 4: identical oligoclonal bands in CSF and serum.
  - Type 5: identical monoclonal bands in CSF and serum.

- Complex calculations of other indices, based on CSF and serum IgG, IgM, and albumin concentrations, and on the IgG synthetic rate have been proposed. They add little information to that obtained from the CSF IgG:albumin ratio, which costs half as much.
- Where unusual infections are suspected, it may be valuable to compare the ratio of specific antiviral titres in the CSF and serum with the equivalent ratio for IgG: if the ratio is higher for the specific antibody, then it suggests that there is a CNS infection.

Fungal precipitins

- Units: semi-quantitative.
- Normal range:
  - may be found in healthy exposed individuals;
  - highest titres in heavily exposed individuals.

Principles of test

- Precipitating IgG antibodies to fungal antigens are usually detected by immunodiffusion, although ELISA, UniCAP®, and fluorescent techniques are also used.

Indications for testing

- Suspected type III hypersensitivity pneumonitis to fungal or other proteins.

Interpretation

- Farmer's lung is typically associated with antibodies to *Aspergillus fumigatus*, *Thermoactinomyces vulgaris*, and *Micropolyspora faeni*.
- Other occupational lung diseases (malt-workers' lung, etc.) may be associated with other fungi, including *Aspergillus clavatus*.
- Antigens are predominantly low molecular weight.
- Antibodies are not diagnostic, but are markers of exposure and should always be interpreted in the light of clinical findings.
- Usually few precipitin lines are present.
- Concentration of the sera may be required to reveal weak lines.
- The antibody response is reduced in smokers.
- When an aspergilloma (fungus ball) is present, often in an old tuberculous cavity, antibodies to high molecular weight antigens may be detected. Here there are multiple precipitin lines and the antibodies are frequently readily detectable, even in unconcentrated sera.
- Allergic bronchopulmonary aspergillosis (ABPA) is an eosinophilic pneumonia, which is also associated with precipitating antibodies to *Aspergillus fumigatus*. Total IgE and *Aspergillus*-specific IgE are elevated.
- Other fungi that are associated with an IgE-mediated response include *Cladosporium*, *Alternaria*, and *Penicillium* species. These are associated mainly with asthmatic symptoms (e.g. in inhabitants of damp, mouldy accommodation).

- Some hypersensitivity pneumonitides (cheese-worker's lung, humidifier fever (*Penicillium*), wood-worker's lung (*Alternaria*)) may be associated with precipitins to these fungi, but the tests are not reliable for diagnoses, as the fungi are ubiquitous and many healthy individuals have antibodies.
- IgG antibodies to *Candida* species may be found in otherwise healthy individuals, indicating the ubiquitous nature of the yeast. These include antibodies against the mannan component (polysaccharide), as well as protein antigens.
- Indeed, absence of antibodies to *Candida albicans* mannan may suggest the possibility of a humoral immune deficiency.
- Patients with chronic mucocutaneous candidiasis (see ⮕ Chapter 1) often have very high levels of IgG precipitins to *Candida*, with multiple precipitin lines, and this is helpful in diagnosis.
- Testing for antibodies to *Candida* in other immunodeficiencies, such as HIV infection, when yeast infection is suspected, is unreliable. Similar constraints apply to detection of antibodies to *Nocardia*.

Haptoglobin

- Units: g/l.
- Normal adult range: 1.0–3.0 g/l.

Principles of test
- Nephelometry/turbidimetry.

Indications for testing
- Suspected haemolysis.

Interpretation
- Haptoglobin is an α_2-globulin that is involved in the recycling of haem iron, by binding free haemoglobin.
- Levels are markedly reduced in the presence of haemolysis.
- Other diseases leading to increased red cell fragility, such as sickle-cell disease, thalassaemia, and G6PD deficiency, are also associated with reduced haptoglobin levels.
- Genetic lack of haptoglobin has been reported.
- Elevated levels are seen in biliary obstruction, aplastic anaemia, and as part of an acute-phase response.
- Haptoglobin exists in polymeric forms, which gives rise to difficulties in measurement by RID.

Interleukin-6

- Known to be involved in inflammatory diseases (rheumatoid arthritis, JIA, Crohn's disease).
- Raised in Castleman's syndrome, but biopsy is diagnostic.
- Assay by electrochemiluminescence via the PRU, Sheffield.

- Reference range < 7 pg/ml.
- Monitoring CRP (driven by IL-6) is more practical, as this can be run daily on automated analysers.

Anti-IgA antibodies

- Units: titre.
- Normal range: not defined.

Principles of test

- ELISA and tanned red cell agglutination are used.
- Assay detects IgM and IgG but not IgE antibodies.

Indications for testing

- Investigation of transfusion reactions including reactions to IVIg.

Interpretation

- Reported in the context of reactions to blood products and immunoglobulins.
- Will only occur in patients with complete absence of IgA (selective IgA deficiency, CVID).
- Expected to be rare in XLA where there is no capacity to produce antibody of any class.
- May be found in healthy IgA-deficient individuals.
- Clinical significance is uncertain; IgE antibodies have been reported and may be more significant in the context of acute transfusion reactions: these are *not* detected by current assays.
- Risk of adverse reactions in IgA-deficient individuals is estimated at 1 in 15 million.
- Similar problems of transfusion reactions have been found in patients with deficiencies of either C4A or C4B (Chido and Rodgers blood groups), as they may also see infused C4 as foreign and make an antibody response.

IgA subclasses and IgD

IgA subclasses

- IgA exists as two subclasses: IgA_1, the predominant serum IgA, and IgA_2, which occurs in secretions with IgA_1 in roughly equal amounts.
- Specific deficiencies of IgA_1 and IgA_2, either alone or in combination with other immunoglobulin abnormalities, have been described.
- There are no routine indications for measurement but it has been suggested that measurement of IgA subclasses may be valuable in the investigation of recurrent *Haemophilus* infection of the respiratory tract.
- May also be valuable in the investigation of transfusion reactions where some IgA is detected, as the patient may be deficient in only one subclass and hence see the other subclass as 'foreign'.

IgD
- Units: kU/l.
- Normal range (adults only):
  - IgD, 2–100 kU/l.
- Rarely measured in clinical practice, as its main function is as a membrane receptor.
- Elevated levels may be seen in the periodic fever syndrome, hyper-IgD syndrome, due to deficiency of mevalonate kinase, and in IgD-secreting myeloma (rare).
- Only 70% of patients with hyper-IgD syndrome will have an IgD > 100 kU/l: a normal IgD does not exclude the diagnosis.
- Measurement is by ELISA.

Immunoglobulins (total serum) 1
- Units: g/l.
- Normal range (adults only):
  - IgG, 5.8–15.4 g/l;
  - IgA, 0.64–2.97 g/l;
  - IgM (males), 0.24–1.90 g/l;
  - IgM (females), 0.75–2.30 g/l.

Principles of assay
- Normally rate nephelometry/turbidimetry.
- Rarely, radial immunodiffusion may be used: this is slow and less accurate.
- For automated analysers, coefficients of variation should be in the 5–10% range. Results are standardized against international standards. In the UK, an EQA scheme operates.
- Laboratories should provide normal ranges, which vary according to age and sex. Unfortunately, many laboratories do not adjust ranges for age and sex, which may lead to confusion.

Indications for testing
Measurement of serum immunoglobulin is indicated in the following conditions:
- Suspected immunodeficiency (primary or secondary): diagnosis and monitoring.
- Suspected myeloma, Waldenström's macroglobulinaemia, plasmacytoma: diagnosis and monitoring.
- Lymphoma.
- Connective tissue disease.
- Liver disease (primary biliary cirrhosis, hepatitis, cirrhosis).
- Sarcoidosis: diagnosis.
- Post-bone marrow/stem cell transplantation: monitoring.
- Measurement of IgA is usually linked to testing for tissue tranglutaminase antibodies (tTG) and endomysial antibodies, as these are IgA-based assays and IgA deficiency is common. IgA deficiency is common (1 in 400–800 depending on racial background).

Interpretation

- Measurement of serum immunoglobulins does not provide categorical diagnosis in any disease.
- Normal serum immunoglobulins do *not* exclude immunodeficiency.
- In all cases, measurement of immunoglobulins *must* be accompanied by serum electrophoresis, and immunofixation to look for paraproteins (see ➲ 'Immunofixation', p. 500).
- Where IgA is low, further tests (Ouchterlony double diffusion; low-level IgA EIA) should be carried out to prove whether IgA is low or absent.
- Transient reductions in all Ig classes are seen in acute bacterial infections: do not act on a single acute measurement—recheck in convalescence.
- IgM normal ranges in adult show a sex difference (lower in males); many laboratories report an average range: this is incorrect.
- Non-white populations have higher normal ranges than white populations.
- Serum IgA levels may be raised in healthy elderly, due to a change in the balance between synthesis and mucosal loss.
- Raised immunoglobulins on a polyclonal background (on electrophoresis) indicates chronic infection/inflammation.

Immunoglobulins (total serum) 2: causes of hypo- and hypergammaglobulinaemia

Causes of hypogammaglobulinaemia

- X-linked agammaglobulinaemia (absent B cells; all immunoglobulins low/absent).
- Common variable immunodeficiency (reduced T/B cells; low immunoglobulins).
- Hyper-IgM syndrome (normal/raised IgM, low/absent IgG, IgA).
- Selective IgA deficiency (absent IgA, normal IgG, IgM).
- Severe combined immunodeficiency (mainly children; all immunoglobulins low; absent T cells).
- Lymphoma (reduced IgM, IgA normal, IgG normal or low; disease, chemotherapy, or radiotherapy).
- SLE (rare).
- Infections:
  - HIV (rare);
  - herpesviruses (rare, Epstein–Barr virus in X-linked lymphoproliferative disease);
  - acute bacterial infections;
  - measles/rubella.
- Drugs (immunosuppressives, e.g. cyclophosphamide, azathioprine, rituximab, chemotherapy, some anticonvulsants, gold, penicillamine).
- Plasmapheresis.
- Renal loss (IgM normal, IgG and IgA reduced).
- Gastrointestinal loss (IgM normal, IgG and IgA reduced).

Causes of hypergammaglobulinaemia

- Chronic infection (all immunoglobulins raised):
  - osteomyelitis;
  - bacterial endocarditis;
  - tuberculosis.
- Chronic inflammation:
  - SLE, rheumatoid arthritis—all immunoglobulins; elevated;
  - Sjögren's syndrome: raised IgG (all IgG_1; normal or reduced IgG_2, IgG_3, IgG_4).
- Sarcoidosis—raised IgG and IgA; IgM usually normal.
- Liver disease:
  - primary biliary cirrhosis (IgM, may be very high (> 30 g/l) with small monoclonal bands on a polyclonally raised background);
  - alcohol-related (increased IgA, polyclonal, $\beta-\gamma$ bridging on electrophoresis);
  - autoimmune hepatitis (increased IgG, IgA; normal IgM).
- Hodgkin's disease—IgE raised (also eosinophilia).
- Viral infections:
  - acute common viral infections: raised IgM; normal IgG and IgA;
  - HIV—all immunoglobulins raised (IgG very high but polyclonal);
  - EBV—all raised.

❶Critical action

- *All* patients with recurrent infections* should be reviewed by an immunologist or paediatric immunologist (as appropriate), irrespective of age. Any patient with recurrent infections and low serum immunoglobulins has an immunological problem until proven otherwise.
- Patients with unusual infections, or with illness caused by opportunist or normally non-pathogenic organism infections, and patients with infections in unusual sites (without good reason) should all be referred for further investigation.

IgG subclasses

- Units: g/l.
- Normal range (adults):
  - IgG_1, 2.2–10.8 g/l;
  - IgG_2, 0.5–8.0 g/l;
  - IgG_3, 0.05–0.9 g/l;
  - IgG_4, 0.0–2.4 g/l.

Principles of test

- Normally measured by nephelometry or turbidimetry.
- Radial immunodiffusion is still occasionally used.
- EQA scheme exists.

---

* Recurrent infections can be pragmatically defined as two or more major microbiologically/virologically proven infections, requiring hospitalization, within 1 year. One major infection and recurrent minor infections should also be referred, where minor are documented infections requiring treatment in the community.

Indications for testing

- No absolute indications for testing, as significant immunodeficiency can occur in the presence of normal subclasses and, conversely, complete genetic absence of a subclass may be completely asymptomatic.
- Measurement usually performed as part of the work-up of patients with recurrent infections.
- Identification of IgG_4 disease.

Interpretation

- Low levels may be significant in the context of presentation with recurrent infections.
- IgG_1 deficiency is essentially similar in effects to CVID, as IgG_1 comprise the bulk of total serum IgG.
- IgG_2 levels are slow to rise to adult levels. Levels are related to Gm allotypes, which are racially determined.
- IgG_2 levels correlate poorly with anti-polysaccharide responses.
- IgG_2 deficiency may be seen in patients with IgA deficiency and may be associated with poor responses to polysaccharide antigens, such as the capsular polysaccharides of bacteria (see ➔ Chapter 1).
- IgG_2 and IgG_4 deficiency frequently coexist.
- Deficiency of IgG_3, which is involved in immunity against viruses, is associated with asthma and intractable epilepsy.
- Isolated IgG_4 deficiency is of uncertain significance: it may be associated with suppurative lung disease.
- Raised IgG_4 has been associated with a range of unusual autoimmune diseases, including autoimmune pancreatitis.
- Care needs to be taken to ensure that the IgG_4 assay is optimized to identify both low/absent IgG_4 and raised IgG_4.
- IgG_4 disease may be associated with a normal serum IgG_4.
- Polyclonal raised IgG_1 with normal or reduced IgG_2, IgG_3, and IgG_4 is seen in Sjögren's syndrome and is a specific pattern, which may occasionally be helpful in diagnosis.
- A high total IgG may mask a low/absent IgG subclass or specific antibody deficiency.

Immune complexes

- No longer recommended for routine use due to difficulties in reproducibility and standardization.
- Many different assays are described, but performance characteristics are all different and there is no gold standard, or EQA.
- Immune complexes may be detected in healthy individuals and form part of the normal immune response.
- Use of more specific markers of complement activation, such as C3 breakdown products or sC5b–C9 complexes, is recommended.

Immunofixation

- Units: qualitative.
- Normal range: no monoclonal bands should be identifiable.

Principles of test

- Immunofixation has replaced immunoelectrophoresis as test of choice for identification of bands on electrophoresis of serum and urine.
- An electrophoretic strip of the test serum in agarose is overlaid with antibodies specific for heavy and light chains (or any other protein of interest, e.g. fibrinogen, CRP) and allowed to react. Unreacted antibody and serum is then washed from the gel and the remaining precipitate stained with a protein-binding dye.

Indications for testing

- Any serum or urine electrophoresis in which bands are identified should undergo immunofixation.

Interpretation

- Bands should be identified with both heavy and light chains.
- Any serum bands with light chain only should undergo fixation with anti-IgD and anti-IgE, to exclude rare myelomas.
- Heavy chain disease (γ, α, μ) is *rare* and it is commoner for there to be failure of reactivity of antisera with the light chain; serum free light chains are commoner.
- Occasionally, paraproteins may react poorly with an antiserum: it may be necessary to re-fix using antiserum from a different source: this is important if heavy chain-only disease is suspected.
- Paired serum and urine electrophoresis is not required if serum free light chains are being measured.
- More than one paraprotein may be identified, with different heavy and light chains.
- IgA paraproteins may show polymerization with multiple 'step-ladder' bands.
- Serum free light chains may show any mobility and may appear in the pre-albumin region.
- A prozone effect may be seen if the paraprotein level is very high, with poor immunofixation. Re-run with serum at several dilutions.
- Fibrinogen and CRP may cause bands if plasma is used or if serum CRP is significantly raised; both run in the β−γ region of the electrophoretic strip. Well-clotted serum will not show fibrinogen bands.

Interleukin-2 receptors, soluble

- Serum levels of soluble IL-2 receptors are useful in monitoring solid organ allograft recipients, as levels rise early in rejection episodes.
- Levels also rise in acute graft-versus-host disease.
- Elevated levels are seen in other conditions associated with lymphocyte activation, but are not, on the whole, clinically useful.

- Measurement is usually by EIA, but this approach is expensive and not easily given to the very rapid turnaround required for monitoring of graft rejection at reasonable cost.

Isohaemagglutinins

- Isohaemagglutinins are mainly of the IgM class, although IgG antibodies may also be detected.
- Measurement of isohaemagglutinins may be helpful but is no longer considered essential in the investigation of suspected immunodeficiency.
- They are the only permanently present IgM antibodies that can be readily measured.
- Test is unusable in individuals of blood group AB, who lack isohaemagglutinins.
- Titres are very low in small infants aged under 1 year.
- Presence of high titres of IgG isohaemagglutinins in IVIg has been associated with significant haemolysis in isolated case reports. Where very high doses are used, it may be appropriate to 'cross-match' the IVIg against the patient's red cells first.

Mannose-binding lectin (MBL)

- Units: ng/ml.
- Range (adults):
  - < 75 ng/ml = homozygous variant alleles and non-functional MBL, associated with highest risk of infection.
  - 75–399.9 ng/ml = functional MBL deficiency associated with increased risk of infection.
  - 400–1300 ng/ml = heterozygous variant alleles; may show evidence of mild deficiency associated with some increased risk of infections.
  - > 1300 ng/ml = wild type alleles showing no deficiency.

Principles of test
- Measurement is usually by EIA; assays for the function of the MBL pathway, analogous to the CH_{100} pathway, are being developed.

Indications for testing
- Patients with unexplained infections, as part of the work-up for immune deficiency; patients with cystic fibrosis and Behçet's disease as prognostic marker.

Interpretation
- MBL is one of the collectin family of carbohydrate-binding proteins. Structurally it strongly resembles C1q and is capable of activating complement directly (collectin or MBL pathway).
- MBL functions as a soluble non-specific opsonin, binding to oligosaccharides.

- It has been suggested that the deficiency is only significant if other aspects of the innate or specific immune system are impaired, when chronic infections, in particular otitis media and chronic diarrhoea, may occur.
- In adults reduced/absent MBL is a cofactor for recurrent infections when other factors are present.
- Risk can be quantitated in terms of the degree of reduction which is linked to genetic status.
- Reduced MBL is associated with increased severity of cystic fibrosis and Behçet's disease.
- Measurement is usually by EIA; assays for the function of the MBL pathway, analogous to the CH_{100} pathway, are being developed.

Neopterin and orosomucoid

Neopterin

- Neopterin is a pteridine that is synthesized predominantly in macrophages, and levels are increased in diseases when macrophages are active.
- It can be measured in CSF and urine in addition to serum.
- It has been proposed to be a useful surrogate marker in HIV disease. However, levels correlate closely with those of β_2-microglobulin and only one or the other need be measured.
- Levels have also been reported to be elevated in other viral, protozoal, and bacterial infections, especially TB, inflammatory bowel disease, tumours, and chronic fatigue syndromes. It is thus not a specific marker of HIV infection or progress.
- Commercial ELISA assays are available.
- Routine diagnostic use is not recommended.

Orosomucoid

- See ➔ 'α_1-Acid glycoprotein', p. 471.

Paraprotein by scanning densitometry

- Units: g/l.
- Normal range: monoclonal proteins should not be detectable.

Principles of test

- Test measures the amount of monoclonal immunoglobulin by scanning a stained electrophoretic strip.
- Measurement of the total protein is also required (measured chemically).
- Some departments quantitate and report all fractions on the electrophoretic strip: this is unnecessary as a routine, but can be a valuable internal check for observational reporting of electrophoresis (absent $\alpha1$, raised $\alpha2$, increased γ, etc.).

Indications for testing

- All patients in whom serum electrophoresis shows a discrete monoclonal protein.
- Serial monitoring of paraprotein provides an excellent check on the progress of myeloma and related conditions.

Interpretation

- Results from paraprotein measurement may not correlate well with the immunochemical measurements, particularly for IgM and IgA paraproteins, where polymerization may occur in the serum and give erroneous results by nephelometry.
- Healthy adults do not have detectable levels of paraproteins, but up to 20% of elderly patients over the age of 75 will have low levels of paraproteins (< 10 g/l = monoclonal gammopathy of uncertain significance, MGUS).
- Cut-offs for myeloma as opposed to MGUS are set at a monoclonal IgG > 15 g/l and IgA > 10 g/l or any concentration of monoclonal IgD/IgE.
- Chronic infections and chronic inflammatory conditions may also cause low levels of paraproteins, usually in a polyclonal background of increased immunoglobulin.
- Transient monoclonal bands may appear after bone marrow transplantation.
- Bands that overlie the β-region cannot be scanned accurately due to interference from other β-proteins: the interference increases as the paraprotein levels drop. Complex correction formulae exist, but do not increase accuracy.

Pneumococcal polysaccharide antibodies

- See ➲ 'Bacterial and viral antibodies', p. 478.

Pyroglobulins

- Pyroglobulins are immunoglobulins that precipitate as the temperature of the body rises above normal.
- They may appear as a consequence of myeloma due to structurally abnormal proteins.
- Investigation requires a cool sample to be taken and separated and the serum is then warmed to 40°C and the precipitate observed.

Salivary IgA and secretory piece

- This is a qualitative test for the presence of mucosal antibody and may be helpful in the work-up of suspected immunodeficiency.
- True secretory piece deficiency is exceptionally rare.
- The usual technique for detection is by double diffusion.

Serum electrophoresis and immunofixation

- Units:
  - not applicable to electrophoresis (qualitative);
  - paraprotein quantitated by scanning densitometry reported in g/l (see ➾ 'Paraprotein by scanning densitometry', p. 502).
- Normal range: not applicable.

Principles of testing

- In serum or urinary electrophoresis, the relevant body fluid is applied to an electrolyte-containing agarose gel. A current is applied across the gel and causes the proteins to migrate through the gel on the basis of their charge, and to a lesser extent size, until they reach a neutral point in the electric field. The proteins are then visualized with a protein-binding stain.
- If the total protein is known, then the electrophoretic strip can be scanned and the absorption by the stain measured, which will be proportional to the amount of protein in the particular region in the gel (scanning densitometry). Thus any monoclonal bands can be directly measured. This is useful for patients with myeloma, as immunochemical methods for measurement of immunoglobulins may be inaccurate in patients with myeloma (see ➾ 'Paraprotein by scanning densitometry', p. 502).
- Immunofixation is the technique by which monoclonal immunoglobulins are identified by overlaying the electrophoresed strips with antisera against heavy and light chains. These precipitate with the monoclonal proteins in the gel and unbound antisera can be washed free prior to staining (see ➾ 'Immunofixation', p. 500).
- The same techniques can be carried out with urine, although this may require concentration to provide the clearest results.
- Cellulose acetate electrophoresis is no longer recommended as it is less sensitive and is not suitable for densitometric scanning.
- High-throughput semi-automated instruments are available (capillary zone electrophoresis, CZE).

Indications for testing

- Electrophoresis and, if necessary, immunofixation of serum is an integral part of measurement of serum immunoglobulins.

❶ALL requests for serum immunoglobulins must have electrophoresis carried out: failure to do so will lead to important abnormalities being missed.
- There is no place for carrying out electrophoresis as a stand-alone test.

Interpretation

- Serum electrophoresis gives valuable information, not only of immunological status but also of other organ systems.
- Reports are often poorly understood by clinicians and not explained by laboratories.
- Monoclonal proteins, typically IgA, may polymerize to give more than one band.

- The restricted mobility of IgG_4 means that elevated polyclonal IgG_4 in IgG_4 disease may be mistaken for a paraprotein.
- Some patients will have more than one clone present producing different immunoglobulins.
- Densitometry cannot be used where the monoclonal protein overlies the beta-region, as the figures include non-immunoglobulin proteins (see ➲ 'Paraproteins by scanning densitometry', p. 502).
- The reports that may be seen and their interpretation are shown in Table 17.5.

Table 17.5 Interpretation of serum electrophoresis reports

Report	Interpretation
Increased albumin	Dehydration
Reduced albumin	Chronic inflammation, nephrotic syndrome, burns, liver disease, pregnancy
Increased α1 band	Pregnancy
Absent α1 band	Absent/reduced α_1-antitrypsin
Increased α2 band	Chronic inflammation/infection; also seen in nephrotic syndrome, due to selective retention of α_2-macroglobulin; adrenal insufficiency, steroid therapy, advanced diabetes
Decreased α2 band	Malnutrition; megaloblastic anaemia; liver disease; Wilson's disease; protein loss
Increased β	Pregnancy (raised β-lipoprotein) and iron deficiency (transferrin); biliary cirrhosis; Cushing's; hypothyroidism; carcinoma
Increased γ	Caused by polyclonal increase in IgG: amyloidosis; cirrhosis infection/inflammation
Faint band(s) on polyclonal background	Caused by monoclonal escape during polyclonal response to infection/inflammation (does *not* indicate myeloma)
Monoclonal band in γ	Due to myeloma, lymphoma, and MGUS*
Absent/reduced γ	Due to inherited or acquired immunoglobulin deficiency (further investigation **essential**)

* MGUS = monoclonal gammopathy of uncertain significance; most evolve to myeloma given time (years).

Serum free light chains (SFLC)

- Units: mg/l.
- Normal range (adults):
  - serum free κ mg/l, 3.3–19.4 mg/l;
  - serum free λ mg/l, 5.7–26.3 mg/l;
  - κ/λ ratio, 0.26–1.65. Renal range 0.37–3.1.

Principles of test

- SFLC are measured by nephelometry. Free λ light chains tend to be dimeric while κ chains are monomeric. Recognition is by polyclonal antisera specific for free, not bound, light chains.

Indications for testing

- Diagnosis and monitoring of myeloma and other paraproteinaemic states, AL amyloid.

Interpretation

- SFLC are a sensitive test for free light chains, usually produced in excess in myeloma.
- SFLC may be the only product of the tumour cells.
- SFLC are nephrotoxic and therefore SFLC may give a more accurate measure of tumour burden than urinary free light chains.
- Ratio and absolute values may need to be corrected in renal impairment (ratio 0.37–3.1).
- SFLC are likely to replace β_2MG as a marker of tumour mass and urine electrophoresis and immunofixation (about 10 times more sensitive).
- Both κ and λ light chains may be elevated in patients with chronic inflammatory conditions and in the elderly.
- Serial monitoring is appropriate.
- SFLC have replaced urine electrophoresis in some guidelines.
- SFLC are useful in determining the prognosis of monoclonal gammopathies of uncertain significance (MGUS).
- Caution is required where there are very high levels to recognize antigen excess.
- Assays may have linearity problems.
- Two major suppliers of assay kits exist in the UK—results may be significantly different between the two assays, and this may affect kappa to a greater extent than lambda.

Transferrin

- Units: g/l.
- Normal adult range: 2.0–4.0 g/l.
- Serum transferrin is increased in iron deficiency and pregnancy.
- It is reduced in anaemia of chronic disease, chronic infections, burns, and rare genetic absence.
- It is a 'negative' acute-phase protein.
- Measurement of transferrin is also used in calculating the urine selectivity (see ❷ 'Urine selectivity', p. 508).

Urine electrophoresis and immunofixation

- Units: not applicable.
- Normal range: no protein detectable.

Principles of test
- See under ➋ 'Serum electrophoresis and immunofixation', p. 504.
- Random urine is usually satisfactory, but a 24-hour urine is more sensitive. It used to be necessary to concentrate urine prior to electrophoresis, but modern electrophoretic systems have increased sensitivity and have rendered this step unnecessary.

Indications
- This is the screening test to detect free light chains in the urine. SFLC is an alternative test and has largely replaced urine electrophoresis.

Interpretation
- Monoclonal free light chains are associated with myeloma, Waldenström's macroglobulinaemia, and, rarely, with lymphoma.
- Polyclonal free light chains may be found in the urine when there is renal tubular damage, and as a consequence of old age and chronic inflammatory conditions (e.g. rheumatoid arthritis).
- Interpretation of urine electrophoresis is difficult as other discrete proteins may be present that give an appearance similar to monoclonal light chains. In particular, prostatic proteins may appear in the urine in older men and give a step-ladder appearance of bands running in the $\beta-\gamma$ region.
- Immunofixation is essential to confirm the nature of any discrete bands found in the urine.
- SFLC has replaced this test, as SLFC are more sensitive and can be quantitated.

Urine free light chains

- Units: g/l.
- Normal ranges: not detectable.

Principles of test
- Usually by nephelometry/turbidimetry.

Indications for testing
- Patients with known or suspected Bence Jones myeloma (producing only light chains).
- Serial monitoring for known patients.
- SFLC measurement has replaced this test.

Interpretation
- There is no generally accepted technique in use.
- Nephelometric assays use antisera that are calibrated for use mainly against bound, not free, light chains, and in serum, not urine, so it is necessary to undertake an arithmetic correction.
- This is based on some assumptions, including that one-sixth of the mass of intact immunoglobulin is light chain and that all the light chain is either free or bound, but not both, and that, if there is whole Ig, it contains only one type of light chain.
- The correction is to multiply the nephelometric result by 0.17. In urines where both free κ and free λ are detected, the κ:λ ratio should be in the range 1.0–4.0. Values outside this range are highly suggestive of the presence of excess free light chains.
- Abnormal renal function, which may itself be caused by the free light chains, will render the test unusable for serial monitoring as the disease progresses.
- Alternatives to nephelometry for light-chain quantitation include scanning densitometry, but this is less accurate in urine than in serum, unless there is significant proteinuria.
- SFLC are a more accurate measure although correction for renal function is required. SFLC should replace urinary quantitation.

Urine selectivity (IgG and transferrin)
- This test may be useful in determining whether the predominant protein in the urine is low molecular weight (as may occur in minimal change disease) or includes higher molecular weight proteins.
- IgG and transferrin are measured and the urine-to-serum ratio of IgG is divided by the urine to serum ratio of transferrin to give the selectivity.
- A value of > 0.15 indicates 'non-selective' proteinuria and is against a diagnosis of minimal change disease.
- This test is only reliable if proteinuria > 1g/l is present.
- It is no longer widely requested by renal physicians.

Viral antibodies
- See under ➋ 'Bacterial and viral antibodies', p. 478.
- Antibodies against exposure and immunization viral antigens should form part of the work-up of patients suspected of having a humoral immune deficiency.
- Absence of detectable antibodies in patients who have a clear exposure or immunization history is highly suspicious.
- The panel should include measles, mumps, rubella, chickenpox, herpes simplex, EBV, CMV, polio, and hepatitis A and B.
- It is important only to select those where exposure/immunization is documented.

❶Remember that test immunization with live vaccines in suspected immunodeficiency is contraindicated!

Viscosity

- Units: as a ratio.
- Normal adult range: 1.4–1.9 (ratio to water).

Principles of test

- For single measurements a manual viscometer is used that compares fluid flow of patient sample against water between two reservoirs connected by a capillary tube.
- In some laboratories measurement of viscosity has replaced measurement of the ESR as a general acute-phase test, as automated viscometers are available.
- Conversely, many laboratories no longer have the facility to measure viscosity!

Indications

- Measurement of serum viscosity is helpful in monitoring Waldenström's macroglobulinaemia and other myelomas where hyperviscosity occurs.

Interpretation

- Hyperviscosity may lead to serious end-organ damage if undetected: cardiac failure, cerebral infarction, retinal vein occlusion, and renal failure being the major complications.
- IgA myelomas are prone to develop hyperviscosity because the IgA paraprotein frequently polymerizes *in vivo*. This is detected on electrophoresis as a step-ladder of multiple bands.
- If a cryoglobulin is present, the viscosity must be measured under warm conditions.
- Serial monitoring is helpful, particularly when plasmapheresis is being undertaken.
- Viscosity is, however, NOT an appropriate acute-phase monitor, as the dynamic range is tiny.

Autoantibodies

Introduction

There are many hundreds of reported autoantibodies, not all of clinical value. The repertoire of the typical regional immunology laboratory will cover most of the ones described within this chapter. Some will only be available through specialist referral laboratories, or through research laboratories.

When requesting tests, the following criteria should be used.

- Decide in advance what clinically useful information will be obtained by carrying out the test.
- Because a test is available does not mean that it is of value under a given circumstance.
- If a test result does not affect clinical management in any way, testing is of no value.

Autoantibodies are divided broadly into two categories

- Organ specific, where the target antigen has a restricted distribution, usually limited to one organ such as the thyroid gland.
- Organ specific, where the target antigen has a wide distribution.
- Organ-non-specific antibodies may be associated with a disease of restricted organ involvement, for example, primary biliary cirrhosis.
  - Target antigen is in the mitochondria, which are widely distributed, but disease is limited to the liver.
  - It is not clear why autoantibodies to a widely distributed antigen should be associated with an organ-specific disease.
  - It is now known that autoantibodies may in some circumstances cross intact cell membranes: tissue-restricted passage may explain selective effects.

Autoantibodies may also be divided into:

- Primary pathogenic antibodies, where the antibody mediates a functional effect by:
  - interfering with a cellular or molecular function, e.g. the blocking of neuromuscular transmission by antibodies to the acetylcholine receptor on muscle endplates;
  - direct damage to tissues, e.g. anti-glomerular basement membrane antibodies.
  - Views on pathogenicity will be modified in the light of known penetration of whole antibodies into intact cells.
- Secondary antibodies, which are not directly involved in the disease process, are markers for the existence of the process, e.g. anti-thyroglobulin antibodies.
  - These may still be useful diagnostic tools.
- Not all autoantibodies are diagnostically useful, as they may have low sensitivity and specificity, e.g.
  - rheumatoid factor;
  - gliadin antibodies.

Techniques: overview

Multiple techniques may be available to test for individual autoantibodies.
- Comparison of different assays is often lacking.
- Results may vary between different laboratories.
- EQA may be widely discrepant.
- No gold standard assay may be identified.

Establishment of a new test requires:
- Review of existing methods (if any).
- Evaluation by comparison with other assays:
  - tested in healthy controls;
  - disease state;
  - other confounding disease states.
- Calculation of sensitivity and specificity.
- Validation of clinical utility.
- Establishment of internal QC material.
- Validation against national/international standard reference material.
- Participation in external QA (if available).
- Evaluation of cost–benefit.

Diagnostic laboratories may use in-house or commercial assays.
- Commercial assays must be CE (Conformité Européenne)-marked (EU regulations).
  - Cost of CE marking has led manufacturers to withdraw low-volume commercial assays, restricting availability.
- In-house assays may apply for CE marking.
  - This requires evidence of utility, a large application form, and lots of money!
  - Non-CE marked assays may not be sold for profit, but may be used within the NHS.

Type of antibodies
- Autoantibodies can be of any class.
- In most circumstances IgG antibodies are usually sought.
- IgM autoantibodies are not normally significant unless persistent and of high titre.
- IgM anti-cardiolipin antibodies are considered significant.
- IgA autoantibodies are rare but may be diagnostically useful, e.g.
  - coeliac disease: IgA endomysial antibodies have the highest sensitivity and specificity.
- Value of other IgA autoantibodies unclear, e.g.
  - IgA rheumatoid factors;
  - IgA ANCA (HSP?).
- Autoantibodies commonly appear after infections, e.g.
  - EBV;
  - adenovirus;
  - HIV;
  - acute and chronic bacterial infections.
  - They will usually disappear after 6 months.
  - They are not usually associated with clinical disease.

- Commonest associations:
  - rheumatoid factor—any infection;
  - anti-nuclear antibodies—adenovirus (children), HIV, Gram-negative bacteria;
  - smooth muscle antibodies—adenovirus;
  - liver–kidney microsomal antibodies—HCV;
  - cardiolipin antibodies—EBV;
  - dsDNA antibodies—rare, HIV.
- Drugs may also induce autoantibodies: these may cause disease and may persist after the drug is withdrawn.
  - Anti-nuclear antibodies (anti-histone): procainamide, hydralazine, ACE inhibitor, chlorpromazine, minocycline.
  - Liver–kidney microsomal antibodies: tienilic acid.
  - Non-M2 mitochondrial antibodies: alcohol.

Particle agglutination assays

- Technique is old and reliable.
- It is cheap, but labour-intensive.
- Use has almost disappeared, apart from low-level screening, e.g. rheumatoid factor, DCT.
- Antigen (either pure or extract) is coated on to an inert carrier particle, usually gelatin or latex but originally tanned red cells.
- When mixed with serum containing the appropriate antibody, the particles are agglutinated.
- The principle is simple but reading the end-point of a particle agglutination titration requires skill.
- IgM antibodies are picked up preferentially because of their pentameric shape, which allows better cross-linking.

Immunoprecipitation assays

- These depend upon the formation of insoluble immune complexes where an antibody encounters the optimum concentration of antigen.
- Prototype assay is the Ouchterlony double-diffusion assay.
  - Antigen and antibody are added to wells cut in agar gels and allowed to diffuse towards one another.
  - Line(s) of precipitation form at the point of equivalence, indicating the presence of an antibody against the antigen.
  - The process is slow and may take up to 72 hours to form lines.
- Technique may be improved by using electrolyte-containing agarose and applying a current across the gel, forcing the antibody and antigen together (countercurrent immunoelectrophoresis, CIE).
  - CIE is used for the detection of antibodies to extractable nuclear antigens.
  - Commercial assays are not available, and CIE tends to be used to complement commercial EIA tests for ENA in specialist centres.
  - It is labour-intensive and time-consuming.

- If the immune complex formation takes place in the liquid phase, then the light absorbing/scattering properties of the solution will be altered and can be measured (nephelometry/turbidimetry).
  - Can be used for antibody detection on automated analysers.
  - Rheumatoid factor, thyroid antibodies.
  - Stability of the immune complex may be poor and agents such as polyethylene glycol (PEG) may be added to ensure a stable reaction.
  - PEG may also be used in gels to enhance and stabilize the immune complex.

Indirect immunofluorescence

Tissue preparation

- Standard technique for the detection of many serum autoantibodies.
- Appropriate tissue block is snap-frozen and is cut on a cryostat to provide sections (usually 4 mm thick) that are mounted on a slide and air-dried.
- Other fixation techniques may be used under special circumstances (e.g. acetone or ethanol).
- Similar methods can be used on cell suspensions prepared on slides using a cytocentrifuge, e.g.
  - neutrophils for ANCA;
  - HEp-2 cells for anti-nuclear antibodies.
- Most laboratories use commercially produced slides (CE marked). The cost is outweighed by convenience.
  - No problems sourcing animal tissues.
  - Staff are not tied up on routine slide production.
  - Quality control of section cutting is better.

Technique

- Slides are incubated with appropriate dilutions of test and control sera, washed, and then incubated with anti-human immunoglobulin (isotype-specific) antiserum which is conjugated with fluorescein isothiocyanate (FITC).
- Technique allows the tissue and intracellular distribution of autoantibody binding to be visualized.
- Alternatives may be used for FITC in the second stage, such as enzymes (immunoperoxidase) that will give a colour reaction when the slides are incubated with an appropriate substrate.
  - Slides can be fixed and counterstained to reveal the tissue structure.
  - Ordinary transmission light microscope is all that is required.
  - Processing has an extra incubation step.

Obtaining reliable results

The following are key features that are essential to obtaining reliable results.
- Good tissue selection and processing.
- Appropriate starting dilution (to avoid non-specific serum binding).
- Use of serum not plasma, as fibrinogen causes non-specific fluorescence.

- Appropriate FITC-conjugated antiserum selection.
  - Commercial antisera are usually used.
  - There may be considerable batch-to-batch variation.
  - Fluorescein molecule-to-protein ratio needs to be between 1 and 4.5 to give reasonable results.
  - If it is too low, the intensity is inadequate.
  - If it is too high, the non-specific fluorescence swamps the specific staining.
  - Optimal dilution needs to be determined by a chequerboard titration.
  - New antisera are tested at serial dilutions on standard tissue sections incubated with serial dilutions of a standard control serum with previously identified titre.
- Appropriate internal/external controls (quantitative as well as qualitative).
- A good-quality fluorescence microscope, properly maintained, with a properly adjusted light source.
- An experienced microscopist who is familiar with the relevant patterns.

Tissue multiblock

For laboratory convenience, it is standard practice to test for the basic auto-antibodies using a tissue multiblock, containing liver, stomach, and kidney (some laboratories also include thyroid), usually rat.

- Commercial slides may have 'chips' containing the separate tissues and HEp-2 cells; this allows the detection of:
  - most anti-nuclear antibodies;
  - smooth muscle antibodies;
  - mitochondrial antibodies;
  - reticulin antibodies; these are not usually reported but may indicate need to check endomysial or tissue transglutaminase antibodies;
  - gastric parietal cell antibodies;
  - ribosomal antibodies;
  - liver–kidney microsomal (LKM) antibodies.
- HEp-2 cells allow detection of cellular staining patterns.
  - HEp-2000 cells have been genetically engineered to express higher levels of Ro antigens: in practice there is little difference.
- The disadvantage of this multiblock screen is that it encourages clinicians to request 'autoantibody screens' without thinking about what they are specifically looking for.
- Always encourage clinicians to request the test they need for diagnosis.

Screening and titration

- Screening will be carried out at a single dilution with a conjugated antiserum that recognizes IgG, IgA, and IgM (polyvalent).
  - Normal adult screening dilution is 1/20.
- Positive samples will then be titrated using a monospecific anti-IgG antiserum.
  - A limited number of steps only are required (twofold dilutions to 1/640, anything higher reported > 1/640).

- Screening dilutions need to be adjusted in children; 1/10 may be appropriate.
- Not all antibodies need to be titrated, e.g. GPC, reticulin.
- Titration is only semi-quantitative.

Other tissues

Same techniques as used for other tissues are used.
- Monkey oesophagus (endomysial, epidermal antibodies).
- Other tissues used are pancreas, adrenal, gonad, small intestine, pituitary, cerebellum, cerebrum, salivary gland.

Alternative techniques

- Some laboratories are now using laser-based array systems or automated EIA screening tools for multiple antigens, to weed out negative samples.
- Array systems are also used to screen for extractable nuclear antigens.
- These supplement but do not replace indirect immunofluorescence (IIF).
- Performance characteristics are variable.
- Systems are available for automation of the dilution and staining of slides.

Direct immunofluorescence

- Technique here is very similar to that used for indirect immunofluorescence, i.e. tissue is obtained directly from the patient, snap-frozen, and sectioned prior to incubation with the FITC-conjugated antiserum.
- This allows the detection of tissue-bound antibody in the patient.
- Tissue-bound antibody may be present even when there is insufficient antibody to be detected free in the serum.
- Other tissue reactants such as complement and fibrinogen may be detected. Patterns of reaction may be absolutely diagnostic, e.g. in bullous skin diseases.
- Direct immunofluorescence is used extensively in the diagnosis of skin diseases (because of the accessibility of the tissue for biopsy) and renal disease.

Radioimmunoassay (RIA)

- These assays are highly sensitive.
- They require pure antigen.
- They require radioistopes.
- Few assays are now done using these techniques as laboratories move away from isotopic tests to enzyme-linked immunoassays.
- RIA is the gold standard for:
  - acetylcholine receptor antibodies;
  - dsDNA antibodies (Farr assay).
- RIA is also used for intrinsic factor antibodies.

Enzyme-linked (EIA) and fluorescent immunoassays (FIA)

- These have taken over from RIA, and to some extent from indirect immunofluorescence.
- Antigen is bound on to a solid phase (bead or plate) which is reacted with serum, washed, and reacted with the antiserum against human immunoglobulin, which is coupled either to an enzyme (EIA) or to a fluorescent dye (FIA).
  - The final stage (EIA) is reaction with the substrate, either directly or via an amplification step to give a colour that can be measured spectrophotometrically.
  - In FIA, the plate can be read directly using an appropriate exciting light source (which will be of a different wavelength to the emitted light).
- Assays tend to be more sensitive than immunofluorescence, but may lose specificity.
- Pure antigen is required: source may be critical to value of tests.
  - Recombinant human tTG gives better results than guinea-pig tTG.
- Commercial assays tend to be expensive.
- Samples may need to be run in duplicate, increasing cost.
- Assays are most cost-effective and accurate when performed on automated instruments.
- Results may differ from those obtained by other methods:
  - dsDNA antibodies by Farr and EIA;
  - ENA antibodies by CIE and EIA.
  - The clinical significance of the different results has not always been established.
- Differences need to be considered when introducing new tests.
  - External quality assurance scheme data may help in comparing methods.

Electrochemiluminescence

- This assay uses luminescence generated during an electrochemical reaction, where a voltage is applied to the reaction cell.
- Advantages include increased sensitivity and decreased background optical signal. Various tags can be used on the antibody reagents including Sulfo-TAG or ruthenium.
- It is replacing conventional ELISA for some assays.

Immunoblotting

- Antigens are either electrophoresed in a matrix or applied to the matrix at specific points, incubated with appropriate dilutions of sera, washed, then incubated with enzyme-conjugated antisera, followed by substrate. This gives a coloured band.
- Assays are often quick, and suitable for urgent screening.
- Staining may be automated (slide-based kits).
- Results are qualitative.
- Commercial kits are available for qualitative detection of antibodies:
  - ENA;
  - ANCA antigens (PR3, MPO);
  - liver antigens (M2, LKM, SLA, LC);
  - neuronal antigens;
  - gangliosides.

Multiplex assays

- Antigens are bound to microspheres and the reaction with serum takes place in solution rather than attached to a solid phase.
- Each microbead can have a specific fluorescent signal, with at least two different fluorochromes attached internally, in varying ratios to give a unique signature. Antigens are attached to beads with specific signatures.
- An externally labelled reporter antibody recognizes the bound autoantibody from serum after incubation and binds to the microspheres.
- Multiple beads can be analysed simultaneously, leading to very rapid and automated analysis for multiple autoantibodies.
- Analysis is essentially a form of high throughput multiparameter flow cytometry.
- Correlation between multiplex assays and solid phase assays such as EIA or immunoblotting is often poor.
- These assays have the advantages of low cost, minimal technical skill to run the assays compared to the interpretation of immunofluorescence, and speed of assay.
- Some centres use the technique to rapidly screen out negative sera.

Proteomics

- This involves using protein microarrays on chips and potentially will allow rapid screening for the presence of autoantibodies to large numbers of protein antigens.
- The chips are incubated with serum, and then developed with a secondary antibody coupled to a fluorescent dye.
- Incubated chips can be rapidly screened by a scanner.

Acetylcholine-receptor antibodies (AChRAb)

- Units: mol/l.
- Normal ranges: $< 2 \times 10^{-10}$ mol/l.

Principles of test
- Antibodies are detected by a quantitative competitive radioimmunoassay.
- No EQA scheme exists.

Indications for testing
- AChRAbs are the marker for myasthenia gravis.

Interpretation
- Two types of antibodies have been described.
  - Those binding to the receptor at sites distinct from the binding site for acetylcholine.
  - Those blocking the binding of the neurotransmitter or α-bungarotoxin.
- Some antibodies are capable of modulating the removal of the receptors from the surface of the muscle through cross-linking followed by internalization.
- Levels above 5×10^{-10} mol/l are regarded as positive.
- Levels of $2–5 \times 10^{-10}$ mol/l are regarded as equivocal, and may be seen in ocular myasthenia.
- Some laboratories report the levels only semi-quantitatively (high, low, etc.).
- Highest levels are seen in young patients (< 40 years with generalized disease).
- Lower levels are seen in:
  - older patients;
  - thymoma;
  - penicillamine-induced myasthenia.
- Approximately 15% of typical myasthenic patients are negative for AChRAb.
- Some may have IgM antibodies (not detected in routine assays).
- In ocular myasthenia, about 20% of patients will be seronegative.
- Antibodies persist in 60% of patients even if the disease is in remission.
- AChRAbs have also been detected in the myasthenic syndrome associated with penicillamine usage (about 1% of treated patients); these antibodies disappear when the drug is stopped.
- Very rarely, they may appear transiently during the immunological reconstitution phase of bone marrow transplantation.

Actin antibodies

See ➲ 'Smooth muscle antibodies', p. 570.

Adrenal cortex autoantibodies

- Units: qualitative.
- Normal adult range: not detected.

Principles of test

- IIF, using a multiblock of primate adrenal gland, ovary, testis, and pituitary.
- EIA or RIA are used in the research setting to look at individual antigens.
- No EQA scheme exists.
- Commercial positive control sera are available.

Indications for testing

- Suspected Addison's disease.
- Screening in polyglandular syndromes.

Interpretation

- Autoantibodies to adrenal cortex (any or all of the three layers) are found in approximately 50% of patients with Addisonian adrenal insufficiency where there are other autoimmune diseases.
- Prevalence drops when the autoimmune adrenalitis occurs alone.
- They are virtually never found in patients with tuberculous adrenal destruction.
- Target antigen is usually adrenal microsomes.
- Antibodies to the ACTH receptor have also been described in a few patients with Cushing's syndrome (paralleling thyroid-stimulating antibodies).
- 21-Hydroxylase (P450c21) is the major target antigen in Addison's disease and type I APGS.
- Frequent cross-reactivity of the antibodies with the steroid-producing cells of the theca interna of the ovary (ovarian failure) and the Leydig cells of the testis.
- Other antigenic enzymes in steroid-producing cells include the P450 side-chain cleavage enzyme (P450scc) and 17α-hydroxylase (P450c17).
  - P450c17 antibodies are associated with type I autoimmune polyendocrinopathy syndrome.
  - P450c21 antibodies are associated with type II autoimmune polyendocrinopathy syndrome.
  - P450scc antibodies are associated with premature ovarian failure.
- Autoimmune adrenal disease is closely associated with other organ-specific autoimmune disease:
  - thyrogastric (Schmidt's syndrome);
  - parathyroid autoimmune disease.
  - It is important to screen also for thyroid antibodies and gastric parietal cell antibodies.
- Multiple endocrine autoantibodies may be found in chronic mucocutaneous candidiasis with endocrinopathy.
  - Screening such patients is important, as the autoantibodies may appear before overt manifestations of endocrine insufficiency.

AMPAR antibodies

- AMPAR antibodies (alpha-amino-3-hydroxy-5-methyl-4-isoxazolepropionic acid receptor) recognize AMPAR, a tetramer comprising subunits GluR1–4.
- Associated with limbic encephalitis.
- Commonly associated tumours are thymus, lung, and breast cancer.
- Relapse is frequent even if there is a good response to immunotherapy whether or not there is tumour recurrence.

Amphiphysin antibodies

- Anti-amphiphysin antibodies bind widely in the brain to pre-synaptic terminals, giving variable cytoplasmic staining.
- Association is with a range of neurological disorders including:
  - subacute sensory neuropathy;
  - sensorimotor peripheral neuropathy;
  - paraneoplastic stiff-person syndrome.
- Commonly associated tumours are small cell lung cancer and breast cancer.

Anti-nuclear antibodies (ANA) and ANCA

Anti-nuclear antibodies (ANA): see ➲ 'Nuclear antibodies (ANA)', p. 557.
ANCA: see ➲ 'Neutrophil cytoplasmic antibodies (ANCA)', p. 555.

Aquaporin antibodies

- IgG antibodies to aquaporin 4 are found in neuromyelitis optica (Devic's disease), a demyelinating disease, with some similarities to multiple sclerosis.
- Brainstem involvement may occur with intractable hiccups.
- Also known as NMO-IgG.
- Found in 60–70% of patients and is a predictor of subsequent relapse.

Auerbach's plexus antibodies

- Antibodies against the myenteric plexus of the oesophagus have been reported to be detected by immunofluorescence in patients with achalasia of the cardia, a motility disorder of the oesophagus.
- The diagnostic role of these antibodies remains to be confirmed.

β₂-GP1 antibodies

- These antibodies have been reported as part of the anti-phospholipid antibody (APS) spectrum (see ➔ 'Cardiolipin antibodies (ACA) and lupus anticoagulant', p. 526).
- Normally measured by EIA/FIA.
- Provided that anti-cardiolipin antibody assays include β_2-GP1 as a cofactor, there is no clinical indication for separate measurement of anti-β_2-GP1 antibodies.
  - Some patients with the APS, negative for ACA, and with a normal dRVVT, are positive for β_2-GP1 antibodies.
  - They can be found in some patients who do not have any other evidence (clinical or laboratory) for APS.
  - Also seen with M5 anti-mitochondrial antibodies.

C1q antibodies

- Normal: < 15 U/ml.
- Assayed by EIA.
- Antibodies to C1q have been described in hypocomplementaemic urticarial vasculitis, rheumatoid vasculitis, and SLE.
  - 70% of patients with Felty's syndrome are positive for C1q antibodies.
  - IgA anti-C1q found in rheumatoid vasculitis.
- In SLE quantitative measurement of C1q antibodies is thought to be a measure of the activity of renal disease.
- Antibodies to the neoantigen formed by activation of C1q have also been associated with types of glomerulonephritis.
- There is no EQA scheme at present and no reference preparation.

C1-esterase inhibitor (C1-inh) antibodies

- Anti-C1-inh autoantibodies block the action of C1-inh and are associated with acquired angioedema (AAE).
- May occur with lymphoma (especially splenic villous lymphoma), SLE, and APS.
- Patients with HAE receiving repeated doses of C1-inhibitor concentrates may also develop blocking antibodies, which reduce treatment effectiveness.
- May be detected by EIA and by functional assays (available from specialist complement laboratories).
- IgG and IgM antibodies occur.

Cardiac antibodies

- These antibodies are positive in:
  - a proportion of patients with Dressler's syndrome after myocardial infarction;
  - cardiac surgery;
  - some cardiomyopathies;
  - after acute rheumatic fever.
- Multiple antigens have been identified.
- Diagnostic value is low.
- Detected by immunofluorescence.

Cardiolipin antibodies (ACA) and lupus anticoagulant

- Units: GPLU/ml; MPLU/ml.
- Normal adult range:
  - IgG, < 10 GPLU/ml (10–20 borderline);
  - IgM, < 10 MPLU/ml (10–20 borderline).

Principles of testing

- EIA.
- International standards exist for IgG and IgM ACA.
- A UK specific standard for IgG ACA.
- An EQA scheme exists in the UK.

Indications for testing

- Suspected anti-phospholipid syndrome:
  - recurrent DVT/PE (as part of thrombophilia screen); major arterial and venous thrombosis;
  - recurrent miscarriages;
  - premature stroke; multi-infarct dementia;
  - severe and/or atypical migraine;
  - vasculitis (Behçet's syndrome);
  - connective tissue disease (SLE, Sjögren's syndrome);
  - livedo reticularis;
  - Sneddon's syndrome (cerebral events and livedo);
  - Budd–Chiari syndrome.

▶Testing *must* include both ACA and a test for lupus anticoagulant (usually dilute Russell's Viper venom test—dRVVT).
- Either or both may be present.
- Clinical significance is the same whichever is present.

Interpretation

- Antibodies to cardiolipin form part of the spectrum of anti-phospholipid antibodies.
- Other related antibodies include:
  - false-positive VDRL;

- lupus anticoagulants;
- antibodies to derived phospholipids.
- Standardization and reproducibility of the assays continue to be a major problem.
  - This is related in part to the requirement for β_2-GP1 (apolipoprotein H) from serum as a cofactor for the binding of cardiolipin antibodies.
  - Autoantibodies have also been detected to the cofactor itself.
  - Cofactor binds anionic phospholipids *in vivo* and its normal function is to inhibit coagulation and platelet aggregation.
- Presence of ACA may be found in the conditions listed previously (see ⊃ 'Indications for testing', p. 526).
- There is no strong correlation with premature myocardial infarction or with cerebral lupus (despite the fact that the brain is full of phospholipid!).
- Symptoms are mainly associated with IgG-class antibodies.
- Rare patients with typical symptoms will be encountered who have only IgM-class antibodies, and never make IgG antibodies.
- Amount of the antibody in units does not seem to relate to the severity of the disease.
- Immunosuppression does not have a significant effect on the level of ACA and does not affect thrombophilic tendency.
- Transient positive antibodies may be found after viral infections (especially EBV).
- Anti-phospholipid antibodies associated with syphilis and other infections do not usually react with β_2-GP1 and are rarely associated with a clotting disorder.
- Lupus anticoagulants are antibodies that interfere with the clotting process *in vitro* and are usually detected by prolongation of the APTT.
  - Test of choice is dilute Russell's Viper venom test (dRVVT).
- Although it has been suggested that lupus anticoagulants are more specific for recurrent fetal loss than cardiolipin antibodies, both may be associated with the syndrome.
- Women with lupus who are planning pregnancy should be screened for both anti-cardiolipin antibodies and lupus anticoagulants, in addition to testing for anti-Ro antibodies.

Cartilage antibodies

- Antibodies to collagens types I, II, and III have been found in a range of inflammatory conditions where there is cartilage damage, including:
  - rheumatoid arthritis;
  - relapsing polychondritis (collagen type II, 60% of patients positive);
  - a range of other connective tissue diseases, e.g. rheumatoid arthritis and juvenile RhA (30–40%).
- Specificity is low and they are of little diagnostic value.

Caspr2 antibodies

- Caspr2 antibodies recognize contactin-associated protein 2. This protein is linked to the voltage-gated potassium channel.
- Associated with neuromyotonia, limbic encephalitis, Morvan's syndrome (neuromyotonia, insomnia, dysautonomia, and neuropathic pain), and a non-neoplastic cerebellar ataxia.
- Associated with thymomas and small-cell lung cancer.

Centriole antibodies

- Centriole antibodies will only be detected if HEp-2 cells are used as the substrate for ANA detection.
- Immunofluorescence will show two brightly staining polar dots.
- Found very rarely in patients with scleroderma and related overlap syndromes.
- May also occur commonly in mycoplasmal pneumonia.

Centromere (kinetochore) antibodies

- Units: qualitative.
- Normal adult range: not detected.

Principles of testing

- Detected by immunofluorescence on HEp-2 cells.
- It is essential that the HEp-2 cells contain adequate numbers of dividing cells.
- EIA and immunoblot assays are available for three main antigens, CENP-A, CENP-B, CENP-C.

Indications for testing

- Indicated in patients with suspected scleroderma, Raynaud's phenomenon, cutaneous calcinosis.
- Patients with severe Raynaud's phenomenon and features of scleroderma should also be screened for the ENA Scl-70, associated with progressive systemic sclerosis (PSS).

Interpretation

- Antibodies can only be detected on HEp-2 cells.
- Also referred to as kinetochore antibodies, as they react with antigens located at the inner and outer kinetochore plates.
- Antigens are 17, 80, and 140 kDa proteins involved in the attachment of the spindle fibres (CENP-A, CENP-B, CENP-C).
- Minor centromere antigens may also be targets (CENP-D, CENP-E, CENP-F).
- CENP-B appears to be the predominant antigen, with five epitopes, some of which are shared with CENP-A and CENP-C.
- Antibodies show diagnostic condensation of fluorescence along the metaphase plate in dividing cells, which distinguishes the staining from other speckled-pattern ANA.

- Found in the CREST syndrome (sometimes referred to as limited scleroderma).
  - About 70–80% of patients with features of CREST will have anti-centromere antibodies.
  - 1% of patients with PSS will be positive.
- Detection of anti-centromere antibodies is of prognostic significance.
- Titration of centromere antibodies is of no value.
- Scl-70 and anti-centromere antibodies seem to be mutually exclusive.
- Up to 12% of patients with PBC may be positive for anti-centromere antibodies, of whom about half will have clinical signs of scleroderma.
- This may be a misinterpretation of the immunofluorescence pattern, as M2-antibody-negative PBC is often positive for a pattern of multiple nuclear dots (see ⟶ 'Multiple nuclear dot antibody', p. 552) which is sometimes referred to as pseudo-centromere, because of its resemblance to the centromere staining. However, the metaphase plate is not stained.

Cold agglutinins

- Often confused with cryoglobulins.
- They are autoantibodies that reversibly agglutinate erythrocytes in the cold.
- Cause small-vessel obstruction in the skin of the extremities, Raynaud's phenomenon, and haemolytic anaemia.
- Most common specificity is anti-i but other specificities such as anti-I or anti-Pr occur.
- Often triggered by infections:
  - *Mycoplasma pneumoniae*;
  - *Rickettsia*;
  - *Listeria monocytogenes*;
  - EBV.
- Usually polyclonal IgMκ, although EBV may be associated with a polyclonal IgMλ anti-i response.
- May also occur in association with lymphoproliferative diseases where the agglutinin is usually monoclonal (invariably IgMκ).
  - This is typically a disease of the elderly.
  - Cold agglutinins may precede the overt development of lymphoma by many years.
- Paroxysmal cold haemoglobinuria is associated with anti-P antibody.
  - Binds to the red cell and fixes complement in the cold.
  - Red cell lysis takes place when the cell is rewarmed.
  - Rare and was originally described in association with syphilis (Donath–Landsteiner antibody).
  - More commonly associated with viral infections such as mumps, measles, and chickenpox.
- As for cryoglobulins, samples must be taken and transported to the laboratory at 37°C.

CV2/CRMP5 antibodies

- Antibodies recognize the collapsin response-mediator brain protein (CRMP) family; CRMP5 is the dominant antigen.
- Staining is seen in the cytoplasm of oligodendrocytes.
- Associated with small-cell lung cancer (SCLC) in 77% and thymoma in 6%.
- Syndrome can include the following:
  - Subacute sensory neuropathy.
  - Limbic encephalopathy.
  - Cerebellar ataxia.
  - Extra-pyramidal syndromes.
  - Myopathy.
- Presence of antibodies to CV2/CRMP5 in SCLC is associated with better prognosis than anti-Hu antibodies.

Cyclic citrullinated peptide (CCP), mutated cyclic vimentin (MCV), cytokeratin, and desmin antibodies

Cyclic citrullinated peptide (CCP) antibodies

- Rheumatoid arthritis has been associated with antibodies to perinuclear factor, keratin, and filaggrin on buccal mucosa and rat oesophagus by IF.
- A synthetic peptic (CCP) can be used in EIA to detect these antibodies.
- Specificity for RhA is said to be 96%.
- It is being increasingly used for early diagnosis of RhA.

Mutated cyclic vimentin antibodies (MCV)

- Antibodies to MCV are a commercially available alternative test to anti-CCP for the diagnosis of rheumatoid arthritis.
- Meta-analysis demonstrates that anti-MCV is more sensitive but less specific and has a lower diagnostic accuracy compared to anti-CCP in rheumatoid arthritis.

Cytokeratin antibodies

- Antibodies to cytokeratin 18 are non-specific and associated with:
  - rheumatoid arthritis;
  - psoriasis and psoriatic arthritis;
  - Crohn's disease;
  - coronary artery disease.
- They are identified by IIF on HEp-2 cells.

Desmin antibodies

- Antibodies to desmin are non-specific and associated with:
  - autoimmune hepatitis;
  - PBC;
  - coronary artery disease;
  - Crohn's disease.
- They are identified by IIF on HEp-2 cells.

dsDNA antibodies

- Units: IU/ml.
- Normal adult range:
  - negative, < 30 IU/ml;
  - borderline, 30–50 IU/ml;
  - positive, 50–300 IU/ml;
  - strongly positive, > 300 IU/ml.
  - May vary according to assay, e.g. Bioplex® assay gives results of negative < 5, borderline 5–9, and positive ≥ 10.

Principles of testing
- Gold standard remains Farr assay (RIA): highly specific and sensitive.
  - dsDNA is precipitated using ammonium sulphate.
  - High avidity antibodies are detected.
- EIA assays available: results may not be concordant with Farr assay, due to presence of ssDNA and Z-DNA.
  - EIA assays are very sensitive but not always specific.
  - Low avidity antibodies of no clinical significance may be detected.
- Staining of the kinetoplast of *Crithidia lucilae* is specific but not sensitive: it cannot be recommended as a screening test.
- Multiplex assays are available that include dsDNA antibodies.

Indications for testing
- Suspected connective tissue disease.
- Suspected autoimmune hepatitis.
- Follow-on test when homogeneous or peripheral fluorescent anti-nuclear antibodies detected.

Interpretation
- Test is confirmatory for SLE.
- Only antibodies to dsDNA are measured.
- Elevated levels occur predominantly in SLE, but also in 'lupoid' chronic active hepatitis.
- Antibodies are not found in other connective tissue diseases, nor in all patients with SLE.
- Because the antibodies have a circulating half-life of 3 weeks, serial measurements are not useful in monitoring the activity of SLE.
- A rising titre may predict clinical relapse, and treatment on a rising titre before symptoms reappear may reduce the total amount of immunosuppression required.
- Titre of high avidity antibody may be associated with progression of renal disease.

ssDNA antibodies
- Antibodies to ssDNA and other forms (Z-DNA) occur in a wide range of connective tissue diseases.
- They have a low sensitivity and specificity.

- Antibodies to ssDNA may occur in drug-induced lupus as well as idiopathic lupus.
- Other diseases in which there is a high prevalence of anti-ssDNA antibodies are:
  - rheumatoid arthritis;
  - scleroderma;
  - polymyositis.
- The antibodies reduce the sensitivity and specificity of EIA assays for dsDNA, because the substrate in assays for the latter may be contaminated with ssDNA, produced during the purification process.
- A number of commercial assays have been shown to be contaminated in this way, leading to erroneous diagnoses of lupus on the basis of false-positive reports of antibodies to dsDNA.
- Assays for antibodies to ssDNA have no clinical role but are used for quality control of assays to dsDNA.

ENA antibodies

- Units: qualitative.
- Normal adult range: see individual antigens.

Principles of testing

- No gold standard test available.
- Originally detected by countercurrent immunoelectrophoresis of serum against saline extracts of cells (thymus, spleen).
- Other techniques include:
  - Ouchterlony double diffusion;
  - immunoblotting;
  - EIA;
  - multiplex assays.
- More than one technique may be required to identify relevant specificities.
- EIA assays have increased sensitivity compared to CIE and double diffusion: clinical significance of this is uncertain.
- Testing should include a six-antigen screen (including Scl-70 and Jo-1): four-antigen screening is not adequate.
- Multiplex assays may include analytes of dubious clinical value, e.g. RNP-A.
- EQA and international standards exist.
- EQA performance can be quite diverse, depending on assays used.

Indications for testing

- Suspected connective tissue disease.
- Investigation of congenital complete heart block.
- Follow-up testing when high-titre speckled ANA detected by IIF.

Interpretation

- These antibodies recognize saline-extracted cellular antigens and cause speckled-pattern anti-nuclear antibody staining.

- Six major specificities are tested for routinely:
  - anti-Ro (associated with Sjögren's, SLE, cutaneous lupus, neonatal lupus, and congenital complete heart block);
  - anti-La (associated with Sjögren's, SLE, and neonatal lupus);
  - anti-Sm (specific for SLE, but common only in West Indians);
  - anti-RNP (associated with SLE and, when occurring alone, said to identify mixed connective tissue disease);
  - anti-Scl-70 (associated with progressive systemic sclerosis);
  - anti-Jo-1 (associated with polymyositis and dermatomyositis).
- The individual antibodies are discussed separately.
- Many other specificities have been identified: clinical utility is variable.
- Where a high-titre speckled ANA is seen but the six-antigen screen is negative, then further investigation by alternative methods may be appropriate if clinically indicated.
- EQA scheme operates.

Endomysial antibodies (EMA)

- Units: qualitative.
- Normal adult range: negative.

Principles of testing

- IIF for IgA EMA on primate oesophagus (preferred substrate) or human umbilical vein.
- Gradually being replaced by EIA for antibodies to tissue transglutaminase (tTG—see ➲ 'Tissue transglutaminase (tTG) antibodies', p. 574).
  - IgA EMA may be a better screening test than IgA tTG.
  - IgA tTG may be better for long-term follow-up.
- Testing should include a screen for IgA deficiency (increased in coeliac disease).
  - Nephelometric assays do not confirm IgA deficiency at lowest detection levels.
  - Ouchterlony double diffusion is more sensitive.
  - However, for lab efficiency, nephelometry/turbidimetry is used to determine low IgA for the purposes of deciding whether to check for IgG-EMA.
- IgG EMA should be sought in IgA-deficient patients.

Indications for testing

- Suspected coeliac disease.
- Suspected dermatitis herpetiformis.
- NICE also recommends regular screening of all children with type I diabetes on an annual basis.
- Any patient with small bowel lymphoma must be screened.
- Monitoring known coeliac patients for dietary compliance.
- NICE has recommended the use of tTG assays for screening in primary care, but this test is too sensitive and generates a lot of false positives that then have to undergo small intestinal biopsy.

Interpretation

- IgA-EMA will be positive in 60–70% of patients with dermatitis herpetiformis and 100% of untreated coeliac patients.
- Monitoring of IgA-EMA is valuable in confirming adherence to a gluten-free diet (GFD), as the antibody disappears, along with anti-gliadin antibodies, on a GFD and returns if there is a gluten challenge, even in the absence of overt symptoms.
- IgA EMA and IgA tTG give entirely comparable results.
- Sensitivity and specificity of IgA EMA and IgA tTG means that jejunal biopsy is no longer compulsory.
- Antibodies may be detected in patients without biopsy evidence of villous atrophy: these may be patients in the early stage of disease. Outcome of early intervention with a GFD is unknown.
- IgA EMA and IgA tTG may be negative in children under the age of 1 year (incomplete development of IgA system); testing for IgG antibodies may be helpful (unproven).
- IgA deficiency increases risk of coeliac disease by 15-fold.
- Patients with coeliac disease may have autoantibodies to the crypt basement membrane of human fetal jejunum. These antibodies appear to be of identical specificity to those detected as endomysial antibodies.
- Also found in children with type I diabetes.

Endothelial antibodies

- Antibodies against a variety of endothelial antigens have been described in a variety of vasculitic syndromes:
  - SLE;
  - rheumatoid vasculitis;
  - systemic sclerosis;
  - haemolytic–uraemic syndrome;
  - Kawasaki syndrome;
  - Wegener's granulomatosis;
  - microscopic polyarteritis;
  - during solid organ graft rejection.
- Diagnostic significance is therefore low.
- Endothelial cell antibodies have been detected by immunofluorescence on rodent kidney, cultured human endothelial cells, and human umbilical vein cell line (Eayh926).
- EIA and immunoblotting and immunoprecipitation have also been used.
- Techniques have been difficult to standardize.
- Titres may correlate with disease activity in vasculitis.
- Test is available through the PRU, Sheffield but is of uncertain clinical value.

Epidermal antibodies (including direct immunofluorescence of skin)

These antibodies are useful in the diagnosis of blistering skin diseases.

Bullous pemphigoid

- Autoantibodies are directed against the basement membrane.
- Autoantibodies recognize two keratinocyte hemidesmosomal proteins, BP230 and BP180.
  - On DIF up to 90% of cases have typical linear IgG deposition.
  - On IIF of serum only 70% will be positive (using monkey oesophagus as a substrate).

Herpes gestationis

- Autoantibody is directed against basement membrane.
- Antigen is the BP180 protein.
- IgG deposition is seen on DIF in only 25% of cases.
- 100% will have C3 deposition.
- Serum is rarely positive.

Epidermolysis bullosa acquisita

- Autoantibody is directed against basement membrane.
- Gives linear IgG and C3 on DIF that has no distinguishing features from other basement membrane staining.
- Diagnostic test is splitting the biopsy between the dermis and epidermis by using high-salt incubation: immunofluorescence appears on the dermal side.
- Antigen is type VII procollagen.

Pemphigus vulgaris

- Antibodies recognize the intercellular substance of the epidermis and give typical chicken-wire staining, by DIF and IIF.
- Antigen is desmoglein-1, an intercellular adhesion molecule of the cadherin family.

Pemphigus foliaceus

- Antibodies recognize the intercellular substance of the epidermis and give typical chicken-wire staining, by DIF and IIF.
- The antigen in pemphigus foliaceus appears to be different from pemphigus vulgaris by immunoblotting.
- The two conditions are not readily distinguishable by routine immunofluorescence.

Paraneoplastic pemphigus

- A paraneoplastic form of pemphigus has been described with autoantibodies to desmoplakin I, a desmosomal protein.

Dermatitis herpetiformis

- DH causes the deposition of granular IgA, and sometimes C3 along the dermal papillae on DIF.
- Endomysial and gliadin antibodies may be present in serum.
- DH must be distinguished from linear IgA disease (a bullous disease).
- Linear IgA deposition, often with IgG and C3, at the dermo-epidermal junction.

SLE

- DIF of the skin from patients with SLE usually shows coarse irregular granular deposition of IgG, IgM, C3, and C4 along the dermo-epidermal junction (lupus band test).
- Similar features may be found in chronically sun-exposed skin from individuals without lupus.

Lichen planus

- DIF of skin from patients with lichen planus shows characteristic flame-shaped deposits of fibrin and IgM in the epidermis.

Solid phase assays are now available for some of the antigens. Salt-split skin DIF can be helpful in localizing the staining.

Erythrocyte antibodies

- Anti-red cell antibodies are investigated to test for:
  - temperature of maximal activity;
  - specificity for red cell antigens;
  - complement binding;
  - agglutination;
  - haemolysis.
- This involves looking at the patient's red cells, serum, and the eluate of the cells.
- Cells may also be treated with enzymes to enhance reactivity with certain antigenic systems (e.g. Ii or Pr).
- In warm haemolytic anaemia the major target antigens are those of the rhesus system, although many other antigens have been reported as involved.
- Warm haemolytic anaemia may be associated with idiopathic haemolysis or be secondary to:
  - SLE;
  - CLL;
  - lymphoma;
  - viral infections.
- In drug-induced haemolysis, there are often antibodies to drug–cell neoantigens (e.g. quinine, penicillins, and cephalosporins).

See also ➔ 'Cold agglutinins', p. 529.

Factor H antibodies

- Factor H autoantibodies have been associated with an acquired autoimmune haemolytic–uraemia syndrome, with functional loss of factor H activity.
- They occur mainly in children and are present in 6–56% of aHUS patients.
- They may be seen in patients with C3 glomerulopathy.
- Measurement should form part of the assessment of atypical HUS.
- Assays available through the supraregional aHUS Service in Newcastle.

GABA-B receptor antibodies

- GABA-B antibodies recognized in patients with limbic encephalitis (seizures, short-term memory loss, and neuropsychiatric symptoms).
  - Reactive against GABA-B1 subunit, rarely against GABA-B2.
- 50% of cases are associated with small-cell lung cancer.

Ganglioside antibodies

- Antibodies to gangliosides (sialylated glycolipids that form part of the myelin sheath) have been associated with a number of neurological diseases.
- Diagnostic value is limited to supporting clinical diagnoses.
- Antibodies to GM1 (and asialo-GM1) and other gangliosides (see ➲ Chapter 5) have been associated with:
  - Guillain–Barré syndrome (GBS);
  - chronic demyelinating polyneuropathy;
  - multifocal motor neuropathy;
  - paraproteinaemic neuropathies (usually monoclonal IgM with anti-GM1 specificity).
- It has been suggested that the presence of anti-GM1 antibodies may be a predictor of response to intravenous immunoglobulin.
- Anti-GD1b is associated with:
  - GBS;
  - sensory neuropathy.
- Anti-GQ1b is associated with:
  - Miller–Fisher variant of GBS (external ophthalmoplegia, ataxia, arreflexia)—most specifically with ophthalmoplegia;
  - chronic ataxic neuropathy (IgM antibodies).
- Anti-GT1a is associated with Miller–Fisher variant of GBS.
- IgM antibodies to GD1b are highly specific for a rare chronic ataxic neuropathy termed CANOMAD (chronic ataxic neuropathy ophthalmoplegia M-protein agglutination disialyl antibody syndrome).

Gastric parietal cell (GPC) antibodies

- Units: semi-quantitative.
- Normal adult range: negative.

Principles of testing

- Indirect immunofluorescence using rodent stomach (tissue multiblock).
- Heterophile antibodies (see ➲ 'Heterophile antibodies', p. 542) may produce false positives on human and rat stomach, but do not react on mouse stomach.
- EIA available.
- There is no international standard.
- In the UK, EQA is provided through the General Autoimmune Serology scheme.

Indications for testing

- Suspected pernicious anaemia.
- Most tests are done without requests as part of 'autoantibody screen'.

Interpretation

- Antibodies to gastric parietal cells are found in almost all patients with pernicious anaemia (PA) in the early stages.
- Frequency diminishes with disease progression.
- Target autoantigens are the α- and β-subunits of the H^+, K^+-ATPase (proton pump).
- Antibodies are associated with atrophic gastritis (type A).
- Antral gastritis (type B) is not associated with GPC antibodies, but may be associated with antibodies to the gastrin-producing cells.
- GPC antibodies may be found in asymptomatic individuals; however, about 3% per annum will go on to develop PA.
- There is a strong association of PA with thyroid disease.
  - 50% of patients with PA will also have anti-thyroid antibodies.
  - 30% of patients with thyroiditis will have GPC antibodies.
- There is no correlation of the titre of antibody with disease.
- Antibodies to gastrin-producing cells and gastrin receptors (blocking gastrin binding) have also been described in patients with pernicious anaemia (8–30%), but these are of no routine clinical value at present.

Gliadin antibodies (AGA) and deamidated gliadin peptide (DGP) antibodies

- Units: qualitative.
- Normal range: 15–20% of children have IgA antibodies to gliadin in the absence of coeliac disease.

Principles of testing

- EIA for IgA and IgG antibodies against alcohol-soluble fraction of gluten.
- Multiplex/EIA assays for anti-DGP antibodies.

Indications for testing

- Higher sensitivity and specificity of IgA EMA and IgA tTG assays mean that these assays are the preferred tests for gluten-sensitive enteropathy.
- Cerebellar ataxic syndromes have a possible weak association with gliadin antibodies: routine testing is not recommended in view of the lack of specificity and sensitivity.

Interpretation

- Gliadin antibodies are found in coeliac disease and dermatitis herpetiformis, but are not specific.
- AGA are found also in Crohn's disease and ulcerative colitis.
- In children IgA-AGA may be seen in cow's milk intolerance and post-infective malabsorption.
- IgG anti-gliadin antibodies occurring alone are of no particular diagnostic significance, and may be present in a wide range of inflammatory and infective bowel conditions.
- The sensitivity and specificity of IgA anti-gliadin antibodies are approximately 100% and 95%, respectively; while the figures for IgG antibodies are 50% and 60%, respectively.
- IgA EMA and IgA tTG are preferred tests for clinical use.
- IgA anti-gliadin antibodies are also found in IgA mesangial glomerulonephritis, and may be useful as a diagnostic test.
  - Disease itself is not affected by adherence to a gluten-free diet.
- Positive results are also seen in:
  - children and adults with diabetes mellitus (type I);
  - first-degree relatives of patients with coeliac disease;
  - patients with Down's syndrome (increased risk of developing coeliac disease).
- IgA anti-DGP antibodies are included in some multiplex systems.
  - They have a lower positive predictive value than IgA tTG antibodies, although are said to be an earlier marker of coeliac disease in children. At present there is no indication for routine reporting of these where IgA EMA and IgA tTG antibody testing is available.

See ➔ 'Endomysial antibodies (EMA)', p. 533, and ➔ 'Tissue transglutaminase (tTG) antibodies', p. 574.

Glomerular basement membrane antibodies

- Units:
  - usually qualitative;
  - quantitative assays available through PRUs.
- Normal adult range: not detectable.

Principles of testing

- Test of choice is EIA, using C-terminal peptide of type IV collagen.

- IIF assays using rodent, primate or group O human kidney are not recommended due to the high rate of false-positive and false-negative reactions.
  - Only 75% of proven cases will show positive IIF.
- Antibodies may be detected by DIF of biopsies of kidney and occasional lung (linear staining on basement membrane).
  - IgG and C3 will be detected.
  - Occasionally IgA will be present.
- Quantitation is useful when plasmapheresis is undertaken.
- An EQA scheme exists in the UK.

Indications for testing

- Investigation of rapid-onset glomerulonephritis.
- Investigation of pulmonary haemorrhage and haemoptysis.

Interpretation

- Anti-GBM antibodies are the marker for GBM disease or Goodpasture's syndrome.
- Antibodies are directed against the non-collagenous domains of type IV collagen.
- There may be other target antigens (entactin/nidogen?).
- Antibodies are examples of primary pathogenic antibodies directly involved in disease processes.
- Complement fixation takes place at sites of antibody localization.
- The same antigen is present in both glomerular and alveolar basement membranes.
- Alveolar haemorrhage is usually limited to patients who smoke or are exposed to other irritants (solvent fumes).
- 10–35% of patients with anti-GBM antibodies may also have anti-neutrophil cytoplasmic antibodies (ANCAs), with a P-ANCA pattern, usually due to myeloperoxidase antibodies. Significance is uncertain.
- Wegener's granulomatosis may present with pulmonary haemorrhage and glomerulonephritis.
- The screen for all patients with glomerulonephritis and/or pulmonary haemorrhage must include both ANCA and GBM antibodies.
- These patients require urgent immunological investigations—one of the few occasions on which this is necessary.

Glutamate receptor (mGluR1) antibodies

- Identified in small numbers of patients with ataxia and cerebellar degeneration.
- Associated with Hodgkin's lymphoma.
- Also identified in patients with stroke and head injury.

Glutamic acid decarboxylase (GAD) antibodies

- Units: AU/ml.
- Normal adult range:
  - negative (< 5 AU/ml).
  - borderline (6–24 AU/ml).
  - positive (> 25 AU/ml).

Principles of testing

- EIA for GAD65 antibodies.
  - Epitopes for IDDM and stiff-person syndrome are different and recognition in EIAs differs between assays.
  - GAD antibodies in stiff-person syndrome recognize linear epitopes, while in diabetes the antibodies recognize conformational epitopes.
- Antibodies to GAD67 also occur but are cross-reactive with GAD65.
  - Separate assays not used clinically.
- Immunoblotting may also be used.
- EQA scheme operates; standard is NIBSC 97/550.

Indications

- Suspected type I diabetes.
  - Screening with islet cell antibodies may be quicker and cheaper.
- Suspected stiff-person syndrome.

Interpretation

- GADI antibodies against conformational epitopes seen in type I diabetes.
  - Only react with native GAD65.
- GADII antibodies against linear epitopes seen in stiff-person syndrome.
- Anti-GAD65 antibodies have been found in more than 60% of patients with stiff-person syndrome.
  - It is known that the enzyme is concentrated in the GABAergic neurons involved in the control of muscle tone.
- Antibodies to GAD67 are not found in type I diabetes.

Glycine receptor (GlyR) antibodies

- Glycine receptor mediates inhibitory transmissions between motor neurons and interneurons in the spinal cord. The receptor is found in other parts of the brain.
- Antibodies are associated with progressive encephalomyelitis, rigidity, and myoclonus (PERM), and also in stiff-person syndrome.
- May be seen in association with lymphoma.

Gut (enterocyte) antibodies

- Antibodies to gut epithelium may occur:
  - in ulcerative colitis: antibodies to brush border have been described in ulcerative colitis and in some patients with *Yersinia enterocolitis*;
  - in ulcerative colitis: antibodies to colonic goblet cells;

- in intractable diarrhoea of infancy and HIV-associated diarrhoea: antibodies to jejunal and ileal enterocytes;
- in IPEX syndrome: antibodies to jejunal and ileal enterocytes;
- in bile salt malabsorption: IgA ileal enterocytes;
- transiently post-BMT.
- Significance of these antibodies is uncertain.
- Detection is by IIF.

Heterophile antibodies

- These are not true 'autoantibodies' but represent a source of confusion with real autoantibodies.
- They are antibodies that may normally be present in serum and bind to tissue sections, particularly rodent tissues (see ➔ 'Gastric parietal cell (GPC) antibodies', p. 538).
- They are particularly common in patients who have been transfused or allo-immunized in other ways (multiple pregnancies, organ grafts).

Histone antibodies

- Antibodies to histones are the marker for drug-induced lupus (95%).
- Also seen in SLE (up to 50%).
- Cause a homogeneous anti-nuclear staining pattern on IIF.
- Target antigens are invariably the histones:
  - H2A–H2B in procainamide-induced lupus;
  - Hs, H4 in hydralazine-induced lupus.
- Virtually all procainamide-treated patients with lupus will have histone antibodies.
- Most cases of drug-induced lupus are negative for antibodies to dsDNA, although antibodies to ssDNA may be present.
- Commercial ELISA assays are available and chromatin antibodies detected in multiplex assays include anti-histone antibodies.
- Histone antibodies can be detected by IIF after acid elution of the cellular substrate.
- It is essential to ensure that the histone is entirely free of contaminating DNA: this is difficult to do, as the DNA has to be digested in the presence of protease inhibitors to prevent damage to the histones.
- There is no EQA scheme.

Hsp-90 antibodies

- Antibodies to the 90 kDa mammalian heat-shock protein have been described in up to 50% of lupus patients and a few patients with polymyositis.
- Antigen is located in the cytoplasm and on the surface membrane.
- They are not sought routinely.

Hu antibodies

- Antibodies specific for neuronal cell nuclei (anti-Hu, ANNA) have been described in some patients with small-cell carcinoma of the lung accompanied by paraneoplastic syndromes of sensory neuropathies or encephalomyelitis.
- Antibodies recognize a 36–42 kDa protein of neuronal nuclei, especially of Purkinje cells, recognizing an RNA binding nuclear proteins (HuD, HuC, Hel-N1, and Hel-N2).
- They must be distinguished from non-neuron-specific anti-nuclear antibodies. The immunofluorescence staining pattern is fine speckled on neuronal nuclei; glial cells are not stained.
- Immunoblotting and EIA may also be used to detect anti-Hu.
- Pathological significance is uncertain, as removal by plasmapheresis does not improve disease and immunization of animals with the antigen does not elicit disease.

IF116 antibodies

- These recognize an autoantigen, which contains pyrin and HIN domains and is involved in cell cycle regulation.
- Detected by EIA.
- Associated with SLE (reduced renal involvement) and limited cutaneous scleroderma (milder disease).

Inner ear antibodies

- Rare cases of progressive deafness may be due to an autoimmune process directed against antigens of the inner ear.
- These can be detected by immunofluorescence on sections of the inner ear (either bovine or guinea-pig), although obtaining suitable material is exceptionally difficult.
- Originally it was thought that antibodies to type II collagen formed the basis of this autoimmune process, but more recently it has been shown that the antigen is a heat-shock protein (Hsp-2).
- A commercial immunoblot system is now available for this antigen.

Insulin antibodies (IAA)

Insulin antibodies may be seen in the following.
- Type I diabetes prior to treatment (40%).
  - They are seen in all young children with type I diabetes.
  - They are seen in few adults with type I diabetes (4%).
  - They disappear with progressive islet cell destruction.
- Autoimmune polyendocrinopathies.
- Detected after treatment with thiol-containing drugs.
- Treatment with exogenous insulins.

- Epitopes recognized differ from those found in type I diabetes pre-treatment.
- Autoantibodies to insulin have been described as a cause of insulin resistance and are highly specific.
- IgE anti-insulin antibodies may be associated with allergic reactions to administered insulin (RAST available).
- Antibodies to the insulin receptor have also been described in insulin resistance, usually associated with acanthosis nigricans.
- Detection is by EIA/FEIA.
- Other diabetes-associated antibodies include:
  - IA2 (see ➋ 'Insulinoma-associated autoantibodies (IA2, ICA512)', see next topic);
  - ZnT8 (see ➋ 'ZnT8 antibodies', p. 576);
  - ICA69;
  - chromogranin A;
  - carboxypeptidase H;
  - ganglioside GM2-1;
  - imogen 38;
  - glima 38;
  - peripherin;
  - Hsp-60.
- The clinical utility of antibodies other than IA2 and ZnT8 is unclear.

Insulinoma-associated autoantibodies (IA2, ICA512)

- IA2 antibodies are found in latent diabetes and in type I diabetes.
- Antibodies recognize an islet tyrosine phosphatase.
- In combination with other antibodies (islet cell antibodies, GAD-65 antibodies, and insulin antibodies) and may provide useful predictive information.
- The presence of 3–4 antibodies gives a risk of progression of 60–100%, although this may be over a long time frame.
- Presence of more than one marker in first-degree relatives of a patient with type I diabetes is a risk factor for autoimmune diabetes.
- The optimum combination of autoantibodies is not defined.

Intrinsic factor antibodies

- Units: qualitative.
- Normal adult range: negative.

Principles of testing

- Radioimmunoassay or EIA.
- There are currently no reliable EQA scheme or international standards.

Indications for testing

- Suspected pernicious anaemia.

- Further investigation of positive gastric parietal cell antibodies.
- Suggest use when GPC antibody pattern obscured.

Interpretation
- Antibodies to intrinsic factor are highly specific for pernicious anaemia and are found in up to 75% of patients (see ➲ Chapter 4).
- Two types of antibodies can be detected:
  - type I: block the binding of vitamin B_{12} to intrinsic factor;
  - type II: block the uptake of the IF–vitamin B_{12} complex.
- Exogenous vitamin B_{12} interferes with RIA for type I antibodies (as the assay is a competitive assay using radiolabelled vitamin B_{12}).
- EIA assays have not been entirely satisfactory.
- Value of testing for IF antibodies is uncertain as negative tests do not exclude the diagnosis. Previously the Schilling test was the gold standard for the diagnosis of PA.
  - Due to concerns about the use of human albumin and porcine intrinsic factor in the Schilling test, the Schilling test is no longer available.

Islet cell antibodies (ICA)

- Units: JDF units.
- Normal adult range: negative.
- > 40 JDF units gives 85% PPV for diabetes.

Principles of testing
- Indirect immunofluorescence using serum on human group O pancreas.
- There is an international standard with a system of units (JDF units).
- No EQA scheme in the UK.

Indications for testing
- Suspected type I diabetes.
- Screening of first-degree relatives.

Interpretation
- Antibodies react with both α- and β-cells.
  - Staining for both is seen in type I diabetes.
  - Staining of β-cells alone is seen in autoimmune polyglandular syndrome.
  - One of the antigens recognized is GAD65.
- May be positive when GAD antibodies are negative.
- May be found early in the course of type I diabetes.
- Detectable within first year of diagnosis.
- > 85% newly diagnosed type I diabetics are positive.
- Gradually disappear with time as islets are destroyed.
- Found in type II diabetes (5–10%).
- A small group of patients with multiple autoimmune endocrine disease maintain their antibody levels.

- Useful for screening first-degree relatives for risk of developing diabetes: their presence increases the relative risk of type I diabetes 75-fold.
  - Prevalence in first-degree relatives is 3–4%. If ICA present and glucose tolerance impaired > 50% risk of developing diabetes within 5 years.
- There is no good evidence that quantitation offers any particularly useful clinical information.
- The role of ICA vis-à-vis direct measurement of GAD-65, IA2, ZnT8, and IAA in the diagnosis of type I diabetes, latent diabetes, and screening of children with coeliac disease has not been defined.

Jo-1 and related anti-transferase antibodies

- Antibodies are found in:
  - approximately 25% of adult patients with autoimmune myositis;
  - 68% in patients with myositis, Raynaud's, arthritis, and interstitial lung disease (anti-synthetase syndrome).
- In sera containing anti-Jo-1, the anti-nuclear antibody may be negative, without the speckled pattern seen with other antibodies to ENA.
- Variable faint cytoplasmic staining may be seen on HEp-2 cells.
- Antibodies to Jo-1 should therefore be included routinely in the six-antigen ENA screen (see ➔ 'ENA antibodies', p. 532).
- Target antigens are aminoacyl-tRNA synthetases; Jo-1 is the major antigen but other specificities have been identified:
  - Jo-1: histidyl-tRNA synthetase;
  - PL-7: threonyl-tRNA synthetase (not reactive in immunoblotting,?conformational epitope);
  - PL-12: alanyl-tRNA synthetase;
  - OJ: isoleucyl-tRNA synthetase;
  - EJ: glycyl-tRNA synthetase;
  - lysyl-tRNA synthetase.
  - All are associated with myositis. Only Jo-1 is common.
- Antibodies to signal recognition particles (SRPs) may also be associated, especially in dermatomyositis and polymyositis without the additional features of the anti-synthetase syndrome.
  - Anti-SRP anti-bodies give a granular cytoplasmic staining on HEp-2 cells.
- Jo-1 antibodies are detected by EIA or immunoblotting.
- Other specificities are detected by immunoprecipitation from cell lysates followed by polyacrylamide gel electrophoresis.
- EQA for ENA covers Jo-1 but not other antigens.
- An international standard is available for Jo-1.

Ki and Ku antibodies

Ki antibodies

- Ki antibodies recognize a 32 kDa protein.
- It used to be thought to be identical to Ku but is now known to be distinct.
- Occur in 10% of SLE and are increased in CNS SLE.
- May be detected by CIE or EIA.

Ku antibodies (also known as PL-2 and SL)

- Ku antibodies recognize 66 and 86 kDa DNA-binding proteins (DNA-dependent protein kinase involved in double-stranded DNA repair).
- Found in patients with SLE, MCTD, Sjögren's syndrome & RA, and scleroderma (often with myositis).
- Patient likely to have Raynaud's phenomenon.
- Also found in primary pulmonary hypertension, polymyositis, Grave's disease, ITP.
- They are of little diagnostic value.
- IIF shows fine speckled nuclear and nucleolar staining, depending on the stage of the cell cycle.

La (SS-B) antibodies

- Antibodies to the ENA La recognize a 48 kDa protein complexed to small RNAs that is probably involved in processing of RNA Pol III transcripts.
- Protein has sequence homology with a retroviral protein.
- Antibody to La is found mainly in primary Sjögren's syndrome.
- It is very rare in Sjögren's syndrome secondary to rheumatoid arthritis, systemic sclerosis, or primary biliary cirrhosis.
- About 15% of patients with SLE will have antibodies to La.
- Antibodies to this specificity have been associated with neonatal congenital complete heart block: this is less common than with anti-Ro antibodies.

For methods of detection, see **⊃** 'ENA antibodies', p. 532.

LGI1 antibodies

- Anti-LGI1 antibodies recognize the leucine-rich glioma inactivated protein (LGI1), involved in regulation of synaptic function.
- Association is with:
  - limbic encephalitis;
  - faciobranchial dystonic seizures.
- Rarely associated with tumours.

Liver cytosol antibodies (LC1)

- LC1 antibodies seen in:
  - autoimmune hepatitis type 2; associated with LKM antibodies;
  - autoimmune cholangitis.
  - Antigen is formiminotransferase cyclodeaminase (FTCD).
- Titre may correlate with disease activity.
- Pattern on IIF similar to that of LKM antibodies.
- Confirm with immunoblot against 58 kDa protein.

Liver–kidney microsomal (LKM) and liver microsomal (LM) antibodies

- Units: titre (semi-quantitative).
- Normal adult range: negative.

Principles of testing

- IIF on tissue multiblock.
- Immunoblotting with purified antigen to confirm.

Indications

- Suspected autoimmune hepatitis.

Interpretation

- LKM antibodies bind to microsomes in the cytoplasm of hepatocytes and the cells of the proximal renal tubules, but do not stain distal renal tubules.
- Often confused with mitochondrial antibodies, but the latter will also stain both the stomach and other tubules in the kidney.
- Three types of LKM antibodies have been described: LKM-1, LKM-2, and LKM-3.
- LKM-1 antibodies recognize the cytochrome P450 2D6 and are associated with types 2a and 2b autoimmune chronic active hepatitis.
  - Type 2a disease begins in childhood in 50% of cases and is associated with autoimmunity to thyroid and gastric parietal cells.
  - Type 2b is associated with antibodies to hepatitis C in addition to the LKM antibodies.
- LKM-2 recognize the cytochrome P450 2C8, C9, C10 and are associated with hepatitis induced by the diuretic ticrynafen (tienilic acid).
- LKM-3 recognize uridine diphosphate glucuronyl tranferase and have been reported in hepatitis.
  - Hepatitis-δ infection is also associated with antibodies to the lamins of the nuclear envelope.
- Liver microsomes (LM antibodies) can be seen, where the target antigen is cytochrome P450 1A2.
  - Fluorescence staining is most marked in perivenous hepatocytes.
  - Associated with hepatitis induced by the drug dihydralazine.

Loop of Henle antibodies and lupus anticoagulant

Loop of Henle antibodies

- This pattern is extremely rare and is probably of low diagnostic value.
- Reported cases have had renal tubular acidosis, pernicious anaemia, and primary biliary cirrhosis.

Lupus anticoagulant

- See **➲** 'Cardiolipin antibodies (ACA) and lupus anticoagulant', p. 526.

Lymphocytotoxic antibodies

- Autoantibodies (as opposed to alloantibodies induced by pregnancy or transfusion) to lymphocytes have been detected in:
  - rheumatoid arthritis;
  - systemic sclerosis;
  - SLE.
- Their role in the generation of lymphopenia is uncertain.
- There is no evidence to support their role in the lymphopenia of common variable immunodeficiency.
- Routine search for these antibodies is probably of little clinical value.

Ma/Ta antibodies

- Antibodies to Ma1 and Ma2 are found in patients with limbic encephalitis in association with germ cell tumours of the testis (78%) and are found in young patients.
- Ma1 and Ma3 antibodies are found in older patients with cerebellar syndromes, in association with tumours (lung, parotid, breast, colon).
- Antibodies react with neuronal nucleolar proteins.

Mi2 antibodies

- Antibodies to this ENA are found typically in patients with a steroid-responsive dermatomyositis, with a favourable course.
- Development of antibodies is associated with HLA-DR7 and UV light exposure, which upregulates Mi2 expression in keratinocytes.
- Antibodies are rare in polymyositis (< 1%).
- Antibodies recognize a 240 kDa nuclear antigen (helicase).
- Homogeneous nuclear staining on HEp-2 cells is usually seen.

Mitochondrial antibodies (AMA)

- Units: titre (semi-quantitative).
- Normal adult range: titre < 1/40.

Principles of testing

- IIF using tissue multiblock.
- Follow-up tests using EIA or immunoblots against purified antigens confirm specificity.

Indications for testing

- Suspected autoimmune liver disease.

Interpretation

- AMA show typical granular staining on the cytoplasm of all cells in the tissue multiblock.
- May be confused with LKM, ribosomal, and signal recognition particle antibodies.
- Nine discrete reactivities have been described, although these are not all detectable on standard tissue sections.
- For those patterns that are detectable, the distinction is dependent on recognizing quantitative differences in the level of staining of different cell populations.
- See Table 18.1.
- Few laboratories report the different specificities by IIF.
- M2 antibodies are strongly associated with primary biliary cirrhosis, and more than 95% of PBC patients will be positive.
- New mitochondrial antibodies should be put up against the E2 antigen in an EIA or immunoblot (see mitochondrial M2 antibodies) to confirm the specificity.

Table 18.1 Interpretation of AMA staining

Antibody	Target antigen	Staining characteristics	Disease associations
M1	Cardiolipin	Distal tubules ++	Syphilis; anti-phospholipid syndrome (1° and 2°)
M2	Pyruvate (2-oxo-acid) dehydrogenase complex	Distal tubules ++ Parietal cells ++	Primary biliary cirrhosis (PBC) Also seen in RhA, SSc
M3	Not known	Proximal P1, P2, P3 ++ Distal tubules ++ Parietal cells ++	Lupus-like disease
M4	Sulphite oxidase	Proximal tubules + Distal tubules ++ Parietal cells ++	PBC (often with M2) PBC–scleroderma overlap
M5	Not known	P1, P2 proximal tubules ++ P3 proximal tubules +	Miscellaneous connective tissue diseases Occur with anti-β_2-GPI antibodies in APS

Table 18.1 (*Contd.*)

Antibody	Target antigen	Staining characteristics	Disease associations
		Parietal cells +	
M6	Monoamine oxidase B	P1 proximal tubules++ Loop of Henle ++ APUD cells, stomach ++	Iproniazid-induced hepatitis
M7	Sarcosine dehydrogenase	Distal tubules ++ P2, P3 proximal tubules +	Myocarditis; cardiomyopathy
M8	Not known	Distal tubules ++ Collecting ducts ++	PBC (often with M2)
M9	Glycogen phosphorylase	Distal tubules ++ Collecting ducts ++	PBC (mild disease?) Autoimmune hepatitis

- M4 and M8 antibodies usually occur with M2 antibodies: this pattern is associated with severe disease.
- M9 antibodies occurring alone are associated with mild disease.
- Patients with type 3 autoimmune chronic active hepatitis (usually associated with antibodies to soluble liver antigens) will often have anti-mitochondrial antibodies and this entity may be an overlap syndrome of CAH and PBC.
- Mitochondrial antibodies are often detected in patients with autoimmune thyroiditis, rheumatoid arthritis, scleroderma, and Sjögren's syndrome, diseases that are associated clinically with PBC.
- Other antibodies have been described in PBC, including antibodies to GW bodies (GWB), GRASP-1 (GRIP associated protein 1), which may have more prognostic value.

Mitochondrial M2 antibodies

- Units: qualitative.
- Normal adult range: negative.

Principles of testing
- EIA using purified E2 antigen.
- Immunoblot/line blot assay.

Indications
- Confirmation of specificity of AMA detected by IIF.

Interpretation
- Antigen of the M2 mitochondrial autoantibodies is now known to be the E2 component of the pyruvate dehydrogenase complex.
- Specificity for PBC approaches 100%.
- Other components, E1-α and E1-β, as well as the E2 subunit of branched-chain dehydrogenase, are target antigens.

- In view of the association of mitochondrial antibodies with diseases other than PBC it is now advisable to screen AMA-positive sera for antibodies to the M2 antigen, to confirm the specificity.
- Screening for PBC in the first instance should be by IIF (non-M2 patterns may be identified).

MuSK antibodies

- Antibodies to muscle-specific receptor tyrosine kinase may be found in acetylcholine receptor antibody-negative myasthenia gravis.
- Antibodies to MuSK interfere with signalling by the nerve-released ligand, agrin. MuSK and agrin are required for the formation of the neuromuscular junction.
- Patients are more likely to be female, have less eye involvement, and are likely to be of African-Caribbean descent.

Multiple nuclear dot antibody

Two patterns of multiple nuclear dots are recognized on HEp-2 cells.
- Nsp-1: pattern of 2–6 dots located close to the nucleolus.
  - Antibodies to p80 coilin (anti-coiled body antibodies).
  - Seen in primary biliary cirrhosis.
- Nsp-2: pattern of 5–10 dots (up to 30).
  - Antibodies to a soluble nuclear protein Sp100.
  - Often called pseudo-centromere, but there is no staining of the metaphase plate as in a true centromere antibody.
  - This pattern is associated with a subgroup of patients with primary biliary cirrhosis, especially those who are anti-M2 antibody negative.

Myelin-associated glycoprotein (MAG) antibodies

- IgM anti-MAG antibodies are associated with paraproteinaemic polyneuropathies where the paraprotein is IgM (but not IgG or IgA).
- Levels of antibody do not correlate with severity of the nerve disease, but removing the antibody by plasma exchange or immunosuppression can improve the neuropathy.
- Rarely, anti-MAG antibodies are found in Guillain–Barré syndrome, MS, and myasthenia gravis.

Myositis-specific antibodies

Multiple antibody specificities are now recognized in myositis and dermatomyositis. These include:
- tRNA synthetase antibodies (see **➜** 'Jo-1 and related anti-synthetase antibodies', p. 546).

- Mi2 (see ➲ 'Mi2 antibodies', p. 549).
- Signal recognition particle (SRP) (see ➲ 'Signal recognition particle (SRP) antibodies', p. 569).
- HMGCR (3-hydroxy-3-methylglutaryl coenzyme A reductase)—associated with necrotizing myopathy and very high CK; seen with statin therapy.
- SAE1 (small ubiquitin-like modifier activating enzyme), associated with amyopathic onset, interstitial lung disease, and rash.
- MDA5 (melanoma differentiation-associated antigen 5), associated with amyopathic onset with rash and interstitial lung disease.
- NXP2 (nuclear matrix protein 2), associated with juvenile polymyositis and dermatomyositis. In adults, may be associated with malignancy (breast, uterus, pancreas).
- TIF1 (transcriptional intermediary factor 1) is seen in cancer associated myositis in adults, but also occurs in juvenile polymyositis and dermatomyositis.
- cN1A (cytosolic 5′ nucleotidase 1A) is seen in inclusion body myositis.
- The PRU in Sheffield offers an extended myositis screen by immunoblot which covers all the key antigens. Apart from Jo-1 there are no EQA scheme and no international standards.

Nephritic factors

Nephritic factors are autoantibodies of either IgG or IgM class that stabilize activated complement components and prevent their normal inactivation by the control proteins. Four types are recognized.

C3 nephritic factor

- An autoantibody to the alternate pathway C3 convertase (C3bBb) that stabilizes the convertase and prevents its natural destruction by factors H and I.
- Antibody recognizes the Bb component of the convertase, allowing continuous and unregulated activation of C3.
- Detected by its effect on C3 mobility on electrophoresis, using immunofixation, and is reported as present or absent.
- Patients with mesangiocapillary glomerulonephritis type II and/or partial lipodystrophy who have a markedly reduced C3 should be screened for the presence of a C3 nephritic factor.
- Not all patients with partial lipodystrophy who have a C3 nephritic factor will have renal disease, although there is an increased risk of them developing it.
- Not all patients with C3 nephritic factor have partial lipodystrophy.

C4 nephritic factor

- A rare autoantibody that stabilizes the active form of C4 (C4bC2a) and leads to increased activation of the first part of the classical pathway.
- Because the normal regulatory processes are intact at the level of C3, the reaction proceeds no further.
- C4 and C3 are usually reduced.

- Associated with SLE and other types of glomerulonephritis.
- Detected by electrophoretic studies of activated serum using immunofixation.

Properdin-dependent nephritic factor
- A nephritic factor of the alternate pathway that slowly cleaves C3, C5, and C9 and is dependent on the presence of properdin.
- It is heat labile.
- It occurs in other types of mesangiocapillary glomerulonephritis.

C1q antibodies
- These antibodies occur in SLE, urticarial vasculitis (hypocomplementaemic urticarial vasculitis), and mesangiocapillary GN.
- They recognize activated C1q (bound to antibody or solid phase).

Neuronal antibodies and neuronal nuclear antibodies (ANNA)

Neuronal antibodies
- These antibodies react with a 96 kDa surface antigen of neuronal cells and occur mainly in patients with neuropsychiatric lupus.
- May be detected by immunofluorescence on cultured human neuroblastoma cell lines or by Western blotting.
- May be found in serum of patients with SLE (11%), even in the absence of neuropsychiatric lupus.
- Approximately 74% of patients with neuropsychiatric lupus will have these antibodies.
- It has been suggested that the titre of antibodies correlates with degree of neuropsychiatric impairment.
- More specific for neuropsychiatric lupus than ribosomal P antibodies.
- Anti-Yo antibodies recognize the cytoplasm of Purkinje cells—see ➔ 'Yo antibodies', p. 575.

Neuronal nuclear antibodies (ANNA)
- ANNA-1 (anti-Hu) react with all neuronal cell nuclei—see ➔ 'Hu antibodies', p. 543.
- ANNA-2 (anti-Ri) react only with central not peripheral neuronal cell nuclei—see ➔ 'Ri antibodies', p. 567.
- ANNA-3 very rare recognizing 170 kDa protein in terminally differentiated neurons and podocytes.
- Anti-Ma1, Ma2 (Ta), Ma3 expressed on neuronal nucleoli—see ➔ p. 549.
- Anti-Zic4—see ➔ 'Zic4 antibodies', p. 576.

Neutrophil antibodies

- Antibodies against neutrophil surface antigens may occur in autoimmune neutropenia.
- Because of the presence of Fc receptors for IgG on neutrophils, it is very difficult to prove unequivocally that anti-neutrophil antibodies are present, and none of the current techniques are entirely satisfactory.
- Tests used include:
  - neutrophil agglutination;
  - antibody-mediated phagocytosis of neutrophils by macrophages;
  - antibody-dependent lysis;
  - flow cytometry.
- Antibodies specific for neutrophil nuclei, reacting with unknown antigens, are found in rheumatoid arthritis with vasculitis, particularly in Felty's syndrome (RhA, splenomegaly, vasculitis and leg ulceration, neutropenia).
  - There is homogeneous nuclear staining present only on neutrophils, but not liver or HEp-2 cells.
  - Their importance is more in their potential to cause misinterpretation in tests for ANCA, where they may be confused, by the inexperienced, with the perinuclear pattern.

Neutrophil cytoplasmic antibodies (ANCA)

- Units: titre (IIF).
- Normal adult range: titre < 1/10.
- EIA and multiplex assays have variable arbitrary units—consult manufacturers' information.

Principles of testing

- ANCA are detected on ethanol-fixed human granulocytes.
- Other fixation methods are *not* recommended by the International Consensus Statement.
- P-ANCA pattern results from a redistribution of certain cytoplasmic antigens when cold ethanol is used as a fixative for the human neutrophils.
- The current International Consensus suggests that assays for anti-PR3 and anti-MPO can be used for primary screening. This can be by EIA or multiplex assay.
- IIF can be used as a secondary assay and for detection of other patterns (X-ANCA—see later in this topic).
- Quantitative monitoring may be valuable.

Indications for testing

- Rapidly progressive glomerulonephritis; pulmonary haemorrhage.
- New patients must always have both ANCA and GBM performed.

Interpretation

- 90% of patient with Wegener's granulomatosis (GPA) will be C-ANCA$^+$.
- 5–10% of GPA patients will be ANCA$^-$.
- Antibodies are present in both the systemic and localized forms of GPA.
- As a test for GPA, meta-analysis of all published data has shown a sensitivity of 66% and a specificity of 98%.
- 30% of patients with microscopic polyarteritis (MPA) and Churg–Strauss syndrome (EGPA) will be C-ANCA$^+$.
- C-ANCA antigen is PR3, a granule protein also expressed on the neutrophil surface.
- Perinuclear (P-ANCA) pattern is found less commonly in GPA and MPA, but mainly in other forms of severe vasculitis, including EGPA, SLE, and rheumatoid vasculitis.
- Atypical ANCA (X-ANCA) may occur in inflammatory bowel disease, particularly where there is liver involvement (primary sclerosing cholangitis (PSC)).
- See Table 18.2.
- Multiple antigens are involved in producing C-ANCA and P-ANCA.
- Antibodies to nuclear antigens and to GBM may coexist with ANCA, making diagnosis difficult.
  - Where there is doubt, check fluorescent pattern on tissue multiblock to exclude ANA.

Table 18.2 Interpretation of ANCA staining

Target antigen	Staining pattern	Clinical association
Proteinase 3	C-ANCA (90%); P-ANCA (2%)	Wegener's (GPA), microscopic polyarteritis (MPA), Churg–Strauss (EGPA) (30%)
Myeloperoxidase	P-ANCA (70%); P-ANCA (5%)	GPA, MPA, EGPA (60%), GBM (30%)
Azuocidin (CAP37)	P-ANCA	Uncertain
β-Glucuronidase	P-ANCA	Uncertain
Bactericidal permeability-increasing protein (BPI)	C-ANCA (4%); atypical 'flat' ANCA	Cystic fibrosis (50%)
Cathepsin G	P-ANCA (5%); X-ANCA	Sclerosing cholangitis, ulcerative colitis
Elastase	P-ANCA (8%); X-ANCA	SLE (neuro-SLE), hydralazine-induced SLE; RhA; ulcerative colitis
Lactoferrin	P-ANCA (10%); X-ANCA	Inflammatory bowel disease, PBC, AIH, SLE, RhA
Lysozyme	C-ANCA; P-ANCA	Uncertain

- Serial monitoring of C-ANCA by IIF or EIA is useful as a rising value may herald a relapse of GPA.
- Patients with treated vasculitis may remain weakly ANCA positive for years in clinical remission.
- Whether there is any value in serial monitoring of P-ANCA is less certain.
- IgA ANCA have been reported in Henoch–Schönlein purpura and can be identified by IIF if an anti-IgA reagent is used.
- Where there is a high clinical probability of ANCA-associated vasculitis and negative results in the PR3/MPO assays, a second-line test should be performed (alternative EIA or IIF).
- An international standard for MPO antibodies exists (ERM-DA476/IFCC) and one for PR3 is being prepared. EQA schemes exist for GBM and ANCA.
- Antibodies to carbonic anhydrase III (detected by immunoblotting) have been associated with vasculitis, typical microscopic polyarteritis.

NMDA (*N*-methyl-D-aspartate) receptor antibodies

- Antibodies to NR1 and NR2 have been associated with limbic encephalitis, SLE, and variant epilepsies.
- Testing is by immunohistochemistry on rat brain sections or by IIF on cell lines. Flow cytometry ('live' NMDAR testing) using cell lines may be more sensitive.
- Patients often have a CSF lymphocytosis.
- There is an association with ovarian or mediastinal teratomas expressing the NMDA receptor, although cases may occur without any evidence of malignancy.

Nuclear antibodies (ANA)

- Units: semi-quantitative.
- Normal ranges:
  - age < 18, titre < 1/20;
  - age 18–65, titre < 1/40;
  - age > 65, titre < 1/80.

Principles of testing

- Testing is undertaken by IIF using a tissue multiblock with HEp-2 cells.
- Genetically modified HEp-2 cells (HEp-2000) are said to express higher levels of Ro antigen; in practice, there is little advantage when the microscopist is experienced.
- Ro antigens may be eluted from rodent liver and give false-negative results ('ANA-negative lupus'); these will be identified by parallel use of HEp-2 cells.
- HEp-2 cells are more sensitive: screening with HEp-2 cells will increase the false-positive rate compared to rodent liver.
- HEp-2 cells are valuable for identification of staining pattern.

- EIA/multiplex screening assays are available to reduce the number of negative immunofluorescent screens performed.
- Only IgG antibodies are of clinical significance: screening should be carried out with anti-human IgG-FITC, not polyvalent antibodies.
- Initial screening dilution for serum must be modified for children.
- Appropriate titratable controls are required.
- Reporting should include significant patterns.
- EQA is available: performance is variable.
  - Modern fluorescent microscopes significantly affect titration results.
- International standards are available.
- An international consensus on reporting patterns has been agreed. This consensus will be used as the basis for the UK EQA scheme. The consensus and further information can be obtained at: ℘ http://www.ANApatterns.org
- Laboratories are advised to use this for clinical reporting.
- Automated titration systems reporting in light intensity units are in clinical use: laboratories must ensure that they have done full mapping against IIF titrations to avoid confusing clinicians.

Indications for testing
- Suspected connective tissue disease.

Interpretation
- See Table 18.3.
- Nuclear antibodies are associated with the connective tissue diseases.
- Only IgG antibodies are significant.
- IgM ANA are non-specific and frequently occur after viral infections.
  - Occasional patients with connective tissue disease produce only IgM ANA.
  - IgM ANA occur in rheumatoid arthritis (cross-reactive IgM RhF).

Table 18.3 Interpretation of ANA staining

HEp-2 staining pattern	Antigen(s)	Disease associations
Nuclear staining		
Homogeneous nuclear/nucleolar	dsDNA, histones, topoisomerase 1, Ku	SLE
Homogeneous nuclear (nucleoli negative)	Histone	SLE, drug-induced SLE
Nuclear membrane	Lamins A, B, C	Autoimmune liver disease; APS; leucocystoclastic vasculitis
Nuclear pore (punctate staining)	gp210 pore protein, lamin B receptor	Primary biliary cirrhosis
Peripheral nuclear	dsDNA	SLE
Nuclear matrix (coarse speckles)	hn-RNP	SLE
Coarse speckled	U1-RNP, Sm, Ki	SLE, MCTD

Table 18.3 (Contd.)

HEp-2 staining pattern	Antigen(s)	Disease associations
Fine speckled	Ro, La, Mi2	SLE, Sjögren's, dermatomyositis
Granular nuclear staining	Topoisomerase 1 (Scl-70)	Systemic sclerosis
Coarse and fine speckles	PCNA	SLE
Centromere (condensed in metaphase plates)	CENP-A, -B, -C	CREST, limited scleroderma
Nuclear dots (2–6) Nsp-1	p80 coilin	PBC
Nuclear dots (6–10, up to 30): pseudo-centromere	Sp100	PBC (AMA negative)
Homogeneous nucleolar	Pm-Scl, Ku, nucleolin	Polymyositis–scleroderma overlap
Clumpy nucleolar	Fibrillarin	Systemic sclerosis
Speckled nucleolar	RNA Pol I	Systemic sclerosis
Nucleolar dots	Nor-90 (nucleolar organizer region)	Scleroderma
Centriole	Centriole	Non-specific (CTDs, post-infective)
Nuclear mitotic spindle apparatus (NuMa, MSA-1)	NuMA protein	Non-specific CTD
Mitotic spindle apparatus-2 (MSA-2)	Midbody	Systemic sclerosis, Raynaud's midbody pattern
Mitotic spindle apparatus -3 (MSA-3)	CENP-F	Respiratory tract tumours
Cytoplasmic		
Mitochondria (large granule staining)	Multiple antigens (M1–M9)	PBC, autoimmune liver disease
Ribosomes	Ribosomal P proteins	SLE
Irregular granular staining	Lysosomes, peroxisomes	Non-specific
Fine speckled	Jo-1, other tRNA synthetases	Polymyositis
Golgi body	Giantin (50%); golgins 245, 160, 95, 97	SLE, Sjögren's, other CTDs, chronic CMV
Actin filaments	Actin	Autoimmune hepatitis
Vimentin	Vimentin	SLE, other CTDs
Cytokeratin	Cytokeratin 18	RhA

- Significance of the titre of IgG ANA is age dependent.
- Low-titre positive ANAs in the elderly must be carefully interpreted in the context of relevant clinical symptoms and signs.
- Pattern of ANA identifies likely antigens and significance.
- Follow-up testing with ENA and dsDNA assays is required to fully investigate antigenic specificities identified by IIF.
- Because of the long circulating half-life of the autoantibodies, measurement does not need to be carried out more frequently than once every 3 weeks (unless the patient has been plasmapheresed).
- Detection of a strong positive ANA is an indicator for confirmatory tests, including dsDNA, ENA, and, if clinically appropriate, histone antibodies.

Nuclear matrix antibodies

- These antibodies give large, coarse speckles on HEp-2 cells.
- Specificity appears to be against heterogeneous nuclear RNA and matrix proteins: by immunoblotting at least four proteins are recognized, of molecular weight 70, 31, 23, and 19 kDa.
  - 70 kDa determinant is U1-RNP.
- The antibodies are rarely seen but occur in lupus as well as in undifferentiated connective tissue diseases.

Nuclear mitotic spindle antibodies

Antibodies will only be seen on HEp-2 cells. They are rare and not specific, being found in:
- SLE;
- rheumatoid arthritis;
- CREST;
- MCTD;
- Sjögren's syndrome.

Described patterns

- NuMA (nuclear mitotic apparatus protein, MSA-1) shows fluorescence concentrated at the spindle poles.
  - Non-specific (CTDs).
- Anti-tubulin antibodies stain the spindle fibres.
  - Post-infective and autoimmune disease.
  - Low titres in normal individuals.

Antibodies to mitotic spindle antigens (MSA) show two patterns of staining:
- MSA-2 does not stain interphase cells and is sometimes referred to as the midbody pattern.
  - Associated with systemic sclerosis and Raynaud's.
- MSA-3 shows fine, dense nuclear staining in some interphase cells and two sets of discrete granules on either side of the metaphase plate in dividing cells.
  - Antigen is CENP-F (p330 protein).
  - Seen rarely with respiratory tract tumours.

Nuclear pore antibodies

- Antibodies to a 210 kDa nuclear pore antigen have been described in up to 27% of cases of primary biliary cirrhosis (in addition to the multiple nuclear dot pattern).
- IIF on HEp-2 cells gives a punctate perinuclear staining pattern.

Nucleolar antibodies

Nucleolar antibodies will be detected on routine screening on rodent liver. They are much easier to see on HEp-2 cells, where three discrete staining patterns may be identified.
- Speckled nucleolar staining with fine, speckled nuclear staining.
  - Antibody recognizes RNA polymerase I.
  - Present in 4% of patients with systemic sclerosis (diffuse disease).
- Homogeneous nucleolar staining.
  - Antibody recognizes PM-Scl and also Ku; see ➲ 'PM-Scl antibodies', p. 563 and ➲ 'Ki and Ku antibodies', p. 547.
- Clumpy nucleolar staining with nuclear dots.
  - Antibody recognizes fibrillarin, component of U3-RNP.
  - Present in 8% of patients with systemic sclerosis, particularly with cardiopulmonary involvement.
- Other nucleolar antigens to which autoantibodies have been detected include:
  - Nor-90, a 90 kDa protein of the nucleolar organizer region (nucleolar dot staining on HEp-2 cells).
  - To, a 40 kDa protein complexed to 7S or 8S RNA, associated with pulmonary hypertension and bowel involvement in scleroderma.
  - An RNP particle that includes RNA polymerase III.

Ovarian antibodies

- Antibodies identified by IIF on multiblock (adrenal, ovary, testis, pituitary).
- Useful for identifying primary autoimmune ovarian failure as a cause of infertility.
- Found in 15–50% of patients with premature ovarian failure.
- Patients may also be positive for adrenal antibodies (cross-reactive steroid cell antibodies) and for thyroid antibodies.
- Ovarian antibodies recognize P450scc enzyme.
- Antibodies to 3β-hydroxysteroid dehydrogenase may be a more sensitive marker of premature (autoimmune) ovarian failure.

See also ➲ 'Adrenal cortex autoantibodies', p. 523.

Parathyroid antibodies

- Found in patients with:
  - idiopathic hypoparathyroidism;
  - hypoparathyoidism associated with other endocrinopathies;
  - chronic mucocutaneous candidiasis.
- Detected on group O human parathyroid by immunofluorescence.
  - They are impossible to detect if ANA or mitochondrial antibodies are present.
  - Testing should therefore be carried out in parallel with testing on the standard tissue multiblock.
  - Control sera are extremely difficult to obtain.

PCNA (proliferating cell nuclear antigen) antibodies

- Antigen recognized by the autoantibody is expressed only at certain times in the cell cycle.
- It is readily detectable only on HEp-2 cells, where it gives variable-sized speckles in only some cells.
- Antigen is a 33 kDa auxiliary protein for DNA polymerase-δ.
- PCNA has erroneously been referred to as cyclin.
- It is seen in about 3% of patients with SLE, but does not appear to identify any particular clinical subgroup.

Phospholipase A2 receptor (PLA2R) antibodies

- Antibodies to PLA2 recognize the transmembrane phospholipase A2 receptor, found in lung, placenta, leukocytes, and on the podocytes of kidneys.
- Associated with idiopathic membranous glomerulonephritis, thought to be due to binding of the antibody in the glomerular membrane with an *in situ* immune complex formation.
- Antibodies to PLA2R may be useful as markers of response to therapy.
- Negative: < 14 RU/ml; borderline 14–20 RU/ml; positive > 20 RU/ml.
- Testing is by ELISA. There is no EQA or standard.

Pituitary gland antibodies

- Antibodies to pituitary components have been described in:
  - a variety of centrally mediated endocrine disorders, including autoimmune lymphocytic hypophysitis (70% positive) and autoimmune hypopituitarism (30% positive);
  - empty sella syndrome;

- some pituitary tumours;
- some patients with type I diabetes mellitus.
- Antibodies are usually detected by immunofluorescence on pituitary sections or on pituitary cell lines.
- Antibodies recognize a cytoplasmic 49 kDa antigen.
- Diagnostic value is uncertain.
- No commercial control sera are available.

Platelet antibodies

- Platelet autoantibodies (as opposed to alloantibodies) are found in patients with ITP.
- Also found in other conditions associated with thrombocytopenia, such as:
  - HIV;
  - connective tissue diseases;
  - thrombotic thrombocytopenic purpura (TTP);
  - heparin-induced thrombocytopenia.
- Many techniques have been described to detect such antibodies, including:
  - phagocytosis by neutrophils;
  - lymphocyte activation;
  - RIA;
  - EIA;
  - flow cytometry.
- Using sensitive techniques, over 90% of patients with ITP will be shown to have platelet-associated IgG.
- There is no consensus on the best technique or on the value of routine testing.
- Target antigens are varied but include platelet GP Ib, IIb, and IIIa.
- Alloantibodies to platelets react with PLA1 antigen.

PM-Scl antibodies (also known as PM-1)

- PM-Scl antibodies are found in the polymyositis–scleroderma overlap syndrome.
- May also be found in patients with dermatomyositis/polymyositis or systemic sclerosis occurring alone.
- There may be an increased risk of renal disease in the overlap patients.
- Target antigen appears to be a complex of 11 proteins occurring in the nucleolus and elsewhere.
  - Two major antigens are PM/Scl-100 and PM/Scl-75.
- The pattern of immunofluorescence on HEp-2 cells is variable, with homogeneous nucleolar staining, with some atypical nuclear speckling and cytoplasmic staining.
- Detection is usually by immunodiffusion or immunoblotting.

Purkinje cell antibodies

- See ➲ 'Yo antibodies', p. 575.

RA-33 antibodies and rheumatoid-associated nuclear antibodies (RANA)

RA-33 antibodies

- These antibodies have been described as specific for rheumatoid arthritis.
- They react with a 33 kDa non-histone nuclear antigen of HeLa cells (heterogeneous nuclear ribonucleoprotein).
- Presence of these antibodies has been linked to radiographic evidence of progression and of therapeutic response to methotrexate.

Rheumatoid-associated nuclear antibodies (RANA)

- If EBV-transformed cell lines are used as a target, antibodies that react only with EBV-infected nuclei but not normal nuclei can be detected in serum of patients with rheumatoid arthritis and other connective tissue diseases.
- There is no routine value to this test.

Recoverin antibodies

- See ➲ 'Retinal S100 and cancer-associated retinopathy (CAR) antibodies', p. 565.

Renal biopsy (direct immunofluorescence)

- Direct immunofluorescence of renal biopsies is an essential part of the evaluation of renal disease.
- DIF should always take place in parallel with examination of biopsies with standard stains and by electron microscopy.
- Staining should include the use of antisera to IgG, IgA, IgM, C3, C4, and fibrinogen.
- Linear deposition of IgG in the glomeruli is a feature of anti-GBM disease.
- IgA deposition is heavy in a segmental pattern in IgA nephropathy.
- Henoch–Schönlein purpura is also associated with IgA deposition, often with fibrin deposition.
- In type II MPGN, associated with a nephritic factor, there is heavy C3 deposition in the GBM, without immunoglobulin.
- Patchy IgG and C3, or C3 alone, is seen in post-streptococcal GN.

- SLE may give any pattern of renal disease, and is usually accompanied by IgG, IgM, and complement deposition with a variable distribution.
- In tubulo-interstitial nephritis, there may be antibodies to the tubular basement membrane.

Reticulin antibodies

- These antibodies are non-specific.
- Found in:
  - coeliac disease;
  - inflammatory bowel disease, particularly where there is concomitant liver disease.
- They may occur in the absence of clinical disease in the elderly.
- They will be detected as part of the 'autoimmune screen' on a tissue multiblock.
- If coeliac disease is suspected, endomysial or tTG antibodies should be requested.
- IgA reticulin antibodies are slightly more specific for coeliac disease than IgG antibodies, but sensitivity and specificity is far lower than for EMA and tTG antibodies.
- Up to five different patterns of anti-reticulin antibodies have been described using immunofluorescence.
  - Only the R1 pattern is associated with coeliac disease.
  - IgA-R1-reticulin antibodies are reported to have a specificity of 98% but a sensitivity of only 25% for coeliac disease.
- Laboratories no longer report reticulin antibodies routinely.
- Detection of strong R1 ARA should trigger EMA or tTG testing automatically in the laboratory.
- See ➋ 'Endomysial antibodies (EMA)', p. 533 and ➋ 'Tissue transglutaminase (tTG) antibodies', p. 574.

Retinal S100 and cancer-associated retinopathy (CAR) antibodies

- Antibodies against retinal antigens (S100) have been identified in many types of chronic inflammatory eye disease affecting the uveal tract, including the Vogt–Koyanagi–Harada syndrome.
- Antibodies are not disease-specific.
- Diagnostic value is uncertain at present.
- The antibodies may induce demyelination of the optic nerve.
- Other anti-retinal antibodies (CAR) have been described as a paraneoplastic phenomenon in patients with a cancer-associated retinopathy syndrome, seen rarely in association with small-cell lung carcinoma.
  - Antibodies bind to small-cell carcinoma cell nuclei.
  - Major antigen is recoverin, a calcium binding protein.

- α-Enolase, carbonic anhydrase, transducin B, TULP1, photoreceptor cell-specific nuclear receptor, heat-shock protein cognate receptor (HSC 70), arrestin, and other proteins are recognized as minor autoantigens.
- CV2/CRMP5 antibodies may be associated with cancer-associated retinopathy.
- Lens-induced uveitis, a rare condition that may follow trauma or surgery, is associated with circulating antibodies to lens proteins.
- Melanoma-associated retinopathy; antigen is not well characterized. Patients present with dazzling photopsia. Autoantibody binds to bipolar cells of the retina.

Rheumatoid factor (RhF)

- Units:
  - titre;
  - IU/ml.
- Normal adult range:
  - titre, < 1/80;
  - <30 IU/ml.

Principles of testing

- Assays detect anti-immunoglobulin antibodies.
- Originally identified by sheep-cell agglutination test (SCAT, Rose–Waaler test)—this test is no longer used.
- Now detected by latex or particle agglutination assays, EIA, nephelometry, or turbidimetry.
- Measurement in IU/ml is preferred, but latex agglutination assays, which are sensitive but not specific, provide a cheap screening tool.
- Semi-quantitative particle agglutination assays are less desirable.
  - These assays may be susceptible to interference by serum fibronectin.
- EQA and international standards exist.

Indications for testing

- The only indication for testing is in patients with clinical rheumatoid arthritis.
- It is *not* a screening test for RhA.
- There is no value in the elderly, as RhF may be found in healthy elderly.

Interpretation

- RhF is a non-specific test; it detects immunoglobulins of any class reactive with the Fc region of other immunoglobulins.
- RhFs occur in a wide variety of conditions, such as:
  - viral infections;
  - chronic bacterial infections (SBE, TB);
  - myeloma;
  - lymphomas;
  - many connective tissue diseases;
  - old age (not associated with disease).

- In myeloma, paraproteins with RhF activity may cause a type II cryoglobulin.
- In infections and connective tissue diseases, polyclonal RhFs may cause a type III cryoglobulin.
- Rheumatoid arthritis patients may be positive or negative for RhFs.
- Those with progressive disease, and with vasculitis, usually have high-titre RhFs.
- There is little value in serial monitoring of RhF, as the titre correlates poorly with disease activity: the CRP is more useful.
- Requesting RhFs in the elderly is not helpful, as positive results do not necessarily indicate disease.
- At present there is no conclusive evidence that detecting IgA RhFs is valuable.

Ri antibodies

- Anti-Ri, a rare anti-neuronal nuclear antibody, has been documented in a few women with breast cancer or small-cell lung cancer, associated with ataxia, myoclonus, and opsoclonus.
- Antibodies recognize 55 kDa and 80 kDa proteins (Nova-1, Nova-2), found in all neuronal cell nuclei.
- Antibodies may be detected by immunofluorescence and immunoblotting.

Ribosomal (ribosomal P) antibodies

- Antibodies to ribosomes, particularly to ribosomal ribonucleoprotein (rRNP), are associated particularly with SLE (about 5–12% of patients).
- Majority of patients with neuropsychiatric lupus will be positive for ribosomal P antibodies: antibody level is reported to correlate with disease activity.
- May also be found in rheumatoid arthritis.
- Antibodies recognize three phosphoproteins (P0, P1, P2).
  - Antigens are distinct from antibodies to nuclear RNPs.
- Ribosomal and ribosomal P antibodies are the same.
- They frequently cause diagnostic confusion as they may be misinterpreted as mitochondrial antibodies by inexperienced microscopists.
  - They react particularly strongly with the chief cells of rodent stomach, and also with pancreatic tissue.
  - On HEp-2 cells there is fine speckled staining of the cytoplasm and some staining of nucleoli.
  - If seen on autoantibody screen, antibody should be titrated and reported.

RNA polymerase III antibodies

- Detected by EIA or FEIA.
- Normal < 7 U/ml.
- Antibodies to RNA pol III are seen in up to 23% of patients with systemic sclerosis.
- Markers for more extensive skin disease and renal involvement.

RNP antibodies

- These antibodies recognize nuclear, rather than ribosomal RNPs.
- There are a number of such complexes (U1–U6-RNPs), which comprise a number of proteins with small nuclear RNAs.
  - The same protein components may occur in more than one RNP complex.
- The most important antibodies are those against the U1-RNP, which recognize the 70 kDa A and C protein components.
  - Give rise to coarse, speckled pattern on IIF on HEp-2 cells.
  - Found in SLE and mixed connective tissue disease (MCTD).
  - When they occur in the absence of antibodies to dsDNA and Sm, this is supposed to indicate MCTD, although some authorities doubt that MCTD is truly a distinct entity and prefer to think of it as a subset of SLE.
  - There is no relation between anti-RNP antibody titres and disease activity.
- Some sera from patients with SLE contain antibodies that react with both Sm and U1-RNP.
- Antibodies have been described that react with both U1- and U2-RNP recognizing the U1-A and U2-B' proteins.
  - These are seen in SLE and SLE overlap syndromes, particularly.

Saccharomyces cerevisiae mannan antibodies (ASCA)

- ASCA are part of a spectrum of anti-glycan antibodies.
- Panels of anti-glycan antibodies are said to be useful in distinguishing Crohn's disease from ulcerative colitis, although only ASCA are routinely available from a few laboratories.

Salivary gland antibodies

- It is not possible to test for these in the presence of anti-nuclear or anti-mitochondrial antibodies.
- These are associated with Sjögren's syndrome and are more likely to occur in secondary rather than primary disease.
- Detected by IIF on rodent salivary gland.

Scl-70 antibodies

- Found in 20–40% of patients with progressive systemic sclerosis (PSS).
- Found in 20% of patients with limited scleroderma.
- Associated particularly with severe skin disease, musculoskeletal disease, and cardiopulmonary disease.
- Antibody may be a marker for the development of carcinoma of the lung in PSS.
- Do not predict the development of renal disease, although their presence in patients with isolated Raynaud's predicts the subsequent development of PSS and hence is a poor prognostic marker.
- Antigen recognized is topoisomerase I, an enzyme involved in supercoiling DNA.
  - Autoantibody interferes with the function of the target antigen.
- Scl-70 and anti-centromere antibodies appear to be mutually exclusive, as only two cases have ever been reported of coexistence of both specificities.
- Scl-70 antibodies give an atypical granular nuclear speckled pattern on HEp-2 cells.
- Definitive proof of their presence is obtained either by immunodiffusion, ELISA, or immunoblotting.
- See ➲ 'ENA antibodies', p. 532 and ➲ 'Nuclear antibodies (ANA)', p. 557.

Signal recognition particle (SRP) antibodies

- These antibodies produce a cytoplasmic staining pattern on HEp-2 cells that may be mistaken for that of mitochondrial antibodies.
- The antigen is a 54 kDa protein complexed with RNA.
- It is associated with polymyositis and dermatomyositis.
- Also seen in a necrotizing myopathy with interstitial lung disease.

Skin and mucosal biopsies (direct immunofluorescence)

- See ➲ 'Epidermal antibodies (including direct immunofluorescence of skin)', p. 535.

Sm (Smith) antibodies

- These antibodies, named after the patient in whom they were first described, are specific for SLE.
- They are seen most frequently in West Indians with SLE.
- Rare in Caucasians.

- Antibodies react with the B′/B and D proteins shared by U1-, U2-, and U4–U6-RNPs.
- These specificities are often seen with antibodies to U1-RNP.
- Whether occurring alone or with anti-RNP, these antibodies are accepted as a diagnostic criterion for lupus.
- They are usually detected by the same techniques as used for other ENAs.
- See ➲ 'ENA antibodies', p. 532.

Smooth muscle antibodies (SMA)

- Units: titre (semi-quantitative).
- Normal adult range: titre, < 1/40.

Principles of testing
- IIF on tissue multiblock.
- Specific subpatterns may be identified on HEp-2 cells.

Indications for testing
- Suspected autoimmune hepatitis.

Interpretation
- SMAs typically stain the muscular coats of arteries and the muscular layer of the stomach section, where there is also staining of the intergastric gland fibres. On HEp-2 cells, a meshwork of fine cytoplasmic fibres may be seen.
- SMA are present in high titre in 50–70% of patients with autoimmune 'lupoid' hepatitis (type 1).
  - 25% of patients may also be positive for nuclear and dsDNA antibodies.
- Also seen in association with hepatitis B surface antigenaemia and adenovirus infection.
- High-titre SMA antibodies against F-actin are seen in type 4 hepatitis, which affects predominantly young children.
- Antibodies to F-actin also seen in subset of PBC patients.
- Other smooth muscle antibodies directed against tropomyosin may be found.

Soluble liver antigen (SLA) antibodies and Sp100 antibodies

Soluble liver antigen (SLA) antibodies
- Predominant marker for type 3 hepatitis.
- May be the only autoantibody in up to 25% of cases.
- Target antigen for SLA antibodies is thought to be a unique enzyme that is a member of the pyridoxal phosphate-dependent transferases.
- SLA is the same as liver–pancreas antibodies.
- Testing is by immunoblot.

Sp100 antibodies

- Antibodies to this antigen of nucleus give rise to the multiple nuclear dot (6–10 dots) pattern of staining on HEp-2 cells (Nsp-2, pseudo-centromere).
- It is found in AMA-negative primary biliary cirrhosis.
- A commercial ELISA assay for antibodies to this antigen is available.
- See ➲ 'Nuclear antibodies (ANA)', p. 557.

Sperm antibodies

Sperm antibodies

- Both agglutinating and immobilizing antibodies have been described.
  - Direct agglutination, indirect agglutination, and EIA are used to detect antibodies.
  - An international standard exists and there is an EQA scheme in the UK.
- Multiple antigens seem to be involved and only some seem to be important in interfering with fertility.
- They are common after vasectomy (50% of men).
- May occur after trauma to the testes.
- Detected in:
  - 1–12% of women;
  - 10–20% of women with infertility.
- Antibodies may be of IgG or IgA class and may be found in serum or seminal/cervical secretions.

Steroid cell antibodies

- See ➲ 'Adrenal cortex autoantibodies', p. 523, and ➲ 'Ovarian antibodies', p. 561.

Striated muscle antibodies

Striated muscle antibodies

- Present in 25–40% of patients with myasthenia gravis.
- Almost all (80–100%) patients with myasthenia with thymoma are positive.
- A subgroup of myasthenic patients under 40 years of age may be positive in the absence of thymoma.
- May be seen in patients on penicillamine.
- May be seen in graft-versus-host disease after BMT.
- Constitute an important simple screening test in myasthenia for the presence of a thymoma and should form part of the diagnostic work-up.
- Antigen is thought to be a protein of the I-band of the myocyte (titin).
- Detected by IIF on primate striated muscle.
  - Rodent striated muscle may give false-positive results.

Thrombospondin type-1 domain containing 7A (THSD7A) antibodies

- Found in idiopathic membranous glomerulonephritis.
- THSD7A is found in the podocytes.
- Antibodies are predominantly IgG$_4$.
- Found in 2.5–10% of patients with primary MG, negative for anti-PLA2R antibodies (see ➔ 'Phospholipase A2 receptor (PLA2R) antibodies', p. 562).
- Detected by indirect immunofluorescence.

Thyroid microsomal (peroxidase) antibodies

- Units:
  - semiquantitative (particle agglutination);
  - kU/l (EIA).
- Normal adult range:
  - titre, < 1/800 (particle agglutination);
  - 0–60 kU/l (EIA; may vary between assays).

Principles of testing

- Particle agglutination assays (thyroid microsomal antibodies) give semi-quantitative results.
  - Particle agglutination assays use either tanned red cells or latex particles.
- EIA for thyroid peroxidase antibodies is preferred assay and gives quantitative results.
- Ideally TPO antibodies should be integrated into thyroid testing strategy, linked to TSH results, on main biochemistry analysers.
- An international standard exists and there is an EQA scheme in the UK.

Indications for testing

- Suspected thyroid disease.
- Autoimmune polyglandular syndromes.

Interpretation

- Present in high titre in:
  - 95% of patients with Hashimoto's thyroiditis;
  - 18% of patients with Graves's disease;
  - 90% of patients with primary myxoedema.
- Present in low titres in patients with:
  - colloidal goitre;
  - thyroid carcinoma;
  - transiently in de Quervain's thyroiditis;
  - occasionally in normal people.

- Positive TPO antibodies have also been associated with increased risks of pre-eclampsia, postnatal depression, and peri-menopausal depression.
- They may also be found in patients with other organ-specific autoimmune diseases, such as pernicious anaemia, Addison's disease, etc.
- Antigen is now known to be thyroid peroxidase.
- There is no diagnostic value in simultaneous testing of thyroglobulin and thyroid microsomal/TPO antibodies.

Thyroglobulin antibodies

- Normal adult range: titre < 1/400 by particle agglutination. Also detected by electrochemiluminescence.
- Occurrence is similar to that of thyroid microsomal (peroxidase) antibodies but thyroglobulin antibodies are less sensitive and specific.
- Some TPO antibody negative patients with thyroid disease will be positive only for thyroglobulin antibodies.
- Little additional information over and above testing for thyroid microsomal/TPO antibodies.
- Main use is to detect interfering antibodies in thryoglobulin assays (used to monitor thyroid cancer).
- EQA scheme operates; an international standard exists.

Thyroid-binding (stimulating/ blocking) antibodies

- Three classes of functional antibodies have also been described:
  - thyroid-stimulating antibodies that increase cAMP levels in thyrocytes;
  - thyroid growth-promoting antibodies that increase tritiated thymidine uptake into DNA by isolated thyrocytes;
  - thyroid-blocking antibodies that block the binding of TSH to its receptor on thyrocytes.
- Several sites of antibody binding to the TSH-R have been demonstrated.
- All three types of antibody have been strongly associated with Graves's disease and rarely occur in other types of thyroid disease.
- They may be of clinical significance through correlation with response to therapy and outcome.
- Their detection involves bioassay with *in vitro* culture of thyrocytes, or competitive RIA.
  - Commercial RIA for thyrotropin receptor antibody (TRAB) does not distinguish the different types of antibodies.
- An international standard exists.

Thyroid orbital antibodies

- These are found in Graves's disease.
- Bind to the retro-orbital fat or fibroblasts, causing hypertrophy and resulting in exophthalmos.
- The antigen(s) is/are unknown.
- Antibodies may persist even when the thyroid disease is treated (exophthalmos may progress).
- There is no routine screen for these antibodies.

Tissue transglutaminase (tTG) antibodies

- tTG is the major autoantigen responsible for anti-endomysial antibody staining pattern by IIF on monkey oesophagus.
- EIA assays for tTG have high sensitivity and specificity for coeliac disease.
- Human recombinant antigen-based assays have superior performance to guinea-pig-derived tTG assays.
- EIA assays have the advantage of automation and rapid throughput.
- Available for multiplex and ImmunoCAP® systems.
- The test is too sensitive for routine screening in primary care, but is excellent for monitoring compliance with a gluten-free diet.
- EIA assays will give quantitative results in arbitrary values.
- See ➔ 'Endomysial antibodies (EMA)', p. 533.

Tr antibodies

- Anti-Tr antibodies are found in paraneoplastic cerebellar ataxia associated with Hodgkin's lymphoma.
- Antibodies can be found in both serum and CSF.
- Staining pattern is similar to anti-Yo antibodies on Purkinje cell cytoplasm.

Tubulin and ubiquitin antibodies

Tubulin antibodies

- IgM antibodies to tubulin are associated with:
  - EBV infection;
  - visceral leishmaniasis;
  - liver disease (PBC, AIH, HBV infection).
- Identified on HEp-2 cells.

Ubiquitin antibodies

- These antibodies occur in up to 80% of cases of SLE and are said to be specific.
- At present, they are not measured routinely.

Voltage-gated calcium-channel (VGCC) antibodies

- IgG antibodies against the presynaptic calcium channel (P-/Q-type) on the nerve terminal cause the Lambert–Eaton myasthenic syndrome (LEMS).
- The number of channels is reduced due to cross-linking and internalization and this impairs release of acetylcholine. Complement is also involved.
- LEMS is usually associated with small-cell lung carcinoma (SCLC).
  - 90% of SCLC-associated LEMS will be positive for antibodies to VGCC.
  - 40% of patients with LEMS have no detectable tumour at presentation, but it may become obvious subsequently.
  - LEMS may also occur in patients who do not have SCLC.
- Several types of calcium channels exist and the antibody is specific for the neuronal (N) type.
- Similar antibodies have also been documented in amyotrophic lateral sclerosis, although the significance is uncertain (anti-ganglioside antibodies may also occur in these patients).
- Antibodies are detected by RIA using precipitation of VGCC with labelled ω-conotoxin.

Voltage-gated potassium-channel (VGKC) antibodies

- Antibody has been associated with acquired neuromyotonia.
- Detected by RIA using precipitation of $_{125}$I-α-dendrotoxin-labelled VGKCs.
- Reported in pM of bound toxin.
  - > 200, pM positive;
  - < 100, pM negative.
- Potassium channels are located on the nerve terminal and control nerve excitability.

Yo antibodies

- Yo antibodies have been associated with paraneoplastic cerebellar degeneration, seen typically with ovarian cancer and, less commonly, with breast cancer or Hodgkin's lymphoma.
- Development of cerebellar syndrome may precede the diagnosis of ovarian tumour.
- Do not occur in the cerebellar syndrome seen in small-cell carcinoma of the lung.
- Antigen is found in the cytoplasm of Purkinje cells, and gives a coarse, granular staining by immunofluorescence.

- The putative target antigen (CDR34) is expressed on epithelial tumours as well as neuronal tissue (cross-reactive anti-tumour antibody).
- Antibodies are detectable in the CSF as well as serum and disappear with successful treatment of the primary tumour.

Zic4 antibodies

- IgG antibodies to Zic4 are found in association with small-cell lung cancer in both CSF and serum.
- Binds to neuronal nuclei on immunofluorescence.
- May occur with anti-Hu, which makes detection difficult.

ZnT8 antibodies

- These antibodies are directed against an islet beta cell granule membrane protein, and are found in type I diabetes.
- Found in up to 80% of new cases and in 26% of GAD65-negative type I diabetics.
- Typically associated with younger age of onset and more severe disease.
- Detected by ELISA (negative < 15 U/ml, positive > 15 U/ml).
- Included in UK-NEQAS Diabetic Markers scheme.

Allergy tests

Introduction

The techniques used for allergy diagnosis *in vitro* are those already discussed in Chapters 17 and 18, and include RIA and EIA. Flow cytometry, as discussed in Chapter 20, may also have a role. The technical principles are identical.

In vitro allergy tests do not substitute for clinical history-taking, examination, and direct patient testing (SPT, patch tests, challenges).

Allergen-specific IgE

- Units: kAU/ml.
- Normal range:
  - < 0.35 = RAST score 0;
  - 0.35–0.70 = RAST score 1;
  - 0.70–3.50 = RAST score 2;
  - 3.50–17.5 = RAST score 3;
  - 17.5–50.0 = RAST score 4;
  - 50.0–100 = RAST score 5;
  - > 100 = RAST score 6.

Principles of testing

- Detection of allergen-specific IgE in the blood is by sensitive RIA, EIA, or fluorescent assay. There are numerous acronyms for this process, depending on the method (RAST, MAST, FAST tests, etc.).
- Radioimmunoassay is now little used.
- Principles of all the tests are identical, with allergen bound on to a solid phase that is then incubated with a labelled anti-IgE antibody.
- Pharmacia UniCAP®/ImmunoCAP® system is most widely used system in the UK.
- Tests are expensive due to costs of purification and standardization of allergen.
- CE marking requirements have reduced the number of commercially available allergens.
- EQA and international standards are available.

Indications for testing

- Skin-prick testing remains the gold standard.
- *In vitro* EIA assays may be used on patients with a high risk of anaphylaxis (SPT contraindicated), on drugs that interfere with SPT (antihistamines, calcium-channel blockers, antidepressants), or with extensive skin disease, and on small children.
- Patients with a total IgE < 20 kU/l have a low (but not zero) probability of having positive specific IgE tests.

Interpretation

- The assays are carried out quantitatively and reported in units.
- There is a trend to reporting units rather than grades, although some laboratories will still report both.

- RAST grades of 0 and 1 are usually considered to indicate a negative result.
- High total IgE levels (> 1000 kU/l) may cause false-positive tests for allergen-specific IgE, due to non-specific binding of IgE to the solid phase: this is less common with newer systems, but applies particularly to food allergens.
- Units are standardized against an international standard for birch pollen allergen, but this cannot validly be applied to reactions with other allergens.
- Attempts are being made to standardize allergens in terms of defined proteins and protein nitrogen. With a potentially limitless list of allergens, this is a slow process.
- The important clinical implication is that the detection of a grade 3 response to two different allergens does not indicate that the same amount of IgE is present against both and that equivalent clinical reactions might be expected.
- There is no close relationship between the grade and the severity of reactions (either past or future).
  - The presence of allergen-specific IgE is a marker only of exposure.
  - Positives may be detected where there is no evidence of any clinical reaction.
- Levels will fall with time if the offending allergen is avoided over a long period, so low or negative results may be obtained even with sensitized patients.
- As with skin-prick tests, if the allergic reaction is highly localized, there may be insufficient spill-over of specific IgE into the circulation to be detected, leading to a false-negative result.
- Results must always be interpreted in the light of the clinical history (blood tests are not a substitute for proper history-taking!).

Limitations
- Few allergens are available for robustly identifying IgE to drugs.
- Reagents for penicillin contain major but not minor determinants: a negative result does not exclude significant allergy, and SPT and IDT are required with a minor determinant mixture.
- Reagents for labile food allergens such as fruits are unreliable: use SPT with the fresh fruit.
  - Recombinant allergens may assist in the diagnosis, where available (see ➲ Table 19.1 and Chapter 3).
- If there is a good history for type I food allergy and an unexpected negative result, consider SPT with fresh food.
- 15% of NRL-allergic patients will be negative by specific IgE testing.

Serial monitoring
- Justified in cystic fibrosis: screen for IgE to *Aspergillus* (marker of colonization and associated with worse prognosis).

Component resolved diagnosis
- Key recombinant allergens are now available for the Phadia systems
- Examples of these are shown in Table 19.1.

Table 19.1 Key recombinant allergens

Recombinant allergens	Substance	Utility
rTri a19	Wheat omega-5-gliadin	Diagnosis of wheat-dependent, exercise-induced anaphylaxis
rAra h1, h2, h3, h8, h9	Peanut allergens	Positives to h2 associated with severe clinical symptoms; responses to h8 and h9 associated with OAS symptoms
rBet v1 (PR-10) rBet v2 (profilin)	Birch	Predictors for OAS
nGal d1(ovomucoid), d2 (ovalbumin), d3 (conalbulin)	Egg	Presence of antibodies to d1 and d2 are predictive of persistence of egg allergy
rHev b1, b3, b5, b6.01, b6.02, b8, b9, b11	Natural rubber latex	Useful back-up for skin-prick tests
rApi m1 (phospholipase A2) rVes v5	Bee Wasp	Main allergens for bee & wasp, don't include cross-reactive carbohydrates (if there is doubt then check for CCD/MUFX3/bromelain IgE antibodies recognizing cross-reactive carbohydrates)
nGal-alpha-1,3-Gal (alpha-Gal) thyroglobulin	Red meat allergen	Diagnostic for tick bite-triggered red meat allergy (on the increase)

- Other recombinant food and inhalant allergens are available, but the precise clinical roles of many still await further clinical studies.
- There may be considerable differences between the results obtained using tests for whole foods, compared to recombinant allergens. For example the standard soybean ImmunoCAP® contains very little of the recombinant allergen rGly m4 (PR10), an important allergen which is a Bet v1 homologue.

Website

This link gives details of all available Phadia allergens with details of their composition and significance:

 http://www.phadia.com/Products/Allergy-testing-products/ImmunoCAP-Allergen-Information/

Allergen-specific IgG antibodies

Principles of testing

- Measured using same techniques as used for specific IgE (CAP, UniCAP®).
- No EQA or standards are available.

Indications for testing

- Uncertain.
- Possibly for following the response to desensitization therapy.

Interpretation

- It has been suggested that desensitization procedures work, in part, by producing blocking IgG antibodies that prevent the allergen binding to cytophilic IgE.
  - These have been identified as IgG_4 subclass.
- Success and duration of desensitization may be determined by measurement of such antibodies. This is controversial!
- It is, however, possible to measure allergen-specific IgG antibodies to allergens such as bee or wasp venom, grass pollen, and house dust mite.
- Whether the results provide any clinically useful information is still unproven.

Basophil activation test

Principles of testing

- Measured by flow cytometric expression of CD63, a membrane tetraspanin (deficiency in Hermansky–Pudlak syndrome), which is increased on degranulated basophils.
- Blood is incubated with IL-3 and allergen (with appropriate controls) and the expression of CD63 detected by FITC-labelled anti-CD63.
- See also ➔ Flow-CAST® assay (p. 590)
- There is no EQA.

Indications for testing

- Uncertain.
- May be useful where direct challenge may be considered too dangerous.
- Widely used in Europe, less so in the UK.
- Testing is available to latex, venoms, beta-lactam antibiotics, aspirin and NSAIDs, and food additives.
- This is a very expensive way to test for allergy!

Interpretation

- Is dependent on proper controls and knowing that there are no non-specific degranulating effects of the allergens.

Bradykinin

- Units: ng/ml.
- Normal range: < 1.

Principles of testing

- EIA.
- EDTA whole blood required and analysed within 2 hours.
- No EQA.

Indications for testing

- Levels will be elevated in hereditary angioedema, acquired angioedema, and ACE-induced angioedema.
- The clinical indication for undertaking measurement is uncertain.

Interpretation

- Levels > 1 ng/ml are associated with active angioedema.

CD23, soluble (Fcε receptor)

- Measurement of soluble CD23, the shed form of the Fcε receptor which has B-cell stimulatory activity, has been proposed as a useful marker of the activity of chronic allergic disease.
- In asthma, elevated sCD23 may denote underlying chronic inflammatory activity even when the peak flow may be near that predicted.
- Measurement of this marker cannot yet be recommended without reservation.
- Assay is by EIA, but is not widely used.

C3a, C4a, and C5a (anaphylotoxins)

- See ⊙ Chapter 17.
- Measurement of the anaphylotoxins may be of value in the investigation of suspected acute allergic reactions, as a marker of complement activation.
- This is particularly valuable in circumstances where IgE is not involved (anaphylactoid reactions).
- Other conditions with raised anaphylotoxins include:
  - SLE;
  - RhA;
  - HSP and IgA nephropathy;
  - ARDS;
  - cardiopulmonary bypass.
- Samples must be collected into Futhan–EDTA, to prevent *in vitro* generation of anaphylotoxins.
  - These tubes are not readily available.
  - Samples need to reach the laboratory quickly, as the breakdown products are labile.
- Value of the tests in clinical practice is limited due to the lack of ready availability of appropriate tubes.
- Other tests for complement activation may be more appropriate.

Challenge tests

Challenge tests form an important part of the diagnosis of allergic disease. Clearly, identification of the site of the reaction is important. Nasal, bronchial, and oral challenges may be performed. It is wise to avoid challenging someone who has had a severe systemic reaction, or who has pre-existent severe asthma, with allergens. As for skin testing, it is essential that patients are not taking antihistamines and have been off treatment for a length of time appropriate to the half-life of their antihistamine (up to 4 weeks in some cases).

- ⓘ Challenge tests are potentially dangerous and should be carried out by experienced staff prepared to deal with any adverse reactions that may arise.
- Informed consent should always be sought from the patient prior to the test.

Nasal challenge tests

- Usually performed by spraying a diluted solution (1:1000 of SPT solution) of the test allergen into one nostril, while spraying a similarly diluted solution of the buffer only into the other nostril.
- Patient's symptoms are recorded (running nose, sneezing, itching eyes, etc.) and the nasal mucosa inspected for signs of inflammation and oedema. Each nostril is inspected.
- Process is limited to one allergen at a time, which restricts its use to confirming sensitivity to a single suspect allergen.
- More complex challenge tests involve measurement of nasal airflow (rhinomanometry), but this is rarely available outside specialist research centres.

Bronchial challenge tests

- Most common bronchial challenge is with methacholine or histamine.
- Carried out by starting with very dilute solutions and gradually increasing the dose, while measuring the forced expired volume (FEV_1) sequentially.
- Reduction of 20% from the control value is viewed as a positive test and is indicative of hyperreactive airways. The dose causing this reduction is the PD_{20}.
- If a 25 mg/ml dose of methacholine is tolerated without achieving a 20% reduction in FEV_1, the test is unequivocally negative.
- Allergen solutions may be substituted for methacholine, but the principles are the same.
- Late reactions may occur 6–8 hours after the challenge, as part of type I response: the patient must be kept under observation for this period.
- Enthusiasts may carry out endobronchial challenge through a bronchoscope, which allows them to observe the changes in the bronchial mucosa and also to carry out bronchoalveolar lavage to look at the release of mediators and the cellular response. This is important in research but not for routine diagnosis.

Food challenge

- Food challenges are complex and must involve an experienced senior dietician.
- Gold standard is double-blind, placebo-controlled (DBPC) challenge: this is time-consuming.

- Initial step is usually withdrawal of the suspect food(s) followed by open challenge.
- For open incremental food challenge, incremental doses of food are given at 15-minute intervals, with monitoring of BP, PEFR, and symptoms before each increment.
  - Steps are: food on lip (may be omitted), 1%, 4%, 10%, 20%, 20%, 20%, 25% of a normal portion (this may be variable!).
  - Over the course of the challenge, 100% of the normal portion size is administered.
  - Shorter protocols may be used, where there is less concern over reactions.
- Where multiple foods are suspected, an oligoallergenic (elimination) diet may be instituted for a period to see whether symptoms remit. If symptoms persist, food allergy/intolerance is not the cause.
- If symptoms improve, foods may then be reintroduced as open challenges one at a time and the patient's symptom response noted.
- This should ideally be followed by a DBPC challenge where the patient, on an oligoallergenic diet, is challenged with the suspect food concealed in opaque gelatin capsules, interspersed with identical capsules containing an innocuous substance, in a random sequence, determined by the dietician but unknown to the patient and doctor.
- This is time-consuming, as some food allergic symptoms may require exposure for several days before they appear and, equally, may take several days to disappear when the food is withdrawn. There needs to be a wash-out period between the placebo and the active capsules.
- A method of scoring symptoms needs to be decided in advance.
- As for bronchial challenges, enthusiasts have directly instilled allergens into the small bowel and watched for inflammatory reactions.

Drug allergy testing

Principles of testing

- Type I reactions are investigated by skin-prick (SPT) and intradermal (IDT) testing.
  - Some drugs are irritant and provoke non-specific reactions on IDT.
  - Some drugs (opiates, radiocontrast media) cause direct histamine release from mast cells.
- There is only a limited range of tests available for *in vitro* testing for IgE to drugs; many of the drug allergens are unvalidated in clinical practice.
- Flow cytometric assays of basophil degranulation/activation are available, but appear to correlate poorly with SPT/IDT testing.
- Type IV reactions are investigated by patch testing.
- Reactions of types II and III are more difficult to investigate.
- Open and blinded challenge tests may be appropriate for atypical reactions.
- :Q: Patients with Stevens–Johnson reactions must *not* be tested—reactions may be severe.
- Testing is time-consuming.

- Table 19.2 (p. 586) shows starting concentrations and usable dilutions for SPT and IDT. Centres vary in their use of IDT, with the aim of reducing the number of dilutions:
  - Morphine, fentanyl, pethidine, and remifentanil are all mast cell degranulating agents; SPT at either 1/10 or neat is sufficient. All opiates when administered quickly in patients are likely to cause generalized urticarial. This is not a good indication for testing.
  - Steroids, including ocular steroids, can be tested neat for SPT and 1/10 for IDT.
  - Local anaesthetics can be tested neat for SPT and 1.10 for IDT. Some Centres go straight to formal challenge, as true IgE-mediated allergy is vanishingly rare!
  - Chlorhexidine can be tested by SPT at 0.05% (neat) and by IDT at 1/100.
  - Gelofusine® and Volpex® can be tested at 40 mg/ml (SPT) and 1/10 by IDT.
  - Antibiotics can be tested by SPT neat and by a single dilution by IDT. Negative tests can then be followed by a challenge.
- Useful information on drug allergy including information on testing can be found at:
  ℘ http://www.phadia.com/Global/A%20Document%20Library/Allergy/Promotion%20Material/Drug%20Allergy/Drug-Book-web.pdf
- Information on concentrations for other drugs, including plasma expanders, antibiotics, and steroids, is available from the Regional Immunology and Allergy Unit, Newcastle-upon-Tyne (+44 191 2820669).
- Increasingly, single-step IDT is being used, to reduce the time taken for testing. Optimum IDT single concentrations are available for some drugs.
- Open drug challenge uses incremental doses:
  - 1%, 4%, 10%, 20%, 20%, 20%, 25% of a standard oral dose at 15-minute intervals, with observation of BP, PEFR, and symptoms before each incremental step.
  - Over the period of the challenge, the challenge administers 100% of the normal dose.
  - Where the risk of reaction is deemed negligible, single-dose open challenge may be used or a reduced number of steps.

Indications for testing

- Suspected drug allergy, where testing will alter clinical management.
- Do not test where there are readily available and safe alternatives (i.e. do not test all 'penicillin-allergic' patients). However, delabelling may be appropriate where the history is poor and repeated antibiotics are required.
- NICE guidance on drug allergy testing (CG183) is available: ℘ https://www.nice.org.uk/guidance/cg183

Table 19.2 Starting concentrations and usable dilutions for SPT and IDT

	SPT at dilution		IDT at dilution			Comment
Drug	1/10 mg/ml	Neat mg/ml	1/1000 µg/ml	1/100 µg/ml	1/10 µg/ml	
Quaternary ammonium compunds						
Succinylcholine (suxamethonium)	5 mg/ml	50 mg/ml	50 µg/ml	–	–	Irritant IDT > 1/1000
Benzylisoquinolones						
Atracurium	1 mg/ml	10 mg/ml	10 µg/ml	–	–	Irritant IDT
Cisatracurium	0.2 mg/ml	2 mg/ml	2 mg/ml	20 µg/ml	200 µg/ml	
Mivacurium	0.2 mg/ml	2 mg/ml	2 µg/ml	–	–	Irritant IDT
Gallamine	4 mg/ml	40 mg/ml	40 µg/ml	400 µg/ml	–	
Doxacurium*						
Aminosteroids						
Pancuronium	0.2 mg/ml	2 mg/ml	2 µg/ml	2 µg/ml	200 µg/ml	
Vecuronium	0.4 mg/ml	4 mg/ml	4 µg/ml	40 µg/ml	400 µg/ml	
Rocuronium*	1 mg/ml	10 mg/ml	10 µg/ml	100 µg/ml	–	
Rapacuronium						
Local anaesthetics						
Articaine	1 mg/ml	10 mg/ml	10 µg/ml	100 µg/ml	1000 µg/ml	

Bupivacaine	0.25 mg/ml	2.5 mg/ml	2.5 µg/ml	25 µg/ml	250 µg/ml	
Citanest with octapressin	3 mg/ml	30 mg/ml	30 µg/ml	300 µg/ml	3000 µg/ml	
Lidocaine	1 mg/ml	10 mg/ml	10 µg/ml	100 µg/ml	1000 µg/ml	
Prilocaine	0.5 mg/ml	5 mg/ml	5 µg/ml	50 µg/ml	500 µg/ml	
Procaine	1 mg/ml	10 mg/ml	10 µg/ml	100 µg/ml	1000 µg/ml	
Induction agents						
Etomidate	0.2 mg/ml	2 mg/ml	2 µg/ml	20 µg/ml	200 µg/ml	
Propofol	1 mg/ml	10 mg/ml	10 µg/ml	100 µg/ml	–	Irritant IDT > 1/100
Thiopental	2.5 mg/ml	25 mg/ml	25 µg/ml	250 µg/ml	2500 µg/ml	
Analgesics						
Alfentanil	50 µg/ml	500 µg/ml	–	–	–	Mast cell degranulator
Fentanyl	5 µg/ml	50 µg/ml	–	–	–	Mast cell degranulator
Morphine	1 mg/ml	10 mg/ml	–	–	–	Mast cell degranulator
Pethidine	5 mg/ml	50 mg/ml	–	–	–	Mast cell degranulator

* Information not available.

Based on information collated by Dr.

Interpretation

- Interpretation of testing requires the demonstration of wheal and flare. Reactions to drugs will usually be much smaller than the typical reactions on SPT/IDT to inhalant antigens.
  - Photographing the results for the medical records is desirable.
- Knowledge of irritant concentrations is required.
  - This may require testing on non-atopic volunteers.
- Clear goals are required for testing:
  - testing to prove causality;
  - testing to prove safety of alternative drugs.
- Information must be provided to patient as well as referring doctor (and GP if referred by other specialist).
- Steps must be taken to ensure that all medical records (paper and electronic) are updated with the outcome of testing, *especially where negative tests result in allergy delabelling*.
- Advice to patient on the use of medical alert bracelets may be required.

Limitations

- Preparation of drug dilutions is time-consuming: assistance from pharmacy is required. Preparation of dilutions in clinical areas is not recommended.
- Where testing is carried out with controlled drugs, appropriate steps must be taken to account for receipt and disposal of the drugs, according to local regulations.

Eosinophil cationic protein (ECP)

- Units: μg/ml.
- Normal range: 1.0–15.0

Principles of testing

- FEIA.
- No EQA.

Indications

- Asthma.
- As it is neurotoxic, may be useful in Churg–Strauss syndrome (EGPA).

Interpretation

- ECP is a granule protein of eosinophils, and its presence in serum is a marker of eosinophil activation.
- It is the neurotoxic agent in Churg–Strauss syndrome.
- Serum levels are elevated in:
  - asthma (valuable as a monitoring tool for allergic inflammation and effectiveness of inhaled steroid therapy?);
  - other allergic diseases, including urticaria;
  - Churg–Strauss syndrome (acute active disease).
- Synovial fluid levels are increased in:
  - rheumatoid arthritis;
  - ankylosing spondylitis.

- Urine levels are increased by carcinoma of the bladder.
- CSF levels are increased by malignant but not benign tumours.
- Levels correlate with the degree of underlying inflammation.
  - ECP may be released during the coagulation process.
  - This significantly limits the usefulness of the test.

Eosinophil count

- Units: cells $\times 10^9$/l.
- Normal range:
  - newborn, $< 0.85 \times 10^9$/l; ·
  - children 1–3 years, $< 0.70 \times 10^9$/l;
  - children > 3 and adults, $< 0.44 \times 10^9$/l.

Principles of testing

- Routinely on the newer automated haematology counters, which are capable of providing a five-part differential. Where older counters are used, an additional manual differential with special stains may be required.

Indications

- Allergic disease, including drug reactions.
- Lymphoma.
- Vasculitis.
- Pulmonary infiltrates.
- Parasitic infection.

Interpretation

- Raised eosinophil counts are not specific for allergic disease; counts $> 10 \times 10^9$/l are *not* due to allergy or parasitic disease.
- Moderate elevations are seen in:
  - parasitic infestations;
  - drug reactions;
  - lymphoma (especially Hodgkin's lymphoma);
  - after radiation therapy;
  - vasculitides (Churg–Strauss vasculitis (EGPA), polyarteritis nodosa);
  - dermatitis herpetiformis;
  - primary immunodeficiencies (Omenn's syndrome, materno-fetal engraftment—see ➲ Chapter 1);
  - hepatic cirrhosis.
- Exceptionally high eosinophil counts are seen in:
  - larva migrans;
  - hypereosinophilic syndromes;
  - severe vasculitis (EGPA, PAN) and occasionally in lymphoma and cirrhosis.
- Eosinophil count is reduced by acute infection, stress, fasting for more than 24 hours, and by corticosteroids.

- Examination of nasal and conjunctival secretions for the presence of eosinophils may provide confirmatory evidence for an allergic cause for local symptoms.
  - Eosinophilia of nasal secretions may be seen in non-allergic rhinitis (NARES).

Flow-CAST® and CAST-ELISA®

- These commercial assays rely on activation of basophils either directly or via specific IgE in the patient's serum.
- CAST-ELISA® measures the release of sulphidoleukotrienes by activated basophils by EIA.
  - Assay is extremely slow and time-consuming and is impractical for a busy diagnostic laboratory.
- The Flow-CAST® uses flow cytometry to identify basophils, labelled with anti-IgE-FITC, and then anti-CD63-PE, a marker of activated basophils, which identifies basophil degranulation.
  - Manufacturer provides an array of specific allergens including food additives and drugs.
- Both assays work well for normal inhalant allergens, but appear less useful for drugs and additives.
- Modification of the Flow-CAST® assay using anti-CD203c in place of anti-CD63 improves the characteristics of the assay.
  - Results for drug allergens compare poorly with those from IDT.
- The assays cannot therefore be recommended as a non-invasive way of testing for drug allergy.
- Assays are more expensive and labour-intensive than standard EIA for routine inhalant allergens.

Histamine-release assays

- *In vitro* release of histamine by basophils in response to stimulation by cytokines or by allergens is a complex test.
  - Measurement of free histamine is required (difficult as it is labile in serum/plasma).
- Assays are of value in the research setting.
- In the clinical setting assays have been used for investigating the histamine-releasing properties of certain drugs.
- Like all bioassays, they suffer from difficulties in standardization.

Immunoglobulin E (total IgE)

- Units: kU/l.
- Normal ranges:
  - age < 1 year, < 11 kU/l;
  - age < 2 years, < 29 kU/l;
  - age 2–3 years, < 42 kU/l;

- age 4–5 years, < 52 kU/l;
- age 6–7 years, < 56 kU/l;
- age 8–10 years, < 63 kU/l;
- age 11–12 years, < 45 kU/l;
- age 13–14 years, < 70 kU/l;
- age > 14 years, < 100 kU/l.

Principles of testing

- Usually the same as for allergen-specific IgE (RIA, EIA).
- Some nephelometers have the capacity to run total IgE.

Indications for testing

- Allergic disease (as screen for atopic tendency).
- Lymphoma.
- Vasculitis (EGPA).
- Primary immunodeficiency.
- Myeloma.

Interpretation

- Measurement of total IgE may be helpful in diagnosing allergic disease.
- Normal range is very wide and levels correlate poorly with clinical disease.
- High level of specific IgE to a single allergen may occur with a total IgE within the 'normal' range.
- In asthmatic patients, a level of > 150 kU/l is suggestive of an allergic basis, while a level < 20 kU/l is very much against it. The severity of asthmatic symptoms correlates very poorly with total IgE (but better with eosinophil count).
- In the investigation of dermatitis, a level of > 400 kU/l is usual while a level of < 20 kU/l is against atopic dermatitis.
- Very high levels of IgE are seen in atopic eczema, allergic bronchopulmonary aspergillosis (ABPA), parasitic infections (larva migrans, hookworm, schistosomiasis, and filariasis), lymphoma (especially Hodgkin's disease), and liver disease.
- Levels may be elevated in EBV infection, the EGPA, systemic sclerosis, and bullous pemphigoid, although this is a poor marker of disease activity.
- Some primary immunodeficiencies are associated with raised IgE, such as Wiskott–Aldrich syndrome and Omenn's syndrome.
- Highest levels are seen in the hyper-IgE syndrome (Job syndrome, Buckley's syndrome): here levels frequently exceed 50 000 kU/l, a level rarely, if ever, seen in atopic disease.
- IgE myeloma is exceedingly rare: diagnosis will have been made on electrophoresis and immunofixation.
- Levels are often higher in Asian people, although it is not clear whether this is just due to a higher prevalence of parasitic diseases.

Limitations
- Specific IgE testing becomes inaccurate with very high levels of IgE (> 1000 kU/l), due to non-specific binding.
- Conversely, where the total IgE is very low, it is not useful to perform tests for specific IgE.

Serial monitoring
- Justified in ABPA (a rise in the level of IgE precedes relapse, and the level falls with appropriate therapy).
- Justified in EGPA (responds to therapy).

IgE autoantibodies/IgE receptor antibodies
- These have been reported in patients with allergic problems.
- Antibodies to the IgE receptor have been reported as a possible cause of chronic urticaria, although the evidence is very weak.
- Routine assays are not available at present and the clinical utility needs to be confirmed in further studies.
- The use of the autologous serum test is said to depend upon these autoantibodies.

IgG to food allergens
- IgG antibodies to food allergens are available (UniCAP®/ImmunoCAP®).
- It has been suggested that these may be valuable in the investigation of irritable bowel syndrome (IgG to wheat, milk).
- IgG to food allergens occur frequently in healthy individuals, especially against bovine, ovine, and porcine proteins.
- Clinical value remains to be determined.

ISAC
- An expensive chip-based test for allergen-specific IgE supplied by Thermo-Fisher.
- Includes a fixed panel of 112 allergens from 51 allergen sources in a microarray, analysed as a single step on 30 μl of serum.
- Precise role in clinical practice is yet to be determined.
- May be valuable in the investigation of polysensitized patients (but will this influence clinical management?)
- May be useful in idiopathic anaphylaxis.
- Sensitivity may be less than standard ImmunoCAP® testing for individual allergens.
- Should *not* be used as a substitute for a proper clinical history.

Mast cell tryptase

- Units: μg/l.
- Normal adult range: 2–14 μg/l.

Sample
- Serum, preferably on several occasions within a 24-hour period after an acute reaction (tryptase is stable in serum).

Principles of testing
- Measured by Thermo-Fisher UniCAP® system (EIA).

Indications for testing
- Confirmation of mast cell degranulation (is a specific marker of mast cell granules).
- Investigation of atypical 'allergic' reactions.

Interpretation
- Does not distinguish between anaphylactic and anaphylactoid reactions.
- False-positive elevations have been reported due to heterophile antibodies (rheumatoid factors).
- Relatively stable in serum, being catabolized in the liver with a half-life of approximately 3 hours.
- Levels may be significantly raised for 24 hours after an acute reaction involving mast cell degranulation.
- Good correlation between plasma histamine and mast cell tryptase makes mast cell tryptase the preferred marker for mast cell activation.
- Persistently elevated levels may be seen in patients with urticaria pigmentosa and systemic mastocytosis.
- Elevated levels may also be detected in nasal and bronchial lavage fluids after allergen challenge.
- In order to assess the significance of a result taken during an acute reaction in a given patient, it is important to have a sample taken when the patient has fully recovered.
- Levels may not be elevated if there is a significant dilution due to administration of IV fluids.
- Post-mortem femoral blood samples may show elevations in anaphylactic deaths. Levels have been reported to be raised in some cases of sudden infant death syndrome, and in blood samples taken from heart as opposed to vein. Asphyxia activates mast cells.
- Levels may be raised due to myocardial infarction, which may cause confusion with post-mortem samples.

Omalizumab monitoring by basophil-bound IgE

Sample
- EDTA. Pre-treatment sample is required to assess baseline expression.

Principles of testing

- Measured by flow cytometry.
- Basophils are identified by using anti-CD45 and anti-CD203c (recognizes the ectoenzyme E-NPP3).
- Anti-IgE to identify basophil bound IgE.
- Baseline measurement pre-treatment is required.

Indications for testing

- Confirmation of satisfactory reduction of basophil-bound IgE.
- Useful where there is concern about response.

Interpretation

- By 2 weeks following infusion, basophil-bound IgE should be approximately 10% of pre-treatment level.

Patch testing

The purpose of patch testing is to identify type IV hypersensitivity, usually in the context of contact hypersensitivity to environmental agents.

Principles of testing

- As for skin-prick testing, an area of normal skin is required: the upper and mid zone of the back is usually appropriate.
- Allergens are made up in petrolatum jelly or in aqueous solution on a filter paper and applied under occlusion in a small metal chamber (Finn chamber), which is secured firmly to the back with hypoallergenic tape.
- Chambers are left in place for 48 hours and the patients are told not to wash the area.
- When the chambers are removed, the application areas are inspected for erythema, vesiculation, and evidence of cellular infiltrate.
  - There may be false positives at this stage due to reactions of types I and III.
  - The sites should be re-read at 72–96 hours.
  - False-positive reactions at 48 hours will have disappeared on the later reading.
- It is usual for a standard panel to be used in the initial screen, unless there are clear indications of the most likely allergens (e.g. through the occupation and exposure history, site of eczema, etc.).
  - Standard panel will include metals (nickel, chromium), preservatives, fragrances, rubber mix, lanolin, formaldehyde, balsam of Peru, and colophony.
- Where there are positive reactions to one of the mixed reagents (rubber mix, fragrances) there are usually supplementary panels of the individual ingredients.
- If the patient is exposed to an unusual substance, then it or its contents may be made into extemporaneous patch tests, provided that appropriate safety data can be obtained from the manufacturers.

- Some allergens only cause reactions when there is concomitant exposure to sunlight. This can be reproduced in the clinic using a photopatch test.
  - Here duplicates of each allergen are applied and, after 24–48 hours, one of the pair is taken off and the back exposed to UV-A light (10 joules).
  - The other one of the pair is then taken off and the sites read as for an ordinary patch test.
  - The unexposed member of the pair serves as the control.

Indications for testing

- Contact eczema or dermatitis.
- Orofacial granulomatosis; oral problems (dental battery).
- Tests are only appropriate for delayed hypersensitivity (type IV).
- Patch testing for drugs may be valuable where reactions are atypical and delayed.
- Patch tests have been used for food allergens in the context of food-protein enterocolitis and eosinophilic gastroenteritis syndromes: the utility is uncertain.

Interpretation

- Results can be roughly graded as:
  - 0, no response;
  - 1+, erythema and oedema;
  - 2+, erythema, papules, and small vesicles;
  - 3+, marked erythema, induration, and large blisters.
- Grades 2+ and 3+ are positive.
- Antihistamines have no effect on the responses, but topical steroids applied to the sites of application or systemic steroids will significantly reduce or abolish the responses.
- Useful information on the European Standard Battery can be seen at: ✍ https://www.dermnetnz.org/topics/baseline-series-of-patch-test-allergens/

Prostaglandins (urinary)

- Units: ng/mmol creatinine.
- Normal adult range: prostaglandin DM < 2300; prostaglandin D2 < 825; prostaglandin F2a < 105.
- (Ranges taken from Sheffield PRU.)

Sample

- 5 ml urine (random or from 24-hour collection).

Principles of testing

- EIA.

Indications for testing

- Tests are said to be useful in investigating mast cell activation syndrome (MCAS), especially when the mast cell tryptase is not elevated.

Interpretation

- The analytes are not stable.
- Ideally baseline and symptomatic samples should be taken.
- Urinary methylhistamine should be measured at the same time.
- Urinary tract infection will cause misleading results.
- There is no EQA and calibration is against manufacturer standards.

Skin-prick testing (SPT)/intradermal testing (IDT) 1

- This remains the most cost-effective method for determining whether someone is sensitized to an allergen.
- SPT is appropriate for most circumstances.
- IDT, using diluted solutions, may be used for drugs and venoms, where SPT gives equivocal or negative responses.

Principles of testing

- SPT has the major advantage that the patient sees the results as they develop, and it takes only 15 minutes to read.
  - Positive and negative reinforcement.
- Testing can either be carried out by SPT or by IDT.
- IDT is more sensitive, but involves the injection of a larger amount of allergen.
  - Adverse reactions are more common.
- Both tests are dependent on the release of histamine from sensitized mast cells.
- Tests will give spurious results in patients taking antihistamines.
  - Short-acting antihistamines should be stopped at least 48 hours before testing.
  - Long-acting antihistamines should be stopped for at least 7 days.
  - Astemizole and terfenadine produce such prolonged blockade that 4 drug-free weeks are required to give meaningful SPT results (both drugs withdrawn in the UK due to effect on QT interval).
  - If there is doubt, run histamine control first to assess response.
- Other drugs that interfere with testing include:
  - tricyclic antidepressants;
  - mirtazapine;
  - calcium-channel blocking drugs.
- Topical steroids do not significantly interfere with testing.
- Preferred site for SPT/IDT testing is the volar aspect of the forearm.
  - Distribution of mast cells is variable and decreases up the arm.
  - The back may be used but reactivity is lower than on the arm.
  - Whealing diminishes with age.
  - Patients with dermographism or extensive skin disease are unsuitable for testing.

- For prick testing, the allergens are applied as a single, small drop, which is pricked through with a slight lifting motion to a uniform depth with a sharp lancet.
  - A separate lancet should be used for each allergen and disposed of immediately.
  - It is poor practice to use a single lancet and wipe it between allergens, as this may give misleading results due to cross-contamination.
  - A histamine control (1 or 10 mg/ml for SPT and 0.01 mg/ml for IDT) and negative control (glycerinated carrier) should always be applied.
  - Tests are read at 15 minutes.
  - The size of the wheal (*not* the surrounding flare) is measured.
  - Positive control should give a response of at least 4 mm.
  - Positive test results require that it be at least 2 mm greater than the negative control.
  - It may be helpful to place a strip of wide Permeable Non-woven Synthetic Adhesive Tape over the test sites and draw round the wheal.
  - This gives a permanent record that can be transferred to the notes, and allows calculation of area when the wheal is an eccentric shape.
  - For irregular wheals, the diameter across the widest part can be measured and then the diameter at right angles.
- IDT exposes patients to doses 100–1000-fold higher than SPT.
  - A dose (0.02 ml) of diluted allergen (a 100-fold dilution of the SPT reagent) is injected intradermally, with the test read at 15–30 minutes.
  - Other dilutions may be used (drugs), often with an incremental scale.
  - If multiple IDTs are carried out at the same time with positive results, the cumulative effect may lead to systemic symptoms.
- There is no agreed standardization of the reagents for SPT/IDT, in terms of reactivity and allergen content.
- Allergen solutions may express the allergen concentration in protein nitrogen units (PNU) or as weight/volume.
- Standardization is best carried out by immunochemical methods such as RAST inhibition which will give a biological potency (BU/ml).
- Consistent results will be obtained if trained staff carry out all tests.

Indications for testing

- SPT is the gold standard for allergy diagnosis and should be considered as the first choice for testing.
- Testing should be driven by clinical symptoms: the use of routine panels of allergens on every patient is wasteful and can be misleading (irrelevant positives).
- Where no commercial antigens are available, direct SPT (prick to prick) with allergens such as foods may be desirable.
  - This is the test of choice for fruit and vegetable allergens that are labile.
- IDT is used to follow-up SPT, particularly for drug allergy investigations.

SPT/IDT 2: interpretation and limitations

Interpretation

- As sensitization is dependent on circulating IgE reaching the mast cells at the test site, it is possible, where the allergic reaction is highly localized, to get negative results, as insufficient IgE is present in the circulation.
- Positive reactions on SPT do not necessarily equate to clinical disease.
  - All results *must* be interpreted in the context of the clinical history.
- If the negative control comes up positive, or if the histamine control produces no reaction, the tests are impossible to interpret.
- Test results greater than the 'positive' negative control might be considered positive: this is risky, and confirmatory blood tests should be undertaken.
- False-positive tests may often be found to food allergens, although the rate is lower with SPT than IDT.
- Where commercial food allergens give an unexpected false-negative, use of the fresh food may be possible.
- Allergen solutions to a wide range of allergens are available commercially from several manufacturers.
- They should be checked regularly to see that they are still within date.

Limitations

- If patients cannot stop their antihistamines, then blood tests may be the only way of diagnosis.
- It is advisable to avoid any form of skin testing in patients known to have had a severe systemic reaction to any of the proposed test agents.
  - The small amount of allergen introduced during SPT may be enough to trigger a reaction in a susceptible individual.

❶Skin testing should only be carried out by staff familiar with resuscitation and with appropriate facilities close at hand.

Unvalidated tests

- A large number of other tests are used for the purported diagnosis of allergic disease, often without conventional medical services.
- These are frequently promoted directly to the public.
- Many of these techniques have not been validated scientifically or use techniques that will not identify allergy as understood by immunologists.
- 'Allergy' therapies may be offered as a result of such testing. Members of the public may be offered 'allergy treatments' based on the results of these tests.
- Publications reviewing these tests include:
  - the Royal College of Physicians: *Allergy—conventional and alternative concepts*;
  - joint publication of RCP, RCPath, and BSACI: *Good allergy practice*;
  - ℘ http://www.quackwatch.com is a valuable website for up-to-date refutation of unscientific testing.

- Tests where there is limited or no current evidence of value in the diagnosis of IgE-mediated allergic disease include:
  - provocation–neutralization;
  - hair analysis;
  - Vega analysis;
  - kinesiology;
  - iridology;
  - auriculo-cardiac reflex;
  - leucocytotoxic testing.

Urinary methyl histamine

- Units: μg/mmol creatinine.
- Normal adult range: < 25 (Sheffield PRU).

Sample

- 5 ml urine (random or from 24-hour collection).

Principles of testing

- Competitive 1-methylhistamine EIA.

Indications for testing

- Tests are said to be useful in investigating anaphylaxis, MCAS, especially when the mast cell tryptase is not elevated.

Interpretation

- The analyte is stable.
- Ideally baseline and symptomatic samples should be taken.
- Histamine release from mast cells is a key feature of acute severe allergic reactions.
- It is rapidly cleared/destroyed in the circulation: measurement of free histamine is therefore difficult and limited to research settings.
- The urinary metabolite, N-methyl histamine, is stable and is therefore useful in determining whether mast cell degranulation has taken place in an acute reaction.
- The Sheffield PRU is now able to offer this test again (along with urinary prostaglandins F2α, D2, and DM).
- Mast cell tryptase is available as an alternative.
- Renal function must also be known to evaluate results.

Venom-specific IgE and IgG

- Measurement of specific IgE to bee and wasp venom is an essential investigation in suspected insect-sting allergy.
- This is carried out as for other allergen-specific IgE tests (see ➜ 'Allergen-specific IgE', p. 578).
- The use of recombinant allergens may assist in diagnosis by excluding reactivity to cross-reactive carbohydrate determinants.

- Negative results may occur with the *in vitro* assays.
- SPT with incremental concentrations of venom may be required.
  - Incremental SPT for bee and wasp venoms can be carried out with solutions of 10, 100, and 300 µg/ml.
- IDT with diluted venom may occasionally be required.
  - 10-fold steps from 0.0001 µg/ml to 1 µg/ml.
- Measurement of venom-specific IgG may be helpful in determining the success of desensitization (see ➲ 'Allergen-specific IgG antibodies', p. 580).

Cellular investigations

Introduction

- Cellular investigations include:
  - identification of cell surface phenotype;
  - identification of intracellular proteins;
  - identification of cellular function, including activation;
  - identification of secreted products (cytokines, chemokines);
  - identification of abnormal cellular constituents (leukaemia/ lymphoma).
- Techniques used include:
  - EIA and RIA (see ➲ Chapters 17 and 18);
  - flow cytometry;
  - tissue culture;
  - PAGE;
  - genetic techniques (see ➲ Chapter 21), mainly PCR-based techniques.
- Few functional assays are standardized and gold standard assays have not been defined.
- EQA exists only for basic lymphocyte phenotyping and then only in the context of testing for HIV.

Flow cytometry

Flow cytometry provides the cornerstone of diagnostic cellular immunology and is dependent upon the availability of monoclonal antibody reagents reactive with human surface and intracellular antigens. Fluorescent intercalating dyes can be used to detect DNA semi-quantitatively (for cell cycle analysis).

- Technique involves the flow of fluorescent-labelled cells past the exciting laser and the subsequent detectors.
  - Method is only applicable to single-cell suspensions, e.g. blood-derived cells or cultured cells.
  - It is possible to use disaggregated solid tissues, such as tumours.
- Modern flow cytometers use a single exciting laser (monochromatic light) and can detect multiple different wavelengths of light emitted by fluorescent dyes.
- There are detectors for forward and 90° light scatter, which are related to size and granularity of the cells, respectively.
- Software permits complex multi-parameter gating and analysis, including real-time data collection and analysis.
- Fluorescent-conjugated monoclonal antibodies are used against surface antigens.
- Cell permeabilization techniques are available to enable staining of intracellular antigens.
- Surface and intracellular stains may be combined.
- Appropriate controls are required to detect non-specific staining.
- The major advantage of flow cytometry for analysis is that it is semi-automated and can analyse very large numbers of cells very rapidly, compared to fluorescence microscopy. It is much more accurate.

- Accurate absolute counts are available on single-platform analysers using bead technology: this obviates the errors from using haematology counter total lymphocyte counts.
- Regular calibration of the instrument is required and it is essential that compensation between the fluorescence detectors is correctly set up: this is done with beads of known fluorescence.

Tissue culture

- *In vitro* functional studies of cells may require purified cells (blood, other fluids).
- This is done by density gradient centrifugation, using Ficol, metrizamide, or dextran solutions.
  - The different buoyant densities of blood cells permits separation when centrifuged through the dense medium.
- Further purification of lymphocyte populations can be undertaken using either:
  - rosetting with sheep red cells; or
  - magnetic separation using monoclonal antibodies coupled to magnetic microspheres.
- The more cells are handled *in vitro*, the more the cells' characteristics are altered.
  - This affects particularly activation parameters.
- Cell culture is usually carried out in tissue-culture medium, supplemented with:
  - antibiotics to prevent contamination with bacteria;
  - fetal calf serum (FCS) or human AB serum (no isoagglutinins);
  - other 'black-box' factors that are required for optimal cell growth (glutamine is added as this is labile).
- Where proliferation assays are being carried out, it is essential to screen the FCS first, as some batches are mitogenic in their own right.
- Good sterile technique is essential.
- Culture is carried out in a 37°C humidified incubator, with a controlled atmosphere (usually 5% CO_2), to maintain pH.
- Many different types of tissue culture media are available: most have pH buffers (bicarbonate) and pH indicators.

Proliferation assays

- There are numerous mitogenic stimuli that can be used (see ➔ 'T-cell function: *in vitro* assays', p. 616).
- These are added at the initiation of the culture.
- Cells are pulsed with tritiated thymidine, which is taken up into newly synthesized DNA in dividing cells: this remains the gold standard.
- Cells are then harvested on to filter papers and exposed to scintillant fluid.
- Counts per minute are determined using a beta-counter.

- Alternative assays have been described using flow cytometers (no radioisotopes).
  - CD69 expression.
  - DNA analysis with intercalating dyes (cell cycle analysis).
  - These do not give comparable results to those from tritiated thymidine uptake and appear less sensitive.

Immunohistology

- Immunoperoxidase and other enzymatic immunostains are used in the diagnosis of lymph-node disease.
- Multiple monoclonal antibodies that recognize different stages of lymphoid development or particular subsets of cells are used.
- Many of the antibodies used will also work on paraffin-embedded sections, but this depends on whether the target antigen is stable under the conditions of fixation. Frozen sections are better at present.
- *In situ* hybridization is used to detect viral nucleic acid (EBV, other herpesviruses).

Cytokine, chemokine, soluble protein assays

- Detection of specific cellular products, such as antibodies, cytokines, and shed surface molecules (soluble CD8, etc.) are usually undertaken using EIA or RIA techniques, as already described in Chapter 18.
- Cytokines may also be detected by bioassays using cell lines that are dependent for their growth on a given cytokine.
  - Strictly, both types of assays should be used, as EIA techniques may give spurious results due to naturally occurring cytokine-binding proteins in serum (soluble receptors, binding factors).
- Bioassays are notoriously difficult to standardize and to reproduce and are not suited to routine diagnostic use.
- Detection of intracellular cytokines with fluorescently labelled monoclonal antibodies in permeabilized cells has been used in conjunction with surface staining.
  - This does not indicate that the cytokines are secreted and therefore does not equate to functional assays of cytokines.

Apoptosis assays

Principles of testing

- Flow cytometric assays exist for identification of degraded DNA in apoptotic cells.
  - Preferred method is the TUNEL method, using enzyme-inserted fluorescent nucleotides into DNA strand breaks present in apoptotic cells. Commercial assays are available.

- Fluorochrome-conjugated annexin V can be used to detect surface phosphatidylserine, exposed on the cell surface in apoptotic cells, but not normal cells.
- Expression of fas and fas-ligand by flow cytometry.
- A functional assay is available using PHA+IL-2 stimulated T cells. These express high levels of fas and can be induced to apoptose by the addition of fas-ligand. Co-staining with annexin V (apoptotic cells) and propidium iodide (identifies dead cells) allows the response of the patient's cells to be compared to a normal control. To improve the reliability of the assay, multiple dilutions of fas-ligand are used.
- Protein and molecular follow-up tests are required to confirm defects: few PID centres have the capacity to run the necessary assays.

Indications for testing

- Suspected apoptotic defect (ALPS, caspase deficiency).
- Increased of Tcr$\alpha\beta^+$ CD4$^-$CD8$^-$ (double negative) T cells is highly suggestive of ALPS where there is evidence of autoimmunity and lymphadenopathy.

Interpretation

- Careful use of controls is required.
- Samples must be run fresh.
- Microscopic confirmation of assay results is advised to exclude artefacts.

Adhesion markers

Principles of testing

- Flow cytometry.
- Analysis should be carried out with CD18, CD11a (LFA-1), CD11b (Mac-1, CR3), and CD11c (CR4) for LAD-1, and CD15 for LAD-2. Neutrophils and lymphocytes should be tested.
- Stimulation studies for upregulation in the presence of PMA or γ-IFN may be required where there is partial expression of CD18.

Indications for testing

- Suspected leucocyte adhesion molecule deficiency (see Chapter 1).

Interpretation

- LAD-1 is associated normally with deficiency of CD18, the common β-chain for the integrins, leading to absence of CD11a, CD11b, and CD11c, as well as CD18.
- CD11b and CD11c deficiency may occur.
- LAD-2 is exceptionally rare and is associated with deficiency of the hapten-X receptor on neutrophils (CD15).
- Under certain circumstances it may be appropriate to look at the expression of the other complement receptors, CR1 (expressed on red cells, eosinophils, and B cells) and CR2 (CD21, EBV receptor, expressed on B cells, NK cells, and follicular dendritic cells).
- Reduction of red cell CR1 has been found in SLE.
- Some patients with CVID may lack CD21 on some of their B cells.

Bronchoalveolar lavage (BAL) studies

- Normal adult values for non-smokers:
  - total cells, 130–180 $\times$ 10^3/ml;
  - macrophages, 80–95%;
  - lymphocytes, < 15%;
  - neutrophils, < 3%;
  - eosinophils, < 0.5%.
- Normal adult values for smokers:
  - total cells, 300–500 $\times$ 10^3/ml;
  - macrophages, 85–98%;
  - lymphocytes, < 10%;
  - neutrophils, < 5%;
  - eosinophils, < 3%.

Principles of testing

- Cells recovered from bronchi by saline lavage during bronchoscopy can be stained and counted, using neat BAL fluid. Total count and percentage differential counts are required.
- Subsets of lymphocytes can be analysed by flow cytometry.

Indications for testing

- Unexplained interstitial lung disease.
- Sarcoidosis.
- Hypersensitivity pneumonitis.
- Idiopathic pulmonary fibrosis (IPF).
- Eosinophilic granuloma.
- Connective tissue diseases.

Interpretation

- In sarcoidosis, there is a marked increase in lymphocytes (to about 30% of the total cells), predominantly CD4$^+$ T cells, giving a CD4:CD8 ratio (which is normally 2:1) of between 4:1 and 10:1.
  - Values improve with treatment, but the levels and the ratio do not predict the severity of the disease.
  - Occasionally there is an increase in neutrophils and mast cells, which is said to indicate a poorer prognosis.
- In hypersensitivity pneumonitis, the BAL lymphocytosis comprises mainly CD8$^+$ cells, with the highest levels occurring in the acutely exposed.
- In IPF, a neutrophilia in excess of 10%, particularly if there is an increase in eosinophils, is associated with a poor prognosis.
  - A lymphocytosis (a rare finding) is associated with a better prognosis and indicates a probable response to steroids.
- In eosinophilic granuloma (histiocytosis X), there is an increase in OKT6-positive (S-100, CD1$^+$) histiocytic cells, up to 20% of total cells, which is diagnostic.

CD40 ligand expression

Principles of testing

- Flow cytometry is used to demonstrate upregulation of expression of CD40 ligand (CD154) upon stimulation of T cells *in vitro* with mitogens (PMA).
- CD69 expression is used as an activation control.

Indications for testing

- Suspected CD40 ligand deficiency.

Interpretation

- Gating stimulated cells can be difficult due to clumping and size changes: this makes the activation control important.
- Variants of CD40 ligand deficiency have been identified in which there is normal upregulation of non-functional ligand. Normal results do not exclude the diagnosis.
- Failure of upregulation is highly suggestive of CD40 ligand deficiency.
- Abnormal results should be followed up with genetic testing for mutations in CD40 and CD40 ligand genes.

Complement membrane regulatory factors

Principles of testing

- Flow cytometry is now used exclusively.
- Functional assays of cell lysis (Ham's test) have been withdrawn.

Indications for testing

- Suspected paroxysmal nocturnal haemoglobinuria.
- Atypical haemolytic–uraemic syndrome (CD46 deficiency).
- Haemolytic anaemia with polyneuropathy (CD59 deficiency).
- Genetic CD55 deficiency.

Interpretation

- Deficiencies of a group of surface proteins, with an unusual glycosyl-phosphatidylinositol membrane binding, are associated with paroxysmal nocturnal haemoglobinuria (PNH). Genetic absence of CD55 is described.
- This is a clonal disorder leading to unusual susceptibility to homologous complement lysis, particularly of red cells.
- The use of FLAER (fluorescent aerolysin, a bacterial toxic aerolysin) reagent is helpful in PNH as it binds directly to the GPI anchor.
- The proteins in question are regulatory proteins that prevent destruction of cells by homologous complement and include:
  - decay accelerating factor (DAF, CD55);
  - homologous restriction factor-20 (HRF20, CD59);
  - membrane attack complex inhibitor (CD59);
  - C8-binding protein (HRF65);
  - membrane cofactor protein (CD46).

Cytokine and cytokine receptor measurement

Principles of testing
- Enzyme immunoassay (serum, cell culture supernatant).
- Bioassay.
- Flow cytometry for intracellular cytokines; surface staining for receptors.
- Immunoblotting.
- *In vitro* stimulation assays with mycobacterial and salmonella antigens may be required to demonstrate defects.
- ELISpot assays can identify specific cellular cytokine production in response to stimulation.

Indications for testing
- Only absolute indication is suspected cytokine/cytokine receptor deficiency (e.g. IL-12, γ-IFN receptor deficiencies).
- Intracellular cytokines have been used to identify functional Th1/Th2 balance.

Interpretation
- EIA assays are unreliable due to presence of natural cytokine binding proteins and soluble receptors.
- Bioassays are difficult to standardize, time-consuming, and unsuitable for routine diagnostic use.
- IL-6 rises very early in acute-phase responses, before a rise in the CRP can be detected. However:
  - CRP is readily available and an acceptable surrogate for IL-6;
  - CRP levels are raised in myeloma, reflecting elevated IL-6;
  - CRP levels are also raised in Castleman's syndrome, reflecting raised IL-6.
- Cytokine and cytokine receptor deficiency is exceptionally rare (see ➔ Chapter 1).
- Flow cytometric tests for intracellular cytokine detection are available.
  - Technique works well for IL-2 and γ-IFN but poorly for IL-4.
  - It has the significant advantage that specific T-cell subpopulations can be studied, using multicolour flow cytometry.

Cytotoxic T cells

- Cytotoxic T cells can be generated during a one-way mixed lymphocyte reaction (sMLR), stimulating the responding cells with irradiated or mitomycin-treated allogeneic target cells and then assessing the ability of the responders to kill ^{51}Cr-labelled targets, in a similar assay to the NK-cell assay (see ➔ 'NK-cell function', p. 621).
- This is a complex and fiddly assay, and has been used mainly as part of the cross-matching procedure (see ➔ Chapter 21).

Dendritic cell assays

- This assay is used for the detection of the MonoMac syndrome (see
  ➲ Chapter 1).
- This syndrome is characterized by complete absence of dendritic
  cells (DC), monocytopenia, together with B- and NK-cell deficiency and
  is caused by mutations in *GATA2*.
- DC can arise for myeloid (CD11c$^+$) and plasmacytoid (CD123$^+$)
  progenitors.
- Normal ranges for CD11c DC are 0.18–0.45% and for CD123$^+$ DC are
  0.09–0.35% of total white cell count.

FOXP3
(regulatory T cells—IPEX syndrome)

Principles of testing

- Flow cytometric test to detect the presence of Tregs by intracellular
  detection of FOXP3.
- This requires a permeabilization step on separated lymphocytes.
- Tregs are FOXP3$^+$ CD4$^+$ CD25^{bright} and CD127^{weak} (CD127 is IL-7
  receptor-α).

Indications for testing

- Investigation of suspected IPEX syndrome (see ➲ Chapter 1).

Interpretation

- Assays that involve permeabilization of separated lymphocytes are
  intrinsically more prone to technical problems.
- The assay must be run on fresh samples with a normal control.
- This is a screening not a quantitative assay and will also pick up non-
  functional FOXP3—essential to do follow-up genetic analysis.

Genetic and protein studies

- Protein and genetic studies are essential for the identification of gene
  defects in primary immunodeficiencies.
- Surface proteins and some intracellular proteins, relevant to the
  diagnosis of primary immune deficiencies, can be identified by flow
  cytometry.
- Protein studies, including surface and intracellular protein detection, are
  frequently used as a screening test prior to genetic testing, e.g. for:
  - XLA (BTK);
  - CGD (phox proteins);
  - CD40 ligand deficiency;
  - IPEX (FOXP3);
  - ICOS deficiency (ICOS);
  - SAP, XIAP;
  - CD3ζ.

- Abnormal protein expression should be followed up by molecular mutation analysis.
- Molecular analysis is also required where there is a high degree of clinical suspicion but apparently normal protein expression (expression of non-functional protein).
- Molecular PID laboratories offer readily accessible genetic panel screens for common defects (GRID Panel (Cambridge, UK); Tiger panel (GOSH, London, UK). ESID will be able to identify other laboratories in Europe.
- Family studies are valuable to identify asymptomatic carriers, who can then receive appropriate counselling.

Leukaemia phenotyping

Leukaemia phenotyping is undertaken to identify the origin of the malignant cell and to identify the presence or absence of markers that are known to be of prognostic significance. This will always be undertaken in conjunction with other studies, including examinations of blood films, bone marrow smears, and trephines, stained for enzymatic cytoplasmic and membrane markers.

Principles of testing
- Flow cytometry of peripheral blood and bone marrow.
  - Surface markers.
  - Intracellular markers.
- Morphology on peripheral blood and bone marrow.
- Enzymatic studies.
- Molecular studies.
  - Oncogene expression.
  - Ig heavy chain and Tcr gene rearrangements.
  - Karyotype and chromosomal abnormalities.

Indications for testing
- Suspected leukaemia or pre-leukaemia.

Interpretation
- Diagnosis is dependent on the use of multiple markers and techniques.
- Follow-up panels may be required (see later in this topic).
- Leukaemic cells often correspond to particular stages of cellular differentiation, which can be matched to normal cell ontogeny.
- Aberrant antigens, expressed out of sequence, may occur.
- This may give rise to biphenotypic leukaemias.
- Bone marrow studies are complex because of the very different light-scatter properties of the cellular constituents.
- Familiarity with the patterns of antigen expression at each stage of differentiation for each lineage is required.
- Re-examination of bone marrow, after treatment, is important to detect the presence of minimal residual disease. This can be done by:
  - flow cytometry, which can detect one leukaemic cell in 10 000 cells;

- polymerase chain reaction (PCR) techniques where the leukaemic cells carry an abnormal genetic marker (oncogene) or have a specific rearrangement of either the immunoglobulin (B lineage) or T-cell receptor (T lineage) genes. These techniques are even more sensitive.
- Flow cytometric karyotyping is now possible as an alternative to molecular techniques.

Leukaemia phenotyping panel

A usual primary panel for acute leukaemias will include the following.
- B lineage:
    - CD10 (CALLA), CD19, CD24, HLA-DR, cytoplasmic Ig (μ heavy chains) and surface Ig.
- T lineage:
    - CD2, cytoplasmic CD3, CD7.
- Lymphoblast:
    - TdT.
- AML lineage:
    - CD13, CD14, CD33.
- Erythroid:
    - glycophorin A.
- Megakaryocyte:
    - CD41.

A secondary panel may be used in difficult cases and may include the following.
- B lineage:
    - cytoplasmic CD22.
- T lineage:
    - CD1, CD3, CD4, CD8.
- AML:
    - CD15, cytoplasmic myeloperoxidase.

For chronic lymphoid disorders the panel will be slightly different, with panels as follows.
- B lineage, primary:
    - CD10, CD20, CD5, surface Ig.
- B lineage, secondary:
    - CD11c, CD25, CD38, and FMC7.
- T lineage, primary:
    - CD3.
- T lineage, secondary:
    - CD4, CD8, CD11b, CD16, CD57.

Lymphocyte subsets

- Normal adult ranges:
    - total T cells (CD3$^+$), 0.69–2.54 $\times$ 10^9/l;
    - CD4$^+$ T cells, 0.41–1.59 $\times$ 10^9/l;
    - CD8$^+$ T cells, 0.19–1.14 $\times$ 10^9/l;
    - total B cells (CD19$^+$), 0.09–0.66 $\times$ 10^9/l;

- NK cells (CD16$^+$ CD56$^+$), 0.09–0.56 $\times$ 10^9/l;
- activated T cells (CD3$^+$ CD25$^+$), 0.1–0.4 $\times$ 10^9/l.

Principles of testing

- Single platform flow cytometry is considered the gold standard.
  - Fluorescence microscopy should not be used.
- Direct conjugation of the fluorochrome to the antibody is preferred.
- Beads are used to calibrate absolute counts.
- Results should be reported as absolute counts: percentages and ratios are not helpful for the basic markers but may be useful for extended panels (see ➲ 'Interpretation: additional markers', see later in this topic).
- Robust EQA schemes exist for common markers.
- Internationally standardized protocols for setting up flow cytometers, quality control, and panel selection have been published. These are dependent on the use of eight-colour flow cytometers.
- For PID, it is doubtful, particularly in the era of genomics, that all the markers recommended are actually of clinical value.

Indications for testing

- Diagnosis and monitoring of immunodeficiency states.
- Monitoring immunotherapeutic agents (anti-T-cell antibodies, cytotoxic drugs).

Interpretation

- Wide availability of commercial reagents with different fluorochromes allows many permutations and combinations, using multichannel flow cytometers.
- Some of the fluorochromes are large molecules and multiple staining of markers on cells may give rise to steric hindrance and reduced binding.
- Correct set-up of compensation for flow cytometer is essential: this must be checked regularly and especially after servicing.
- Regular quality control checks should be carried out with commercial fluorochrome-coupled beads.
- A basic panel for primary immunodeficiency work should include:
  - T cells: CD3, CD4, CD8;
  - B cells: CD19 or CD20;
  - NK cells: CD16 and CD56;
  - activated cells: CD25, MHC class II.
- Additional markers may include:
  - CD45RA, CD45RO, CD27 (naïve and effector T cells);
  - CD4$^+$CD45RA$^+$CD27$^+$ = naïve T cells;
  - CD4$^-$CD45RA$^+$CD27$^+$ = naïve T cells;
  - CD4$^-$CD45RA$^+$CD27$^-$ = effector T cells;
  - CD27, sIgM, sIgD (naïve, memory, and class-switch memory);
  - CD27$^-$sIgM$^+$sIgD$^+$ = naïve B cells;
  - CD27$^+$sIgM$^+$sIgD$^+$ = memory B cells;
  - CD27$^+$sIgM$^-$sIgD$^-$ = class-switch memory B cells;
  - Tcr $\alpha\beta$ and $\gamma\delta$;
  - leucocyte adhesion and complement receptors (see ➲ 'Adhesion markers; complement receptors', p. 605);
  - MHC class I (bare lymphocyte syndrome).

- Lymphocyte numbers have a marked circadian rhythm: for serial monitoring, samples must be taken at the same time of day.
- In a baby with suspected SCID, the presence of mainly activated CD8$^+$ T cells is suspicious of materno-fetal engraftment, while the presence of activated CD4$^+$ T cells, in the presence of large numbers of eosinophils, is suggestive of Omenn's syndrome.
  - T-cell receptor gene rearrangements will show an oligoclonal response.
- Absence of CD8$^+$ T cells is a feature of ZAP-70 kinase deficiency.
- Abnormalities of T- and B-cell populations are also seen in CVID, with CD4$^+$ T-cell lymphopenia, affecting particularly CD45RA$^+$ T cells, and absence of class-switch memory B cells.
- After HSCT, high levels of activated T cells often indicate GvHD.
- Very low CD4$^+$ T-cell counts are *not* a diagnostic feature of HIV disease.
  - Temporary reductions in the CD4$^+$ T-cell count are seen with a number of trivial viral infections, particularly in the acute phase.
  - This is often accompanied by an elevation of the CD8$^+$ T cells and NK cells.
  - Lymphocyte phenotyping must not be used as a surrogate for HIV testing without consent.
  - CD4:CD8 ratio is of little value: risk of opportunist infections is determined by absolute CD4 count.
  - Basic panel of CD3, CD4, and CD8 is all that is required (with viral load monitoring).
  - Significant recovery of cell numbers may be seen with HAART in HIV.
- Persistent CD4$^+$ T-cell lymphopenia has also been reported as a cause of opportunistic infections in the absence of any evidence for infection with either HIV-1 or HIV-2 (idiopathic CD4$^+$ T-cell lymphopenia).
- Rare deficiency of the binding site for the anti-CD4 mAb OKT3 is recognized giving spuriously low CD4 counts: this variant CD4 appears functionally normal.
- Abnormal lymphocyte profiles are also seen in:
  - lymphoma;
  - malignancy;
  - chronic fatigue syndromes;
  - protein-losing enteropathy;
  - overtraining syndrome.
- Generalized proportionate reductions in lymphocyte counts are seen with long-term immunosuppressive therapy.
- CD4/CD8 double-negative Tcr $\alpha\beta^+$ $^+$T cells are increased in ALPS (see ➲ Chapter 1).

B-cell function: *in vivo* assays

Principles of testing

- *In vivo* antibody production is measured by detection of serum antibody levels and rise in titre after deliberate test immunization.
- Antibody levels should be measured to exposure and immunization antigens.

- Testing should include protein and polysaccharide antigens.
- Subclass-specific responses can be measured to some antigens.
- Serotype-specific responses can be measured to pneumococcal polysaccharides (not all serotypes are equally immunogenic).
- Isohaemagglutinins, in appropriate blood group patients, allow detection of IgM responses. Despite the utility of this test, consensus suggests that it is not required in the diagnosis of immune deficiency.
- In the USA, the bacteriophage ΦX174 has been used as an immunogen: this neoantigen permits detection of primary and secondary antibody responses.
- Antibodies will normally be detected by EIA on serum, or by complement-fixation assays (viral antibodies).
- ELISpot assays allow the detection of specific antibody-producing B cells.
- EQA schemes exist for viral and bacterial antibodies.
- Common antigens are shown in Table 20.1.

Indications for testing
- Suspected antibody deficiency.

Interpretation
- Full infection and immunization history is required to evaluate responses.
- Dynamic responses after immunization give a better view of B-cell function.

Table 20.1 Common antigens used to evaluate *in vivo* B-cell function

Antigen	Type of antigen	Isotype/subclass	Robust assays available?
Pneumovax® 23	Polysaccharide	IgG, IgG$_2$	Yes?
Salmonella Vi	Polysaccharide	IgG, IgG$_2$	Yes
Tetanus toxoid	Protein	IgG, IgG$_1$	Yes
Diphtheria toxoid	Protein	IgG, IgG$_1$	No (poor CV & EQA)
Hib capsular polysaccharide	Polysaccharide	IgG, IgG$_1$ (when conjugated to protein), IgG$_2$	Yes
Meningococcal group C capsular polysaccharide	Polysaccharide	IgG, IgG$_1$ (when conjugated to protein), IgG$_2$	No
Poliovirus	Protein	IgG, IgM, IgG$_1$, IgG$_3$	Yes
MMR	Multiple proteins	IgG, IgM, IgG$_1$, IgG$_2$	Yes
Hepatitis B virus surface antigen	Protein	IgG, IgG$_1$, IgG$_3$	Yes
Isohaemagglutinins	Polysaccharides	IgM	Yes

- Target should be a rise into the normal/protective range with a minimum of a fourfold rise in titre.
- Assays for bacterial antibodies are poor with CVs of 15–25%: pre- and post-immunization samples should be run on the same assay.
- Assays must be interpreted with caution.
- Only killed or subunit vaccines should be given to patients with suspected immunodeficiency.
- Role of subclass- and serotype-specific assays is uncertain at present. Multiplex assays may be valuable for rapid screening of responses to multiple serotypes.
- Move to conjugated pneumococcal polysaccharide vaccines may lead to loss of a useful and safe, well documented, *in vivo* test of B-cell function. Salmonella Vi antigen may be a valid alternative and a commercial assay exists for measuring the antibody response.

B-cell function: *in vitro* assays

Principles of testing
- *In vitro* B-cell function is usually tested by stimulation of purified mononuclear cells by:
  - pokeweed mitogen (PWM);
  - anti-IgM + IL-2;
  - *Staphylococcus* strain A Cowan (SAC);
  - Epstein–Barr virus (EBV).
- IgG, IgA, and IgM production can be measured at 7 days by sensitive ELISA of the supernatant.
- Testing is time-consuming.

Indications for testing
- There are few routine clinical indications for this type of testing.
- Flow cytometric detection of class-switch memory B cells is quicker and easier than using anti-IgM + IL-2 system to identify prognostically important subgroups of common variable immunodeficiency (see ➲ Chapter 1).

Interpretation
- Interpretation is dependent on the type of assay used and the establishment of appropriate ranges for age and sex.

T-cell function: *in vivo* assays

Principles of testing
- T-cell function *in vivo* is tested by delayed-type hypersensitivity.
- Antigens are pricked through the skin (Merieux Multitest CMI®) or injected intradermally.
- Most useful antigens include PPD, *Candida*, mumps, tetanus, and streptokinase/streptodornase, which are available (some with difficulty) as single antigens, or are part of the battery in the Multitest.

Indications for testing

- Testing is of limited value except in the circumstance of chronic mucocutaneous candidiasis, where there is often specific anergy to *Candida*, with reasonable responses to other antigens.

Interpretation

- There may be early reactions but these are due to mechanisms not involving T cells.
- At 72–96 hours, in a positive reaction, there will be a cellular infiltrate that is palpable, with overlying erythema.
- Reactivity to the panel is low in early childhood and increases with age.
- Poor responses are seen in:
  - T-cell immune deficiencies (primary and secondary);
  - combined immune deficiency;
  - some patients with CVID;
  - leukaemias;
  - lymphomas;
  - other malignant disease;
  - renal failure;
  - during some chronic infections (late HIV).

T-cell function: *in vitro* assays

Principles of testing

- *In vitro* T-cell function testing is carried out by inducing the T cells to proliferate by exposure to either mitogens or antigens.
- Mononuclear cells are separated from neutrophils by density gradient centrifugation (Ficoll®).
- Proliferation of the T cells is measured by the incorporation into DNA of tritiated thymidine in replicating cells.
- Other methods used to study T-cell function *in vitro* include flow cytometric tests for:
  - measurement of calcium flux;
  - DNA replication (a non-isotopic alternative to the standard proliferation assay);
  - changes in surface antigen expression in response to activation (IL-2 receptor, CD25, transferrin receptor, CD71, CD69, and the nuclear antigen Ki-67);
  - intracellular cytokines: cytokine production in culture can be measured, but this is not done routinely, and the flow cytometric determination of intracellular cytokine is likely to be of more value.
- There is little value in the MLR as a test of T-cell function, although it forms a part of cross-matching bone marrow.
- ELISpot assays can be used to measure cytokine production in response to antigens and will also give a precursor frequency.

Indications for testing
- Suspected primary T-cell or combined immune deficiency.
- Functional assays are rarely required in secondary T-cell immunodeficiency.
- Monitoring of the T-cell proliferative response after HSCT provides a useful marker of returning function that will determine safe release from laminar flow.

Interpretation
- Results will be reported as counts per minute (cpm) for the unstimulated and stimulated cells and as a stimulation index.
- For PHA-stimulated cells the uptake should be > 5000 cpm and the increment over the unstimulated cells should be > 4000 cpm; the stimulation index should be > 10.
- For antigens such as *Candida*, the response is smaller and an increment of 2000 cpm and a stimulation index of 3.0 are satisfactory.
- The requesting clinician must also arrange a control sample from a healthy volunteer, where possible of the same age/sex as the patient.
  - This is necessary, as there are wide variations of individual responses, even in healthy individuals, and there are variations with age.
- Each laboratory should establish its own age and sex-specific normal ranges for each mitogen.
- The most useful stimuli are the following.
  - **Phytohaemagglutinin (PHA)**, a lectin (sugar-binding molecule) derived from kidney beans. This binds to sugar residues on a number of surface molecules, thus activating cells by several pathways simultaneously, including via the CD3–Tcr complex.
  - **Concanavalin A (ConA)**, a lectin derived from jack beans. Its effect is similar to that of PHA except that it is dependent on normal monocyte accessory function.
  - **Mitogenic anti-CD3 monoclonal antibodies**. Soluble and immobilized anti-CD3 cause specific stimulation of T cells via the CD3–Tcr complex, mimicking antigen.
  - **Phorbol esters (phorbol myristate acetate, PMA)**. This molecule activates protein kinase C directly in cells, bypassing the need for membrane events. The addition of a calcium ionophore, which raises the intracellular calcium by inserting unregulated calcium channels in the membrane, increases the effect of PMA as it is a calcium-dependent enzyme.
  - **Interleukin-2**. This has very little effect on its own but is synergistic with anti-CD3. Restoration of proliferative responses to other stimuli by the addition of IL-2 suggests a downstream defect leading to reduced/absent IL-2 production.
  - **Antigens**. Many antigens can be used but the most useful are *Candida*, tetanus, PPD, and viral antigens (CMV, HSV, rubella), as patients are likely to have been exposed or immunized. Responses are lower, as the frequency of T cells with the correct Tcr will be small.

Lymphoma diagnosis

Principles of testing

- Diagnosis of lymphoma follows principles similar to those of leukaemia typing, except that the cells are in a solid organ.
- Single-cell suspensions produced by disaggregating the tissue can be used.
- Most information is gained from looking at tissue sections.
- Staining is usually done with monoclonal antibodies followed by anti-mouse antibody conjugated to a reagent for developing a colour reaction (peroxidase, alkaline phosphatase–anti-alkaline phosphatase, etc.).
- Most studies can now be carried out on paraffin sections.
- Immunophenotyping will normally be undertaken in parallel with morphological, virological, and enzymatic studies.
- The primary panel usually includes:
  - CD45 (leucocyte common antigen);
  - CD45RA (minority of T cells and B cells);
  - CD3 (T cells);
  - CD4 (T-helper cells plus macrophages and dendritic cells);
  - CD8;
  - C3bR (follicular dendritic cells, B cells, macrophages);
  - HLA-DR (B cells, activated T cells);
  - surface immunoglobulins (heavy and light chains);
  - Ki-67 (nuclear antigen expressed in proliferating cells).
- The secondary panel for T-cell antigens includes:
  - CD2, CD5, CD7, and CD1, although the latter is also expressed on dendritic cells and macrophages.
- The secondary panel for B-lineage antigens includes CD10, CD21, CD22, CD23, CD24, CD79a, and CD5 (also expressed on T cells).
- Confirmation of the presence of Reed–Sternberg cells can be obtained by using CD30 and CD15.
- Histiocytes are reactive with CD68.
- LMP-1 is a surface marker of EBV+ cells and is expressed on Reed–Sternberg cells.
- *In situ* hybridization can be used to detect oncogene expression and viral genes.
- Initial and supplementary antibody panels will be used.
- Extracted material can be used as a source of DNA for molecular studies of T-cell receptor and Ig heavy chain gene rearrangements, as markers of clonality.
- EQA systems exist.

Indications for testing

- Any excised lymphoid tissue where lymphadenopathy is a feature should be examined for evidence of lymphoma.

Interpretation

- In the differential diagnosis of an abnormal lymph node the question must be answered: 'Is this a malignant process or a reactive process?'

- Lymphomas often express aberrant patterns of surface and cellular antigens:
  - κ:λ ratios > 10:1;
  - sIg negative, B-lineage antigen positive;
  - co-expression of B-lineage antigens and CD5, CD10, CD43, or CD6;
  - loss of an expected T-lineage antigen;
  - dual expression of CD4 and CD8 (outside the thymus);
  - expression of terminal deoxytransferase (TdT) or CD1a (outside thymus).
- Lymphoid tumours need to be distinguished from other (metastatic) malignancy.
  - Cells of lymphoid origin usually express CD45.
  - Other markers are available to distinguish cells from other sources, including carcinoembryonic antigen, cytokeratin, chromogranin, desmin, and S-100.
- Hodgkin's disease is distinguished by the presence of characteristic Reed–Sternberg cells.
  - Usually detectable by standard histology, although they may be sparse.
  - Can be identified by their reaction with CD30 and CD15, without reactivity with CD45 or T/B-lineage antigens.
- Evidence of clonality can now be obtained by studies of Ig and Tcr gene rearrangements by molecular techniques.
  - This can be carried out even on DNA extracted from paraffin sections.
  - Because of the use of PCR techniques to amplify DNA of interest, very small samples can be analysed.
- Abnormal expression of oncogenes and tumour suppressor genes can be detected by *in situ* hybridization; oncogenes routinely screened for include:
  - Bcl-2
  - Cyclin D1
  - p53
  - Bcl-6
  - CD99 (myc-2)
  - c-myc.
- Viral screens include EBV, CMV, HHV6, HHV8.
- The classification of lymphomas is constantly being revised in the light of new findings: readers are advised to consult an up-to-date detailed text to understand the process.

Neutrophil function testing

Principles of testing

- First test is neutrophil count (serial counts required for cyclic neutropenia—three times weekly for 6 weeks).
- Screening test for defects of oxidative metabolism (CGD) is nitroblue tetrazolium reduction test, in which a colourless intracellular dye

is reduced to an insoluble blue compound, formazan, when the neutrophil's oxidative machinery is activated.
- Usually done as a simple slide test.
- Can be done as a quantitative assay, with extraction of the formazan and quantitation by colorimetry.
- Flow cytometry using dye reduction (dihydrorhodamine, DHR) allows more cells to be analysed more quickly.
  - Both NBT and DHR tests should be done in parallel, as there are examples of neutrophil deficiencies where one test is abnormal but not the other.
- Other tests of the oxidative machinery include chemiluminescence (amplified by luminol), and the iodination test, which relates to hydrogen peroxide production.
- Phagocytosis can be measured by simply counting the number of latex beads or yeasts ingested by neutrophils or, more accurately, by flow cytometry using labelled bacteria.
- Bacterial killing assays allow the whole process to be tested, including opsonization, phagocytosis, and oxidative metabolism.
  - Test organism is incubated with patient's serum or control serum and then each is incubated with either normal or patient's neutrophils.
  - At a fixed time thereafter, the cells are lysed and the lysate plated out to allow residual live bacteria to grow.
  - Normally all bacteria will be killed within 30 minutes.
- Chemotaxis assays are usually carried out by measuring migration under agarose or by the Boyden chamber method, in which cells migrate into a microporous filter, which is examined under a microscope with a vernier gauge on the focusing ring, allowing the distance travelled to the leading edge to be measured.
- Monocytes can be studied on flow cytometers at the same time as neutrophils.
  - Specific defects include absence of γ-IFN receptors, IL-12.
- No EQA schemes exist: laboratories must therefore establish their own normal ranges and set up normal controls in parallel with patient samples for all assays.

Indications for testing
- Any patient with suspected neutrophil disorder:
  - recurrent abscesses, especially if deep-seated (liver);
  - extensive oral ulceration/gingivitis;
  - atypical granulomatous disease;
  - unusual bacterial or fungal infections—especially catalase-positive organisms (*Aspergillus*, *Staphylococcus*).

Interpretation
- Slide NBT tests may miss some cases of chronic granulomatous disease and it is essential, if there is a high degree of suspicion, to perform a more sensitive flow cytometric assay.
- With sensitive flow cytometric assays, heterozygotes for CGD mutations may have half normal activity.

- Bacterial killing assays may be abnormal in healthy children under the age of two.
- Chemotaxis is an important part of the process and rare defects due to the lack of anaphylotoxin receptors have been reported.
  - Both methods for chemotaxis give wide ranges even for normal individuals, so determining what is abnormal is often difficult.
- Neutrophil function testing should always include testing for adhesion molecule deficiency (see ➲ 'Adhesion markers', p. 605) and for neutrophil enzymes, especially myeloperoxidase (a common deficiency of doubtful significance), G6PD, and alkaline phosphatase (reduced in specific granule deficiency).
- Neutrophil assays absolutely require fresh samples.
- Any intercurrent infection will cause abnormal function.
- Follow-up protein studies and genetic investigations are required where defects of oxidative metabolism are identified in screening tests.

NK-cell function

Principles of testing

- Activity of MHC non-restricted killer cells (NK) cells can be assessed *in vitro*.
- Erythroleukaemia cell line K562 is known to be susceptible to lysis by NK cells.
- Assay is carried out by incubating mononuclear cells with labelled K562 cells at varying effector target cell ratios and then identifying the death of the targets.
  - Conventional way is to surface label the targets with ^{51}Cr, and then measure the release of the isotope into the medium on cell death.
  - Appropriate controls are required to identify spontaneous release of the isotope and target cell death unrelated to effector cell activity (should be less than 5%).
  - Flow cytometric assay uses a green fluorescent, membrane-bound dye to label the targets.
  - Cell death is identified by the uptake of propidium iodide, which gives a red fluorescence.
  - Live and dead targets can thus be separated by their staining from the unlabelled effector cells.
- The assays can be modified using different targets to look at antibody-dependent cell-mediated cytotoxicity (ADCC) and lymphokine-activated killer (LAK) activity.
- No EQA exists: laboratories must establish normal ranges and run normal controls with each assay.
- The test is dependent on high-quality K562 cells being available: long-term cell culture must be meticulous.

Indications for testing

- Indications are limited.
- NK-cell deficiency has been reported (rarely), causing severe infections with herpesviruses.

- Routine screening of patients with simple cold sores is not justified.
- NK-cell function may be relevant in graft rejection and in assessment of rare NK-cell leukaemias.

Interpretation

- Flow cytometric assay is more sensitive to minor target-cell damage, permeabilizing the cell to the red dye: oversensitivity is therefore a problem.
- Chromium-release assay depends on the complete disintegration of the cell.
- Clinical diagnostic value of the NK assay remains to be fully evaluated; routine evaluation of ADCC and LAK activity is not undertaken.
- Excessive NK-cell activity has been associated with an increased risk of graft loss in mismatched bone marrow transplants (particularly host NK-cell activity).
- Low/absent NK-cell activity has been reported in rare patients with recurrent infections with herpes family viruses.
- Very high activity may be found in NK cell leukaemias.
- Number of NK cells identified by flow cytometry does not necessarily correlate with the activity.

NK granule release

Principles of testing

- CD107a (lysosomal-associated membrane protein 1 (LAMP1)) is expressed on the surface of NK cells that have degranulated.
- K562 cells are used as a target for NK cells to stimulate degranulation, as they do not express MHC class I antigens.
- Expression of CD107a on NK cells (CD3$^+$ CD56$^+$) is detected by flow cytometry after incubation of separated PBMNC with K562 cells.
- PHA is also used as a non-specific activator of degranulation.

Indications for testing

- Suspected familial haemophagocytic lymphohistiocytosis.

Interpretation

- Patients with familial haemophagocytic lymphohistiocytosis due to Munc 13-4 and Syntaxin 11 deficiency will have absent degranulation.
- Patients with perforin deficiency will have normal granule release.
- A normal control is required with each run.
- Very few NK cells should express CD107a unstimulated; > 7% should express it when stimulated.
- Assay is dependent on ready access to high-quality K562 cells.
- Genetic testing is more valuable.

Perforin expression

Principles of testing

* Flow cytometric detection of intracellular perforin, using a permeabilization technique on separated PBMNC.
* Perforin is expressed in the granules of NK cells, some CD8+ T cells, CD56+ T cells, and γδ T cells.

Indications for testing

* Suspected FLH—see ➲ Chapter 1.

Interpretation

* Only 30% of patients with FLH will have a perforin defect; follow-up degranulation assays should be carried out if perforin expression is normal and there is a high degree of suspicion (see ➲ 'NK granule release', p. 622).
* XLPS should be excluded in males.

Toll-like receptors (TLRs)

Principles of testing

* Flow cytometric assay based on the shedding of CD62L (L-selectin) by neutrophils when activated.
* All 10 TLRs identified signal via MyD88 and IRAK-4 (clinical deficiencies of both are described—see ➲ Chapter 1); four TLRs signal via UNC-93B (TLR3, TLR7, TLR8, & TLR9).
* Activation of neutrophils via TLRs will lead to loss of CD62L.
* Lipopolysaccharide (LPS) is the ligand for TLR4; CL097 (an imidazoquinoline) is a ligand for TLR7/8. PMA is used as a positive control (bypasses TLRs to activate neutrophils).

Indications for testing

* Suspected deficiency of IRAK-4, MyD88, or UNC-93B.

Interpretation

* IRAK-4- and MyD88-deficient patients will shed CD62L normally with PMA but not with LPS or CL097.
* UNC-93B-deficient patients will shed CD62L normally with PMA and LPS but not with CL097.

TRECs

- Analysis of T-cell receptor excision circles (TRECs) is valuable in assessing thymic output, e.g. post HSCT, in HIV patients on HAART (low levels may predict disease progression).
- As TRECs do not replicate during cell division, progressive dilution occurs post-emigration.
- Assays are not yet widely available for routine use.
- TRECs can be detected on magnetic bead-separated T-cell subpopulations by quantitative PCR techniques.

T-cell receptor and immunoglobulin heavy chain gene rearrangements

- Testing is carried out by multiplex PCR amplification followed by PAGE.
- Panels of Tcr Vβ-specific labelled monoclonal antibodies can be used to carry out testing by flow cytometry.
- This enables monoclonal expansions in the T-cell repertoire (lymphoma, response to chronic infection) and selective clonal loss (e.g. Omenn's syndrome, DiGeorge syndrome) to be identified.
- Spectratype of Tcr Vβ and IgH gene usage can be constructed to demonstrate polyclonal, oligoclonal, and monoclonal gene usage, using fluorescent PCR products.
- This type of testing is crucial in lymphoma diagnosis, and in the diagnosis of oligoclonal states such as Omenn's syndrome.

Tissue typing

Introduction

Key elements

- Key elements for successful transplantation are:
  - ability to correctly identify tissue types of recipients and donors;
  - prediction of graft rejection (host-vs-graft);
  - in the case of a bone marrow transplant, prediction of graft-versus-host disease (GvHD).
- Antigens of the MHC system are defined and reviewed by the WHO to ensure there is a common approach to nomenclature and typing.
- Ideal match is an identical twin: few individuals requiring transplantation have such a donor.
- Most transplants are from matched unrelated donors (MUDs) or parents/siblings with a close but not identical match.
- In the case of a parental donor, this will usually only be a haplo-identical match (half identical) unless there is consanguinity in the family, in which case the match may be better.
- Not all transplantation is affected identically by HLA matching.
  - For renal and bone marrow transplantation, the better the match, the better the graft function and the fewer the complications.
  - For liver transplantation, HLA matching is not beneficial.
  - For cardiac transplantation, HLA matching is impractical due to time constraints and door limitations.
  - Matching for living related donors is less critical than for cadaveric transplants.
- If a poorly matched solid organ is transplanted, the recipient may require considerable immunosuppressive therapy to prevent rejection, increasing risks of secondary malignancies and of opportunist infections.

Historical approach

- Requirement for a high-resolution match in BMT and HSCT has led to the generation of highly specific techniques capable of identifying very minor changes in histocompatibility antigens.
- Tissue typing used to be undertaken by two techniques:
  - HLA class I antigens were identified (and in many cases defined) by serology, using sera derived from multiparous women who often develop anti-HLA antibodies;
  - as this technique does not identify all class II antigens, cellular tests had to be used.

Current approach

Molecular biological techniques are now used.

- Where antigens have previously been defined serologically, it is now clear from molecular genotyping that some antigens classed as completely distinct by serology are more closely related to each other than some specificities thought, on serological grounds, to be part of a closely related family ('splits' of an antigen).
- Nomenclature has been changed to reflect the differences.
- Molecular typing is critical in deciding whether a donor is a good match for a given recipient, as two different HLA-B antigens, defined

serologically, may differ by only one amino acid, and therefore represent a better match than two splits of the same antigen that may differ by five or more amino acids.

- Under the right circumstances even a one-amino-acid change is enough to generate a detectable specific CTL response, while a five-amino-acid difference may lead to irretrievable graft rejection or GvHD.

Process

- In transplant matching there are two main steps:
  - tissue types of recipient (and donor) must be established;
  - cross-match stage, in which the suitability of the proposed match is tested.
- For renal transplantation, donor will be tissue typed and blood grouped (ABO and rhesus) and the recipient screened at regular intervals for the presence of anti-HLA antibodies.
  - If there are potential living related donors, then these will be tissue typed and blood grouped and then the recipient's sera will be tested against donor cells for anti-donor antibodies.
  - A good donor will be ABO compatible, with the best match of HLA antigens, and the recipient will lack anti-donor antibodies (pre-formed antibodies are a cause of hyperacute rejection).
  - If there is no suitable living related donor, then the patients will be listed to receive a cadaver organ, with their clinical and immunological details stored on a central register.
  - This allows best use of cadaver organs across the country, as cadaver organs can be given to the best-matched recipients, who are likely to derive most benefit.
  - The cadaver organ will have been ABO/Rh and HLA typed and recipients chosen on the best match if they have no pre-formed antibodies against the identified HLA antigens.
  - Immediately before transplant takes place, a fresh sample of the patient's serum will be cross-matched against donor lymphocytes, to check that no new antibodies have developed.
  - Normally, to ensure that there are sufficient donor lymphocytes to cross-match (as this may have to be done several times against different potential recipients), the spleen is removed to provide a source of cells.
  - Patients who have had previous grafts are often highly sensitized, and have high levels of antibodies, which can cause difficulty in identifying suitable donors.

Matching procedures: detecting pre-formed circulating antibodies

- Cross-match allows detection of antibodies in the recipient that may affect graft viability.
- Used in the case of solid organs, where the patient's serum is tested against donor cells.

- Antibodies of interest are mainly IgG anti-HLA class I and anti-HLA class II antibodies.
- IgM antibodies are often (but not always) considered to be autoantibodies that may cause false-positive responses that are not deemed significant to the outcome of the transplant unless there has been a recent sensitizing event.

Microlymphocytotoxicity

- Recipient's serum incubated with donor cells in the presence of complement and wells scored for cytotoxicity.
- To control for autoantibodies, donor's cells are also tested.
- To distinguish anti-HLA class I and anti-HLA class II antibodies, T cells and B cells are run separately since B cells express higher levels of HLA class I antigens.
- Positive IgG anti-T-cell antibody is generally regarded as a contraindication to transplantation because of risk of hyperacute rejection and increased incidence of early vascular rejection.
- B-cell reactivity may occur in the absence of a positive T-cell match.
- IgM antibodies can be detected by performing the assay in the presence of dithiothreitol or dithioerythritol to disrupt pentameric IgM.
  - If a positive cross-match becomes negative in the presence of these agents, then an IgM antibody is likely.
- Performing tests at 37°C helps eliminate cold-reactive antibodies that are often non-specific.

ELISA

- ELISA can be used to identify antibodies to HLA classes I and II.
- Purified HLA class I or class II antigens are coated on to microtitre wells and patient's serum added.
- Bound antibody identified using labelled anti-human IgG ± IgM antibodies.
- Less sensitive and specific than flow cytometry but more suitable for testing large numbers of samples.

Flow cytometry

- Flow cytometry can be used to sensitively and specifically identify antibodies to HLA classes I and II.
- Donor lymphocytes are incubated with patient serum and then washed.
- They are then incubated with fluoresceinated anti-human IgG or IgM and anti-CD3 or anti-CD19 antibodies conjugated to a different fluorochrome.
- Analysed on flow cytometer using dual-colour fluorescence.

Magnetic bead technique

- Newer and quicker method using magnetic beads coated with specific class I and class II antigens ('Luminex®' technology).
- Beads are incubated with recipient serum and then fluoresceinated anti-human IgG or IgM, separated with a magnet, and analysed in flow cytometer.

- Beads can be coated with single recombinant HLA molecules.
- This is much more sensitive and also much faster.
- Positive reactions may be diluted to assess titre of antibodies.
- Allows distinction between IgG and IgM antibodies.
- Identifies both complement-fixing and non-complement-fixing antibodies.
  - Complement-fixing antibodies more likely to have a major deleterious effect.
- Increased sensitivity picks up weaker antibodies making positive results harder to interpret.
- Excludes non-HLA antibodies, which may cause false-positive lymphocytotoxic cross-matches but do not affect graft suitability.
- Specific assays have been developed that demonstrate whether the antibodies detected bind C1q or C3d.
- The use of epitope matching (where epitopes are shared) may allow 'acceptable' transplants, where previously the cross-match would be rejected.

Epigenetics

- The role of epigenetics in transplantation is being studied.
- This includes DNA methylation, histone modifications, and microRNAs (miRNAs).
- It is thought that these changes may contribute to graft success/failure.
- Techniques are being developed to study miRNAs as a tool for predicting rejection in renal transplantation.
- Urinary miRNAs may be useful to monitor post-graft renal function.

Virtual crossmatch

- This uses a paper-based cross-match, based on the known highly accurate HLA type of the donor and recipient and accurate recipient HLA antibody testing of the donor.
- This is allows more rapid transplantation (e.g. cardiac transplantation, which is very time critical).

Monitoring

- Patients on waiting lists for renal transplants will be screened at intervals by microcytotoxicity and other antibody screening techniques, which should be as sensitive as the cross-matching technique against panels of pre-typed cells to identify the presence of any anti-HLA antibodies.
- This speeds up the cross-matching, as cadaver grafts can be selected that lack the antigens recognized.
- Donor-specific cross-matching has limited relevance to liver transplants since they are relatively resistant to humoral rejection.
- Liver allograft may even protect a subsequent kidney transplant from hyperacute rejection.

Mixed lymphocyte reaction (MLR)

- MLR is an *in vitro* reaction to analyse recipient T-cell response to foreign HLA and non-HLA molecules predicting likelihood of T-cell-mediated graft rejection, which may not be predicted from HLA typing alone. This has been used in the assessment of potential bone marrow donors but is now no longer in routine use.
- Peripheral blood mononuclear cells (PBMC) from both donor and recipient are cultured together.
- If donor and recipient have differing MHC and non-MHC alleles then the mononuclear cells will proliferate.
- The proliferation assay takes 4–7 days to reach peak proliferation.
- Proliferation is usually identified by tritiated thymidine incorporation, as for other T-cell proliferative assays (see ➲ Chapter 20).
- If donor and recipient lymphocytes are cultured together, then both sets of cells will proliferate (two-way MLR), confusing the results.
- Cells from donor may be prevented from proliferating by exposing them to mitomycin or irradiation, so that only the recipient lymphocytes will proliferate (one-way MLR).
- In bone marrow transplantation a one-way MLR is performed in both directions, as the graft will also be immunologically active.
- Results are reported as a stimulation index or relative response.
- In detecting differences in class II antigens, the MLR is much more sensitive than serology: T cells may respond to allelic variants differing in a single amino acid.

HTLp and CTLp frequency

- Variant on the mixed lymphocyte reaction allowing identification of number and functional capacity of responding T cells. It is now no longer in routine use.
- Limiting dilution step to identify the frequency of helper T lymphocytes (HTLp) and cytotoxic T lymphocytes (CTLp) precursors.
- HTLp and CTLp assay may be performed in a combined assay.
- A stimulatory one-way MLR is run; effector cells are removed and assessed for cytotoxic activity (to assess CTLp frequency) and IL-2 activity in supernatants is analysed (to assess cytokine-generating HTLp frequency).
- More sensitive than ordinary MLR, as the quantitation is more accurate and allows different recipient–donor combinations to be compared.
- Increased frequency of precursors may increase likelihood of *in vivo* reactivity, although clinical utility to predict graft-versus-host and host-versus-graft unclear.

Tissue typing: serological methods

- Purpose of tissue typing is to identify the phenotype, i.e. expression of HLA on cells. More than one method may be required to give a complete picture.
- Now molecular testing identifies genotype, and phenotype is inferred.

HLA class I antigens

- For class I antigens (HLA-A, -B, -C), the standard technique is the microcytotoxicity assay carried out in 20 µl Terasaki plates.
- Patient's mononuclear cells are plated out and typing sera, derived from multiparous women, with known reactivity are added in the presence of a source of fresh complement (normally rabbit).
- A panel of sera, up to 200, may be used to cover all the specificities.
- Each serum usually has more than one specificity and some of the antibodies will be against more than one antigen (cross-reacting antigen group), while others will be against a single monospecific private antigen.
- A dye such as propidium iodide that enters only dead cells is added and the plate is then viewed under fluorescence, so that dead cells show up as red.
- Other dye systems exist for visualizing the cells (eosin Y).
- Each well is then scored for the amount of cell death.
- The pattern of killing is then correlated with the known specificities of the sera to identify the probable pattern.

HLA class II antigens

- Typing for class II antigens serologically has been difficult, as the antigens are only expressed on a minority of the mononuclear cell fraction (B cells, monocytes, and activated T cells).
- In order to carry out the tests, purified B cells are required, which can either be obtained by nylon wool adherence (B cells adhere but T cells do not) or by using a monoclonal antibody against a B-cell antigen coupled to a magnetic bead, allowing the B cells to be purified with a magnet.
- Obtaining adequate anti-HLA class II typing sera is also difficult, as these antibodies tend to be weaker than the HLA class I antibodies.
  - Anti-HLA class I antibodies can be removed by absorption with pooled human platelets, which express class I antigens only.
  - As B cells express more class I than class II antigens, the need for reagents free of anti-class I antibodies is obvious if false-positive reactions are to be avoided.
- As a result, serological techniques have been of limited value in defining HLA class II polymorphisms.
- Molecular techniques have replaced both serological and cellular techniques for class II typing and are also being used for more accurate class I typing.

Molecular HLA typing

- Determination of the HLA type by genotyping has revolutionized tissue typing and also revealed that the designation of specificities on the basis of serology has been misleading.
- A variety of methods are in use: which to choose depends on the speed with which an answer is required.

RFLP

- This technique uses the ability of certain endonucleases to cut DNA at sites of fixed sequences.
- By using several endonucleases specific for different sequences, DNA will be reduced to fragments of different lengths.
- Differences in the lengths will be determined by the underlying genetic structure.
- This technique, which is very slow (2–3 weeks), also requires significant amounts of DNA and is not sensitive enough to identify all the alleles of class II antigens identified now by other techniques.
- It is therefore of very limited value and is no longer in routine use.

PCR

- The development of the polymerase chain reaction, based on a cyclical synthetic reaction catalysed by the *Thermus aquaticus* (Taq) polymerase, has been to molecular biology what the monoclonal antibody has been to immunology.
- Upstream and downstream primers are used to start off the reaction by binding to the denatured single-stranded DNA, which is then re-annealed and allowed to complete synthesis.
- The new chains then act as the templates for further cycles.
- Rapidly, in about 25–30 cycles, many millions of copies of the desired piece of DNA can be produced.
- Probes can be directed at generic sequences, e.g. the flanking regions of a gene, or more specific probes can be derived.

Sequence-specific primer (SSP)

- This uses probes specific for allelic variants of HLA genes, where the probes are specific for the allelic variant sequence and therefore only amplify that sequence.
- This is known as sequence-specific primer PCR or SSP-PCR.
- It is a rapid technique (3 hours) but is of relatively low resolution.
- Higher resolution may be achieved at the cost of large numbers of PCRs, expense, and complexity.
- It requires minimal amounts of DNA to start with.

Sequence-specific oligonucleotide probes (SSOPs)

- The target DNA sequence is amplified by PCR and immobilized on filter.
- Labelled SSOPs specific for individual alleles are hybridized to the immobilized DNA.

- The oligonucleotide probes (18–24 nucleotides long) carry a radioactive tracer and the pattern of binding with the panel of probes identifies the sequences present and hence the genotype.
- Technique is relatively slow and also requires a large number of probes to cover all the possible allelic variants (e.g. 22 probes are required for the DR52 family (DR3, DR5, and DR6) alone).
- If it is a previously unrecognized allele, there will be no reaction, as no probe will be available.
- Reverse SSOP can be performed by hybridizing target biotinylated DNA with immobilized oligonucleotide probes.
- This technique is faster and is more suitable for routine diagnostic use.

Sequence-based typing
- The nucleotide sequence of the HLA gene DNA is identified directly.
- RNA is used as the original template, to avoid amplifying pseudogenes.
- DNA is made initially by reverse transcription.
- This technique is fast (16–24 hours) and very accurate.
- It will identify previously unknown alleles and has revealed a degree of heterogeneity within the HLA genes that had not previously been recognized.

Other techniques
- Reference-strand-mediated conformation analysis (RSCA) is a conformational method that offers high resolution.
  - The HLA type is assigned on the basis of accurate measurement of conformation-dependent DNA mobility in gel electrophoresis.
  - This allows the discrimination of HLA alleles that differ by one nucleotide.
  - Variable number tandem repeat (VNTR) analysis looks for polymorphisms in the non-coding repeated DNA and can be used for detecting and monitoring microchimerism post transplant.
  - Fluorescently labelled PCR primers amplifying short tandem repeat loci are employed to obtain a 'VNTR profile' for patient and donor to assess the chimeric status of the patient.

Next-generation sequencing
- More advanced combinations of next-generation sequencing have speeded up analysis considerably.
- Several systems are available including the Roche 454 platform, Life Technologies/Ion Torrent platform, and the Illumina/MiSeq system, all of which involve automated multi-stage processing.
- Pacific Biosciences system uses single molecule real-time sequencing (SMRT).

KIR testing

- Increasing recognition of the importance of the NK-cell receptors in transplantation (as well as autoimmunity and response to infection) has led to interest in typing for these, using molecular techniques.
- The KIR receptor family (killer inhibitory receptor) comprises 15 genes and 2 pseudogenes. They recognize a limited spectrum of HLA class I molecules.
- CD94/NKG2 family comprises 4 genes plus NKG2D and recognize unconventional HLA class I-like molecules.

HLA testing as a disease marker

- Many diseases are associated with HLA antigens, the best known being the association of ankylosing spondylitis (AS) with HLA-B27.
- Requests are often submitted for tissue typing to identify this particular antigen.
- It is not a diagnostic test, as HLA-B27 is a relatively common antigen (8% of Caucasians) and not every positive patient develops the disease.
- 90% of patients with AS will be HLA-B27$^+$, but 10% will have other antigens.
- The relative risk of developing AS is 100 times greater in HLA-B27$^+$ individuals compared to HLA-B27$^-$ individuals.
- It is most useful as a marker of probable exclusion of AS.
- In rheumatoid arthritis, the presence of DR4 (particularly DRB1*0401 and *0404 alleles) is associated with a greater risk of developing erosions and extra-articular disease and a worse prognosis.
- Typing may therefore provide useful prognostic information that may alter the approach to using disease-modifying drugs (e.g. anti-TNFα therapeutics).
- In the absence of full tissue typing facilities, HLA-B27 can be detected by a more economical, simple flow cytometric test, although this is less accurate.

Human anti-animal antibodies

- Circulating anti-animal antibodies are an often unrecognized and unsuspected cause of interference in immunological assays (anti-bovidae).
- These must be distinguished from heterophile antibodies that have a broader reactivity.
- Circulating anti-animal antibodies can arise from iatrogenic (diagnostic or pharmaceutical agents) and non-iatrogenic (including animal husbandry and pets) causes.
- Immunoassays may give false-positive or -negative results and should be considered where results do not match the clinical picture, particularly if the patient has been exposed to animal-derived agents.
- Interference may be overcome by blocking agents or assay redesign (e.g. use of chimeric antibodies).

Anti-mouse antibody

- These are the most common human anti-animal antibodies.
- The main reason is the increased use of murine monoclonal antibodies.
- OKT3, an anti-CD3 monoclonal antibody used as an immunosuppressant in transplantation, has been associated with the development of anti-mouse antibodies.
- These can interfere with its therapeutic effects when used subsequently and therefore monitoring of the development of antibodies is useful clinically.

Anti-rabbit antibody

- Rabbit anti-thymocyte globulin (ATG) may be used as an immunosuppressant and development of anti-rabbit antibodies has been associated with decreased therapeutic efficacy.
- False-positive immunoassays have been associated with unnecessary invasive diagnostic procedures.

Anti-chimera antibodies

- Antibodies to recombinant humanized fusion proteins and chimeric proteins, which interfere with function, have been described.

Chimerism studies

- Chimerism studies are valuable after HSCT. Mixed chimerism of different lineages is common.
- Magnetic beads coupled to specific antibodies can be used to separate key haematopoeitic cells for analysis with high purity.
- Where the donor is of the opposite sex, probes for X and Y chromosome-specific genes can be used.
- Otherwise donor and recipient polymorphisms in short tandem repeats (STR) are used (as previously described).
- After HSCT for CGD, the profile of the neutrophil oxidative burst by flow cytometer gives an accurate measure of donor neutrophils.

Useful websites

British Society of Histocompatibilty and Immunogenetics: ✍ www.bshi.org.uk

HLA databases: ✍ www.ebi.ac.uk\imgt\hla

National Marrow Donor Program: ✍ www.marrow.org

Quality and managerial issues

Introduction

Clinical and laboratory services do not operate in isolation but are integrated into the clinical and managerial framework of a hospital, and in the UK into a nationwide network (the NHS). This provides a constraint in both managerial and financial terms and also provides a legal framework in which services are delivered. It is essential that, no matter where the patient is treated, the right diagnosis is reached and the appropriate treatment is given.

NHS service providers in England are now subject to rigorous central direction by the Department of Health and by NHS-England (NHS-E) and inspection by the quasi-autonomous Care Quality Commission (CQC)—previously known as the Healthcare Commission and before that the Commission for Healthcare Improvement, CHI (see ℘ http://www.cqc.org.uk/). For mainstream therapeutics and procedures, the National Institute for Health and Care Excellence (NICE) determines whether therapies (drugs, procedures) should be available on the NHS, supposedly to eliminate postcode prescribing (see ℘ http://www.nice.org.uk/).

The severe constraints on funding have meant both covert and overt restrictions on funding of expensive treatments. For many drugs, individual funding requests (IFRs) are required, which have to demonstrate exceptionality (to avoid setting precedents for common conditions). These require a detailed, referenced application by a clinician, and scrutiny by local drug and therapeutics committees, before being sent to unaccountable and frequently non-specialist committees, where they are rejected. The cost in manpower terms at all stages is probably thousands of pounds in lost productivity by highly qualified clinicians and pharmacists.

With devolution, the healthcare systems in Wales, Scotland, and Northern Ireland have now diverged substantially from the model in operation in England, despite the anachronistic term of a 'National Health Service'. This has become progressively more marked. The following description relates to healthcare in England (space precludes discussion in detail of the healthcare systems in the devolved administrations).

Scotland has retained a system of Health Boards which manage all services including Hospitals and Primary Care. There is no system where money follows patients. This is less bureaucratic. There has been divergence in service provision, with some services not available in Scotland, and there are different approvals of drugs, so a new drug may be available in England but not Scotland and vice versa.

Structure of the NHS and the NHS plan (England)

Department of Health

- The Department of Health (DH) is responsible for leading the NHS on social care as well as improving standards of public health.
- The Secretary of State for Health and Social Care currently works with five ministers for health and the Permanent Secretary of DH.

- The NHS has a chief executive, accountable to the DH and to Parliament.
- The Secretary of State for Health and Social Care is accountable to Parliament for the functioning of the NHS.
- The role of the DHSC is to focus on providing strategic leadership to the NHS.
- Examples include:
  - setting overall direction;
  - ensuring national standards are set;
  - securing resources.
  - It also interferes by attempting to micromanage services directly!
- In 2012, a new Health & Social Care Bill was passed in England. This bill:
  - allows GP-led commissioning;
  - enshrines a right to a level playing field (which means that any qualified provider can bid to run services, including private sector, charities, etc.);
  - claims to provide a greater voice for patients (very unlikely, as patients' wishes are always ignored!);
  - removes the NHS from the direct control of the Secretary of State (so politicians can't be blamed when it all goes wrong!);
  - potentially privatizes the NHS by the back door.
  - The impact of these is difficult to assess: mass privatization has not taken place and there have been significant failures of privately run services, most spectacularly when Circle handed back the running of Hinchingbrooke Hospital to the NHS and walked away!
  - The current Secretary of State for Health for England (2019) is now reviewing this plan, recognizing the increased cost of the bureaucracy. Purchaser-provider splits and competition are likely to be reviewed.

Delegated responsibilities

Previous DH responsibilities have been now devolved to other organizations, including the following.

- Overall regulation and inspection of the NHS is now the responsibility of the Care Quality Commission (CQC).
- The running of the NHS is in the hands of NHS England. It has a medical director. It includes the NHS Quality Board.
- Regional planning and modernization have been devolved to the Strategic Health Authorities.
- Accountable Care organizations have delegated responsibilities, but have no legal framework and their existence has been challenged in the Courts.
- Evaluation of therapies, devolved to NICE. Theoretically if NICE approves a drug/therapy it should be available. However, NHS-E has taken to making its own decisions about therapies and withdrawing funding from some therapies, even when NICE is still considering them.
- National Patient Safety Agency (NPSA, Special Health Authority): responsible for identifying and learning from risks to patients. Now incorporated into NHS Improvements.

- NHS Litigation Authority (NHSLA, Special Health Authority), responsible for all litigation against the NHS. Operates as NHS Resolution.
- National Clinical Assessment Authority (NCAA) responsible for dealing with poorly performing doctors; part of NHSLA.
- NHS Improvements, which has subsumed the role of Monitor, and effectively becomes responsible for failing Trusts.

Strategic Health Authorities (StHAs)

Below the Secretary of State for Health there were 28 StHAs (replacing the regional health authorities) who managed the NHS locally. Their roles included the following.

- Coherency and developing strategies to improve the local health service.
- Ensuring high-quality performance of local health service.
- Building capacity.
- Making sure national priorities are integrated into local health plans.
- Implementation of modernization programmes, such as the Sustainability & Transformation Partnerships (STPs). These include rationalization of pathology services. Most STPs have failed on the funding required to support radical change.
- In England some of the functions have been devolved to the GP-led Clinical Commissioning Groups (CCGs)

Clinical Commissioning Groups (CCGs)

- CCGs manage a budget of approximately £65bn.
- They have replaced Primary Care Trusts (PCTs), but the process have led to more CCGs than there were PCTs (more not less bureaucracy!)
- They are responsible for:
  - planning and securing services for the local population's needs;
  - improving health of local population;
  - integrating health and local care socially working with local authorities.
- They are required to spend part of their budgets on commissioning services from the independent sector, via independent treatment centres: this has proven highly destabilizing to NHS services, with wards being closed and staff laid off.
- As well as commissioning services they also acted as providers of services, which many viewed as a conflict of interest.
- As part of the Health Service reforms (2012), PCTs have been abolished. Their provider functions have been transferred to other provider units (often Foundation Trusts) and their commissioning role has been transferred to CCGs.
- Senior staff have been laid off, with loss of key expertise. Some have been re-engaged by the CCGs (after receiving redundancy pay-offs!).

Clinical Networks

- Clinical Networks have been established to work across organizational boundaries (e.g. in cancer).

Specialist commissioning

- Clinical Immunology and Allergy are separately commissioned in England, by regional specialist commissioning teams.
- In 2013, the regional commissioning was replaced by central specialized commissioning.
- A national advisory process has been set in place.
- Services for SCID and other rare diseases or low-volume expensive procedures (e.g. lung transplantation) are commissioned nationally already with only 1–2 sites in England. For SCID, these sites (Great Ormond Street Hospital (GOSH) and Great North Childrens' Hospital, Newcastle) also provide services for Scotland, Wales, and Ireland.
- A new national programme for adult HSCT in PID is being established, with transplants to take place either in Newcastle or the Royal Free Hospital (which includes GOSH) to begin with.
- Other expensive services such as immunoglobulin therapy, treatment for HAE, amongst others, are also centrally commissioned. NHS-E issues guidelines on the permitted use separately from NICE, but not as thoroughly evidence based.

NHS trusts

- NHS trusts continue to run some hospitals, usually where there have been major financial issues affecting stability.
- They will usually be working with NHS Improvements.
- Their budget is derived predominantly from contracts with CCGs.
- Trusts also receive funding from medical schools to undertake medical student training—this replaces the old SIFT (service increment for teaching) arrangements, which have now been dismantled.
- The chief executive is now legally responsible for activities within his/her trust: he/she can be dismissed by the trust board.

Foundation trusts

- Established in April 2004, they are freestanding organizations with greater freedom within the NHS, including the freedom to borrow money in commercial markets.
- They now comprise the majority of NHS hospitals in England.
- They are considered as separate non-profit making organizations.
- They are owned by their members who are local people, employees, and other key stake-holders.
- A board of governors must be elected by members of the foundation trust including local people, patients, and employees.
- The board of governors works with the management board to ensure that the foundation trust acts in a way that is consistent with its objectives.
- The Secretary of State for Health does not have power to direct NHS foundation trusts or appoint board members.
- They are accountable to an independent regulator, NHS Improvements (which has taken over Monitor's function) that is responsible for approving their application for foundation status and which may remove that status if they do not manage their affairs satisfactorily.

- They are accountable externally though inspection by the Care Quality Commission.
- Income is derived through legally enforceable contracts with CCGs.
- Few NHS foundation trusts are now running budget surpluses and more and more are requiring direct intervention by NHS Improvements, with bail-outs and replacement of management teams, or takeovers by other foundation trusts.

Franchise hospitals
- One hospital in England with long-standing problems (Hinchingbrooke) was handed over in its entirety to the private sector to be run as an NHS franchise.
- As noted earlier, this failed.
- It is unlikely that this is a model that will be rolled out more widely, as private companies are unwilling to take on the risk.

Opted-out services
- Current legislation in England allows services to opt out of direct NHS control, while continuing to provide contractual services to NHS patients.
- There are a number of financial models for this.
- So far this has mainly involved therapy services in the community, but could in the future include clinical services in secondary and tertiary care.
- This could include the development of doctors' chambers.

Funding of pathology services
- Pathology laboratories receive funding from Primary Care (via CCGs). This is usually a block contract or cost and volume.
- Within the hospital, there will be funding supplied for inpatient and outpatient work, which is either block funding, roughly determined by expenditure, or by internal service level agreements, whereby patient service delivery directorates are recharged according to their usage. The cost of the laboratory services is then incorporated into the clinical contracts.
- It is essential that, where new work is taken on or clinical services expand, provision of extra resources for the laboratory is agreed.
- Laboratories may also provide services to other laboratories, for which invoices are raised. All NHS organizations must be charged the same price by the laboratory, i.e. one hospital cannot negotiate a discounted rate.
- Other income will be derived from private patient work and research, where the laboratory is free to determine the price.
- Costing of laboratory tests needs to accurately reflect the true costs, which include fixed overheads (heat, light, accommodation), equipment costs (rental, depreciation), variable costs (reagents), and staff time (costed according to the grade). Doing this correctly is time-consuming, and once base costs are established, prices tend to be adjusted to account for wage and reagent cost inflation.
- All directorates will also have cost improvement targets: a fixed % of their agreed budget that must be saved (doing more for less!).

- As this has been going on for 20 or more years, the amount of fat that can be cut now is limited. The usual tricks are as follows.
  - Skill mix review (doing the same work with lower-banded staff). Downside is loss of senior experienced staff.
  - Demand management, i.e. rationing clinicians' access to tests. This is not usually cost-effective, because of the time taken by senior laboratory staff dealing with disgruntled clinicians. Electronic ordering systems do make it easier to block requests.
  - Changing technologies to cheaper alternatives (may require capital expenditure = spend-to-save).
  - Outsourcing work that can be done more cheaply elsewhere. Conversely bringing work in house where capacity exists and it is cost-effective.
  - Marketing services to external users, to bring in income.

Regulatory bodies

- There are multiple bodies that have oversight of pathology laboratories and clinical services. The key ones are covered in the following sections. Readers are advised to consult the organizations' websites to ensure that they have the most up-to-date information.
- In the UK, medical staff are regulated by the GMC, while scientific and technical staff are regulated by the HPC. Nurses are regulated by the NMC.
- Education is now the responsibility of Health Education England (HEE), with regional offices, covering both medical and non-medical training. Curricula for medical trainees and examinations are generated by the relevant Royal College bodies but must be approved by the GMC.

UK Accreditation Service (UKAS)

- UKAS (⌦ https://www.ukas.com/), which is the only internationally approved accreditation service in the UK (under the Accreditation Regulations 2009), has now subsumed all the functions previously carried out by CPA.
- Laboratories need to provide documentary evidence to meet an extensive set of standards covering personnel, premises, equipment, and pre- and post-analytical phases of the sample.
- Laboratory inspection is now measured against ISO 15189:2012, the international standard for diagnostic laboratories.
- The original CPA structure of shareholding ownership by the professional bodies has been wound up.

Process

- The DH has decreed that enrolment with the UKAS is now mandatory for all NHS laboratories.
- Despite laboratory accreditation being available since 1990, some laboratories remain uninspected. As of March 2017, 75% of laboratories had been assessed against ISO 15189:2012.

- Once a laboratory applies for enrolment, inspection will automatically follow.
- The laboratory initially applies for accreditation by submitting an application defining the laboratory's scope of practice.
- Unlike CPA, UKAS accredits tests not laboratories. Laboratories may continue to offer non-accredited tests, as long as their status is clearly identified on reports.
- A UKAS-employed regional assessor will review applications and will liaise with the laboratory concerning the timing of inspection.
- Before the inspection, the regional assessor will identify which areas/ tests will be inspected.
- The regional assessor is responsible for assessing the quality management system, including quality manual and document control.
- UKAS will usually send one or two inspectors, one clinician or scientist and one senior BMS.
  - Where a laboratory has a small repertoire a single inspector may be used.
  - After the inspection the laboratory will receive a detailed report of any non-conformities and will be given a relatively short period to correct these and provide supporting documentation. Failure to complete within the timescale will require re-application and starting the process from scratch.
- Paid assessors, with expertise in audit and quality systems management, are now employed by UKAS to carry out the horizontal and vertical audits.
- UKAS Central Office, who may still insist on further changes and/ or documentation before the scope of practice is approved for accreditation, gives the final approval.
- The regional assessor, assisted by discipline-specific assessors, carries out annual surveillance visits. This will include checks on documentation, QMS, and identified tests.
- UKAS accredits EQA Schemes to ISO 17043 and point-of-care testing to ISO 22870. Similar systems of documentation and inspection apply.

Medicines & Healthcare products Regulatory Agency (MHRA)

- MHRA is responsible for licensing drugs and medical devices, and products made by genetic engineering for clinical use, and also regulates blood transfusion services (with inspections of both production facilities and blood banks that are separate from UKAS).
- Licensing drugs is now regulated by Directives of the European Union, but this will change after Brexit.
- Laboratories that create their own tests may be subject to MHRA regulations and thus subject to inspection.
- See ℘ http://www.mhra.gov.uk/Aboutus/index.htm for more information.

Health & Safety Executive (HSE)

- HSE regulates all working environments in the NHS, including laboratories.
- This includes the use of ionizing radiation and radiation protection.
- They may inspect at any time and with no notice, to ensure that the working environment is compliant with legislation.
- See ➲ 'Health and safety' p. 656 for more details.

Human Tissue Authority (HTA)

- HTA regulates all post-mortem, transplantation, and research with human tissues.
- Organizations licensed by the HTA will have a designated individual who has statutory responsibility for all activities carried out under the licence.
- The HTA publishes a list of standards and evidence required to fulfil the standards.
- It carries out inspections and its work overlaps with UKAS.

Royal College of Physicians (London)

- The RCP now has responsibility for the standards and inspections of clinical services in Primary Immunodeficiency and Allergy (among others).
- QPIDS is the PID accreditation scheme, and uses the standards originally developed by UK Primary Immunodeficiency Network, which in turn were based on the original CPA standards, before assimilation to ISO 56189. Uptake has been good, with all centres registered and many entering their third cycle of inspections.
- IQAS is the Allergy scheme, and rather than adapting the tried and tested standards from UKPIN it has developed different standards which are less well defined. Uptake has been poor.
- Convergence of standards to more generic quality standards is now happening.

Quality management system (QMS)

- QMS defines the process by which a laboratory ensures that all aspects of its function achieve the highest possible quality.
- QMS requires documentation of all functions undertaken, both to meet statutory requirements (COSHH) and to provide the framework for staff to function effectively.
- Effective QMS is required to meet ISO standards.
- QMS must include robust document control, so that only current versions of policies are available to staff.
- It is expected that a senior member of the technical staff will act as quality manager.

Quality manual

- The quality manual defines how the laboratory meets ISO15189.
- It includes the management structure and operational procedures for the laboratory.
- It will cross-reference trust policies on health and safety, personnel (training, induction), visitors, standing financial instructions, IT, etc.

Laboratory handbook

- The laboratory handbook provides essential information on services to users, including repertoire, sample requirements, normal ranges, on-call services, and contact details.
- The handbook must be accessible to all users including primary care: intranet, internet, and hard copy may be available but inspectors will check that they all match!

Annual management review

- It is desirable that laboratories undertake an annual management review. This is not mandatory under UKAS. However, it provides an opportunity for the laboratory to review objectives, quality management processes, incidents, and complaints. Review of operations against the RCPath key performance indicators (KPIs) is desirable.

Getting it right first time (GIRFT)

- GIRFT aims to improve patient pathways and improve patient experience and patient outcomes.
- It requires verifiable data from provider organizations that can be related to professionally agreed outcomes.
- It includes (for pathology) demand management and not repeating tests when they have been carried out elsewhere.

Royal College of Pathologists—key performance indicators (KPIs)

- RCPath has published a list of key performance indicators for laboratories.
- As part of their QMS, laboratories should review and audit their performance against these standards.
- See 🔗 https://www.rcpath.org/profession/clinical-effectiveness/key-performance-indicators-kpi.html

Concepts of quality assurance in the laboratory

- The primary goal of all clinical diagnostic laboratories is to generate accurate and reproducible laboratory test results.
- All activities performed to monitor the quality of laboratory testing are referred to as quality control (QC), which should include both internal and external processes.
- Quality assurance (QA) is a broader term encompassing not only QC but also referring to every stage from venesection to correct delivery of the final report.
  - It includes physician ordering practices, maintenance of incubators and glassware, clarity of reports, and appropriateness of testing methods.
  - The purpose of QA is to ensure that the right test is carried out on the right sample and that the correct result is delivered to the requesting clinician with the appropriate interpretation.

Definitions

- **Sensitivity.** Incidence of positive results obtained when the test is used for patients known to have the disease or condition = (number of true positives/sum of true positives and false negatives) × 100.
- **Specificity.** Ability of a test to indicate a negative result in the absence of disease = (number of true negatives/sum of true negatives and false positives) × 100.
- **Precision.** Closeness of replicate analyses.
- **Accuracy.** Closeness to true value.
- **Coefficient of variation (CV)** is defined as the standard deviation expressed as a percentage of the mean.
- **Positive predictive value (PPV)** is defined as number of true positives/ number of true positive + number of false positives.
- **Negative predictive value (NPV)** is defined as number of true negatives/number of true negatives + number of false negatives.

Quality control (internal)

Internal QC consists of those procedures used by laboratory staff for the continual assessment of laboratory work in order to decide if the results are reliable. The main objectives are to ensure day-to-day consistency of measurements and to quantify random variation.

Internal QC samples

- To ensure that the test is carried out correctly it is essential practice that internal QC samples are included in each run.
- Control sera must:
  - be stable;
  - be stored for long periods without loss of activity;

- be similar in composition to patient's sera and treated in the same way;
- be standardized against international (WHO) or national reference materials where available;
- test negative for HIV and HBV.
- Depending on the assay, ideally more than one control should be used.
  - They should be high, low, and at the cut-off level of the assay.
  - For automated analysers that include an automatic further dilution step, a control should be included at a level that requires dilution.
- All values for the internal QC sample must be recorded, which will allow running plots to be produced that give warning of deterioration in assay performance or running bias.

Recording internal QC data
There are a number of ways in which these can be plotted.
- The Shewart chart plots the value of the internal control in absolute values against time, with one and two standard deviations and the mean marked out.
  - The values should be arrayed equally either side of the mean.
  - Usually, action will be taken if more than four points are on the same side of the mean or if two sequential points are beyond 2 SD (although this should also result in run rejection) (Westgard rules).
- The Youden chart has a high and a low standard and the plot is the same as for the Shewart plot but in two dimensions. Here one value is plotted with its mean horizontal and the other with its mean vertical. Each point represents the value for the high sample plotted against the value for the low sample.
  - The points should be randomly arrayed around the intersection of the means.
- The Cusum chart plots the difference of the day's result from the calculated mean value (with sign included). This plot will reveal whether the mean has been set correctly and will also reveal changes in accuracy.

Standard operating procedure
- The standard operating procedure (SOP) is a detailed recipe by which tests are carried out. The SOP must identify:
  - the name and purpose of the test and all the reagents used;
  - a detailed method that someone with normal laboratory competence should be able to follow successfully;
  - hazards of the reagents, as required by COSHH regulations;
  - how and by whom the test results will be reported;
  - normal ranges;
  - which internal control samples should be used;
  - run rejection criteria;
  - author of the document;
  - sources of information (normal ranges) and references;
  - revision date for the document (normally annually).
- SOPs are controlled documents and all copies must be numbered.

- Use of an electronic-based document-control system such as Q-Pulse®️ is strongly recommended.
- Old SOPs must be archived for medicolegal reasons. The RCPath gives advice on how long archived documents should be stored.

Evaluation of reagents

Another important facet of internal QC is the evaluation of reagents. This applies particularly to any fluorescence reagents.

- The conjugated anti-human immunoglobulin reagents used in direct and indirect immunofluorescence need to be titrated to determine the optimum (and most economical) working dilution.
- This is done by a chequerboard titration, where serial dilutions of the conjugate are titrated against serial dilutions of a serum of known specificity and titre.
- Reagents for use of the flow cytometer should also be titrated against increasing cell numbers.
- This process should be carried out each time a new batch is purchased.

Evaluation of new tests

- If a new test or methodology is considered for use in the laboratory, features to consider include:
  - cost;
  - ease of operation;
  - utilization of existing resources;
  - accuracy, precision, sensitivity, and specificity;
  - comparison with gold-standard test;
  - evidence of clinical utility.
  - There should be a clear understanding of the predictive value of the test (PPV, NPV) and this needs an understanding of the pre- and post-test probabilities for the test and clinical condition.
- An analyte should be repeatedly assayed on at least 20 runs to determine the mean value and SD.
- The coefficient of variation (CV) is more useful than the SD as several QC samples at different levels in the result span may be used and the assay variability will change.
  - Comparison should be made with the established or reference method.
- New test evaluations require the parallel testing of large numbers of samples.
- End users must be warned of this change.
- Acceptable assay CVs will also vary depending on the nature of the assay. Between-run CVs for nephelometry assays are 4–6%, whereas for ELISA they are 10–20%.
- Accurate reference ranges are of prime importance in laboratory practice.
- This should involve sampling the appropriate population of normal individuals.

- The larger the group, the more reliable this should be. A minimum sample of 100 is required. The reference interval is set by including 2 SD each side of the mean.
- ROC curves (receiver operating characteristics) are used to show the connection between clinical sensitivity and specificity, and the area under the curve gives an idea about test benefit.

Evaluation of new tests: evaluation, verification, and validation

- An important aspect of QC is the assessment of tests. This includes the following.
  - Evaluation: an internal comparison of old and new tests, comparing performance parameters.
  - Validation: this is a more extensive assessment of a test and must be performed for all in-house tests. Manufacturers of CE-marked tests will have carried out the validation of the test. Data must include objective evidence that the test is fit for the purpose proposed.
  - Verification: this is local assessment of a test/kit to ensure that it performs as per specification, when carried out following the manufacturer's instructions. New batches require verification and should be compared against the previous batch before being introduced into routine use.
- Any modifications to a manufacturer's assay will invalidate its CE marker, and mean that full responsibility for the assay and any defects will fall on the laboratory. Accordingly, full validation will be required!

Evaluation of new tests: uncertainty of measurement (UoM)

- As part of compliance with the ISO15189 standards, clinical laboratories are expected to calculate the uncertainty of measurement of their assays, and document this in their SOPs.
- The UoM should be reviewed for acceptability and reviewed at least annually.
- This information should be available to users if requested.
- The UoM is calculated from IQC data (minimum recommended = 6 months) and is either expressed as SD or CV for quantitative tests.
- For qualitative tests the UoM is based on the diagnostic efficiency, which is determined from the true and false positives and true and false negatives.
- For further information see White, G.H. and Farrance, I. (2004). Uncertainty of measurement in quantitative medical testing—a laboratory implementation guide. *Clin. Biochem. Rev.* **25**, Suppl. 1 ᔕ https://www.ncbi.nlm.nih.gov/pmc/articles/PMC1934961/

Quality control (external) 1: EQA schemes

- External QC is an essential tool for ensuring that the laboratory is performing satisfactorily and obtaining the same answers as other laboratories.
- Satisfactory participation in external QC is a mandatory standard for UKAS accreditation.
- UKAS accredits EQA schemes in the same way as it accredits laboratories.
- Responsibility for EQA matters at UKAS is assumed by the professional advisory committee (PAC) with three lead EQA members.
- EQA schemes fall under the remit of NEQAS—see 🕮 http://www.ukneqas.org.uk/

Process of EQA

- The essential element is the distribution of unknown samples at regular intervals.
- Obtaining appropriate samples can be difficult and in some cases samples must be modified in order to be stable and reproducible (e.g. cellular samples for flow cytometric analysis).
- It is important that the samples are treated in the same way as normal patient samples for the results to be meaningful.
- Once the returned results have been analysed, participants are sent a summary showing their performance and how it compares with that of other laboratories.
  - This will often be broken down by method used, which allows laboratories to see whether a method is performing particularly well or badly.

Quantitative schemes

For quantitative analytes such as specific proteins, the method used is the ABC of EQA where each analyte is given an A, B, or C score. Scores are derived from specimen % bias, calculated as:

$$\text{specimen \% bias} = (\text{result} - \text{target})/\text{target} \times 100$$

Each of the three scores is calculated over a rolling time window of six distributions.

Score A: accuracy. This tells you how good your overall performance is. It has been transformed to make it comparable across analytes. The median is set at 100. It is calculated as follows.

- Specimen % bias is transformed by a 'degree of difficulty' factor, to get specimen transformed bias (positive or negative).
- Modulus of this is taken to give specimen accuracy index (no sign).
- A score is calculated as the trimmed mean of specimen accuracy indices in the rolling time window.
- Degree of difficulty is derived from examination of coefficient of variations between laboratories in relation to target values and concentration-dependent factors, normalized to a median A score of 100.

Score B: bias. This tells you how far away from the target on average you are. It is calculated as follows.
- Trimmed mean of all individual specimen % biases (including sign) in rolling time window.

Score C: consistency of bias. This tells you if you have the same bias pattern on average. It is calculated as follows.
- Standard deviation of B score data, with allowances for trimming.

Older scoring schemes (gradually being replaced). These rely on variance index scoring.
- For each sample there will be a designated value (DV).
- For quantitative analytes (i.e. protein chemistries), this is usually the trimmed mean (i.e. the mean recalculated with outliers excluded).
- For qualitative analytes (e.g. ENAs) the designated value is determined by the consensus of a small group of specialist reference laboratories.
- Performance is assessed by calculating the variance index (VI) from the difference of the obtained value from the designated value corrected by the chosen coefficient of variance (CCV), a scaling factor dependent on the type of assay being used, according to the formula:
- For the variance index, the sign is ignored, but for the bias index the sign is kept.
- The variance (VIS) and bias index (BIS) scores are calculated as VIS (or BIS) = VI where VI < 400. If VI > 400 then the maximum score of 400 is applied.
- For many analytes, these are plotted graphically as running performance scores by using the mean running VIS (MRVIS) or mean running BIS (MRBIS), which are calculated by taking the mean of the last 10 VISs or BISs.

Qualitative schemes
- For qualitative reporting, overall performance is judged by scoring 1 point for each misclassification compared to a designated value (misclassification score, MIS).
- The running performance is looked at by adding the scores of the preceding 10 circulations to give the overall misclassification score (OMIS), which will have a maximum dependent on the maximum number of answers that can be given wrongly. Perfect performance gives a score of zero. Acceptable and unacceptable scores are defined by NEQAS for each analyte.

Weaknesses of EQA
- The problem about this type of EQA scheme is in the determination of the 'right' answer.
- If in a quantitative scheme 90% of the laboratories use a method that gives the 'wrong' answer and 10% use a method that gives a different but correct answer, then the apparent performance of the 10% will appear poor as the mean and SD will be determined largely by the majority.

- This is difficult to address, although the Department of Health does sponsor methodological evaluations that are published as 'blue book' reports.
- Interpretation of immunofluorescence can be particularly subjective, so many laboratories are also members of regional QA schemes. Sera are regularly distributed and participants meet and discuss the results and problems.

Poor performance

- NEQAS will only intervene if performance is persistently poor over a long period, and according to pre-determined standards will report failing laboratories to the chairman of the relevant National Quality Assurance Advisory Panel (NQAAP).
- The chairman of NQAAP will then write to the head of the laboratory pointing out the problem and asking what steps are being taken to remedy the problem, as well as offering help (usually a visit from a panel member).
- Lack of a response or an inappropriate response to this letter will lead to a report direct to UKAS so that the laboratory's accreditation status can be reviewed.

Quality control (external) 2: benchmarking and CE marking

Benchmarking

- Benchmarking is another method by which labs can demonstrate the quality and cost-effectiveness of their service.
- It is a process of measuring products, services, and practices against leaders in a field allowing the identification of best practices that will lead to improved performance.
- In the UK the Clinical Benchmarking scheme for pathology has been running for many years. The report analyses 10 areas of lab performance.
- Weaknesses include (for immunology) lack of comparability between laboratories (repertoires, staffing, etc.).
- The College of American Pathologists offers a Q-Probes scheme.
- However, benchmarking does not necessarily provide the 'right' answer.
- The most productive laboratory may not provide the best quality.

CE marking

- In 2003 a third European Medical Device Directive was introduced stating that all diagnostic products must carry the CE mark (kite mark) following registration with the Medicine & Healthcare products Regulatory Agency (MHRA) in the UK.
- This requires submission of data about the product (and a large fee!).
- The CE mark can also be seen on electrical toys and goods.

- The cost of complying with these laws has led to the withdrawal of some products that were no longer commercially viable due to the additional expense of registration.
- This law may have a significant impact upon immunology where conventionally many tests have been developed in-house.
- Provided that tests are not commercially marketed, an exemption has been obtained for in-house NHS assays.
- By December 2005 all laboratories offering a commercial testing service or making kits for commercial resale had to comply with the new rules.
- What will happen after Brexit is unknown, possibly a separate mark from British Standards Institute.

Clinical standards and audit

Clinical work has been less amenable to such detailed quality assessment However, several organizations now exist that produce guidelines of 'best practice' against which the audit cycle can be carried out.

National Institute for Health and Care Excellence (NICE)

- NICE is an independent organization responsible for providing national guidance on the promotion of good health and the prevention and treatment of ill health (see ✎ http://www.nice.org.uk/).
- Currently, NICE produces three kinds of guidance:
  - technology appraisals—guidance on the use of new and existing medicines and treatments within the NHS in England and Wales;
  - clinical guidelines—guidance on the appropriate treatment and care of people with specific diseases and conditions within the NHS in England and Wales;
  - interventional procedures—guidance on whether interventional procedures used for diagnosis or treatment are safe enough and work well enough for routine use in England, Wales, and Scotland.
- NICE and the National Service Frameworks (produced by the Department of Health) are responsible for setting clear national standards for NHS services and treatments.
- In 2004 the Department of Health published a document, *Standards for better health*, which sets out how NHS organizations should respond to NICE guidance.

Care Quality Commission

The Commission regularly reviews the performance of trusts, healthcare providers, and social care providers against the standards set down by NICE and the National Service Frameworks. The functions of the Care Quality Commission are to:

- regulate the independent healthcare sector through annual registration and inspection in England;
- publish regular ratings of NHS hospitals and trusts, and publish information about the state of healthcare across the NHS and independent sector;
- coordinate its NHS inspections with a range of other healthcare organizations in order to minimize disruption to healthcare staff;

- identify how effectively funds are used within healthcare—particularly whether tax payers are getting good value for money;
- investigate serious failures in healthcare services.

It has also taken over responsibility for handling the independent review process for complaints about treatment within the NHS, and it works closely with NHS Improvements.

UK Primary Immunodeficiency Network

The UK Primary Immunodeficiency Network (see ℘ http://www.ukpin.org.uk/home/) is a multidisciplinary organization of those caring for patients with primary immunodeficiencies. All nurses, scientists, and medical practitioners involved in the healthcare of patients with primary immune deficiencies, or in research into these diseases, are deemed to be members. The aims of UKPIN are:

- development of common approaches to management by means of setting consensus standards of care;
- peer review accreditation scheme for PID centres—this is now managed by the Royal College of Physicians (➜ QPIDS—see p. 645);
- provision of generic protocols based on common practice;
- organizing a biennial conference.

The website has approved and draft clinical guidelines for the management of PIDs.

Management of clinical incidents

Every hospital should have a process for investigating incidents and recording these. Data from this process is inspected by CQC and by NHSLA.

Pathology laboratories should have a robust mechanism for investigating errors and incidents. This will usually be led by the quality manager, and/or a clinical quality lead, reporting to the head of department/clinical director.

Root cause analysis (RCA)

- This is the bedrock of incident investigation.
- This is based on the 'Five whys': actually, five is deemed a minimum not a required number! It aims to peel away the layers of a problem until you reach the root cause. However, if you don't see the right questions to ask, you won't get the right answer!
- Identification of key individuals is essential.
- The answers can be incorporated into a 'fishbone analysis'.
- Consultants and scientists should be familiar with RCA and preferably be trained in its use.
- The process should not be vindictive or punitive, nor should it seek to attribute blame.
- NHS Improvements have a section on resources which provides a starting point:
  ℘ https://improvement.nhs.uk/resources/?publishingbody=advancing-change-team

Health and safety

Hospitals, and particularly laboratories, are subject in most countries to a significant legal framework. In practice this means that the employers are responsible in law for ensuring that this legal framework is implemented.

- In the UK, a number of organizations have the right to make unannounced inspections to ensure compliance.
- The Health and Safety Executive (see ℘ http://www.hse.gov.uk/) has wide powers regarding the workplace, including, as a last resort, the power to close an installation down and to bring prosecutions.
- Heads of departments can be held accountable directly for breaches.
- Particularly important are the regulations regarding all chemical and biological materials (COSHH regulations), which require a full safety assessment to be carried out on any substance in use or held in the laboratory.
  - These must be held in a written form and read by all employees using the substances.
  - This information must contain information on dealing with spills.
  - There are commercially available directories (Croner) from which this information can be obtained and most manufacturers include such information in the packaging.
- Strict regulations apply to the use and handling of radioisotopes, in particular the route of disposal and the amount of permitted discharges.
- Every hospital will have a radiation protection officer, usually a member of the medical physics team, who will provide guidance and monitor local compliance.
- Breaches of the legislation are viewed seriously and both hospitals and individuals have been prosecuted by HM Inspectorate of Pollution.
- The handling of biological high-risk samples is governed by the guidance produced by the Advisory Committee on Dangerous Pathogens, under the auspices of HSE (see ℘ http://www.hse.gov.uk/aboutus/meetings/committees/acdp/).
- In the guidance, pathogens are graded according to the potential risk to workers, and handling facilities and other precautions are laid down.
- Those working in laboratories should treat all samples as being potentially high risk and take sensible precautions, i.e. wearing gloves, appropriate laboratory coats (Howie coats, properly buttoned up!), and disposing of samples safely via an autoclave (universal precautions).
- The use of latex products, i.e. gloves, is covered by COSHH, as latex is considered a substance hazardous to health—full risk assessment is required.
- All staff should be fully immunized, particularly against hepatitis B.
- All staff (including doctors!), as part of their induction, should read the necessary statutory documentation and also local policies, which need to be fully documented as one of the CPA accreditation standards.
- The induction should also include annual fire safety training (a mandatory requirement). This training should be documented for all staff and is included in the logbooks for trainee clinicians and scientists.

Laboratory and clinical organization

- In the UK, UKAS-accredited immunology laboratories must have a clear management structure with evidence of regular meetings and consultation.
- A clinician or top-grade scientist must lead the department, assisted by a laboratory manager (senior BMS or scientist). These two will be responsible for the management of the department.
- The laboratory will usually be part of a directorate of laboratory medicine, with a clinical director (either a clinician or top-grade scientist) who has overall responsibility for the directorate and will usually be a part of the trust hospital's higher management structure.
- Heads of department will usually be responsible for a devolved budget and should be involved in the negotiation of contracts, budget setting, and personnel matters, with appropriate support from finance and personnel departments.
- Management of staff is a major role and heads of department need to be aware of the employment legislation, particularly in regard to equal opportunities and discrimination.
- Staff development is important and UKAS expects to see performance appraisal for all grades in place.
- Clinical heads of department will now also be responsible for all types of staff, usually assisted by a senior nurse.
- All junior clinical staff will have nominated consultants who are responsible for the supervision of their training. Regular appraisal meetings for junior medical staff are required.

Funding

- See 'Funding of pathology services', p. 642.
- Pathology managers need to ensure that new developments at a clinical level include sufficient funding to cover additional laboratory costs.

Managing change

- Services never stand still—change is inevitable.
- Pathology managers need to ensure that they are familiar with best practice in managing change.
- Key elements include the following.
  - Early and continuous open communication with staff (no 'mushroom management' = keep people in the dark and cover them with manure).
  - Early involvement of Human Resources.
  - Identify stakeholders, key leaders for change, and key resisters to change, and work with all groups.
  - Support staff.
  - Effective leadership
  - Implementation plan.
  - Rumour scotching!
  - Evaluate outcome.

Training

Training in immunology in the UK takes place at both a clinical and technical level (biomedical scientists (BMS) and clinical scientists).

Medical training

- Basic medical training has changed with the introduction of 'foundation schools'.
  - All medical graduates will initially enter a 2-year foundation programme.
  - In order to gain experience of immunology, it may be possible to arrange a 'taster' attachment to immunology during the foundation years.
  - This will be followed (for a time at least) by core medical training posts (CMT).
- Following foundation and CMT, trainees will compete for specialist training posts (specialist registrar).
- 'Shape of Training' is changing how specialisms are incorporated and this may be by post-CCT training. For immunology, for now little change is envisaged.
- At the stage of selection into immunology, possession of the MRCP or MRCPCH (or equivalent training abroad approved by JRCPTB) is an explicit entry criterion.
- Core training currently includes basic science, clinical practice related to immunology, and laboratory practice, culminating in the part I examination of the FRCPath, comprising two written papers. Trainees in immunology must also complete the FRCPath part II, which may be in the form of a thesis (this may have been submitted for a PhD or MD or may be specifically written for the FRCPath), a casebook, or submission of a collection of published papers. This is followed by a practical exam and an oral examination. Details are on the college website (see ℳ https://www.rcpath.org/trainees/examinations/examinations-by-specialty/immunology.html).
- Whether the FRCPath is adequate in identifying competence to run a diagnostic immunology laboratory is debatable. Clinical scientists sit a slightly modified exam with less emphasis on clinical skills.
- Completion of training will be certified by the award of a certificate of completion of training (CCT) issued by GMC, on receipt of a large fee!

BMS training

- BMS training may be entered through an approved degree in biological sciences followed by a year in-service training. Sandwich degrees exist and a co-terminus programme is being developed, whereby state registration and award of degree occur simultaneously.
- After 1 year, candidates are required to submit a log-book or training with a portfolio followed by an oral examination to obtain state registration with the Health Professions Council (HPC).
- Additional specialist qualifications, including submission of a specialist portfolio and advanced practitioner status may be obtained.
- Further progress up the career scale is dependent upon the acquisition of further qualifications such as an MSc.

Clinical scientists

- Clinical scientist trainees will usually start as junior scientists having undertaken a primary degree in a relevant subject at university and currently go through a structured programme of training lasting 3 years.
- Scientists who have undertaken their training in academic departments and obtained PhDs are often employed directly into the middle scientist grades.
- Registration with the HPC is required.
- Progression to consultant scientist level is usually dependent on acquisition of the FRCPath in the appropriate discipline, although there is no written rule requiring this at present.
- As a result of Modernising Scientific Careers, new Scientific Training Programmes (STP) and Higher Scientific Training Programmes (HSTP) have been established, with the curricula set by Health Education England (HEE).

Agenda for Change

- The concept of 'Agenda for Change' is that all staff are paid equally for work of equal value.
- It applies to all directly employed NHS staff except doctors, dentists, and senior managers.
- Agenda for Change was rolled out nationally in December 2004.
- There are two pay spines, one for nursing and other health professions, and a second for all other directly employed NHS staff.
- Detailed assessment of each post using the job evaluation scheme determines the correct pay band for each post and therefore the correct basic pay.
- In each pay band there are a number of points in which there should be progress through each year as skills and knowledge are successfully developed (KSF: knowledge and skills framework).
- The already grey area of distinction between clinical scientists and BMS staff has become even more blurred. The opportunity for 'consultant BMS' staff exists.
- It is accepted that Band 7 posts will normally be filled by BMS with an MSc, while Band 8 posts require a PhD (or equivalent such as FRCPath).
- Old Grade C scientist posts are mostly Band 8 or occasionally Band 9.

Writing a business case

All NHS trusts are required to submit annual plans outlining the organization's plans over the next 3 years. These aim to establish the organization's priorities as determined by national and local policies. Directorate business plans contribute to the development of the organization's business plan. On an annual basis, each directorate outlines the financial and other resources that it requires to deliver its service, what is expected by the commissioners, and proposals for service and capital development. A business case is a document that supports the proposals for a new service development or a capital project.

Within pathology, one of the most common reasons for developing a business case is a response to increasing workload or a need to introduce new tests into the service. The first step is informal discussions with colleagues such as the clinical director and business manager. It is important to identify any financial threshold below which directorates will be expected to fund the developments themselves.

A business case should address three questions:
- Where are we now?
- Where do we want to be?
- How do we get there?

Suggested outline of a written business case

- Executive summary (at the beginning for those too busy/idle to read long documents!).
- Introduction.
  - Describe current service. Identify any national or local policies that impact on service provision (national service frameworks, recommendations by UKAS/MHRA/HSE/HTA) and need for change based on differences between existing service and future needs.
- Aims.
  - Should be SMART (specific, measurable, achievable, relevant, and with a time element).
- Option appraisal.
  - State 'do nothing' as one option.
  - Describe long list of options and then cut down to a short list of the most appropriate options.
  - Assess each option for benefits and costs.
- Proposal.
  - Main section of the business plan.
  - Identify the preferred option.
  - Summarize why it is superior to other options and the cost–benefit analysis.
  - Identify any risks and how they should be managed.
  - Assess the impact of the proposal on pathology and other clinical directorates.
- Conclusions and recommendations.
- The business case is more likely to be successful if:
  - it is a statutory/national requirement that must be implemented;
  - the development is part of an existing strategy;
  - it requires relatively simple management action with few/small capital or revenue consequences;
  - it has support in clinical directorates outside pathology;
  - it has a positive impact on waiting times and waiting lists.

Further reading

Galloway, M.J. (2004). ACP best practice guideline: writing a business case for service development in pathology. *J. Clin. Pathol.* 57:337–43.

Applying for a consultant post

Basic information

- Start looking in the *British Medical Journal* and NHS Jobs websites at least 6 months before you are going to apply.
- Has the post been advertised before (how often)?
- If possible, get experience.
  - Enquire about acting-up as a consultant or doing a locum.
- Think about what sort of job you want (clinical, laboratory, research, location).
- Is this a new post or a replacement following a departure or retirement?
- Use colleagues to obtain background information about jobs available or likely to become available.

Responding to the advert

- The information pack should include job description and information on office accommodation and secretarial support, job plan, personal specification, and terms and conditions of service. Organizational information should include business plan, annual report, and healthcare commission report.
- Ask around among colleagues about the job.
- If there is doubt about the terms and conditions, check with the BMA (if a member).
  - It is a good idea to be a member of either the BMA or the Hospital Consultants and Specialists Association (HCSA) *before* applying for posts.

First visit

- Arrange to meet consultant colleagues, clinical director, business manager, medical director, chief executive (if possible!).
- Make sure you have read the information supplied carefully.
- Have a list of questions for those you are going to meet.
- Don't be taken in by people talking-up the job.
- Be suspicious of promises to do things—look for evidence that they will happen!
- On the way home, list the good points and bad points of the job—do you still want to apply?
- Be sure your application is received on time.
- Remember to ask your referees' permission to use them!

Second visit (after short listing)

- Ask:
  - What is the management structure?
  - Outcome of last Care Quality Commission inspection?
  - Is there any induction for new consultants?
  - Any plans for rationalization of services?
  - Outcome of last UKAS visit?
  - Sample audit trail?
  - Travel between sites yourself using normal means of transport.
  - Who is the budget holder for your department?

- What are the arrangements for out- and in-patient services?
- Has a QPIDS inspection been carried out?
- What are the teaching commitments?
- Ask the same question of different people.
- Smile—remember at this point you are trying to sell yourself as a desirable colleague!

Preparing for the interview

- Who will be on the committee? Appointments committees may be very large and will always include a management representative and have a lay chairperson.
- Is a presentation required? If so try to keep a local focus.
- Be up to date on current hot topics.
- Prepare answers for key questions: have a plan of what you would like to achieve over your first few years in post.
- If you don't think you will accept an offer of the post, don't go to the interview: it causes enormous upset, and word will spread.
- If you drop out, make sure you telephone the personnel officer well in advance.

At the interview

- Arrive in plenty of time (don't rely on public transport to get you there in the nick of time!).
- Wear appropriate sober dress.
- Again, you are there as a salesman, selling yourself.
- Direct your answers to the questioner. Think before speaking and speak clearly.

After acceptance

- Once you have accepted and before you take up the post is the only time when you have power to influence terms and conditions.
- Check which point on the salary scale you have been offered—if they have had difficulty in filling a post or you have longer than usual training, you can negotiate a higher starting salary.
- Check contract for unusual terms (check it out with BMA/HCSA if necessary).
- Check the terms for relocation expenses.
- Appointment is subject to clearance checks with the Disclosure & Barring Service (DBS) and Occupational Health: do *not* hand in your notice until you have a satisfactory written offer and confirmation of DBS/Occupational Health clearance.

Further reading

ACP guide: applying for a consultant post in pathology.

Consultant contract and private practice

- A new consultant contract has been negotiated. It is time-based rather than professional.
- A basic 40-hour week is divided into 10 programmed activities (PAs), of which 7.5 will be direct clinical care and 2.5 supporting activities (SPAs)—administration, teaching, CPD. Trusts have however been driving down the time allowed for SPAs to 1.5, or even 1. This is not supported by professional bodies.
- Additional PAs may be offered by trusts on a temporary basis to meet specified clinical needs.
- Additional payments are made for on-call commitments according to intensity and frequency.
- Most trusts have found that the work currently delivered exceeds the PAs for which they are funded!
- Under the new contract, limitations are placed on consultants' private practice, which must not overlap with defined NHS PAs.
- The job plan forms the basis of determining work patterns and remuneration and is separate from appraisal.
- Pay progression is subject to satisfactory appraisal and an agreed job plan and is no longer automatic.
- Annual appraisal is now required and must be documented both by the trust and also by the individual.
- Revamped appraisal is part of the revalidation process with the GMC, required to maintain a licence to practise, which has to be renewed every 5 years.
  - This will include 5-yearly multi-source feedback and patient feedback.
  - A GMC-approved responsible officer (usually a trust medical director) will be required to sign off the appraisals as indicating that the doctor is fit to continue practising.
- Participation in continuing professional development, with documentary evidence, is a mandatory requirement, usually through a Royal College.
- Trusts may award additional discretionary salary increments for meritorious service.
- Consultants may apply for higher clinical excellence awards (CEAs) on a national basis. At least 5 years as a consultant in the NHS is expected. Applications must be accompanied by a supporting form from the chief executive. Colleges and professional bodies may make nominations.
- CEAs are renewable every 5 years and may be withdrawn if performance declines.
- Many doctors believe that the extra work (unpaid) required for a CEA award is not worth the aggravation and loss of free time.
- This means that much unpaid work for the NHS and for Royal Colleges etc. is now unpopular and it is difficult to get people to serve on committees.
- The future of clinical excellence awards is still in doubt (rewarding doctors for performance is not seen to be desirable).
- The combination of pension changes (lifetime limit and scheme changes) and general aggravation from working in the NHS is leading to an exodus of senior and experienced consultants and GPs.

- Establishing private practice needs to be considered carefully: where, how often, secretarial and nursing support, time to be spent on billing and chasing bad debt.
- Registration with private health insurers is required. They frequently set maximum allowable fees and limit costs for investigations. They do not recognize consultants until they have been in post for a certain number of years.
- Medical indemnity insurance is required.
- Professional bodies can provide advice, and run courses.
- Consultants planning to undertake medicolegal work should undertake specific training (courses are available) and must have indemnity insurance that covers medicolegal work.
- Further advice is available from the British Medical Association (BMA) and from the Hospital Consultants and Specialists Association (HCSA).

Websites

Association of Clinical Pathologists: ℘ www.pathologists.org.uk/
BMA: ℘ www.bma.org.uk
Department of Health: ℘ www.dh.gov.uk
HCSA: ℘ www.hcsa.com

Index

For the benefit of digital users, indexed terms that span two pages (e.g., 52–53) may, on occasion, appear on only one of those pages.

Note: Tables are indicated by an italic t, following the page number.

.

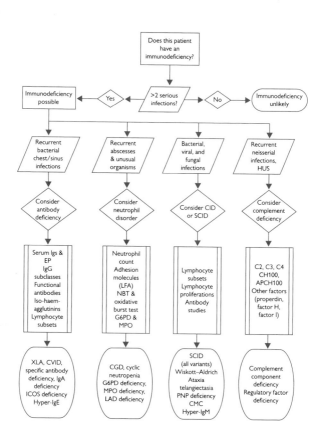